Health Survey for England:
Cardiovascular Disease '98

Volume 1: Findings

A survey carried out on behalf of The Department of Health

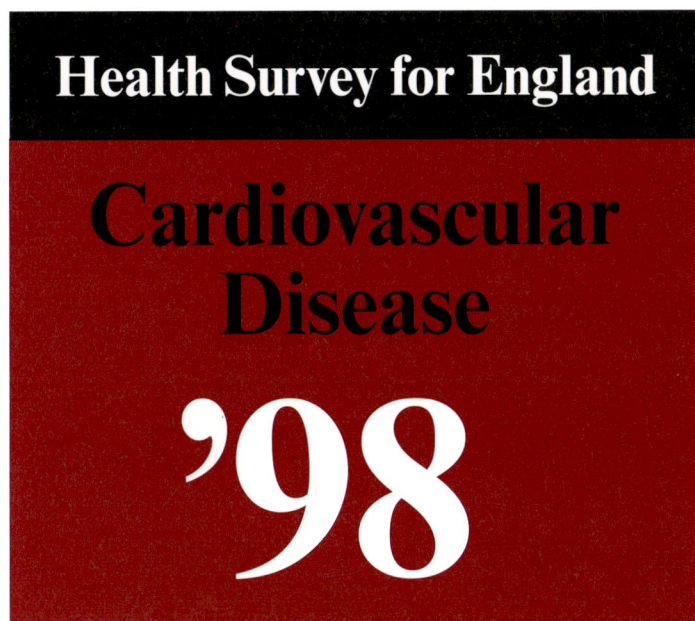

Health Survey for England

Cardiovascular Disease

'98

Volume 1: Findings

Edited by
Bob Erens
Paola Primatesta

Principal Authors
Madhavi Bajekal, Richard Boreham
Bob Erens, Emanuela Falaschetti
Vasant Hirani, Paola Primatesta
Gillian Prior, Clare Tait

Joint Health Surveys Unit
National Centre for Social Research
Department of Epidemiology and Public Health
at the Royal Free and University College Medical School

LONDON: THE STATIONERY OFFICE

Designed by Davenport Associates
Printed in the United Kingdom for The Stationery Office
J99580 C8 12/99 9385 11747

Contents

Volume 1: Findings

Contents

Volume 2: Methodology and Documentation

Editors' acknowledgements

We would first like to acknowledge the debt the survey's success owes to the commitment and professionalism of the interviewers and nurses who worked on the survey throughout the year. We also wish to express our gratitude to all those who gave up their time to be interviewed and who welcomed these interviewers and nurses into their homes.

We would like to thank all those colleagues who contributed to the survey and this report. In particular, we would like to thank:

- The chapter authors: Madhavi Bajekal, Richard Boreham, Marion Brookes, Emanuela Falaschetti, Vasant Hirani, Johanna Laiho, Gillian Prior and Clare Tait

- Other research colleagues, in particular Professor Michael Marmot, Andrea Nove and Professor Neil Poulter

- Operations staff, especially Marion Bolden, Loretta Curtis, Audrey Hale, Pam Huggett, Kerrie Stuart, and the Area Managers

- The principal programmers: Jo Periam and Sven Sjodin

- Liane Roe, who devised the DINE questionnaire, for advice on the design of the eating habits questionnaire and commenting on the analysis.

We would also like to express our thanks to the staff of the Department of Clinical Biochemistry at the Royal Victoria Infirmary in Newcastle upon Tyne for their helpfulness and efficiency.

We would also like to take this opportunity to acknowledge the invaluable contribution made to the Health Survey by Patricia Prescott-Clarke, who was co-director of the project from 1994 until her retirement in 1998.

Last, but certainly not least, we wish to express our appreciation of the work of Department of Health staff at all stages of the project and in particular the contribution made by Antonia Roberts, Dr. Sunjai Gupta, Tony Boucher and Richard Bond.

Bob Erens and Paola Primatesta

Notes

1. The following conventions have been used within tables:

   - no observations (zero value)

   0 non-zero values of less than 0.5% and thus rounded to zero

   [] used to warn of small sample bases, if the base is less than 50.

2. Because of rounding, row or column percentages may not add exactly to 100%.

3. A percentage may be quoted in the text for a single category that aggregates two or more of the percentages shown in a table. The percentage for the single category has been recalculated, and because of rounding may differ by one percentage point from the sum of the percentages in the table.

4. Values for means, medians, percentiles and standard errors are shown to an appropriate number of decimal places. Standard Error may sometimes be abbreviated to SE for space reasons, and Standard Deviation to SD.

5. 'Missing values' occur for several reasons. They include refusal or inability to answer a particular question; refusal to co-operate in an entire section of the survey (such as the nurse visit or a self-completion questionnaire); and cases where the question is not applicable to the informant. In general, missing values have been omitted from all tables and analyses.

6. Most tables in the report show a 'dependent' variable (comprising the rows of the table) cross-analysed by an 'independent' variable (comprising the columns). The percentage base for the values of the dependent variable is normally at the foot of each column. It excludes missing values. Informants with a missing value on the independent variable are not shown as a separate column, but are normally included in the total column (unless they also have a missing value on the dependent variable).

7. The population sub-group to whom each table refers is stated at the upper left corner of the table, and the reference year is stated at the upper right corner.

8. The term 'significant' refers to statistical significance and is not intended to imply substantive importance.

Summary

Introduction

The Health Survey for England comprises a series of annual surveys, of which the 1998 survey is the eighth. All eight surveys have covered the adult population aged 16 and over living in private households in England. The four most recent surveys, 1995-1998, have also covered children aged 2 to 15 living in households selected for the survey, and the 1997 report was focused on young persons aged 16-24. Results for children in 1998 are not presented in the present report, but tables will be found on the Department of Health's website (see Chapter 1, Section 1.6.6). Information about response rates and other technical matters is detailed in Volume II of the present report, in Chapter 8 Survey Methodology.

The Health Survey series is part of an overall programme of surveys commissioned by the Department of Health and designed to provide regular information on various aspects of the nation's health which cannot be obtained from other sources. The Health Survey series was designed to achieve the following aims:

1. To provide annual data for nationally representative samples to monitor trends in the nation's health

2. To estimate the proportion of people in England who have specified health conditions

3. To estimate the prevalence of certain risk factors associated with these conditions

4. To examine differences between subgroups of the population (including regional populations) in their likelihood of having specified conditions or risk factors

5. To assess the frequency with which particular combinations of risk factors are found, and in which groups these combinations most commonly occur

6. To monitor progress towards selected health targets

7. (From 1995) to measure the height of children at different ages, replacing the National Study of Health and Growth.

Each survey in the series consists of core questions and measurements (for example, anthropometric and blood pressure measurements and analysis of blood samples), plus modules of questions on specific issues that change periodically.

Since 1994, the Health Survey for England has been carried out by the Joint Health Surveys Unit of the *National Centre for Social Research* (formerly Social and Community Planning Research) and the Department of Epidemiology and Public Health at the Royal Free and University College Medical School.

The 1998 Health Survey

During the first four years of the Health Survey, the focus was on cardiovascular disease (CVD). The focus shifted to other topics in 1995 to 1997, but in 1998 the topic of CVD was revisited so that any changes since the last survey on CVD, in 1994, could be examined.

Questions on CVD in 1998 were very similar to those asked in 1994, and included the Medical Research Council (MRC) respiratory questionnaire. In addition to a number of 'core' topics repeated every year (cigarette smoking, alcohol consumption, general health, prescribed medication, use of services), other topics covered in 1998 included physical activity, eating habits, psychosocial health and social support.

As noted above, the survey included children aged 2-15 as well as adults. Methodological description in the present report covers both children and adults, but results are reported for adults only, results for children being separately posted on the Department of Health's website. All results reported in this summary and in individual chapters thus refer only to adults aged 16 and over, living in private households in England.

Cardiovascular disease (CVD)

The White Paper 'Saving Lives: Our Healthier Nation' recognised that the United Kingdom is at present one of the worst countries for deaths from circulatory disease, and identified heart disease and stroke as among the four priority areas to tackle. The target was set of reducing the death rate from coronary heart disease and stroke amongst people aged under 75 years by at least two fifths (based on 1996 data) by the year 2010.

For the purpose of this report, informants were classified as having a cardiovascular (CVD) condition if they reported having had any of the following conditions diagnosed by a doctor (or by a nurse in the case of blood pressure): angina, heart attack, stroke, heart murmur, abnormal heart rhythm, 'other heart trouble', diabetes and high blood pressure.

Including self-reported high blood pressure among the CVD conditions, 27.9% of men and 27.8% of women reported having been diagnosed as having a CVD condition. CVD prevalence increased with age in both sexes. Overall, 5.3% of men and 3.9% of women reported having had angina. A similar number of women (3.1%) but fewer men (2.6%) were classified as having angina according to the Rose Questionnaire, which is based on perceived symptoms rather than a previous diagnosis. Men had a higher prevalence of heart attack (4.2%), stroke (2.3%) and diabetes (3.3%) than women (1.8%, 2.1% and 2.5% respectively). Ischaemic heart disease (IHD) was defined as a history of reported angina or heart attack: 7.1% of men and 4.6% of women reported IHD. The prevalence of IHD or stroke combined was 8.5% in men and 6.2% in women.

The prevalence of CVD, IHD and IHD or stroke by socio-economic characteristics was examined in informants aged 35 and over only, given the low prevalence of CVD among younger people. The prevalence of any CVD condition showed a significant association in women only, while IHD and IHD or stroke showed a gradient according to social class and income in both sexes; for instance, the age-standardised prevalence of IHD was 5.2% in men in Social Class I and 11.3% in Social Class IV (for women it was 5.7% in Social Class II and 10.0% in Social Class V).

Small changes over the period 1994 to 1998 were observed for IHD, IHD or stroke, diabetes and Rose Angina symptoms in both sexes. Even though the changes were statistically significant for some of the conditions (e.g. IHD or stroke), caution is recommended in the interpretation of results from these cross-sectional data and a longer time series is needed for a more robust interpretation.

Risk factors for CVD

Alcohol consumption

High consumption of alcohol is a risk factor for cardiovascular disease (CVD), though low levels of consumption are considered to have a protective effect. Men reported considerably higher alcohol consumption than women, but the gap narrowed slightly between 1994 and 1998, with women's consumption showing an increase while men's remained unchanged. However, in 1998 men's estimated weekly consumption remained well over double that of women. In both sexes, consumption decreased sharply after about age 50.

Younger drinkers had more irregular drinking patterns than older drinkers, in terms of both frequency and amounts per occasion. Older drinkers were more likely to drink small amounts regularly.

Women's estimated consumption increased from Social Classes IV and V to Social Classes I and II, but men's did not.

Cigarette smoking

No overall trend in cigarette smoking prevalence was discernible between 1994 and 1998, but there was evidence of an increase in smoking prevalence in those aged 16-24.

In both sexes, cigarette smoking prevalence decreased with age. The number of cigarettes per smoker per day increased into middle age and then decreased in later life. The initial increase is likely to reflect smoking cessation by lighter smokers, and higher death rates among heavier smokers are likely to have contributed to the subsequent decrease with age.

Cigarette smoking was much more prevalent among those in manual social classes and in lower income groups.

A higher proportion of men than of women smoked roll-ups. The proportion smoking roll-ups was also higher in Social Classes IV and V, and in lower income groups.

Among smokers of branded cigarettes, men smoked brands with higher tar levels than women. The tar yield of branded cigarettes also increased from Social Classes I and II to Social Classes IV and V and, for women but not for men, was higher in lower income groups.

Eating habits

The Health Survey collected information on frequency of consumption of various groups of food, and derived scores for fat and fibre consumption using a modified version of the Dietary Instrument for Nutrition Education (DINE) questionnaire. The prevalence of high fat and low fibre consumption was notably higher amongst the youngest age group (16-24); a higher proportion of men in this age group (38%) than of women (16%) had high fat consumption. There was less difference between the sexes in fibre consumption. The proportion with low fibre consumption was also high in this age group (65% of men aged 16-24, compared with 53% of all men, and 72% of women aged 16-24 compared with 60% of all women).

There was a clear socio-economic gradient in age-standardised high fat and low fibre intakes in both sexes. The prevalence of high fat intake was highest in men (38%) and women (17%) from Social Class V and it was also highest in men (33%) and women (18%) in the lowest income quintile. There was a strong social class gradient in the prevalence of low fibre intake, which increased steadily in both men and women from Social Class I (45%, 47%) to Social Class V (59%, 68%); the increase was greater in women. Both men and women in the lowest income quintile had the highest prevalence of low fibre intake (59% and 67% respectively).

Physical activity

Respondents were asked about a range of physical activities, including activity at work. Combining all activity types, 80% of men and 76% of women reported at least one occasion of physical activity (of at least 15 minutes' duration) in the last four weeks. This proportion tended to fall with age, particularly after age 35.

Participation in physical activities was summarised into activity groups; Group 3 is the level that fulfils the current activity guidelines, which are that adults should take part in physical activities of at least moderate intensity and of at least 30 minutes' duration, on most days (at least five days a week). Men overall were far more likely to be classified in Group 3 (37%) than were women (25%).

Among men, the proportion in Group 3 fell steadily with age from 58% of those aged 16-24 to 7% of those aged 75 and over.

Among women, the proportion in Group 3 was fairly level at 30%-32% in women aged 16-54, before falling with age to just 4% among women aged 75 and over.

Among men, there was no change since 1994 in the proportion in Group 3. Among women, there was a small increase, from 22% in 1994 to 25% in 1998.

Participation in physical activities overall tended to increase with increasing household income, particularly among men. Participation in sports and exercise and walking was strongly related to household income, with men and women in higher income quintiles being more likely to take part in these activities.

However, because of the greater contribution of occupational activity in the manual social classes, the proportion of men in activity Group 3 was highest in Social Class V, and lower in the non-manual social classes. Similarly the proportion of men in Group 3 was lower in the lowest and highest income quintiles than in the middle incomes. Among women there was no clear pattern according to income or social class in the proportions in Group 3. These findings were confirmed by logistic regression.

Body mass

The Body Mass Index (BMI), defined as weight (kg) divided by the square of height (m^2), was calculated for informants who had a valid height and weight measurement. Mean BMI was 26.5 kg/m^2 in men and 26.4 kg/m^2 in women.

Obesity was defined as having a BMI greater than 30 kg/m^2. The obese category was split further into categories of 30-40 kg/m^2 and 40 kg/m^2 or above, the latter being defined as morbid obesity. Obesity was more prevalent in women (21.2%) than in men (17.3%), and the prevalence of morbid obesity among women (1.9%) was also higher than in men (0.6%). Mean BMI and the prevalence of obesity have continued to increase in both sexes since 1994.

There were body mass differences by socio-economic status. The prevalence of obesity (over 30 kg/m^2) and of morbid obesity (over 40 kg/m^2) was higher in manual than non-manual social classes in both sexes; in women, there was a progressive increase in obesity and morbid obesity from Social Class I (14.4%, 0.7%) to Social Class V (28.1, 3.3%) respectively. The gradient was less evident in men.

In men, the prevalence of obesity increased from the highest (14.5%) to the lowest (20.3%) equivalised income quintile, and similar differences were seen in women (15.9% and 26.3% respectively). The prevalence of morbid obesity also showed a strong gradient for equivalised income, in both sexes. In men it increased from 0.6% in the highest income quintile to 1.2% in the lowest income quintile and in women from 0.9% to 3.7%.

Blood pressure

As in previous rounds of the Health Survey, blood pressure was measured using an automated device, the Dinamap 8100 monitor.

There was a general tendency for mean systolic blood pressure (SBP) to decrease between 1994 and 1998. In 1998 mean SBP was 136.8 mmHg in men and 132.5 mmHg in women. The corresponding values in 1994 were 137.6 mmHg and 134.3 mmHg. Mean diastolic blood pressure (DBP) was 76.2 mmHg in men and 72.3 mmHg in women (in 1994 76.3 mmHg in men and 72.8 mmHg in women).

Adult informants were classified in one of four groups on the basis of their systolic (SBP) and diastolic (DBP) readings and their current use of anti-hypertensive medication. In 1998 the survey's SBP and DBP thresholds for hypertension were changed, in accordance with the latest guidelines on hypertension management. The four groups were defined in 1998 as follows:

Normotensive - untreated	SBP<140 mmHg and DBP<90 mmHg , not currently taking drug prescribed for high blood pressure
Normotensive - treated	SBP<140 mmHg and DBP<90 mmHg, currently taking drug prescribed for high blood pressure
Hypertensive - treated	SBP≥140 mmHg and DBP≥90 mmHg, currently taking drug prescribed for high blood pressure
Hypertensive - untreated	SBP≥140 mmHg and DBP≥90 mmHg, not currently taking drug prescribed for high blood pressure.

The three latter categories together are considered as 'hypertensive' for the purpose of this report. According to this definition the prevalence of high blood pressure was 40.8% for men and 32.9% for women and increased with age.

Significant differences in high blood pressure between socio-economic groups (with higher prevalence in more deprived groups) were seen in women only: the age-standardised prevalence of high blood pressure was 30.1% in the highest income group and 37.3% in the lowest.

Blood analytes

The blood analytes that were investigated were total cholesterol, HDL-cholesterol, C-reactive protein and fibrinogen. All of these have been shown to be independently associated with cardiovascular disease and are therefore important in the determination of cardiovascular risk profile.

Mean cholesterol was 5.5 mmol/l for men and 5.6 mmol/l for women. It was slightly lower than in 1994 for all age groups in both men and women. Caution is nevertheless needed when interpreting these results, since the laboratory used in 1998 was different from that used in 1994. Overall, 18.0% of men and 22.4% of women in 1998 had a cholesterol level of 6.5 mmol/l or above. Total cholesterol showed very little social class, income and area variation.

Women had higher mean HDL-cholesterol than men (1.6 mmol/l vs 1.3 mmol/l). The proportion of informants with an HDL-cholesterol level of 0.9 mmol/l or less was much higher in men (16.9%) than in women (5.4%). No difference in age-adjusted mean HDL-cholesterol levels was found between social classes among men, while women in manual social classes tended to have a lower mean level than those in non-manual social classes. Mean HDL-cholesterol tended to increase as income increased in both sexes, after adjustment for age.

In the literature there is no recommendation for a C-reactive protein (CRP) threshold and quintile distributions are presented in this report. CRP increased with age in both sexes, but this increase was more marked among men. An income gradient was observed: high levels of CRP were more prevalent in people in low income households.

Mean fibrinogen was 2.6 g/l for men and 2.8 g/l for women and increased with age. Fibrinogen levels were higher in women than in men in all age groups. A social class gradient was observed: mean fibrinogen value adjusted for age was higher in manual than non-manual social classes in both sexes, and negatively associated with income in both men and women.

Relationship of CVD to risk factors and socio-demographic factors

The relationship between CVD and various risk factors was investigated. Plasma cholesterol, cigarette smoking and hypertension, established as major risk factors for CVD, were considered together with many other risk factors, looking at their association with CVD individually initially, then at the contribution of each risk factor after the others were simultaneously taken into account.

In both men and women, the mean age of those with CVD was 60.4. The mean age of those without CVD was 43.8 in men and 45.2 in women. After age standardisation, the prevalences of the main CVD risk factors in both groups were compared: 49% of men with CVD had high blood pressure compared with 39% of those without CVD (in women 44% vs 33% respectively). In both sexes, current cigarette smoking prevalence was no higher in those with CVD than in those without. This was not unexpected, as many people may have decreased their consumption after having been diagnosed. It is nevertheless worth noting that between a fifth and a quarter (21% of men and 23% of women overall) of people with CVD were still smoking cigarettes. Levels of total cholesterol did not differ significantly between those with and without CVD, but a higher proportion of those with CVD than of those without had low HDL-cholesterol (0.9 mmol/l or less): 23% of men with CVD had low HDL-cholesterol, compared with 16% of men without CVD; in women 8% vs 5% respectively. 25% of men with CVD were physically inactive, compared with 17% of those without CVD (in women 33% vs 22%). Other risk factors that were found to be positively associated with CVD were a family history of CVD, high GHQ12 scores (scores of 4 or more, indicative of possible psychiatric morbidity), a raised waist-hip ratio (0.95 or more in men, 0.85 or more in women), high levels of C-reactive protein. In women, an association between manual social classes and CVD was also seen.

Hypertension is a major risk factor for CVD. On the whole, a higher proportion of informants with high blood pressure were physically inactive, were overweight or obese, had high total cholesterol and low HDL-cholesterol than of those without high blood pressure.

Further analyses were carried out on informants aged 35 and over with IHD or stroke. Multiple regression models assessed the contribution of each risk factor once the others were simultaneously taken into account. In men, high blood pressure, high levels of fibrinogen and high GHQ12 scores (indicative of possible psychiatric morbidity) remained independently associated with IHD or stroke, while the relation between social class and IHD or stroke was eliminated by simultaneous adjustment for age and biological, behavioural and psychological risk factors. For women, low physical activity and high GHQ12 scores, in addition to manual social class, remained associated with the disease.

Self-reported health and psychosocial well-being

44% of both men and women reported a longstanding illness. This is an increase since 1994, when prevalence was 39% among men and 40% among women. Prevalence increased with age, as did the number of illnesses reported. 25% of men and 27% of women reported a longstanding illness that limited their activities in some way.

The age-standardised prevalence of longstanding illness increased with decreasing household income and was higher in manual social classes. Differences in the prevalence of limiting longstanding illness by social class and household income were similar to those for longstanding illness overall, but were more strongly marked.

15% of men and 19% of women reported acute sickness in the two weeks before the interview. Prevalence was higher in 1998 than in 1994 (increasing from 12% to 15% among men and 15% to 19% among women).

Among men, the prevalence of acute sickness was inversely related to household income, and was higher among manual social classes. Among women, there was no clear relationship with social class or household income.

75% of men and 73% of women rated their health as 'good' or 'very good', a decline from 78% of men and 75% of women in 1994. 19% of men and 20% of women rated their health 'fair'. 7% of each sex rated it as 'bad' or 'very bad'.

The proportion rating their health as 'good' or 'very good' declined with increasing age, and (less markedly) with decreasing household income. It was lower in manual social classes, and was below average in Inner London.

The General Health Questionnaire (GHQ12) is a measure of psychiatric morbidity and a GHQ12 score of four or more is used to identify informants with a possible psychiatric disorder. Women (18%) were more likely than men (13%) to have a high GHQ12 score (of 4 or more). No trend since 1994 was seen.

The prevalence of high GHQ12 did not appear to be related to social class. Among men, but not among women, it was inversely related to household income. The prevalence of a high GHQ12 score was higher in Inner London than other areas.

Men (16%) were more likely than women (11%) to report a severe lack of social support. No clear trend since 1994 was observed. There was a higher prevalence of severe lack of social support in lower income quintiles, manual social classes, and in Inner London.

Use of services and prescribed medication

13% of men and 18% of women had contacted their (NHS) GP in the two weeks before interview.

In the year preceding the interview, a third of each sex had visited an outpatient or casualty department, 6% of each sex had had a day patient stay, and 8% of men and 11% of women had been admitted as inpatients.

The use of health services increased with age for both men and women. Compared to men, women in the reproductively active ages of 16-44 had consistently higher rates of GP consultation and inpatient attendance, probably due to pregnancy and childbirth. From the age of 45 onwards and for services not related to maternity, such as day patient and outpatient attendance (which exclude ante-natal visits), the pattern of service use for men and women was similar.

About two in five men (39%) and half of all women (49%) were taking prescribed medicines. From age 45, use of prescribed medicines rose steeply with age. From age 75, 81% of men and 86% of women were on prescribed medication, with more than two in five of those on medication taking four or more drugs.

Overall, there has been a slight upward trend since 1994 in the proportions of adults who took any medication. There was no significant change in the distribution of medicines taken by broad British National Formulary (BNF) categories over the period 1995 to 1998.

9% of women were on hormone replacement therapy (HRT) when interviewed and 6% had been users in the past. A significantly higher proportion of women in Social Class I households reported having used HRT (31%) than of women in Social Class V households (20%). Similarly, women in households in the highest income quintile were more likely to have used HRT (33%) than women in the lowest income quintile (20%).

Introduction

1.1 The Health Survey for England

The Health Survey for England comprises a series of annual surveys, of which the 1998 survey is the eighth. All eight surveys have covered the adult population aged 16 and over living in private households in England. The four most recent surveys, 1995-1998, have also covered children aged 2 to 15 living in households selected for the survey.

The series is part of an overall programme of surveys commissioned by the Department of Health and designed to provide regular information on various aspects of the nation's health which cannot be obtained from other sources. The Health Survey series was designed to achieve the following aims:

1. To provide annual data for nationally representative samples to monitor trends in the nation's health

2. To estimate the proportion of people in England who have specified health conditions

3. To estimate the prevalence of certain risk factors associated with these conditions

4. To examine differences between subgroups of the population (including regional populations) in their likelihood of having specified conditions or risk factors

5. To assess the frequency with which particular combinations of risk factors are found, and in which groups these combinations most commonly occur

6. To monitor progress towards selected health targets

7. (From 1995) to measure the height of children at different ages, replacing the National Study of Health and Growth.[1]

Each survey in the series consists of core questions and measurements (for example, anthropometric and blood pressure measurements and analysis of blood samples), plus modules of questions on specific issues that change periodically.

Since 1994, the Health Survey for England has been carried out by the Joint Health Surveys Unit of the *National Centre for Social Research* (formerly Social and Community Planning Research)[2] and the Department of Epidemiology and Public Health at the Royal Free and University College Medical School.

1.2 The 1998 Health Survey for England

During the first four years of the Health Survey, the focus was on cardiovascular disease (CVD). The focus shifted to other topics in 1995 to 1997, but in 1998 the topic of CVD was revisited so that any changes since the last survey on CVD, in 1994, could be examined.

Questions on CVD in 1998 were very similar to those asked in 1994, and included the Medical Research Council (MRC) respiratory questionnaire. In addition to a number of 'core' topics repeated every year (cigarette smoking, alcohol consumption, general health, prescribed medication, use of services), other topics covered in 1998 included physical activity, eating habits, psychosocial health and social support.

A brief outline of survey methodology follows. Further details are given in Chapter 8.

1.3 Ethical clearance

Ethical approval for the 1998 survey was obtained from the North Thames Multi-centre Research Ethics Committee (MREC) and from all Local Research Ethics Committees (LRECs) in England.

1.4 This report

The 1998 report presents results only for adults. Comparisons are made with the findings from the last survey focusing on CVD (1994), in which only adults were interviewed.

Tables containing data about children for 1998, and also summarising selected trends among children since 1995, will be found on the Department of Health website referenced in Section 1.6.6 below. To assist users of these child data tables, the present report provides a full description of the methods of sampling, interviewing and taking measurements among children, as well as those relating to adults.

1.5 Overview of the survey design

1.5.1 Sample design

The survey was designed to provide a representative sample of the population of England aged two and over living in private households. Those living in institutions were outside the scope of the survey. This should be borne in mind when considering survey findings; the institutional population is likely to be older and, on average, less healthy than those living in private households.

A random sample of 13,680 addresses was selected from the Postcode Address File, using a multi-stage sample design with appropriate stratification. 720 postcode sectors were selected and 19 addresses were selected within each sector.

At each household contacted, all persons aged two and over were eligible for the survey. However, where there were more than two children, only two (selected randomly) were interviewed, in order to avoid an excessive burden on individual households.[3]

A full account of the sample design is given Chapter 8.

1.5.2 Weighting of children

None of the surveys in the series prior to 1995 involved weighting, the achieved samples being judged to reflect the shape of the population sufficiently closely to make this unnecessary. It was, however, necessary to introduce weighting for the sample of children, in surveys from 1995, in order to compensate for the limitation to two per household (see Chapter 8, Section 8.8.2 for a description of the weighting method). The adult data, however, have continued not to be weighted (except that in 1997 special weighting was required for those aged 16-24 as well as for children).[4]

1.5.3 Interviewing children

Children aged 13 to 15 were interviewed in person, with the permission of a parent or guardian. Where the child was aged 2 to 12, one of the child's parents or guardians answered the questions on the child's behalf, with the child present during the interview. Because of children's need for privacy in respect of some of their responses, self-completion questionnaires were provided to children aged 8 to 15 for topics such as drinking and smoking. (This was also the case for young adults aged 16 and 17.)

1.5.4 Fieldwork design

Each sampled address was sent an advance letter and then visited by an interviewer. The interviewer sought the agreement of each adult in the household to an interview, and sought parents' and children's permissions to interview children. The content of the interview is detailed in Chapter 8, Section 8.3, and the questions asked are given in

Appendix A. After obtaining information on general health, psychosocial health, social support, CVD conditions, eating habits, smoking and drinking behaviour, physical activity, use of services, and socio-demographic characteristics, the interviewer measured the informant's height and weight. At the end of the interview, the interviewer sought agreement for a visit by a nurse. At all stages of the survey informants were given the opportunity to opt out.

The nurse obtained information on prescribed medication, took the blood pressure of those aged 5 and over, made a number of other measurements - mid-upper arm circumference for children, waist and hip for those aged 16 and over, and demi-span for those aged 65 and over - and obtained a sample of saliva (for all those aged 4 and over).

Informants aged 18 and over and, in sample points selected for the second half of the survey year, those aged 11 to 17 were asked to provide a small sample of blood by venepuncture (see Chapter 8, Section 8.3.4, in Volume II). Written consent was obtained prior to taking a sample. Informants aged 11-17 were offered the option of an anaesthetic cream prior to venepuncture.

The blood and saliva samples were analysed for the following analytes (see Chapter 8 and Appendix B):

saliva   cotinine

blood   total cholesterol, HDL cholesterol, haemoglobin, ferritin (in children and adults), fibrinogen, C-reactive protein (in adults only).

Computer-assisted methods were used by interviewers, as in the three preceding surveys, and, for the first time, by nurses.

1.5.5   Survey response

Interviews were obtained with 19,654 persons: 15,908 with those aged 16 and over and 3,746 with those aged 2-15. 16,799 saw a nurse (13,586 aged 16 and over and 3,213 aged 2-15). A blood sample was obtained from 10,773 of those aged 16 and over and from 268 children aged 11 to 15.

Response to the survey can be calculated in two ways: at a household and at an individual level. A summary of responses obtained to each component of the survey is given below.

Interviews were carried out at 74% of sampled households. Interviews were obtained with 92 % of adults and 96% of (sampled) children living in these households.

Assuming that households where the number of adults and children was not known contained, on average, the same number as in households where it was known, the individual response rate was 69% among adults and 75% among (sampled) children.

Not all those interviewed agreed to all other stages of the survey. For example, 59% of adults and 64% of (sampled) children saw a nurse. The table below gives further details. Columns 1 and 2 give the proportion of adults and (sampled) children in sampled eligible households who responded to each stage of the survey. Columns 3 and 4 give the proportion of adults and children in co-operating households who responded to each stage of the survey. Where a stage is age-specific, the base for the percentage is the total number of adults or (sampled) children in that age group in co-operating households. Chapter 8, Section 8.6, provides a fuller response analysis.

	Adults in eligible households	Sampled children in eligible households	Adults in co-operating households	Children in co-operating households
	%	%	%	%
Interviewed	69	75	92	96
Height measured	66	72	89	92
Weight measured	64	71	86	91
Saw nurse	59	64	79	83
Demi-span measured (aged 65 and over)	*	na	*	na
Upper arm circumference measured (aged 2-15)	na	64	na	82
Blood pressure measured (aged 5 and over)	58	62	77	81
Saliva sample obtained (aged 4 and over)	57	61	77	81
Blood sample obtained (aged 11-15)	na	32	na	41
Blood sample obtained (aged 16 and over)**	47	na	62	na

* Not calculated, as number of persons aged 65 and over in non-co-operating eligible households is not known.

** 5% of sampled adults were not eligible to give a sample.

na Not applicable.

1.6 Data analysis

1.6.1 Introduction

The Health Survey is a cross-sectional survey of the population. It examines associations between health states, personal characteristics and behaviour, but such associations do not necessarily imply causality. In particular, associations between current health states and current behaviour need careful interpretation, as current health may reflect past, rather than present, behaviour. Although the survey includes questions about past behaviour, these are necessarily limited and subject to memory and other forms of error.

1.6.2 Age standardisation

Age-standardised tables focusing on categories of particular interest (for example, household income groups) are presented in the report. In comparing such groups, age standardisation reweights the sample in each household income group so as to give it the same age profile as the total population,[5] thereby removing the effect of age from income group comparisons in respect of the health variable concerned. (See also Appendix E: Glossary.)

1.6.3 The treatment of age as an analysis variable

Age is a continuous variable. The presentation of tabular data involves classifying the sample into year bands. This can be been done in two ways:

● *Age last birthday*

● *'Rounded age',* rounded to the nearest integer.

In the present report, age always refers to age last birthday.

1.6.4 Trend analysis

The two earliest surveys (1991 and 1992) have not been included in trend analysis because of their smaller size and the limitation of their fieldwork to one quarter of the year. Of the two following full-scale surveys (1993 and 1994) that also focused on CVD, the more recent (1994) was chosen as the baseline for examining trends in the present report. Trend analysis thus covers a five year period, 1994 to 1998 inclusive.

1.6.5 Regional and area analyses

This report contains tables giving analyses by NHS regional offices. While the four northern regions remained unaltered, the boundaries and names of the four southern regions were changed in 1999.[6] However, to permit comparisons with previous years of the Health Survey, the regional tables are based on the pre-1999 boundaries. Regional differences are not reported in the commentary.

In addition to the regional analysis, analyses will also be found by Health Authority (HA) area type, using the Office of National Statistics (ONS) grouping of HAs into a number of types using cluster analysis of socio-demographic data from the 1991 Census. There are several levels of classification, but the one used in this report is that relating to the six 'families' of HAs,[7] which are referred to as 'area types'.

1.6.6 Availability of published data

As in the case of previous surveys, a copy of the 1998 Health Survey data will be deposited at The Data Archive at the University of Essex. Copies of anonymised data files can be made available for specific research projects through the Archive (telephone 01206 872001).

In addition, data is available on the Department of Health's website at www.doh.gov.uk/public/summary.htm, where it is planned to post a wider range of tables, and on the website of the Joint Health Surveys Unit, which can be accessed from the UCL website at: www.ucl.ac.uk/epidemiology/jhsu/jhsu.html.

1.7 The content of this report

The report is in two volumes. Volume I presents the survey findings in Chapters 2 to 7. Tables are presented at the end of each chapter. Some tables are included for reference purposes only and are not commented on in the text.

Methodological issues are covered in Volume II (Chapter 8 and Appendices). Notes on the conventions adopted for tables will be found at the front of Volume I.

VOLUME I

Chapter 2   Prevalence of cardiovascular conditions (CVD)

This chapter deals with the prevalence of cardiovascular disease (CVD), investigating the prevalence of self-reported conditions: angina, heart attack, stroke, heart murmur, abnormal heart rhythm, 'other heart trouble', diabetes and high blood pressure. For angina and heart attack the prevalence according to the Rose Angina Questionnaire is also presented. This chapter also examines these conditions by socio-economic characteristics, and investigates differences in specific conditions between 1994 and 1998. The prevalence of some respiratory symptoms, namely breathlessness, phlegm and wheezing as assessed by the MRC Respiratory Questionnaire, is also reported on.

Chapter 3   Cardiovascular risk factors

This chapter presents results relating to a number of cardiovascular risk factors - alcohol consumption, cigarette smoking, eating habits, physical activity levels, body mass, blood pressure and selected blood analytes. Current prevalences are indicated, as are variations between socio-economic groups. Trends over time are also noted.

Chapter 4   Relationship of CVD to risk factors and socio-demographics

This chapter considers the associations between CVD and a variety of risk factors (including those discussed in Chapter 3) and socio-economic characteristics. The association between CVD and socio-economic status is examined, taking into account the contribution of the other various risk factors.

Chapter 5   Physical activity

This chapter reports on the different types of physical activities undertaken (housework, manual work, walking, sports and exercise, and also including physical activity at work), the time spent on them, and the intensity level involved. A summary measure of overall physical activity is derived. Trends since 1994 are commented on.

Chapter 6   Self-reported health and psychosocial well-being

The first part of this chapter examines self-report of general health, longstanding illness and acute sickness. The second part looks at two measures of psychosocial well-being (the GHQ12 and a social support scale).

Chapter 7 Use of health services and prescribed medicines

The first part of this chapter reports on levels of use of various health services (GP consultations, outpatient, day patient and inpatient visits), including information on where GP consultations took place and the duration of inpatient stays. The second part of the chapter analyses informants' reports of any prescribed medicines they take, with a particular focus this year on hormone replacement therapy (HRT). Women's use of contraception is also examined.

VOLUME II

Chapter 8 Survey methodology and response rates

A full account of the survey design is provided, with an analysis of response to the various stages of the survey. Sampling errors associated with many of the estimates shown in this report are presented. There is also an analysis of non-response. Information about the laboratory technique and quality control of blood analytes is also presented here.

Appendix A

Provides a list of the questions included in the computer assisted interviews (interviewers and nurses) and copies of other key fieldwork documents.

Appendix B

Protocols used for making measurements of height, weight, demi-span, mid-upper arm circumference and blood pressure, and for taking blood and saliva samples.

Appendix C

Summarises the system used to classify prescribed medicines.

Appendix D

Provides a map of the areas covered, as at 1998, by the eight regional offices of the NHS Executive.

Appendix E

Is a glossary which contains descriptions and definitions of analysis techniques and terms used frequently in the report.

References and notes

1 The National Study of Health and Growth was set up in 1972 to monitor the growth of primary school children. For example, see Chinn S, Price CE, Rona RJ. *The need for new reference curves for height.* Archives of Disease in Childhood 1989; **64**:1545-1553.

2 Social and Community Planning Research (SCPR) changed its name in 1999, on the occasion of the thirtieth anniversary of its founding, to the *National Centre for Social Research.*

3 For similar reasons, a maximum of ten adult interviews was imposed, but there was no case where this applied.

4 The reason for this is that in 1997 those aged under 16 were oversampled relative to those aged 16 and over, in order to provide a larger sample of children. In the report, which was confined to those aged under 25, it was thus necessary to weight the 16-24 sample in order to bring them into proper balance with those under 16.

5 The population used for age-standardising is the mid-year 1997 population estimate for England. No adjustment is made for the fact that the survey covers only that part of the population that is resident in private households.

6 The four new regions introduced in 1999 are Eastern, London, South East and South West; they replaced the previous regions of Anglia and Oxford, North Thames, South Thames and South West. The northern regions of Northern and Yorkshire, Trent, North West and West Midlands were not affected by the 1999 changes.

7 Wallace M, Denham C. *Classification of local and health authorities of Great Britain.* Studies on Medical and Population Studies No. 59. HMSO, London, 1996.

Prevalence of cardiovascular disease

2

Paola Primatesta

SUMMARY

- Including self-reported high blood pressure among the CVD conditions, 27.9% of men and 27.8% of women reported having been diagnosed as having a CVD condition.

- CVD prevalence increased with age in both sexes. Men had a higher prevalence of CVD conditions than women. In particular, the prevalence of angina (5.3% vs 3.9%), heart attack (4.2% vs 1.8%), stroke (2.3% vs 2.1%) and diabetes (3.3% vs 2.5%) was higher in men than in women.

- The prevalence of the most severe category of CVD conditions (i.e. heart attack or stroke) was twice as high in men as in women.

- The overall prevalence of angina and possible myocardial infarction symptoms as shown by the Rose Questionnaire were different from the prevalence of reported doctor-diagnosed conditions; the prevalence of angina was higher in women (3.1%) than in men (2.6%).

- The MRC Respiratory Questionnaire was used in order to ask about various respiratory symptoms, namely breathlessness, phlegm and wheeze. The prevalence of breathlessness was higher in women (26.4%) than in men (19.8%) while the prevalence of phlegm production was higher in men (13.1%) than in women (7.9%). About a fifth of both men and women reported wheeze symptoms.

- The prevalence of CVD, ischaemic heart disease (IHD) and IHD or stroke by socio-economic characteristics was examined in informants aged 35 and over only. The prevalence of any CVD condition showed a significant association in women only, while IHD and IHD or stroke showed a gradient according to social class and income in both sexes; for instance, the age-standardised prevalence of IHD was 5.2% in men in Social Class I and 11.3% in Social Class IV (for women it was 5.7% in Social Class II and 10.0% in Social Class V).

- Small changes over the period 1994 to 1998 were observed for IHD, IHD or stroke, diabetes and Rose Angina symptoms in both sexes. Even though the changes were statistically significant for some of the conditions (IHD or stroke), caution is needed in the interpretation of results from these cross-sectional data and a longer time series is needed for a more robust interpretation of the results.

2.1 Introduction

This chapter deals with the prevalence of cardiovascular disease (CVD). Despite the reduction in mortality from CVD since the 1970's in most industrialised countries, cardiovascular disease, and in particular coronary heart disease, is still the leading cause of death in the western world.[1,2] The White Paper 'Saving Lives: Our Healthier Nation' recognised that the United Kingdom is at present one of the worst countries for deaths from circulatory disease, and identified heart disease and stroke as among the four priority areas to tackle.[3] The target was set of reducing the death rate from coronary heart disease and stroke amongst people aged under 75 by at least two fifths (based on 1996 data) by the year 2010.

CVD was the main focus of the Health Survey series from its inception in 1991 until 1994. This chapter reports the prevalence of self-reported CVD conditions, examines CVD by socio-economic characteristics in 1998 and investigates differences in specific conditions between 1994 and 1998.

The prevalence of some respiratory symptoms, namely breathlessness, phlegm and wheezing as assessed by the Medical Research Council (MRC) Respiratory Questionnaire, is also reported on.

This chapter does not cover the relationship between various risk factors and CVD: this is examined in Chapter 4.

2.2 Methods and definitions

2.2.1 Methods

Informants were asked whether they suffered from any of the following conditions: angina, heart attack, stroke, heart murmur, abnormal heart rhythm, 'other heart trouble', diabetes and high blood pressure, and (if they responded affirmatively) if they had ever been told they had the condition by a doctor. For the purpose of this report, informants were classified as having a particular condition only if they reported that the diagnosis was confirmed by a doctor (or by a nurse in the case of blood pressure). Those informants who reported having a particular condition were also asked if they had it in the last 12 months (referred to in the tables as 'currently'), with the exception of high blood pressure (where they were asked if they still had it and if they were taking medication for it) and diabetes (where it was assumed that the condition is chronic and irreversible).

It should be noted that high blood pressure and diabetes are generally considered to be predisposing factors rather than cardiovascular conditions per se. They have been included in this chapter for comparability with previous surveys, but blood pressure is not dealt with in this chapter. (See Chapter 3, Section 3.6.3 for blood pressure distribution and prevalence of high blood pressure and Chapter 4 for the relationship between high blood pressure and CVD.)

It should also be stressed that no attempt was made to assess these self-reported diagnoses objectively. There is therefore the possibility that some misclassification may have occurred, because some informants may not have remembered (or not remembered correctly) the diagnosis made by their doctor.

2.2.2 Definitions used in this survey

Based on conditions mentioned above, the following definitions were used:

Any CVD condition

Informants were classified as having any CVD condition if they reported ever having any of the following conditions confirmed by a doctor (or a nurse in case of blood pressure): angina, heart attack, stroke, heart murmur, irregular heart rhythm, 'other heart trouble', high blood pressure or diabetes.

Ischaemic heart disease

Informants were classified as having ischaemic heart disease (IHD) if they reported ever having angina or a heart attack confirmed by a doctor.

Ischaemic heart disease or stroke

Informants were classified as having ischaemic heart disease or stroke (IHD or stroke) if they reported ever having angina, or a heart attack or a stroke, confirmed by a doctor.

'Severity' of CVD conditions

As in previous Health Survey reports, a hierarchical measure of 'severity' of CVD conditions was used, considering the categories as mutually exclusive. This definition of severity is somewhat arbitrary, and it is used for descriptive purposes only. It does not necessarily correlate with quality of life or risk of death. The hierarchy is defined below, from greatest severity to least.

● Heart attack or stroke

● Angina (but not a heart attack or stroke)

● High blood pressure or diabetes (but none of the above)

● Murmur or irregular heart rhythm or other heart trouble (but none of the above)

2.2.3 Rose Angina Questionnaire

In addition to the self-reported prevalence of angina and heart attack, the Rose questionnaire on angina and heart attack ('Rose Angina Questionnaire') was used as an alternative means of estimating the prevalence of these conditions. The Rose Angina Questionnaire was originally developed to identify the characteristic symptom complex known as angina in a standard way.[4] Its validity has been established predominantly by studies that compared the questionnaire to clinical diagnosis.[5,6]

From this questionnaire, informants were classified as having angina symptoms based on standard criteria.[7] Angina was then classified as grade 1 or grade 2, with grade 2 being the most severe.

Based on the Rose Angina Questionnaire, informants were classified as having had a possible myocardial infarction (heart attack) if they reported having ever had an attack of severe pain across the front of the chest, lasting for half an hour or more. This is referred to in this chapter as 'possible myocardial infarction'.

2.2.4 MRC Respiratory Questionnaire

The MRC Respiratory Questionnaire was developed in the 1950s and subsequently updated, to identify people with emphysema and chronic bronchitis, based on the prevalence of cough, sputum and breathlessness as predictors of chronic respiratory disability.[8]

Breathlessness was defined as shortness of breath brought on by exertion.[9] Wheeze was classified as attacks of wheezing or whistling in the chest at any time in the past 12 months, or attacks of breathlessness at night.

2.3 Prevalence and severity of CVD

2.3.1 Angina

Overall, 5.3% of men reported having ever had angina and 3.2% reported having it currently. Among women the corresponding figures were 3.9% and 2.5%, lower than in men in all age groups. In both sexes the prevalence increased with age, from being almost negligible in those aged under 35 to almost 1 in 5 in those aged 75 and over (18.3% of men and 17.0% of women aged 75 and older reported having ever been diagnosed by a doctor with the condition).

2.3.2 Heart attack

Overall, 4.2% of men reported having had a heart attack and 0.6% reported having it in the last 12 months. Among women prevalence was less than half of that in men (1.8% and 0.3% respectively). In both sexes prevalence increased with age: among men aged 65 and over more than 10% had had an heart attack, a tenth of them in the last 12 months.

2.3.3 Stroke

Stroke was a rarer condition than heart attack or angina. The differences between men and women were also smaller: overall 2.3% of men and 2.1% of women reported having had a stroke. Prevalence rose from 1.2% in men aged 45-54 (0.7% in women) to 6.2% in those aged 65-74 and 10.3% in those aged 75 and over (5.0% and 8.8% in women). Overall, 0.6% of men and 0.4% of women reported having had a stroke in the previous 12 months.

2.3.4 Diabetes

Overall, 3.3% of men and 2.5% of women reported being diabetic. The question did not make any attempt to differentiate between insulin-dependent (type I) and non insulin-dependent (type II) diabetes. Higher rates of disease were reported by older people (7.0% and 8.7% in men aged 65-74 and 75 and over, and 6.6% in women in both age groups), almost three times the rates reported by those aged 45-54 in men and more than four times in women.

2.3.5 Heart murmur, abnormal heart rhythm and 'other' heart trouble

Overall, 3.0% of men and 3.3% of women reported having had a heart murmur. The prevalence was higher in women than in men from age 35 to 64. For this condition the differences between the sexes, however, were not large.

Overall, 5.0% of men and 4.8% of women reported an abnormal heart rhythm. Prevalence increased markedly with age and was slightly higher in men than in women in all age groups. This, as a symptom of CVD, was often present in association with other CVD conditions: 24% of both men and women with an abnormal heart rhythm also reported angina, 17% heart attack, 24% heart murmur. (Data not shown.)

When the informant reported a heart condition that could not be placed in any of the above-mentioned categories they were considered as having 'other' heart trouble. Overall, 1.6% of men and 1.4% of women reported ever having had 'other' heart trouble.

In summary, CVD prevalence increased with age in both sexes. This was true for each condition with the exception of heart murmur, where no clear age pattern emerged. Men had in general a higher prevalence of CVD than women did; in particular the prevalence of angina, heart attack, stroke and diabetes was higher in men than in women.   **Table 2.1**

2.3.6 Ischaemic heart disease

The prevalence of ischaemic heart disease (angina or heart attack) was 7.1% in men and 4.6% in women. It was more than three times as high among those aged 55-64 (13.6% in men, 6.3% in women), as among those aged 45-54 (4.3% in men, 1.8% in women), and continued to increase with age to 23.4% in men and 18.4% in women aged 75 years and over.

2.3.7 IHD or stroke

The prevalence of ischaemic heart disease or stroke combined was 8.5% in men and 6.2% in women. The increase with age was steep and similar to that for ischaemic heart disease only. From age 65 onwards between a quarter and a third of men reported having had IHD or stroke: 24.2% of those aged 65-74 and 29.9% of those aged 75 and over. In women the corresponding figures were 15.6% and 24.7%.   **Table 2.2**

2.3.8 Severity

Including self-reported high blood pressure among the CVD conditions, 27.9% of men and 27.8% of women reported having been diagnosed as having a CVD condition. Excluding reported high blood pressure, the prevalence of reported CVD conditions almost halved to 15.7% of men and 14.1% of women overall. As can be seen by comparing Figures 2A and 2B, high blood pressure alone accounted for about two thirds of the reported CVD conditions in Table 2.3 and Figure 2A. The high absolute prevalence of high blood pressure and the fact that high blood pressure was more prevalent among women than men explain the small overall difference between men and women in the prevalence of CVD conditions.

For the most severe category (ie heart attack or stroke) the difference between men and women was larger, with men's rates almost double women's. Heart attack or stroke was the second most frequent category of CVD after high blood pressure or diabetes in men and women after 55 years of age. A further 2.6% of men and 2.5% of women had had angina but not heart attack or stroke. Once again the difference in prevalence between men and women was smaller than that presented in Table 2.1; when angina alone was present, without heart attack or stroke, women had comparatively higher rates than men.

Table 2.3, Figures 2A, 2B

Figure 2A

Proportion with any CVD condition (including self-reported high BP), by age

■ Men
■ Women

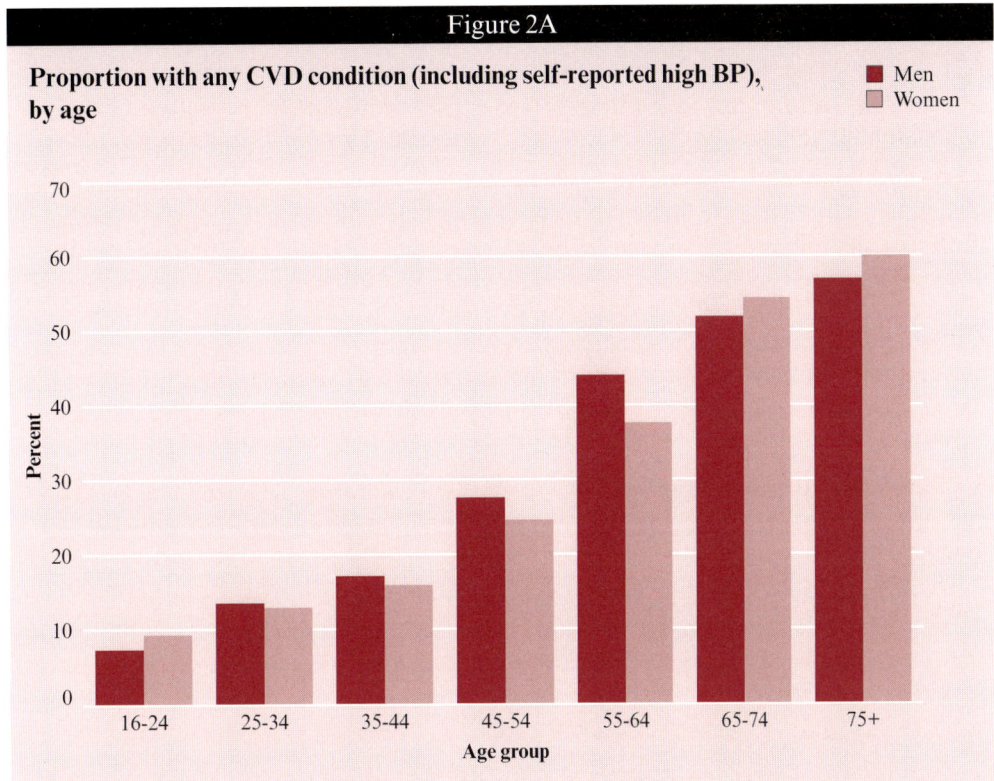

Figure 2B

Proportion with any CVD condition (excluding self-reported high BP), by age

■ Men
■ Women

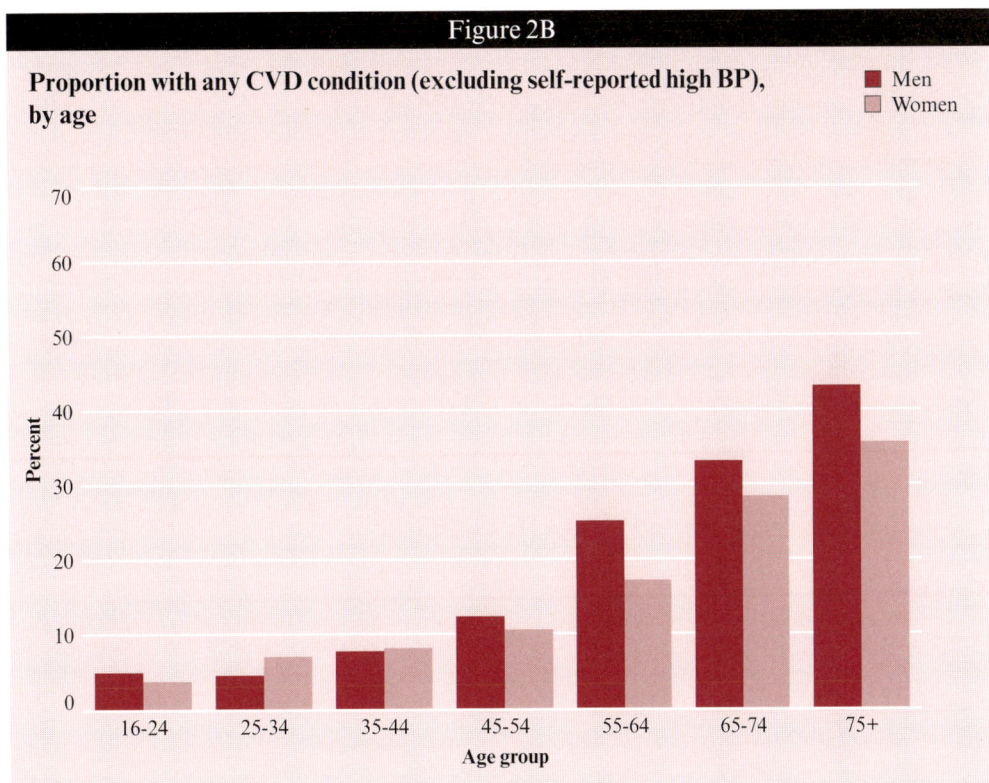

2.3.9 Rose Angina Questionnaire

Angina

The overall prevalence of angina symptoms by the Rose Questionnaire (grade 1 angina and grade 2 angina) was 2.6% in men and 3.1% in women. It was higher in women than in men in all age groups except for those aged 75 and over, where 7.3% of men and 5.9% of women reported the symptoms. The prevalence of angina symptoms as assessed by the Rose Questionnaire showed a different pattern to reported doctor-diagnosed angina (see Table 2.1): the overall prevalence was lower than for reported doctor-diagnosed angina, and women reported more symptoms than men. Also, the Rose Questionnaire gave higher estimates in the younger age groups and lower estimates in the older age groups than the self-reported prevalence.   **Table 2.4**

An attempt was made to measure the sensitivity, specificity and positive predictive value of the Rose Questionnaire in this population by comparing the Rose Questionnaire to the doctor-diagnosed condition, assuming the reported doctor-diagnosed condition to be representative of the actual rates of the condition in the population. The overall sensitivity was low, reflecting a high number of 'false negatives'; ie people who were not identified as having angina by the Rose Questionnaire but who reported doctor-diagnosed angina (24% in men, 25% in women). It improved slightly when Rose Angina was compared to self-reported angina in the last 12 months (32% in men, 29% in women). (Data not shown.)

Specificity was high, around 98%, reflecting the small number of 'false positives'; ie people who were classified as having angina by the Rose Questionnaire but did not report a diagnosis of angina.

The positive predictive value of the Rose Questionnaire (ie the proportion of people with doctor-diagnosed angina among those positive to the Rose Questionnaire) was 49% in men and 31% in women. The positive predictive value increased with age: it was 62% in men and 51% in women aged 65 and over. (Data not shown.)

Possible myocardial infarction

The overall prevalence of possible myocardial infarction symptoms according to the Rose Questionnaire was 8.6% in men and 5.6% in women. These rates were higher than the reported doctor-diagnosed heart attack rates; in men it was more than double the prevalence of doctor-diagnosed heart attack, while in women (where doctor-diagnosed heart attack was reported overall by 1.8%) the differences were even larger.   **Table 2.4**

2.3.10 Respiratory conditions

The MRC Respiratory Questionnaire was used in order to ask about various respiratory symptoms, namely breathlessness, phlegm and wheeze. The prevalence of breathlessness was higher in women than in men, and increased with age in both sexes. The prevalence of phlegm production was higher in men than in women, being more directly linked to symptoms of chronic bronchitis, which is generally more prevalent in men than in women. A fifth of women of all ages reported wheezing (20.1%), as did 21.0% of men. In women prevalence remained fairly constant with age, whereas in men it rose sharply from age 45-54 to age 55-64, and continued to increase to 28.8% in those aged 75 and over.   **Table 2.5**

2.4 CVD by socio-economic characteristics

2.4.1 Introduction

A gradient in CVD morbidity and mortality according to social class and other indicators of socio-economic status has been demonstrated in several studies. Mortality from IHD for men aged 20-64 in England & Wales in 1991-93 in Social Class V was nearly three times higher than in Social Class I; for stroke the difference was slightly over three.[10]

This section examines differences in the prevalence of CVD, IHD and IHD or stroke by social class, equivalised household income and Health Authority area type. Given the low prevalence of CVD among young people, the observed and age-standardised figures are presented in this section for informants aged 35 and over only. The overall prevalence of any CVD, IHD and IHD or stroke in this age group was as follows:

	Men %	Women %
CVD	36.3	35.5
IHD	10.4	6.7
IHD or stroke	12.5	8.9

2.4.2 Social class of head of household

The age-standardised prevalence of any CVD condition (including high blood pressure) was generally higher in manual than non-manual social classes in both sexes. In men prevalence was lowest in Social Class I (28.6%) and highest in Social Class V (38.2%) but the gradient was not consistent. In women the prevalence of CVD increased steadily from Social Class I (31.8%) to Social Class IV (39.7%), then decreased to 36.6% in Social Class V. In a logistic regression analysis, after adjusting for age differences were significant in women (p=0.001) but not in men.

For IHD and IHD or stroke a social class gradient was observed in both sexes. The age-standardised prevalence of IHD doubled in men from 5.2% in Social Class I to 11.3% in Social Class IV and 10.2% in Social Class V. In women there was a marked increase from Social Class II (5.7%) to Social Class V (10.0%), while the age-standardised prevalence in Social Class I was higher than in the other non-manual social classes (8.2%). The differences relative to average were statistically significant in both sexes (p<0.01).

The social classes most likely to be associated with IHD or stroke were IIINM (13.1%) and IV (13.4%) in men (p<0.01 statistically significant difference from Social Class I), and Social Class V in women (14%, p<0.001 statistically significant difference from Social Class I).

Table 2.6, Figure 2C

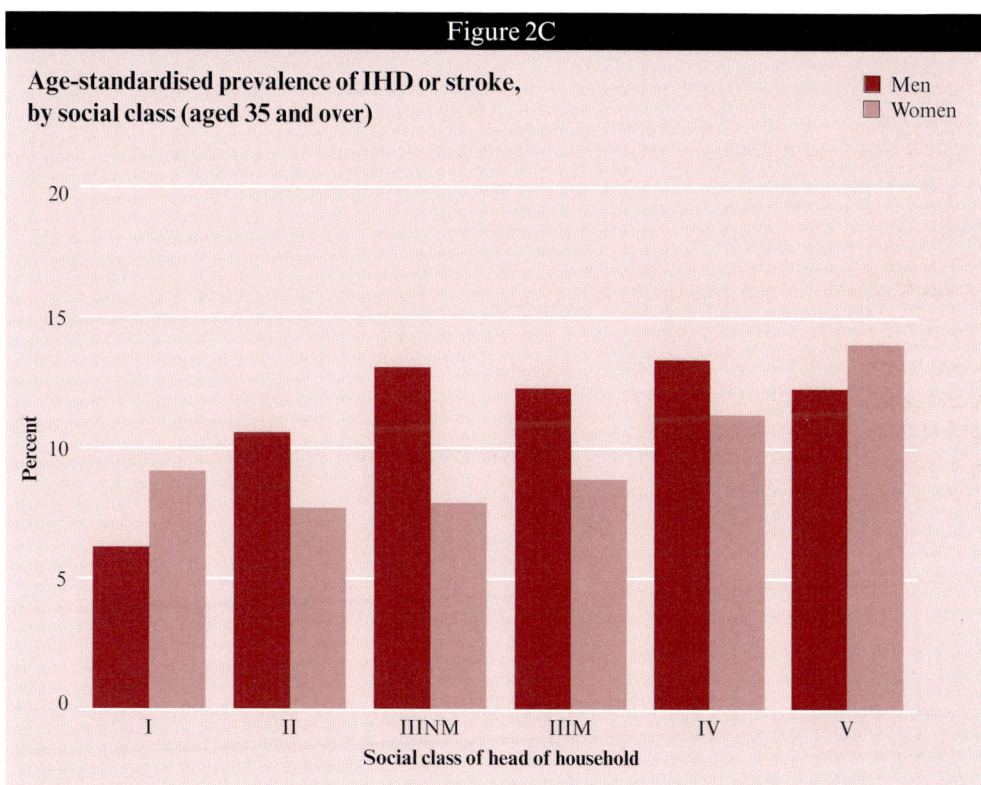

Figure 2C

Age-standardised prevalence of IHD or stroke, by social class (aged 35 and over)

■ Men
■ Women

Social class of head of household

2.4.3 Equivalised household income

Equivalised income differences were similar to differences in social class, CVD prevalence being inversely related to equivalised income. Both men and women in the lowest income quintile had a prevalence of any CVD condition almost 50% higher than those in the highest income quintile. For IHD and IHD or stroke men in the lowest income quintile had almost twice as high a prevalence as those in the highest quintile (13.7% vs 7.0% for IHD, and 16.0% vs 9.4% for IHD or stroke). In women the gradient was steeper for IHD or stroke

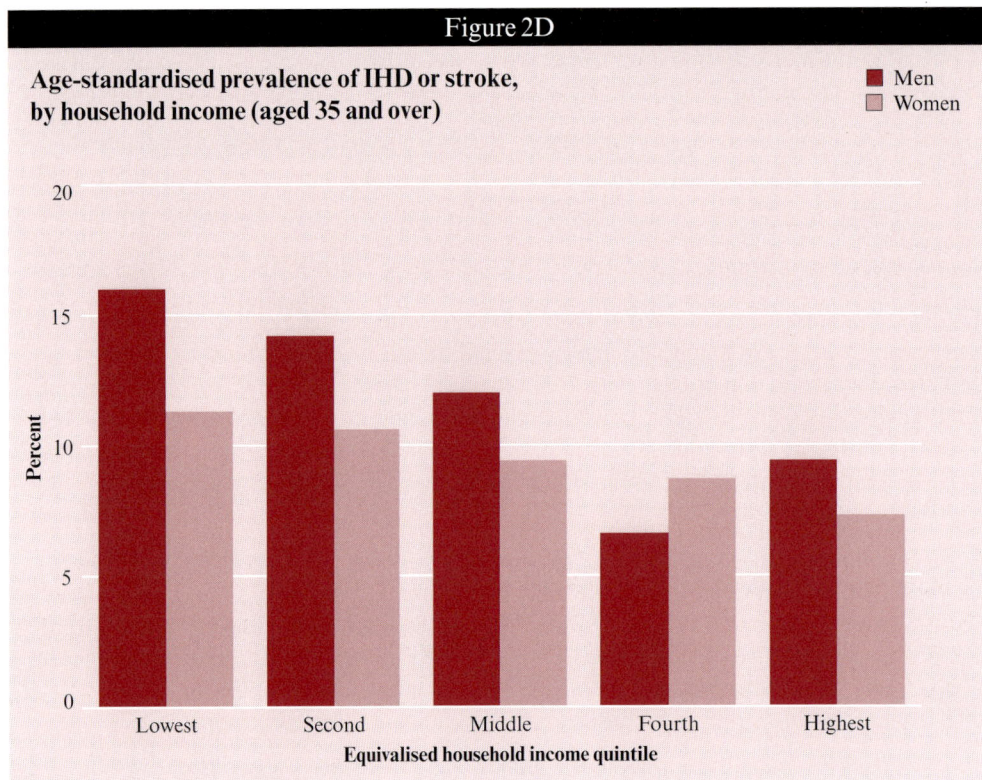

Figure 2D

Age-standardised prevalence of IHD or stroke, by household income (aged 35 and over)

■ Men
■ Women

Equivalised household income quintile

(11.3% in the lowest and 7.3% in the highest quintile) than for IHD alone (8.4% in the lowest vs 6.2% in the highest income quintile). **Table 2.7, Figure 2D**

2.4.4 Health Authority area type

The age-adjusted prevalence of CVD did not show great variation between the different area types. Urban and Mining and Industrial areas had higher prevalence than Rural areas in both sexes and for all conditions, but the differences were small. Inner London men had the lowest prevalence of IHD and IHD or stroke, while this was not true in women. **Table 2.8**

In summary, the prevalence of any CVD condition (including high blood pressure) showed a significant association with socio-economic status in women but not in men. This difference may be partly due to the fact that high blood pressure tends to show a social class gradient in women but not in men (see Chapter 3, Section 3.6.4). IHD and IHD or stroke showed a gradient according to social class and income in both sexes, confirming previous reports documenting social inequalities in the ischaemic heart disease profile.[11] Whether social class differences in risk factors for CVD can explain the excess burden in groups with low socio-economic status is still uncertain. The association between socio-economic characteristics and ischaemic heart disease and stroke after adjustment for other known risk factors is examined in Chapter 4.

2.5 Trends over time in CVD and respiratory conditions (1994-98)

This section considers variations in self-reported IHD, IHD or stroke, diabetes, angina and possible myocardial infarction symptoms according to the Rose Questionnaire, and wheezing (according to the MRC Questionnaire), between 1994 and 1998. Trends in blood pressure are reported in Chapter 3 Section 3.6.3.

Overall, the prevalence of IHD increased between 1994 and 1998. In men the prevalence was 6.0% in 1994 and 7.1% in 1998, with a small percent increase in most age groups. Once age was adjusted for in a regression analysis this increase was not statistically significant. In women the overall increase (observed in most age groups) was smaller, from 4.1% to 4.6%.

An increase was also seen in the overall prevalence of IHD or stroke. In men it rose from 7.1% to 8.5%; this increase was significant after adjustment for age (p<0.05). In women the increase was larger than in men in most age groups, with the overall prevalence increasing from 5.2% to 6.2% (p<0.01).

An analysis of change by age group is complicated by the low prevalence in the younger age groups, but the increase, which was observed across most of the age range, seems to have been more marked among younger people (aged under 45) than people aged 45 and over.

It should be emphasised that the data analysed are from cross-sectional, independent samples of the population in England; therefore the observed increase in prevalence refers to differences over time between different groups of people rather than longitudinal data in the same individuals. More robust results from longitudinal studies are needed to confirm these trends. If confirmed, the observed increase in prevalence could be due to an increase in the incidence (i.e. the new cases of disease) or to better management of the disease, which increased the survival rates of incident cases.

The self-reported symptoms as assessed by the Rose Questionnaire showed small, not significant changes between the two survey years: in men angina showed a slight decrease (from 3.2% to 2.6%) and in women the prevalence was unchanged at 3.2% in both years. The other symptoms assessed by the Rose Questionnaire, those of possible myocardial infarction, increased slightly in both sexes.

The prevalence of diabetes also increased slightly overall, although the increase seemed to be more marked in the older age groups (65 years and over): it increased from 5.8% to 7.0% in men aged 65-74 and from 7.5% to 8.7% in those aged 75 and over. In women it increased from 4.8% to 6.6% and from 5.2% to 6.6% respectively.

The prevalence of wheezing symptoms did not change appreciably. **Table 2.10**

References and notes

1 American Heart Association. *Heart and Stroke Facts.* 1994 Statistical Supplement. Dallas, Texas: American Heart Association, 1994.

2 Thorn TJ. *International mortality from heart disease: rates and trends.* Int J Epidemiol 1989; **18**:S20-8.

3 Department of Health. *Saving lives: our healthier nation.* The Stationery Office, London, 1999.

4 Rose GA, Blackburn H. *Cardiovascular survey methods.* World Health Organization Monograph 1986; **56**:1-188.

5 Bass EB, Follansbee WP, Orchard TJ. *Comparison of supplemented Rose Questionnaire to exercise tallium testing in men and in women.* J Clin Epidemiol 1981; **42**:385-94.

6 Blackwalder WC, Kagan A, Gordon T, Rhoads GG. *Comparisons of methods for diagnosing angina pectoris: the Honolulu heart study.* Int J Epidemiol 1981; **10**:211-15.

7 Rose defined angina as a chest pain or discomfort with the following characteristics:

   1. The site must include *either* the sternum (any level) *or* the left arm and left anterior chest (defined as the anterior chest wall between the levels of clavicle and lower end sternum);

   2. It must be provoked by either hurrying or walking uphill (or by walking on the level, for those who never attempt more);

   3. When it occurs on walking it must make the subject either stop or slacken pace, unless nitroglycerin is taken;

   4. It must disappear on a majority of occasions in 10 minutes or less from the time when the subject stands still.

   Grade 1 angina occurs when the subject only experiences the chest pain when walking uphill or hurrying.

   Grade 2 angina occurs when the subject experiences the chest pain even when walking at an ordinary pace on the level.

8 Fletcher CM, Peto R, Tinker C, Speizer F. *The natural history of chronic bronchitis and emphysema.* Oxford University Press, 1978.

9 The MRC identifies two categories of breathlessness:

   Grade 1: if breathlessness occurred when hurrying on level ground or walking up a hill.

   Grade 2: if breathlessness occurred when walking on level ground at the informant's own pace or at the pace of the informant's peers.

10 Drever F, Whitehead M (eds). *Health inequalities. Decennial Supplement.* ONS Series DS no. 15, The Stationery Office, London, 1997.

11 Iribarren C, Luepker RV, McGovern PG, Arnett DK, Blackburn H. *Twelve-year trends in cardiovascular disease risk factors in the Minnesota Heart Survey. Are socioeconomic differences widening?* Arch Intern Med 1997; **157**:873-81.

Tables

Table 2.1

Prevalence of CVD conditions (ever and currently), by age and sex

Aged 16 and over								*1998*
CVD conditions	**Age**							**Total**
	16-24	25-34	35-44	45-54	55-64	65-74	75 +	
	%	%	%	%	%	%	%	%
Men								
Angina								
Ever	-	0.1	0.7	2.8	10.5	15.6	18.3	5.3
Currently	-	0.1	0.5	1.9	7.1	8.2	11.3	3.2
Heart attack								
Ever	0.1	0.2	0.5	2.7	8.4	11.6	13.5	4.2
Currently	0.1	-	0.2	0.5	0.8	1.8	1.2	0.6
Heart murmur								
Ever	3.4	1.7	2.5	2.9	3.1	4.9	3.9	3.0
Currently	0.7	0.4	0.5	0.9	1.4	2.0	1.4	1.0
Abnormal heart rhythm								
Ever	1.9	1.8	3.4	3.9	8.5	9.1	11.6	5.0
Currently	0.8	0.7	1.8	1.9	5.2	4.5	7.0	2.7
'Other' heart trouble								
Ever	0.2	0.6	1.0	1.4	2.7	3.2	3.6	1.6
Currently	0.1	0.2	0.6	0.5	1.6	2.0	1.8	0.8
Stroke								
Ever	0.1	-	0.4	1.2	3.3	6.2	10.3	2.3
Currently	-	-	-	0.2	0.8	1.4	3.4	0.6
Diabetes								
Ever	0.1	0.7	1.6	2.9	5.8	7.0	8.7	3.3
Women								
Angina								
Ever	-	0.2	0.4	1.4	5.5	9.9	17.0	3.9
Currently	-	-	0.3	1.0	3.7	6.7	10.3	2.5
Heart attack								
Ever	-	0.1	0.3	0.8	2.4	5.5	6.5	1.8
Currently	-	-	-	0.1	0.7	1.0	0.8	0.3
Heart murmur								
Ever	2.2	3.0	2.9	3.5	3.7	4.9	3.6	3.3
Currently	0.9	1.0	1.0	1.8	1.6	1.6	1.5	1.3
Abnormal heart rhythm								
Ever	0.8	3.1	3.7	4.9	5.8	8.8	8.8	4.8
Currently	0.5	1.7	1.9	2.4	3.3	4.7	5.1	2.6
'Other' heart trouble								
Ever	0.1	0.7	0.6	0.9	2.7	2.6	3.4	1.4
Currently	-	0.2	0.3	0.5	1.0	1.8	2.4	0.8
Stroke								
Ever	0.4	0.4	0.6	0.7	2.2	5.0	8.8	2.1
Currently	-	0.1	-	0.1	0.7	0.5	1.7	0.4
Diabetes								
Ever	0.8	0.7	0.9	1.6	3.1	6.6	6.6	2.5
Bases[a]								
Men	*875*	*1338*	*1305*	*1289*	*987*	*837*	*562*	*7193*
Women	*1006*	*1630*	*1573*	*1484*	*1148*	*967*	*907*	*8715*

[a] Bases vary: those shown are for the overall sample.

Table 2.2

Prevalence of IHD,[a] and of IHD or stroke, by age and sex

Aged 16 and over   *1998*

IHD/IHD or stroke	Age							Total
	16-24	25-34	35-44	45-54	55-64	65-74	75 +	
	%	%	%	%	%	%	%	%
Men								
IHD	0.1	0.4	0.9	4.3	13.6	20.2	23.4	7.1
IHD or stroke	0.2	0.4	1.3	5.1	15.4	24.2	29.9	8.5
Women								
IHD	-	0.3	0.6	1.8	6.3	12.5	18.4	4.6
IHD or stroke	0.4	0.7	1.2	2.6	8.1	15.6	24.7	6.2
Bases								
Men	*875*	*1337*	*1305*	*1289*	*987*	*836*	*561*	*7190*
Women	*1006*	*1630*	*1573*	*1483*	*1148*	*967*	*907*	*8714*

[a] Ischaemic heart disease, reported as doctor-diagnosed heart attack or angina.

Table 2.3

Severity of CVD conditions, by age and sex

Aged 16 and over   *1998*

Severity of CVD conditions	Age							Total
	16-24	25-34	35-44	45-54	55-64	65-74	75 +	
	%	%	%	%	%	%	%	%
Men								
Heart attack or stroke	0.2	0.2	0.8	3.6	10.8	16.2	21.7	6.0
Angina but not heart attack or stroke	-	0.1	0.5	1.5	4.6	7.9	8.2	2.6
Only high blood pressure or diabetes	2.7	10.2	12.0	18.9	25.4	24.9	23.0	16.0
Only heart murmur, irregular heart rhythm or other heart trouble	4.3	2.9	3.8	3.5	3.2	2.9	4.1	3.5
Any CVD condition	7.3	13.5	17.1	27.6	44.0	51.8	56.9	27.9
No CVD condition	92.7	86.5	82.9	72.4	56.0	48.2	43.1	72.1
Women								
Heart attack or stroke	0.4	0.5	0.8	1.5	4.4	9.7	14.6	3.7
Angina but not heart attack or stroke	-	0.2	0.4	1.0	3.7	5.9	10.2	2.5
Only high blood pressure or diabetes	6.6	7.3	9.9	17.1	25.5	34.7	32.0	17.4
Only heart murmur, irregular heart rhythm or other heart trouble	2.4	4.9	4.9	5.1	3.9	3.9	3.3	4.2
Any CVD condition	9.3	12.9	15.9	24.6	37.6	54.3	60.0	27.8
No CVD condition	90.7	87.1	84.1	75.4	62.4	45.7	40.0	72.2
Bases[a]								
Men	*875*	*1338*	*1305*	*1289*	*987*	*837*	*562*	*7193*
Women	*1006*	*1630*	*1573*	*1484*	*1148*	*967*	*907*	*8715*

[a] Bases vary: those shown are for the overall sample.

Table 2.4

Prevalence of angina and MI symptoms (using the Rose Angina Questionnaire), by age and sex

Aged 16 and over   *1998*

Angina or myocardial infarction symptoms	Age							Total
	16-24	25-34	35-44	45-54	55-64	65-74	75 +	
	%	%	%	%	%	%	%	%
Men								
Grade 1 angina	0.7	0.6	0.8	1.6	2.3	4.1	5.9	1.9
Grade 2 angina	0.1	-	0.3	0.9	1.5	1.2	1.4	0.7
No angina symptoms	99.2	99.4	98.8	97.6	96.1	94.7	92.7	97.4
Symptoms of possible MI	3.2	5.2	6.9	8.5	13.9	14.2	11.9	8.6
No symptoms of possible MI	96.8	94.8	93.1	91.5	86.1	85.8	88.1	91.4
Women								
Grade 1 angina	0.8	1.8	1.3	2.4	3.1	5.1	3.9	2.4
Grade 2 angina	0.1	0.2	0.3	0.2	1.7	1.7	2.0	0.7
No angina symptoms	99.1	98.0	98.5	97.4	95.3	93.3	94.2	96.8
Symptoms of possible MI	2.9	3.3	4.6	5.5	7.9	7.7	9.6	5.6
No symptoms of possible MI	97.1	96.7	95.4	94.5	92.1	92.3	90.4	94.4
Bases								
Men	*874*	*1337*	*1303*	*1283*	*984*	*837*	*562*	*7180*
Women	*1006*	*1628*	*1571*	*1481*	*1147*	*967*	*904*	*8704*

Table 2.5

Respiratory conditions (using the MRC Respiratory Questionnaire), by age and sex

Aged 16 and over 1998

Respiratory conditions	Age							Total
	16-24	25-34	35-44	45-54	55-64	65-74	75 +	
	%	%	%	%	%	%	%	%
Men								
Breathlessness								
Grade 1 breathlessness	6.6	7.0	7.8	12.0	17.8	19.3	21.4	12.0
Grade 2 breathlessness	2.1	3.3	4.3	6.2	13.2	14.7	19.6	7.8
No breathlessness	91.3	89.7	87.9	81.8	69.0	66.0	59.1	80.2
Phlegm production								
Morning phlegm	11.1	9.5	9.4	10.0	14.1	17.0	20.6	12.2
Other phlegm	0.9	0.4	0.6	0.4	1.3	1.9	1.1	0.9
No phlegm	88.0	90.0	90.0	89.6	84.6	81.1	78.3	87.0
Wheeze symptoms[a]								
Wheeze symptoms	18.0	18.3	19.3	19.3	24.3	24.7	28.8	21.0
No wheeze	82.0	81.7	80.7	80.7	75.7	75.3	71.2	79.0
Women								
Breathlessness								
Grade 1 breathlessness	13.4	10.2	11.3	15.9	18.9	22.7	25.2	15.8
Grade 2 breathlessness	8.3	7.0	7.2	8.9	13.0	16.1	19.6	10.6
No breathlessness	78.3	82.8	81.5	75.3	68.1	61.2	55.3	73.6
Phlegm production								
Morning phlegm	7.0	6.0	5.9	5.9	8.8	11.2	12.0	7.6
Other phlegm	0.4	0.2	0.2	0.5	0.1	0.4	0.7	0.3
No phlegm	92.6	93.8	94.0	93.7	91.1	88.4	87.4	92.1
Wheeze symptoms[a]								
Wheeze symptoms	24.3	19.8	18.5	17.9	21.3	20.1	21.2	20.1
No wheeze	75.7	80.2	81.5	82.1	78.7	79.9	78.8	79.9
Bases								
Men	*874*	*1337*	*1305*	*1287*	*987*	*837*	*562*	*7189*
Women	*1006*	*1630*	*1572*	*1483*	*1148*	*967*	*906*	*8712*

[a] Informants were classified as having wheezed if they reported having had attacks of wheezing or whistling in the chest at any time in the past 12 months, or if they had been woken at night by attacks of breathlessness.

Table 2.6

Prevalence of CVD/IHD/IHD or stroke in informants aged 35 and over (observed and age-standardised), by social class and sex

Aged 35 and over   1998

CVD/ IHD / IHD or stroke	Social class of head of household						Social class of head of household					
	I	II	IIINM	IIIM	IV	V	I	II	IIINM	IIIM	IV	V
	%	%	%	%	%	%	%	%	%	%	%	%
	Men						**Women**					
CVD												
Observed	28.5	35.2	36.5	35.8	37.5	39.9	26.5	29.4	37.9	35.2	41.5	40.1
Standardised	28.6	35.5	35.4	34.4	34.9	38.2	31.8	32.9	35.0	37.7	39.7	36.6
IHD												
Observed	5.2	8.7	11.6	10.9	12.8	11.0	4.6	4.4	7.1	5.9	9.3	11.7
Standardised	5.2	8.8	11.1	10.1	11.3	10.2	8.2	5.7	6.0	6.7	8.4	10.0
IHD or stroke												
Observed	6.3	10.4	14.1	13.2	15.3	13.2	5.5	5.9	9.2	7.7	12.3	16.3
Standardised	6.2	10.6	13.1	12.3	13.4	12.3	9.1	7.7	7.9	8.8	11.3	14.0
Bases[a]	*368*	*1577*	*455*	*1603*	*689*	*228*	*347*	*1814*	*935*	*1512*	*934*	*370*

[a] Bases vary: those shown are for those aged 35 and over in the overall sample.

Table 2.7

Prevalence of CVD/IHD/IHD or stroke in informants aged 35 and over (observed and age-standardised), by equivalised household income and sex

Aged 35 and over   1998

CVD/ IHD / IHD or stroke	Equivalised annual household income quintile				
	Up to £7,186	Over £7,186 to £10,834	Over £10,834 to £17,890	Over £17,890 to £27,705	Over £27,705
	%	%	%	%	%
Men					
CVD					
Observed	44.0	41.5	37.3	31.6	25.0
Standardised	39.1	35.7	36.7	34.2	29.2
IHD					
Observed	17.1	14.8	10.3	4.6	4.7
Standardised	13.7	11.1	10.1	5.8	7.0
IHD or stroke					
Observed	20.3	18.7	12.3	5.4	5.9
Standardised	16.0	14.2	12.0	6.6	9.4
Women					
CVD					
Observed	42.2	46.4	31.7	25.9	22.8
Standardised	41.2	39.0	34.9	33.5	32.8
IHD					
Observed	8.9	11.4	5.1	3.4	1.6
Standardised	8.4	8.1	6.3	6.2	6.2
IHD or stroke					
Observed	11.9	14.2	7.2	4.6	2.2
Standardised	11.3	10.6	9.4	8.7	7.3
Bases[a]					
Men	*671*	*767*	*1026*	*913*	*921*
Women	*909*	*1177*	*1154*	*983*	*881*

[a] Bases vary: those shown are for those aged 35 and over in the overall sample.

Table 2.8

Prevalence of CVD/IHD/IHD or stroke in informants aged 35 and over (observed and age-standardised), by Health Authority area type and sex

Aged 35 and over   *1998*

CVD/ IHD / IHD or stroke	Health Authority area type					
	Inner London	Mining & Industrial	Urban	Mature	Prosperous	Rural
	%	%	%	%	%	%
Men						
CVD						
Observed	33.1	35.9	39.4	35.9	35.0	33.3
Standardised	35.3	35.4	38.7	34.8	33.8	32.3
IHD						
Observed	7.7	10.7	12.1	9.7	9.0	10.3
Standardised	8.1	10.4	11.7	9.0	8.4	9.6
IHD or stroke						
Observed	8.5	13.5	14.6	11.9	10.5	12.2
Standardised	8.8	13.1	14.0	11.1	9.9	11.5
Women						
CVD						
Observed	37.7	36.5	36.9	35.6	32.6	34.1
Standardised	40.6	36.7	36.7	35.8	34.4	35.4
IHD						
Observed	7.4	7.5	8.3	6.0	5.5	6.3
Standardised	8.4	7.5	8.2	6.0	6.3	6.8
IHD or stroke						
Observed	9.1	9.8	10.6	8.1	7.4	8.4
Standardised	10.5	9.8	10.5	8.1	8.4	9.1
Bases[a]						
Men	*130*	*793*	*718*	*757*	*1363*	*1219*
Women	*176*	*923*	*907*	*914*	*1677*	*1482*

[a] Bases vary: those shown are for those aged 35 and over in the overall sample.

Table 2.9

Prevalence of CVD/IHD/IHD or stroke in informants aged 35 and over (observed and age-standardised), by region and sex

Aged 35 and over   *1998*

CVD/ IHD / IHD or stroke	Region							
	Northern & Yorkshire	North West	Trent	West Midlands	Anglia & Oxford	North Thames	South Thames	South & West
	%	%	%	%	%	%	%	%
Men								
CVD								
Observed	37.6	32.5	36.2	34.2	33.0	36.2	35.8	37.2
Standardised	36.6	32.9	35.4	33.4	33.2	34.2	35.3	35.3
IHD								
Observed	12.1	9.5	10.2	10.6	8.8	10.6	8.2	10.3
Standardised	11.4	9.6	9.9	10.0	8.6	9.7	8.0	9.1
IHD or stroke								
Observed	15.1	11.4	12.5	12.4	10.8	12.2	10.0	12.3
Standardised	14.3	11.5	12.0	11.5	10.8	11.1	9.7	10.9
Women								
CVD								
Observed	36.5	36.7	35.0	33.9	34.1	34.3	33.5	34.1
Standardised	35.9	37.7	36.0	34.9	36.9	35.4	35.0	34.2
IHD								
Observed	7.3	7.3	7.0	7.9	6.0	4.7	6.6	5.6
Standardised	7.0	7.8	7.4	8.2	7.2	5.0	7.4	5.7
IHD or stroke								
Observed	9.7	9.3	9.4	10.8	7.9	6.4	7.9	8.0
Standardised	9.4	9.9	9.9	11.2	9.2	6.9	8.9	8.1
Bases[a]								
Men	*727*	*676*	*561*	*528*	*536*	*632*	*611*	*709*
Women	*886*	*776*	*670*	*658*	*655*	*771*	*808*	*855*

[a] Bases vary: those shown are for those aged 35 and over in the overall sample.

Table 2.10

Prevalence of CVD and respiratory conditions in 1994 and 1998, by age and sex

Aged 16 and over   *1998*

Condition	Age							Total
	16-24	25-34	35-44	45-54	55-64	65-74	75 +	
	%	%	%	%	%	%	%	%
Men								
IHD								
1994	-	0.3	0.5	3.0	10.3	21.0	22.7	6.0
1998	0.1	0.4	0.9	4.3	13.6	20.2	23.4	7.1
IHD or stroke								
1994	-	0.3	0.6	3.2	12.3	25.0	27.7	7.1
1998	0.2	0.4	1.3	5.1	15.4	24.2	29.9	8.5
Angina (by the Rose Questionnaire)								
1994	1.1	0.7	1.1	2.6	5.8	7.8	8.8	3.2
1998	0.8	0.6	1.1	2.4	3.9	5.3	7.3	2.6
Possible MI (by the Rose Questionnaire)								
1994	3.2	3.2	6.1	8.3	12.0	15.3	15.2	8.0
1998	3.2	5.2	6.9	8.5	13.9	14.2	11.9	8.6
Diabetes								
1994	0.8	0.8	1.0	2.5	6.4	5.8	7.5	2.9
1998	0.1	0.7	1.6	2.9	5.8	7.0	8.7	3.3
Respiratory conditions (wheeze)								
1994	21.9	17.6	18.5	17.4	24.5	26.5	29.0	21.1
1998	17.9	18.3	19.3	19.3	24.3	24.7	28.8	21.0
Women								
IHD								
1994	0.2	0.1	0.3	2.3	5.9	10.5	15.9	4.1
1998	-	0.3	0.6	1.8	6.3	12.5	18.4	4.6
IHD or stroke								
1994	0.2	0.3	0.5	2.8	7.5	13.4	20.2	5.2
1998	0.4	0.7	1.2	2.6	8.1	15.6	24.7	6.2
Angina (by the Rose Questionnaire)								
1994	1.4	1.6	2.2	2.7	4.9	5.8	6.1	3.2
1998	0.9	2.0	1.5	2.6	4.7	6.7	5.8	3.2
Possible MI (by the Rose Questionnaire)								
1994	2.6	2.6	4.1	5.2	6.3	6.5	8.6	4.8
1998	2.9	3.3	4.6	5.5	7.9	7.7	9.6	5.6
Diabetes								
1994	0.6	0.3	0.9	1.5	2.5	4.8	5.2	1.9
1998	0.8	0.7	0.9	1.6	3.1	6.6	6.6	2.5
Respiratory conditions (wheeze)								
1994	22.2	18.7	18.6	20.1	19.7	20.8	23.2	20.2
1998	24.3	19.8	18.5	17.9	21.3	20.1	21.2	20.1
Bases[a]								
Men								
1994	*968*	*1434*	*1329*	*1127*	*1001*	*877*	*441*	*7177*
1998	*875*	*1338*	*1305*	*1289*	*987*	*837*	*562*	*7193*
Women								
1994	*1080*	*1723*	*1520*	*1300*	*1059*	*1120*	*825*	*8627*
1998	*1006*	*1630*	*1573*	*1484*	*1148*	*967*	*907*	*8715*

[a] Bases vary: those shown are for the overall sample.

Risk factors for cardiovascular disease

3

Richard Boreham, Bob Erens, Emanuela Falaschetti,
Vasant Hirani, Paola Primatesta[1]

SUMMARY

Alcohol consumption

- There was a significant increase in alcohol consumption by women between 1994 and 1998, estimated mean weekly consumption increasing from 6.3 to 7.2 units, but men's alcohol consumption showed no significant change over this period (17.8 and 18.0 units). Nevertheless, as in 1994, men's estimated consumption was considerably in excess of women's, by a factor of more than two to one.

- Women's alcohol consumption progressively increased from Social Classes IV and V to Social Classes I and II, but men's did not. In both sexes consumption increased with household income. Consumption by both sexes decreased sharply with age after about the age of 50.

- Younger drinkers had more irregular drinking patterns than older drinkers, in terms both of frequency and of amounts per occasion. Older drinkers were more likely to drink regularly, and to drink the same amount each time.

Cigarette smoking

- Women's cigarette smoking prevalence remained the same (at 27%) over the five years 1994 to 1998. Men's fluctuated around 28%/29%, but did not exhibit any overall trend. However, among those aged 16-24 cigarette smoking prevalence was higher in 1998 than in 1994 (young men increasing from 35% to 41%, young women from 34% to 38%).

- For women, cigarette smoking prevalence as estimated by cotinine levels was the same as estimated by self-report of cigarette smoking, but for men it was higher than self-report of cigarette smoking, owing in part to pipe and cigar smoking.

- Cigarette smoking prevalence decreased with age, but the number of cigarettes per smoker per day increased into middle age before decreasing in later years.

- Cigarette smoking was much more prevalent among those in manual social classes and lower income groups. For example, age-standardised prevalence among men was 42% in the lowest income quintile and 21% in the highest. Those in lower income groups who smoked also smoked more cigarettes per day.

- The proportion smoking roll-ups was higher among men than women, and higher in Social Classes IV and V than in Social Classes I and II. It was also higher in lower income groups.

- Among branded cigarette smokers, men smoked brands with higher tar levels than women. The tar yield of branded cigarettes increased from Social Classes I and II to Social Classes IV and V, and - for women but not for men - was higher in the lower income groups .

Eating habits

- The Health Survey collected information on frequency of consumption of various groups of food and derived scores for fat and fibre consumption using a modified version of the DINE questionnaire. The prevalence of high fat and low fibre consumption was notably higher amongst the youngest age group (16-24); men in this age group had a higher prevalence of high fat consumption (38%) than women (16%). The prevalence of low fibre consumption was also high in this age group in men (65%) and women (72%).

- There was a clear socio-economic gradient in fat and fibre intake in both sexes; the prevalence of high fat and low fibre intake was higher in men and women in Social Class V and in the lowest income quintile.

Body mass

- Mean Body Mass Index (BMI) was 26.5 kg/m^2 in men and 26.4 kg/m^2 in women. Overall, obesity (BMI over 30 kg/m^2) was more prevalent in women (21.2%) than in men (17.3%); in particular, morbid obesity (BMI over 40 kg/m^2) was 30% higher in women than men. Mean BMI and the prevalence of obesity have continued to increase in both sexes since 1994.

- The prevalence of obesity and morbid obesity was higher in manual than in non-manual social classes in both sexes; in women, there was a progressive increase from Social Class I (14.4%, 0.7%) to Social Class V (28.1%, 3.3%) respectively. The gradient was less evident in men. The prevalence of obesity increased from the highest to the lowest income quintile in both men (14.5%, 20.3%) and women (15.9%, 26.3%).

Blood pressure

- Mean systolic blood pressure (SBP) was 136.8 mmHg in men and 132.5 mmHg in women. Mean diastolic blood pressure (DBP) was 76.2 mmHg in men and 72.3 mmHg in women. There was a decrease in mean SBP between 1994 and 1998. Mean DBP showed a slight decrease, mainly in the older age groups.

- High blood pressure (SBP≥140 mmHg or DBP≥90 mmHg or taking drug prescribed for high blood pressure) was found in 40.8% of men and 32.9% of women. Significant differences in high blood pressure between socio-economic groups (with higher prevalence in more deprived groups) were seen only in women, where the prevalence was 30.1% in the highest income quintile and 37.3% in the lowest.

Blood analytes

- 18.0% of men and 22.4% of women had a cholesterol level of 6.5 mmol/l or above. Small, not significant variations in mean total cholesterol by social class and equivalised income groups were seen in both sexes. The proportion of informants with an HDL-cholesterol level of 0.9 mmol/l or less was much higher in men (16.9%) than in women (5.4%). While total cholesterol did not show a gradient for socio-economic status, the proportion with low HDL-cholesterol (0.9 mmol/l or less) was higher in lower income quintiles. Age-standardised proportions in the lowest income quintile were 19.2% for men, 7.9% for women, compared with 14.9% and 2.9% respectively in the highest income quintile.

- C-reactive protein (CRP) is a marker of cardiovascular risk. CRP increased with age in both sexes, but this increase was more marked among men. High levels of CRP were more prevalent in people in lower income groups and manual social classes.

- Prospective population studies have established that fibrinogen is an independent predictor for ischaemic heart disease and stroke. Mean fibrinogen was 2.6 g/l for men and 2.8 g/l for women and increased with age. Mean fibrinogen value adjusted for age was higher in manual than non-manual social classes in both sexes.

3.1 Introduction

This chapter reviews the current prevalence among adults of a number of risk factors for cardiovascular disease (CVD), and, for those where comparative data are available, examines changes in their prevalence since 1994.

The risk factors reviewed are:

- Alcohol consumption (3.2)
- Cigarette smoking (3.3)
- Eating habits (3.4)
- Body mass (3.5)
- Blood pressure (3.6)
- Blood analytes: total cholesterol, HDL cholesterol, C-reactive protein and fibrinogen (3.7).

Another risk factor, physical activity level, was treated in considerable depth in a module of the questionnaire, and is reported on in a separate chapter of this report (Chapter 5).

3.2 Alcohol consumption

3.2.1 Background

Alcohol is a significant component of the diet, in this as in other countries. Epidemiological studies have suggested that heavy drinking constitutes a severe risk for cardiovascular disease, but that low levels of consumption can have a protective effect against coronary heart disease (CHD) mortality. A U- or J-shaped association between alcohol consumption and various types of ischaemic illnesses, including myocardial infarction and stroke, was demonstrated in several studies, with heavy drinkers and abstainers most at risk, while light and moderate drinkers showed the lowest risk.[2,3]

Since its inception in 1991, the Health Survey has carried a set of questions on alcohol consumption (the same questions as in the General Household Survey (GHS)). These questions were designed to provide an estimate of average weekly consumption. Until the end of 1995, advice about sensible drinking was given in terms of weekly amounts, men being advised not to exceed 21 units per week and women 14 units. In late 1995, an inter-departmental Working Group recommended that advice on sensible drinking should be expressed in terms of daily, rather than weekly, consumption, and that it should reflect evidence that moderate consumption can be beneficial for certain groups of the population.[4] Advice about sensible drinking was revised as follows:

> There is no significant health risk for men (of all ages) who regularly consume between 3 and 4 units a day and for women (of all ages) who regularly consume between 2 and 3 units a day
>
> Regular drinking of 4 or more units a day for men, or 3 or more for women, is likely to result in increasing health risk and is not advised
>
> The health of men aged over 40 and of post-menopausal women can benefit from drinking between 1 and 2 units a day.

The main series of questions in the Health Survey and in the GHS was designed to estimate average weekly consumption rather than daily drinking patterns. To provide continuity with earlier reports, the results given in this chapter include weekly consumption estimates and show the proportions of men and women exceeding the weekly levels advised before 1996. But the chapter also briefly reports some findings from new questions intended to throw more light on daily consumption. The 1997 survey had already included some questions with similar aims,[5] but these were revised for the 1998 survey.

3.2.2 Weekly consumption patterns

Previous reports have stressed the well-known finding that surveys tend to underestimate alcohol consumption, and have suggested that the results should be used primarily to compare the consumption of different population groups and to monitor change over time, rather than as absolute estimates of actual consumption. They have also described in some detail the way in which estimates of weekly consumption were derived from the responses.[6]

Several changes were made to the module of questions on drinking in the 1998 survey. The biggest innovation was the distinction made for the first time between normal (alcoholic strength less than 6%) and strong (6% or more) beer, lager and cider.[7] The separate question on shandy, which had been asked in all previous Health Surveys, was dropped, and shandy was included with normal strength beer. Also, a question on alcoholic lemonades, colas, and fruit drinks was added to the adult interview for the first time. (Previously it had only been included in the self-completion booklets for those aged 13-17, beginning with the 1997 Health Survey.) Finally, a new series of questions on drinking behaviour over the seven days before the interview was added (and is described in section 3.2.4).

The weekly consumption tables annexed to this chapter show patterns of variation by age and social class in 1998 that were similar to those discussed in previous Health Survey reports. There are two convenient summary measures: the proportion drinking more than the weekly levels advised before 1996 (21 units for men, 14 units for women), and estimated mean weekly units. In 1998, the proportion was 31% for men and 18% for women; the mean was 18.0 units for men and 7.2 units for women.

Variations in estimated weekly consumption by age

Among both men and women, the general pattern emerging from the surveys since 1994 has shown mean weekly consumption decreasing slightly from age 16-24 until age 45-54, and thereafter decreasing rapidly with increasing age. For men in 1998, mean weekly units was estimated at 23.9 units at age 16-24, decreasing to 9.0 units at age 75 and over. Comparable figures for women were 10.8 decreasing to 3.4.

The proportion whose weekly consumption was above the levels advised before 1996 showed a broadly similar pattern to the mean. For men, it decreased from 41% in the youngest group to 13% in the oldest, and for women from 27% to 7%.   **Table 3.1**

Variations in estimated weekly consumption by social class of head of household

Among women, estimated alcohol consumption in the Health Survey series has generally been found to increase from Social Classes IV and V to Social Classes I and II. Among men the social class pattern is different. In the surveys since 1994, there has been a persistent tendency for men in Social Class II to have the highest proportion drinking above the pre-1996 advised levels, with some evidence of a below-average proportion in Social Class IV (though this latter feature is not seen in the 1998 results). Estimated mean weekly units showed a similar pattern, but with the difference that mean consumption among men was high in Social Class V as well as in Social Class II. Social Class V thus does not contain a particularly high proportion of men drinking above the pre-1996 advised levels, but those who are drinkers in Social Class V have heavier consumption that increases the overall mean for this group.   **Table 3.2**

Variations in estimated weekly consumption by equivalised household income

The tables annexed to this chapter present analyses of weekly consumption not featured in earlier reports, by (equivalised) household income and Health Authority area type. Regional tables will also be found among those annexed, but are not commented on.

Among both men and women, the (age-standardised) proportion drinking above the pre-1996 advised levels increased markedly with income from the lowest two income quintiles to the top quintile. The increase for men in the 1998 sample was from 26% in both the lowest quintiles to 38% in the highest, and for women from 13% in both the lowest quintiles to 26% in the highest.

(Age-standardised) estimated mean weekly consumption followed the same pattern, rising among men from the two lowest income quintiles (16.5 and 17.3 units) to the highest (21.1 units), with the corresponding increase for women being 5.7 to 9.8 units.   **Table 3.3**

Variations in estimated weekly consumption by Health Authority area type

The (age-standardised) proportion drinking above the pre-1996 advised levels was highest for men in the two Health Authority area types labelled Mining and Industrial (34%) and Urban (35%), and lowest in Inner London (26%). A similar pattern was found in estimated mean weekly units, which was 19.7 both in Mining and Industrial and in Urban areas, compared with 14.2 in Inner London.

Among women there was less variation both in the proportion drinking above pre-1996 advised levels (the higher figure for Inner London is not statistically significant), and in estimated mean weekly units.   **Table 3.4**

3.2.3 Trends in weekly consumption

There is evidence of an upward trend in alcohol consumption among women. Women's estimated mean weekly units were 6.3 in 1994 and 6.2 in 1995, increasing to 6.6 in 1996, 6.7 in 1997 and 7.2 in 1998. In the same five years, the proportion of women drinking more than the levels advised prior to 1996 were respectively 14%, 14% 15%, 16% and 18%. The increase appears to have occurred mainly among younger adults (those aged 16-24).

Among men, figures for 1998 were not very different from those for 1994, and there is no evidence of a consistent trend.   **Table 3.6**

Questions asked in 1998 were changed in some respects from those in earlier Health Surveys, and this could affect comparability. For the first time, a distinction was made between normal and strong beer, and a separate question was added on alcoholic lemonades. Strong beer and alcoholic lemonades are most commonly drunk by the youngest age group, so the change in methodology would be likely to affect this group more than others.

3.2.4 The heaviest day's drinking in the previous week

Informants were asked whether they had drunk alcohol in the past seven days; if so, on how many days and, if on more than one, whether they had drunk the same amount on each such day or more on one day than others. If they had drunk more on one day than others, they were asked how much they drank on that day. If they had drunk the same on several days, they were asked how much they drank on the most recent of those days. If they had drunk on only one day, they were asked how much they had drunk on that day. In each case, the questioning obtained details of amounts drunk of each type of drink (similar to those obtained for establishing average weekly consumption), rather than a direct estimate of units consumed.

The proportions claiming to have drunk alcohol in the previous seven days were 78% for men and 62% for women. Of men who had drunk alcohol in the past seven days, 21% had drunk on only one day and 20% on two days, with decreasing proportions on three (15%), four (10%), five (7%) and six days (6%), and then increasing again to 21% on all seven days. The distribution (which had a mean of 3.6 days) was thus to some extent polarised between every day drinking and drinking on only a few days. This was also true of women, though with a lower mean (3.0 days) the distribution was more skewed towards the lower end: 33% of women who had drunk alcohol in the past seven days drank on only one day, 22% on two days and 15% on all seven days.

The proportion of past seven day drinkers who drank on all seven days increased with age. Figures for the youngest and oldest groups respectively were 9% and 38% for men, 4% and 32% for women. This is consistent with patterns commented on (using evidence from other questions) in earlier Health Survey reports.[8]   **Table 3.7**

As noted above, those who drank on more than one day were asked whether they had drunk the same on each day or different amounts. The results showed very marked differences by age, with younger people tending to drink different amounts and older people the same amounts. Figures for the youngest and oldest groups were as follows:

	Men		Women	
	16-24	75 and over	16-24	75 and over
Proportion of those drinking on more than one day who drank:	%	%	%	%
The same amount each day	33	87	35	89
A different amount each day	67	13	65	11

Thus the tendency is for drinking habits to become more regular with increasing age: as noted above, daily drinking is common among older people, and the amounts consumed per occasion are more uniform than among younger people.

Where amounts differed between days within the last seven, consumption estimates were obtained for the heaviest day. Amalgamating these with estimates where there had been a uniform sequence of days and also with estimates where there had been drinking on only one day, it is possible to derive an estimate of the heaviest day's consumption out of the previous seven, the base being all drinking in the past seven days.

Amounts consumed on the heaviest (or only) day are shown in Table 3.8. The table does not give sufficient information to allow a full assessment of whether current advice on sensible drinking, quoted earlier in this chapter, is being followed, since the advice refers to regular consumption rather than consumption on a single day. 'Binge' drinking - drinking an excessive amount on a single occasion - is thought to be less healthy than drinking moderate amounts more regularly.[9] The table throws some light on this by indicating whether 'binge-level' amounts are being consumed, though there is no medically-specified criterion for such amounts. The level chosen for the analysis that follows is over 8 units for men and over 6 for women - that is, double the daily amounts that people are advised not to exceed on a regular basis.   Table 3.8

It was found that 33% of men who had drunk alcohol in the past week had drunk more than 8 units on their heaviest drinking day. This proportion decreased with age, from 58% of men aged 16-24 to 6% of men aged 75 and over. A similar pattern was seen among women, though at a lower overall level of consumption, with 38% of women aged 16-24 drinking more than 6 units, compared with 2% of women aged 75 and over.

The heaviest day's amount was highly correlated with estimated weekly consumption: mean weekly units varied from 8.5 among men whose heaviest day's consumption was under 2 units to 37.0 among men with a heaviest day's consumption of 8 or more units. Comparable figures for women were 5.4 units rising to 24.2 units. (Table not shown.)

Variations in heaviest day's consumption by social class of head of household

The social class pattern was similar for men and women, with drinkers in Social Classes IV and V more likely to exceed these amounts than drinkers in Social Classes I and II.

These figures contrast with drinking prevalence and estimated weekly mean consumption for the sample as a whole. For women, the prevalence of drinking more than the pre-1996 advised amounts, and overall mean consumption, was higher in Social Classes I and II than in IV and V, but drinkers in Social Classes IV and V had heavier drinking days than those in Social Classes I and II.[10]   Table 3.9, Figure 3A

Variations in heaviest day's consumption by equivalised household income

Among women, the drinkers most likely to exceed the specified levels were those in the lowest income quintile. There was very little difference among the other four quintiles. No clear pattern was seen among men.   Table 3.10

Variations in heaviest day's consumption by Health Authority area type

The pattern by Health Authority area type was similar to that described for weekly consumption, with the two area types of Mining and Industrial and Urban showing the highest proportions of men and women drinkers likely to exceed the specified levels (8 units for men, 6 for women) in a single day.   Table 3.11

3.3 Cigarette smoking

3.3.1 Introduction

Government White Papers

The importance attached by the government to reductions in levels of smoking in all social classes is emphasised in the White Paper 'Smoking Kills'.[11] One of the targets is:

> To reduce adult smoking in all social classes so that the overall rate falls from 28% to 24% or less by the year 2010; with a fall to 26% by the year 2005.

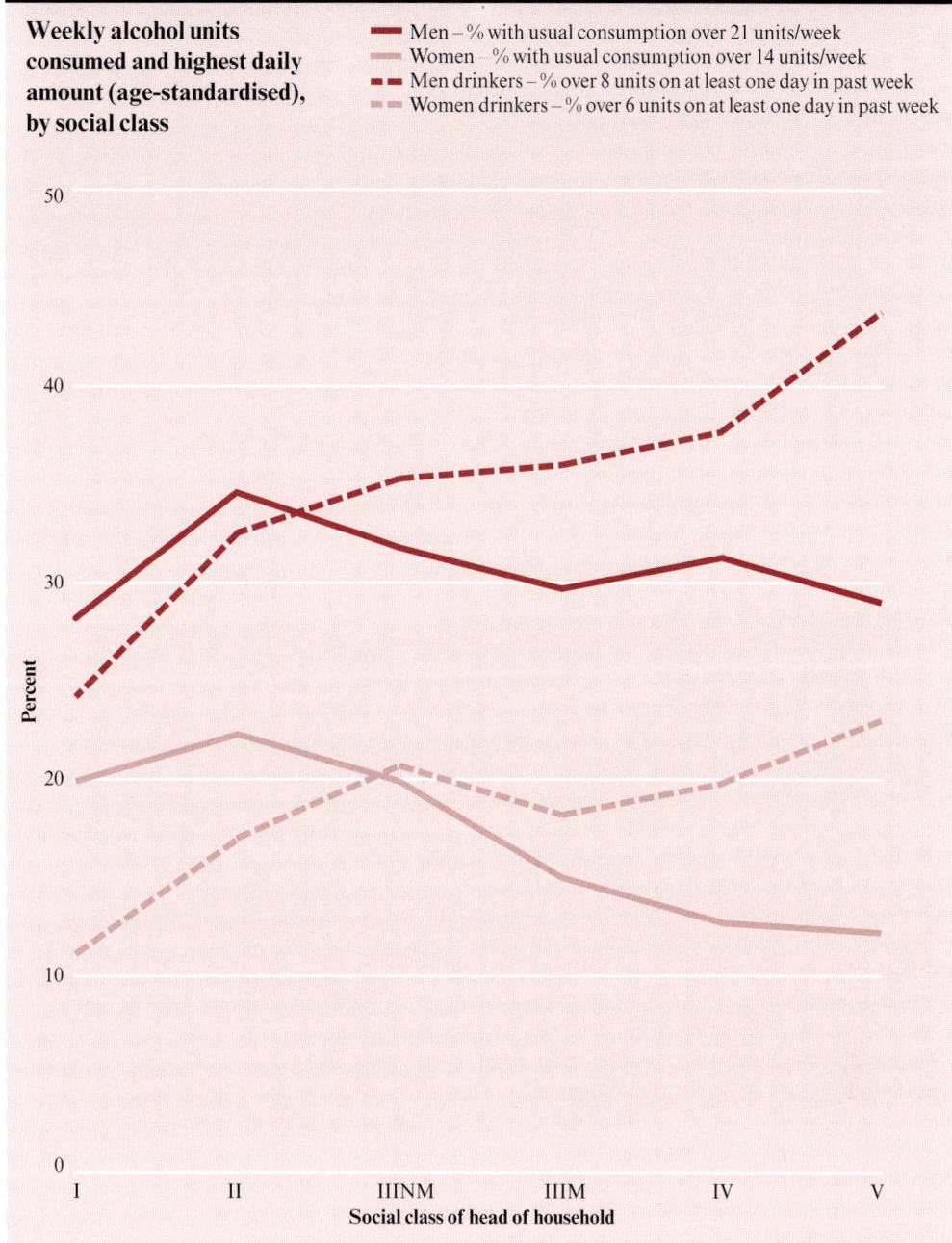

Figure 3A

Weekly alcohol units consumed and highest daily amount (age-standardised), by social class

— Men – % with usual consumption over 21 units/week
— Women – % with usual consumption over 14 units/week
■ ■ Men drinkers – % over 8 units on at least one day in past week
■ ■ Women drinkers – % over 6 units on at least one day in past week

Percent

Social class of head of household

I   II   IIINM   IIIM   IV   V

The White Paper 'Our Healthier Nation'[12] identifies smoking as a major risk factor for deaths from cancer and coronary heart disease and stroke - two of the four health targets set.

Questions asked about cigarette smoking in the Health Surveys

Since its inception in 1991, the Health Survey series has collected information about smoking. It uses essentially the same questions as the General Household Survey (GHS), which is the source for the Smoking Kills prevalence targets. An analysis of levels of smoking reported by informants in the GHS and the Health Survey for England has shown that the measurements in the two surveys are comparable in spite of their different contexts.[13] In 1998, as in previous surveys, information about cigarette smoking was collected from those aged 16 and 17 by means of a self-completion questionnaire, while for those aged 18 or over[14] it was collected as part of the main interview. Questions about the main brand of cigarette smoked were added in the 1998 survey.

Cotinine

Before 1998, cotinine levels in the Health Survey were measured in serum in adults, but in 1998 were measured in saliva, primarily to increase the number of people being measured as more people refuse to give a blood sample than a saliva sample.

Cotinine is a metabolite of nicotine. It is one of several biological markers that are indicators of smoking (others include carbon monoxide and thiocyanate), and is generally considered the most useful. It can be measured in, among other things, saliva or serum. Cotinine has a half-life in the body of between 16 and 20 hours, which means that it will detect regular smoking but will not detect occasional smoking if the last occasion was several days ago.

Tar, nicotine and carbon monoxide content of cigarettes smoked

New information is provided in the present report, which utilises analyses of cigarette content by the Laboratory of Government Chemists for the Department of Health. This is examined in Section 3.3.5 .

3.3.2 Cigarette smoking prevalence

Cigarette smoking prevalence is measured in two ways in the Health Survey for England. Informants are asked directly whether they smoke cigarettes nowadays, and cotinine levels in saliva are measured for those providing a saliva sample at the nurse interview. A saliva cotinine level of 15 ng/ml and over is taken as an indication that the informant currently smokes (those who use other nicotine products are excluded).

The measurement of cotinine levels in the Health Survey series provides an objective cross-check on self-reports of smoking behaviour, which are known not always to be accurate. Inaccuracies in reporting arise in part from difficulties informants may experience in providing quantitative summaries of variable behaviour patterns, but in some cases arise from a desire to conceal the truth from other people, such as household members who may be present during the interview.

However, previous Health Survey reports have shown a very high level of agreement between self-report and cotinine levels. Systematic differences are mostly minor, and are due to under-reporting for the reasons given above, or to alternative sources of nicotine, notably pipe or cigar smoking or the use of other nicotine products, or to passive smoking, though nicotine levels due to passive smoking are normally not high enough to result in the informant's misclassification as a smoker. Cotinine-based estimates of prevalence were more or less the same as self-report for women (27% overall in either case), but for men they were higher (32%) than self-report (28%), due to some extent to pipe and cigar smoking.

Given the close resemblance between patterns shown by self-report and those shown by cotinine analysis, the present report deals mainly with self-report. But Table 3.20 presents saliva cotinine levels by age and sex, and Table 3.21 presents a logistic regression in which a saliva cotinine level of 15 ng/ml is the dependent variable, while Table 3.28 explores the determinants of particularly high cotinine levels among smokers.

Analysis of self-reported cigarette smoking prevalence was conducted using cross-tabulations (age-standardised where appropriate) and logistic regression models. Separate logistic regressions were run for men and women in SPSS with the following independent variables: age, social class of head of household, equivalised household income, Health Authority area type and highest level of educational qualification. The odds ratios shown in the tables are relative to average. An odds ratio of less than one means that the group was less likely than average to smoke cigarettes currently, and an odds ratio greater than one indicates a greater than average likelihood of smoking.

Cigarette smoking prevalence by sex and age

As in previous reports, the 1998 survey showed that similar proportions of men (28%) and women (27%) reported smoking cigarettes.

Cigarette smoking prevalence was highest among those aged 16-24 (41% among men aged 16-24, 38% among women aged 16-24), and declined with increasing age to levels of 9% among men aged 75 and over and 10% among women aged 75 and over. The decrease in prevalence with age is likely to be due in part to higher death rates among smokers than non-smokers.[15]   **Tables 3.13, 3.20**

Cigarette smoking prevalence by social class of head of household

The 1998 survey results again showed the well-documented social class gradient in cigarette smoking. The (age-standardised) prevalence of cigarette smoking by men in Social Class I was 15%, rising to 42% in Social Class V. Corresponding proportions of women were 14% to 37%.   **Table 3.14**

Cigarette smoking prevalence by equivalised household income

Cigarette smoking prevalence increased as equivalised household income decreased. The age-standardised proportion of men and women who were current smokers rose consistently from 21% of men and 18% of women in the highest income quintile to 42% of men and 37% of women in the lowest income quintile.   **Table 3.15, Figure 3B**

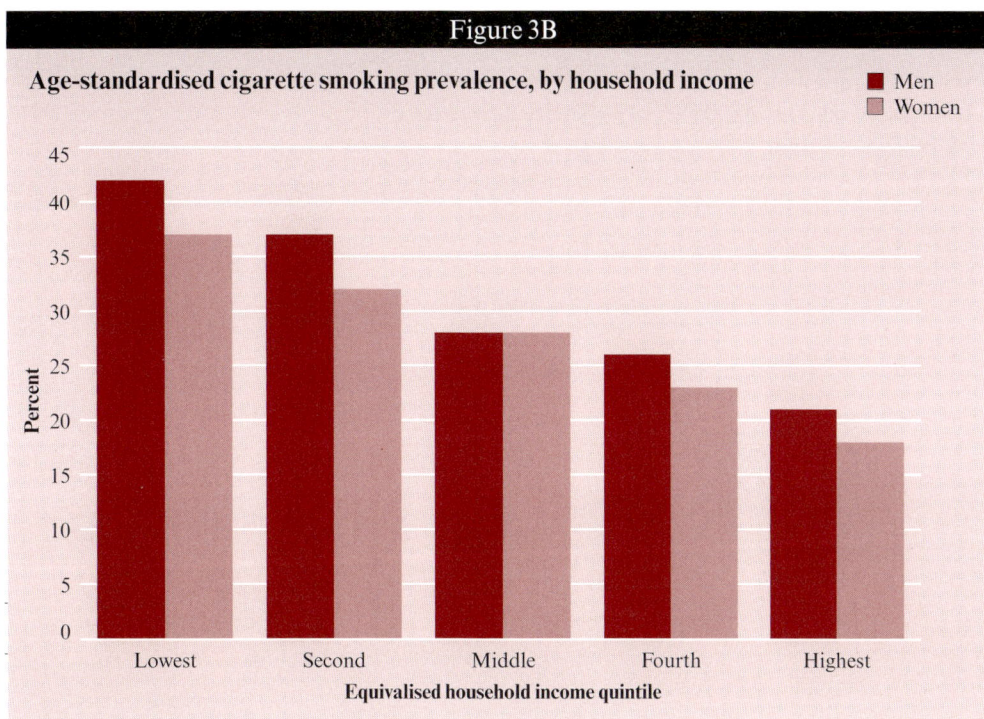

Figure 3B

Age-standardised cigarette smoking prevalence, by household income   ■ Men ■ Women

Cigarette smoking prevalence by Health Authority area type

There was much less variation between area types than between age, class and income groups, and no clear overall pattern.   **Table 3.16**

Logistic regression models predicting cigarette smoking and cotinine levels

After adjusting for the other variables in the model, age was still a strong predictor of cigarette smoking, and of saliva cotinine levels of 15 ng/ml or more. The odds of cigarette smoking decreased as age increased, being nine times as great at age 16-24 as at age 75 and over for both men and women.   **Figure 3C**

Socio-economic variables were also strong predictors of cigarette smoking. The odds of smoking showed social class, income and educational qualification gradients. After adjustment for the other factors in the model, men in Social Class V were $2^1/_2$ times as likely to smoke as men in Social Class I, men in the lowest income quintile were 58% more likely to smoke than men in the top income quintile, and men with no qualifications were more than twice as likely to smoke as men with a degree. Similar results were found for women.   **Tables 3.19, 3.21**

3.3.3 Trends over time in self-reported cigarette smoking

There has been no consistent overall trend in cigarette smoking prevalence between 1994 and 1998. The proportion of men reporting cigarette smoking varied between 28% and 30%, while the proportion of women reporting cigarette smoking remained constant at 27%. Early indicators of an increase in smoking prevalence among young adults[16] were not confirmed in the 1997 survey, but prevalence in 1998 among those aged 16-24 supports the hypothesis of an upward trend among young people. The proportions of men aged 16-24 who reported current cigarette smoking in each of the five years from 1994 to 1998 were 35%, 36%, 38%, 36%, 41%. Corresponding proportions of women were 34%, 37%, 35%, 38% 38%.   **Table 3.18**

3.3.4 Number of cigarettes smoked by smokers

Those who smoked cigarettes were asked how many cigarettes they smoked during the week and at the weekend. Analysis was conducted using cross-tabulations and logistic regression.

Number of cigarettes smoked per day by sex and age

Reported daily consumption was higher among men smokers (15.7 cigarettes a day) than among women smokers (13.6 per day).

Among men smokers, the number smoked per day was highest among those aged 45-54 and 55-64 (18.2 cigarettes per day). Among women smokers, it was highest among those aged 45-54 (16.0 cigarettes per day).

Table 3.22

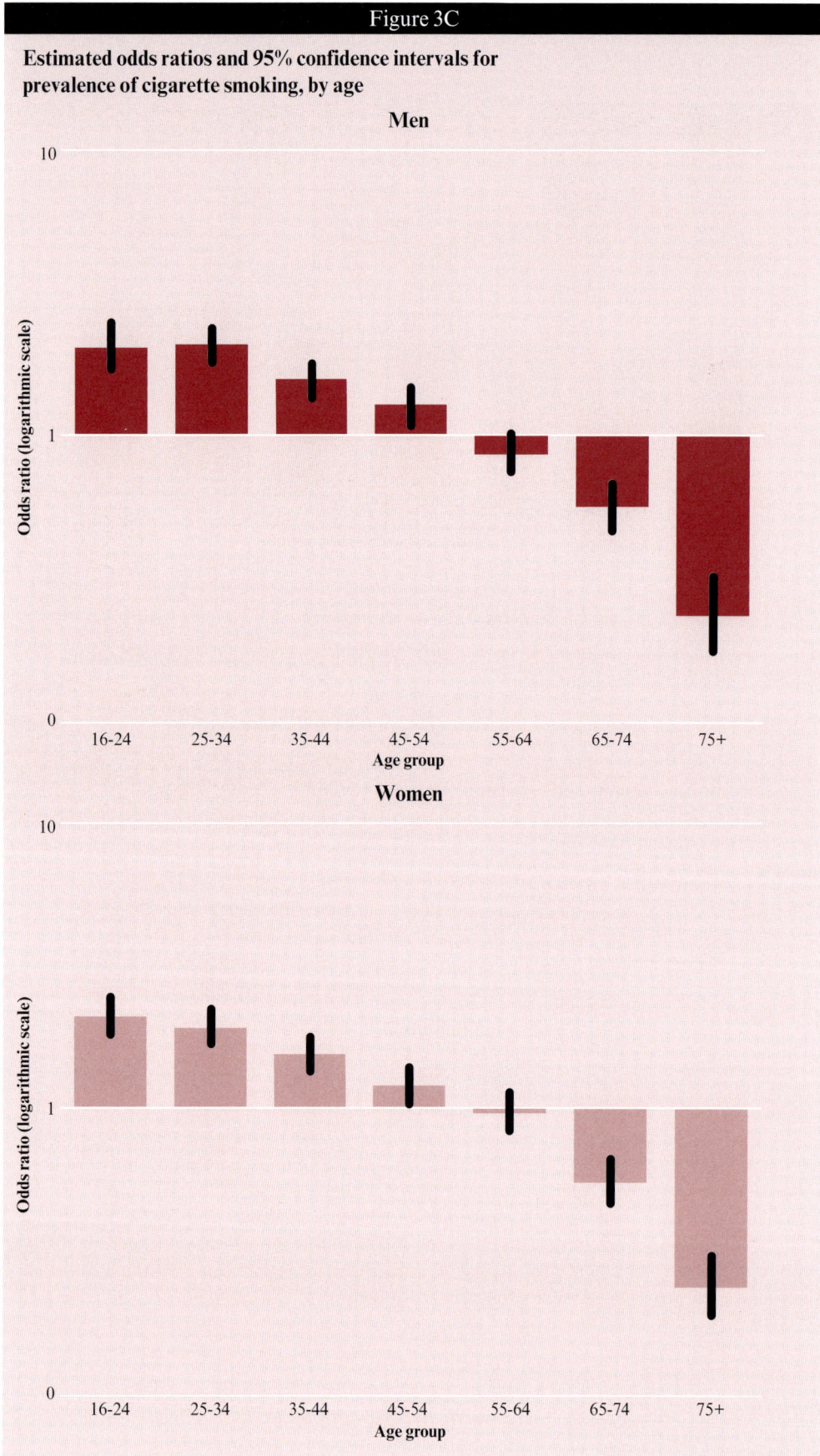

Figure 3C

Estimated odds ratios and 95% confidence intervals for prevalence of cigarette smoking, by age

HSE '98 / 3 RISK FACTORS FOR CARDIOVASCULAR DISEASE

Number of cigarettes smoked per day by social class of head of household

There was a clear social class gradient in number of cigarettes smoked per day, with smokers in Social Classes I and II smoking least and smokers in Social Classes IV and V smoking most, among both men and women. However, there was no social class gradient once the effects of age, educational qualifications and income were taken into account using logistic regression.

Tables 3.23, 3.27

Number of cigarettes smoked per day by equivalised household income

Among those who smoked cigarettes, the mean number of cigarettes per day tended to increase as income decreased, although the gradient was not consistent. Among men

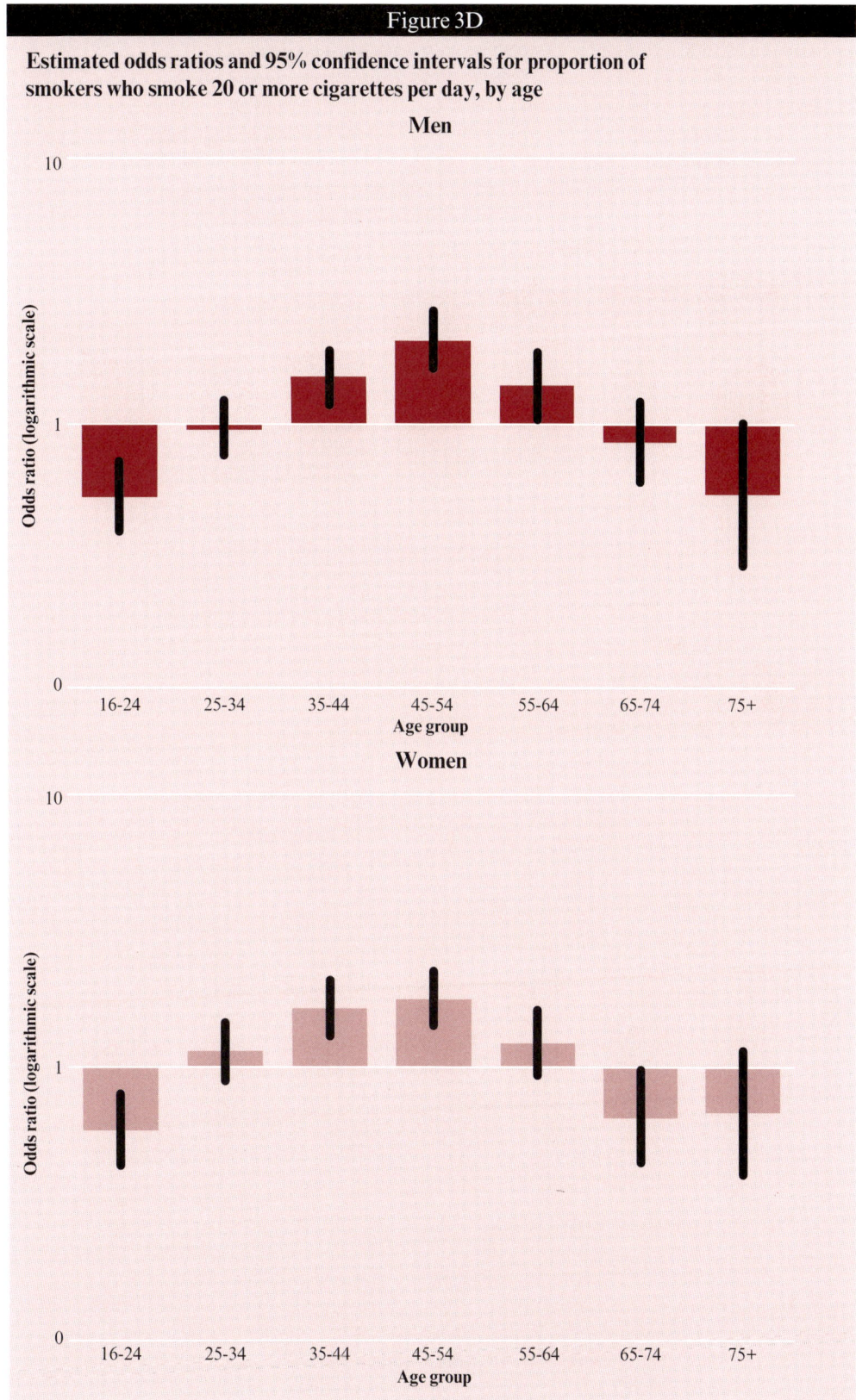

Figure 3D

Estimated odds ratios and 95% confidence intervals for proportion of smokers who smoke 20 or more cigarettes per day, by age

smokers, the highest average reported daily consumption figure (16.8 cigarettes a day) was found in the second lowest income quintile, and the lowest average consumption figure in the highest income quintile (14.3 cigarettes/day). The same pattern was found for women smokers (those in the second lowest income quintile smoked 14.3 cigarettes per day, and those in the highest income quintile smoked 11.6 cigarettes per day).   **Table 3.24**

Logistic regression model predicting heavy cigarette smoking

The dependent variable for the logistic regression model was heavy smokers, those who smoked 20 or more cigarettes per day.

As well as being a main predictor of cigarette smoking prevalence, age was also a main predictor, among current cigarette smokers, of heavy smoking (20 or more cigarettes per day), but the relationship between age and heavy smoking was different from that between age and cigarette smoking prevalence. For men who smoked, the odds of being a heavy smoker increased with age to reach a maximum among those aged 45-54 (odds ratio 2.06 relative to average), but then decreased with age, the odds among men aged 65 and over of being heavy smokers not being significantly different from those of men aged 16-24 (odds ratio relative to average 0.54 for men aged 16-24, odds ratio relative to average 0.53 for men aged 75 and over). For women the pattern was the same, but the differences were not as pronounced. Among women smokers, those aged 45-54 had an odds ratio of 1.76 (relative to average) of being heavy smokers, those aged 16-24 an odds ratio of 0.59 and those aged 75 and over an odds ratio of 0.67. The contrasting patterns of cigarette smoking prevalence and of heavy smoking among smokers can be seen by comparing Figure 3D with Figure 3C.

Smoking prevalence decreases with age, and smoking cessation increases. Those who stop smoking are likely to be lighter smokers, so that people who remain smokers tend to be heavier smokers. This probably accounts, at least in part, for the increase into middle age in the odds of smokers being heavy smokers. In addition, heavy smokers have higher death rates, and this may explain why the odds of being a heavy smoker decrease with increasing age from the peak at 45-54.   **Table 3.27, Figure 3D**

Social class was not a significant predictor of heavy smoking once adjusted for other factors in the model.

For men smokers, there was no clear relationship between household income and the odds of being a heavy smoker. In contrast, for women smokers, the odds of being heavy smokers increased as income decreased, so that women in the lowest income quintile were nearly twice as likely to be heavy smokers as smokers in the top income quintile (odds ratios relative to average: top quintile 0.74 bottom quintile 1.41).

The highest educational qualification achieved was a significant predictor of heavy smoking among men and women smokers. Smokers with no educational qualifications were more likely to be heavy smokers (odds ratio relative to average 1.37 for men, 1.34 for women).   **Table 3.27**

3.3.5 Type of cigarettes smoked

Tar, nicotine and carbon monoxide yields

The Laboratory of Government Chemists (LGC) conducts an annual survey for the Department of Health to determine the tar, nicotine and carbon monoxide yields of brands of cigarettes available in the UK. This data was linked to the Health Survey data using the information collected about the main brand of cigarette smoked by informants. Yields of tar, nicotine and carbon monoxide are highly correlated, so to avoid repetition, this section, after an initial discussion of cigarette content, considers tar yields only. Those who roll their own cigarettes, for whom information about content was not available, were included as a separate category.

Tar describes the particulate matter inhaled when the smoker draws on a lighted cigarette, and tar levels have been linked to prevalence of CVD.[17] Nicotine, an alkaloid, is a powerful drug which stimulates the central nervous system, increasing the heart rate and blood pressure, leading to the heart needing more oxygen. Its effects are related to mode of delivery. Cigarette smoking is the optimal delivery system, producing effects on the brain within seconds and peak blood levels not achieved by tobacco dependence products.[18] In a report published in March 1998, the Government's Scientific Committee on Tobacco and

Health said: 'Over the past decade there has been increasing recognition that underlying smoking behaviour and its remarkable intractability to change is addiction to the drug nicotine. Nicotine has been shown to have effects on brain dopamine systems similar to those of drugs such as heroin and cocaine.'[19] Carbon monoxide, the main poisonous gas in car exhausts, is present in all cigarette smoke. It binds to haemoglobin much more readily than oxygen does, thus raising the blood carboxyhaemoglobin levels, particularly in heavy smokers.

Reliability and validity of tar, nicotine and carbon monoxide yield data

The LGC data was derived from tests of packs sampled between January and December 1997,[20] the year preceding the 1998 Health Survey for England fieldwork. At the end of 1997 new legislation affecting the permitted tar levels of cigarettes came into effect. From January 1st 1998 the maximum tar yield for new production of cigarettes was reduced to 12 mg/cigarette. Between January 1st 1998 and December 31st 1998 existing production stock with declared tar yields in the range 12-15 mg/cigarette was allowed to be retailed. From January 1st 1999 it was illegal to sell any cigarettes with declared tar yield over 12 mg/cigarette. The analysis of tar yields may thus slightly overestimate the actual yields of tar in the cigarettes that informants were smoking at the time they were interviewed.

There are concerns whether measured tar, nicotine and carbon monoxide yields have much relevance to actual smokers' exposures. The yields used in the analysis were those determined by smoking machines.[21] It is known that there is variation in the way people smoke cigarettes, and that smokers may compensate for low nicotine content in cigarettes by inhaling more, or by blocking ventilation holes in the filter with fingers, saliva or lips. Thus people may receive higher tar and nicotine levels than those indicated by the machine test and there may also be considerable variation between smokers.

Cigarette type smoked by sex and age

Men were more likely than women to smoke roll-ups (26% of men, 7% of women), and less likely to smoke cigarettes with a tar yield of under 10 mg/cigarette (20% of men, 37% of women).

Among men smokers, the proportion smoking roll-ups increased with age, from 15% of those aged 16-24 to 31% of those aged 45 and over. For women, the proportion smoking roll-ups did not vary greatly by age, but the proportion smoking cigarettes with a tar content of 10 mg/cigarette or more decreased from 52% of those aged 16-24 to 33% of those aged 55 and over. **Table 3.29, Figure 3E**

Cigarette type smoked by social class

Compared to men in non-manual classes, men in manual classes were more likely to smoke roll-ups (age-standardised proportion 35% in Social Classes IV & V, 16% in Social Classes I & II), and less likely to smoke cigarettes with a tar yield of under 10 mg/cigarette (12% in Social Classes IV & V, 32% in Social Classes I & II). Among women, those in Social Classes I & II were more likely to smoke cigarettes with a tar content of under 10 mg/cigarette than those in manual classes (age-standardised proportion 53% in Social Classes I & II, 30% in Social Classes IV & V). **Table 3.30**

Cigarette type smoked by income

Among men smokers, the proportion smoking roll-ups decreased as income increased, from 34% (age-standardised) among the bottom income quintile to 12% among the top income quintile. The reverse was true for cigarettes with a tar yield of under 10 mg/cigarette, where prevalence increased with increasing income from 13% in the bottom income quintile to 38% in the top income quintile. Men in higher income groups were thus more likely to smoke branded cigarettes and to smoke those with lower tar levels.
Table 3.31, Figure 3F
Women smokers in the bottom income quintile were more likely to smoke cigarettes with a higher tar yield (51% with tar yield of 10 mg/cigarette or more, 28% with tar yield of under 10 mg/cigarette), while the reverse was true for women in the top income quintile (28% with tar yield of 10 mg/cigarette or more, 60% with tar yield of under 10 mg/cigarette). **Table 3.31**

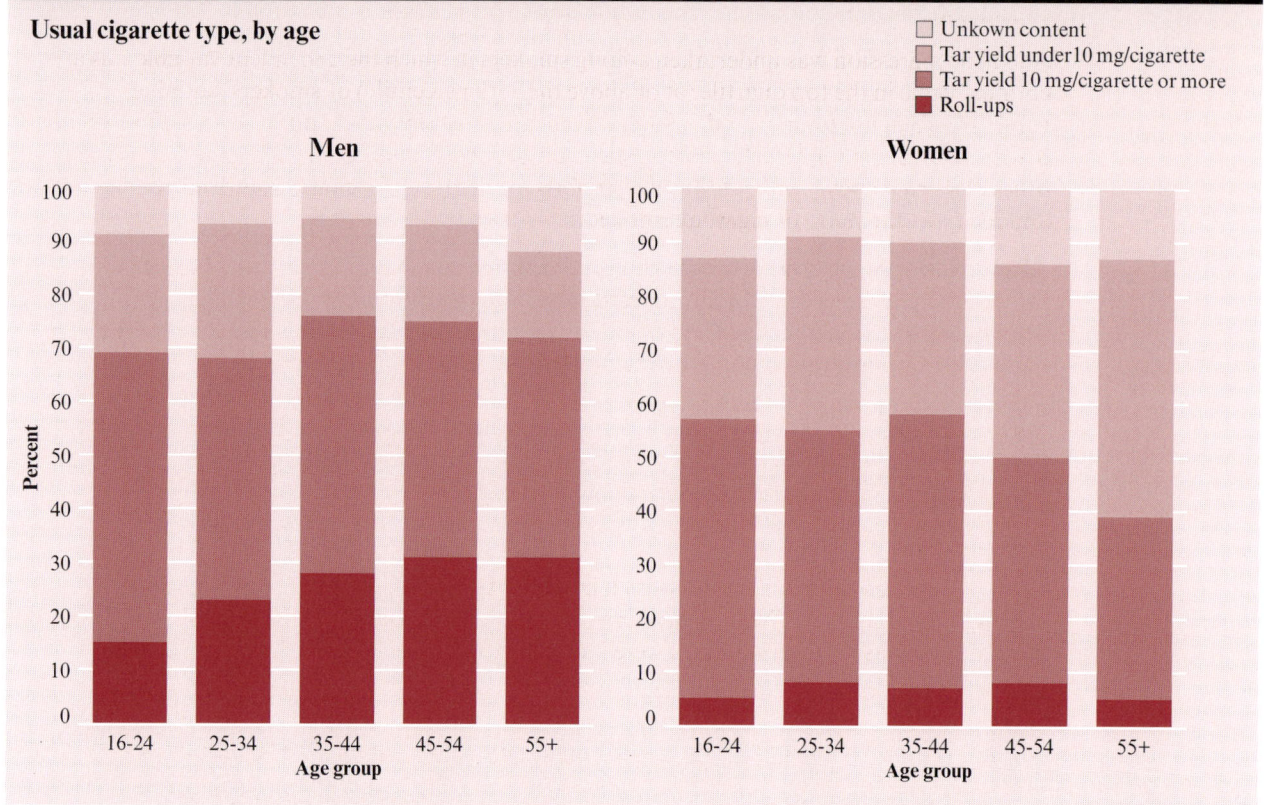

Figure 3E

Usual cigarette type, by age

Legend:
☐ Unkown content
☐ Tar yield under10 mg/cigarette
☐ Tar yield 10 mg/cigarette or more
☐ Roll-ups

Men

Women

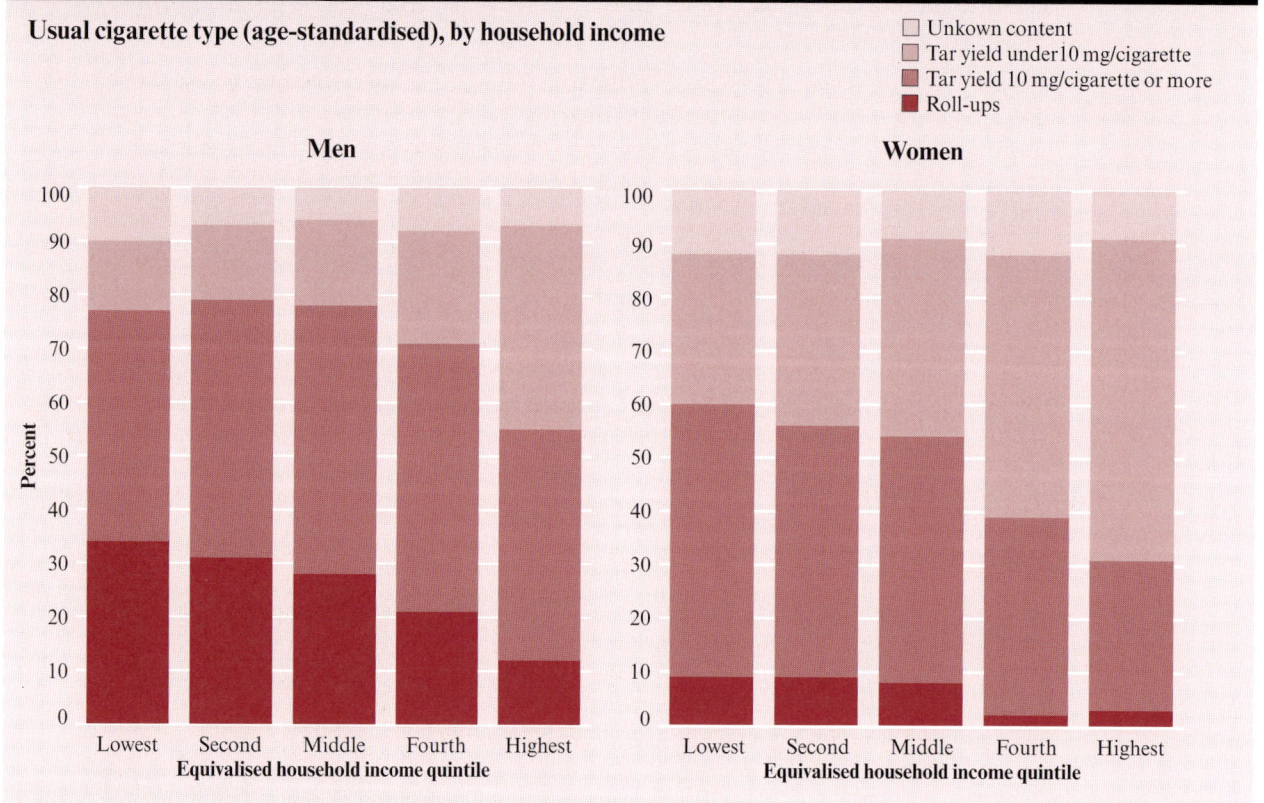

Figure 3F

Usual cigarette type (age-standardised), by household income

Legend:
☐ Unkown content
☐ Tar yield under10 mg/cigarette
☐ Tar yield 10 mg/cigarette or more
☐ Roll-ups

Men

Women

3.3.6 Levels of saliva cotinine among smokers

Previous research[22] has shown that people with high scores on a measure of deprivation[23] tend to have higher cotinine levels, even when controlling for the number of cigarettes smoked, but that analysis could not control for the brand of cigarette smoked. The addition of cigarette brand questions to the 1998 survey allows a further investigation of the relationship between deprivation or socio-economic factors and high cotinine levels when both the number of cigarettes smoked and the nicotine yield are taken into consideration.

A logistic regression was undertaken among smokers in which the dependent variable was a cotinine value in the top quartile (at or above the 75th percentile) of smokers' cotinine values (431.5 ng/ml for men and 369.0 for women). Values in the top quartile are referred to below as 'high' cotinine levels. The logistic regression was conducted in the same way as the others reported above, with additional variables for number of cigarettes smoked per day, and the type (tar yield) of cigarette smoked.

Not surprisingly, the odds of a high cotinine level increased with the number of cigarettes smoked per day. The odds of high cotinine were only one-third of average among those smoking under ten per day, but $2^1/_2$ times average among those smoking 20 or more a day, these results being similar for both men and women.

Age was also an important predictor of high cotinine levels. Men smokers aged 16-24 were the least likely to be in the top cotinine quartile (odds ratio 0.43 relative to average), and men smokers aged between 35 and 54 were the most likely to be in the top quartile (odds ratio relative to average 1.53 for those aged 35-44, 1.63 for those aged 45-54). Similar results were found for women.

Level of educational qualification was an important predictor of high cotinine levels among women smokers. Women smokers with no qualifications or whose highest qualification was 'O' level standard were more likely than average to be in the top cotinine quartile (odds ratios relative to average 1.36 for no qualifications, 1.56 for 'O' levels), whilst women with a degree had an odds ratio of 0.55 relative to average. There was no significant relationship between educational qualifications and high saliva cotinine levels among men.

The type of cigarette smoked was a predictor of high cotinine levels for both men and women. Men smokers who smoked roll-ups were 48% more likely than average to be in the top cotinine quartile. Chapter 7 of the Scientific Committee report already referred to[19] commented that hand-rolled cigarettes have on average higher yields of nicotine than manufactured cigarettes.

For men (in cases where the tar level of the cigarette smoked was known), the odds of high cotinine levels were not significantly different between those smoking branded cigarettes with tar yields of 10 mg/cigarette or more and those smoking cigarettes with under 10 mg/cigarette.

The odds ratio for women who smoked branded cigarettes with a tar yield of 10 mg/cigarette or more was 1.34, compared to an odds ratio of 0.79 for women who smoked cigarettes with a tar yield of under 10 mg/cigarette.

There were no additional effects due to income or social class once other variables were taken into consideration, but it should be borne in mind that all the variables identified as significant predictors are themselves highly correlated with both income and social class.

Table 3.28

3.4 Eating habits

3.4.1 Introduction

The White Paper 'Our Healthier Nation' states that a good diet is an important way of protecting health.[24] Unhealthy diets have been linked to cardiovascular disease (CVD), cancers and dental decay. One of the targets of 'Our Healthier Nation' is to improve the diet of the population by educating and providing information about diet and health to groups at risk, and to ensure that there is adequate access to, and availability of, a wide range of healthy foods. An increase in the intake of fruit and vegetables and a reduction in the consumption of fats and salt can have a beneficial influence on health. Dietary modifications which reduce fat intake,[25] increase fibre intake from fruits and vegetables (in particular from cereals and grains[26]) and reduce salt intake[27] can aid in reducing the risk of developing CVD.[28,29,30] Increased fat intake is directly related to obesity,[31,32] a major risk factor for CVD. There are many studies which suggest that antioxidant vitamins from dietary sources such as fruits and vegetables have a preventive role in the development of atherosclerosis (a condition where fatty plaques are deposited on the walls of arteries causing hardening and narrowing) which is associated with CVD.[33,34]

There is evidence to suggest that there are significant associations between greater sodium intake and high blood pressure.[30,35] A diet rich in fruits, vegetables, and low-fat dairy foods and with reduced saturated and total fat can substantially lower blood pressure, a major risk factor for CVD.[36] It is therefore important to develop strategies aimed at offering an additional nutritional approach to preventing and treating hypertension alongside the more traditional pharmacological treatment.

The Health Survey for England included questions on eating habits in the years 1994 and 1997 and focused on the behavioural patterns relating to a few 'healthy eating' messages. The interview included questions about the types and frequency of categories of foods eaten. This was a simplified version of a food frequency questionnaire aimed at getting a broad view on the general eating habits of the population in England. Detailed information on the British diet is collected in other surveys, the National Food Survey[37] and the National Diet and Nutrition Surveys[38] carried out among different age cohorts.

3.4.2 **Methods**

In 1998 the eating habits questionnaire underwent substantial changes. The modified version was based on the Dietary Instrument for Nutrition Education (DINE) questionnaire, developed by the Imperial Cancer Research Fund's General Practice Research Group to assess dietary fat and fibre intake.[39,40] The DINE consists of a weighted food frequency questionnaire of 19 groups of food which together accounted for 70% of the fat and fibre in the typical UK diet according to the National Food Survey, together with measures of the types of spread, frying and cooking fat used.[39] Scores were assigned to food groups proportionally to the fat and fibre content of a standard portion size. The DINE provides a quick assessment of an individual's diet by adding the scores relevant to the frequency of consumption of the groups of foods to give a total fat and a total fibre score. For both fat and fibre, three categories are then derived grouping the scores: low intake (less than 30), medium intake (30-40) and high intake (more than 40). A total fat score of 30 or less on the DINE is estimated to represent a fat intake of 83g/day or less, which corresponds to about 35% of the energy recommended dietary allowance (RDA) for adults in the UK.[41] A score of 40 or more indicates a fat intake greater than 122g/day or about 40% of energy RDA.

Fibre intake was assessed from sub-scores for fruit and vegetable intake, breakfast cereal, and bread. A total fibre score of 30 or less is estimated to correspond to a dietary fibre intake of 20g/day or less, which is about the national average, and the high fibre score of 40 or more represents more than 30g/day.

The DINE scores for fat and fibre consumption measure absolute intakes, not intakes relative to recommended daily allowances, or to individual differences in size. This should be taken into account when interpreting the results.

The DINE questionnaire was adapted for use on the Health Survey (See Appendix A for a copy of the questionnaire used). Some food categories, such as pasta or rice and potatoes, which were separated categories in the original DINE within the vegetables sub-section, were combined in the Health Survey questionnaire into one question covering all three foods. The same applied to the meat and meat products sub-sections, where questions on beefburgers or sausages, beef, pork or lamb, bacon, meat pies and processed meat were combined into one question covering all these foods. The scores for the combined foods question were assigned by comparison with results obtained from the Oxford and Collaborators Health Check (OXCHECK) data.[42] Moreover, the frequency of consuming a serving of particular foods was kept the same as DINE but a 'Rarely or never' category was added for most food groups. This category was scored the same as the lowest frequency group in the original DINE questionnaire. Cases where people did not consume the 'usual types of food' specified were excluded from the analysis.

Every attempt was made to ensure that the Health Survey yielded results comparable to those from DINE, but given the differences in the questionnaires, the correspondence may not be exact. It has been assumed in this chapter that it is close enough to justify imputing to the Health Survey categories the same actual intakes as the equivalent DINE categories, but it should be noted that the correspondence is an assumption that has not been verified.

The questionnaire was administered by the interviewer only to informants aged 16 and over. Informants were also asked whether salt was added to prepared foods at the table.

Fat, fibre and salt consumption and socio-economic variations (by social class, equivalised household income, Health Authority area type) in fat and fibre consumption are reported in this chapter. Tables of fat and fibre scores by region are also appended, but are not commented on.

3.4.3 Fat and fibre consumption, and addition of salt to food, by age

Fat consumption

Fat consumption was notably higher among men than women. The mean fat score was 34.0 for men, 28.3 for women. The prevalence of high fat scores (over 40) was 26% among men and 11% among women. In men, the youngest age group (16-24) had the highest mean fat score (38.7). This was also the age group with the highest prevalence of high fat consumption (38%): more than one in three men in this age group were in the high fat intake category, while in the middle age groups (25-64) this proportion was less than 25%. Prevalence of high fat consumption increased to 27% in those aged 65-74 and 28% in those aged 75 and over.

In women too, fat consumption was higher in the extreme age groups than in the middle age groups, nevertheless a difference from the pattern for men was seen; the highest mean fat score (31.8) was in those aged 75 and over, amongst whom about a fifth were in the high fat consumption category (18%). Young women aged 16-24 were in the second highest fat consumption category (16%).The prevalence of high fat was much lower for women than for men in all age groups.

Fibre consumption

There was less difference between the sexes in fibre consumption than in fat consumption. 53% of men and 60% of women had low fibre scores.

In both sexes, there was a steady increase in fibre intake with age. Fibre intake was thus lowest among the youngest age group. About two thirds of young men aged 16-24 (65%) and more than two thirds of women in the same age group (72%) had low fibre intake.

It is therefore the youngest group who appear at most risk, having diets that are relatively high in fat and low in fibre. **Table 3.34**

Salt consumption

Slightly over a third of men (35%) stated they added salt to food without tasting it first. Men aged 55 and over were more likely than those aged 16-54 to 'add salt to food without tasting it first'. The proportion of women adding salt without tasting was lower, at 24%. Contrary to what was observed in men, this eating pattern was more likely to be present in those aged 16-44 years than in the older age groups. **Table 3.35**

3.4.4 Socio-economic variations in fat and fibre consumption

The report of the Independent Inquiry into Inequalities in Health raised important issues about the link between diet and inequalities in health.[43] There is increasing evidence suggesting that nutrition-related diseases cluster in disadvantaged groups. People in lower socio-economic groups buy more foods that are high in fat, tend to eat less fruit and vegetables, and less food which is high in fibre. The report highlighted the differences in dietary intake with social class, income, and areas of residence (disadvantaged vs affluent). These issues are investigated below by examining differences in the prevalence of high fat and low fibre intake by social class, equivalised income and Health Authority area type. All prevalences quoted are age standardised. As noted above, the DINE questionnaire estimates absolute fat and fibre intakes, not taking into account differences in overall energy intake, which may vary between socio-economic groups.

Social class of head of household

There was a clear social class gradient in age-standardised high fat intakes in both sexes; the prevalence of high fat intake increased steadily from Social Class I to Social Class V in both sexes. In men, the increase was from 19% in Social Class I to 38% in Social Class V and in women from 7% in Social Class I to 17% in Social Class V. In all social classes, the prevalence of high fat intake was much higher in men than in women.

There was a strong social class gradient in the prevalence of low fibre intake, increasing steadily in both men and women from Social Class I (45%, 47%) to Social Class V (59%, 68%) although the increase was greater in women. **Table 3.36, Figure 3G**

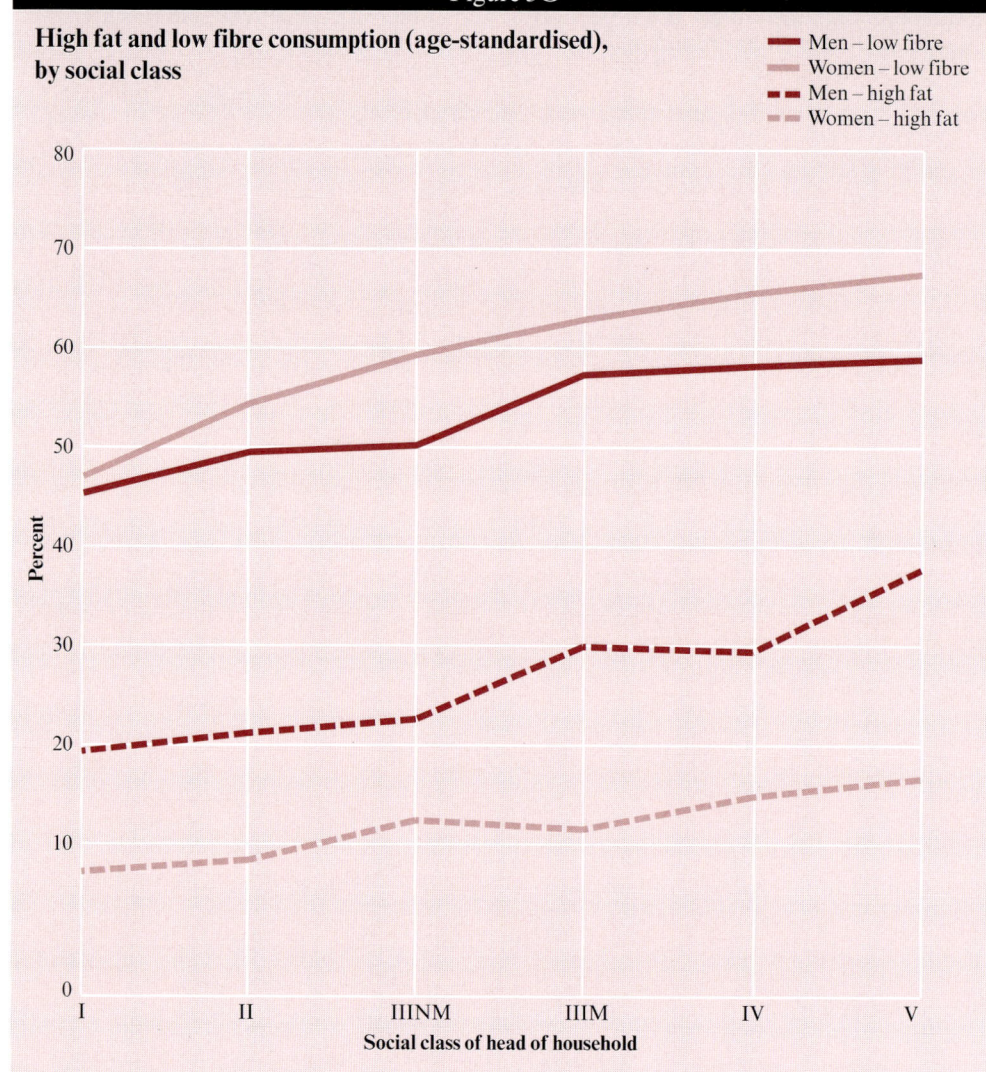

Figure 3G

High fat and low fibre consumption (age-standardised), by social class

Legend:
- Men – low fibre
- Women – low fibre
- Men – high fat
- Women – high fat

Y-axis: Percent (0–80)

X-axis: Social class of head of household (I, II, IIINM, IIIM, IV, V)

Equivalised household income

In men, the prevalence of high fat intake was highest (33%) in the lowest income quintile and lowest in those in the highest income quintile (19%). In women the prevalence of high fat intake also increased from the highest income quintile (6%) to the lowest income quintile (18%).

Unlike the prevalence of high fat intake, the prevalence of low fibre intake did not show a clear overall relationship to income in either sex, but both men and women in the lowest income quintile had the highest prevalence of low fibre intake (59% and 67% respectively).

Table 3.37, Figure 3H

Health Authority area type

High fat intakes were highest in men from Rural areas (30%) and lowest in men living in Inner London (19%). This did not appear to be true for women, among whom the highest prevalence of high fat intake (14%) was in Inner London. High prevalence was observed among women living in Mining and Industrial (13%) and Rural areas (13%).

Table 3.38

3.5 Body mass

3.5.1 Introduction

Obesity, a major risk factor for cardiovascular disease, diabetes, hypertension and premature death,[44,45,46,47,48,49,50] is increasing amongst adults in England ,[51,52,53] and in other western populations.[48,54] In particular, the abdominal or android type of obesity (see section on waist-hip ratio in Section 3.5.2) has been generally recognised as a risk factor in relation to these chronic diseases.[50,54,55]

Figure 3H

High fat and low fibre consumption (age-standardised), by household income

Legend:
- Men - low fibre
- Women - low fibre
- Men - high fat
- Women - high fat

Y-axis: Percent (0 to 80)
X-axis: Equivalised household income quintile (Lowest, Second, Middle, Fourth, Highest)

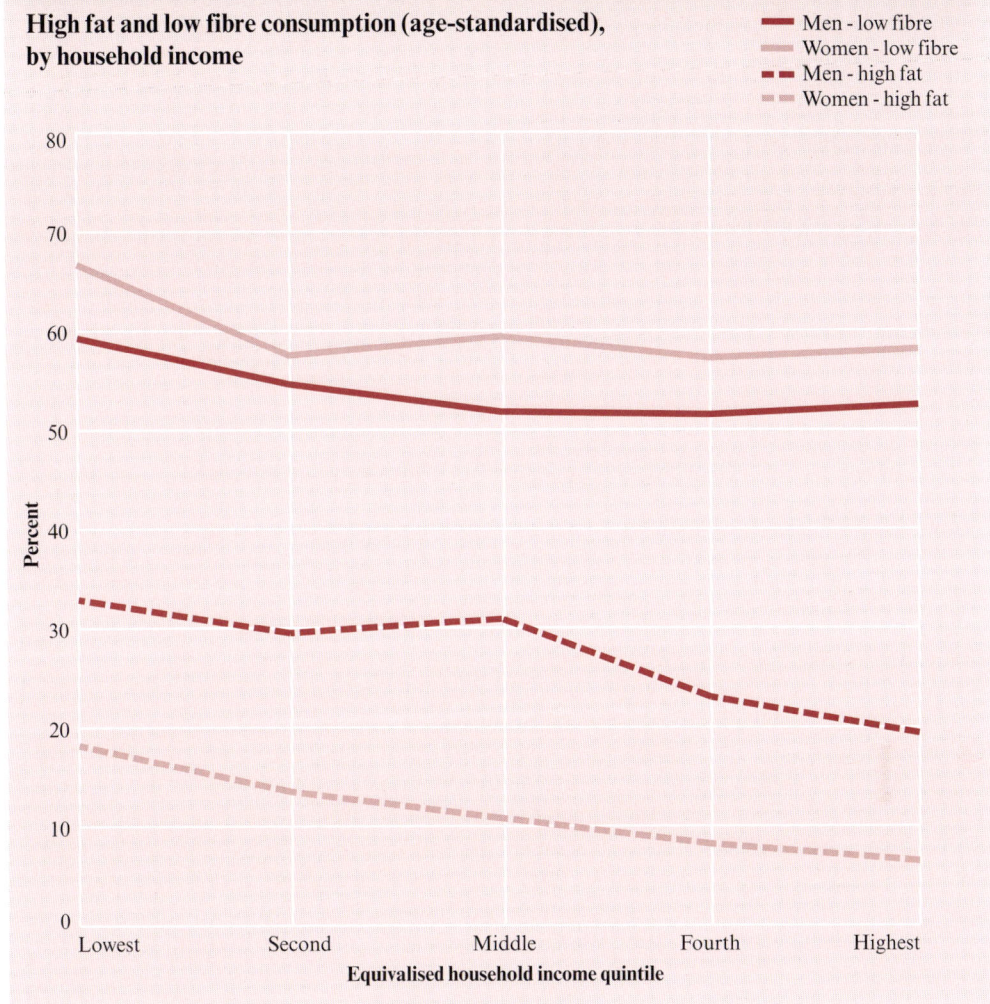

The anthropometric measures presented in this chapter for adults (aged 16 and over) focus on measurements relevant to obesity. Height and weight data used to calculate body mass index (BMI) were collected in each year of the Health Survey series. Waist and hip data, used to calculate waist-hip ratio (WHR), were collected in 1994, 1997 and 1998. Firstly, the methods and definitions of these measurements are described. The distributions and trends over time of these measurements are then reported. Finally, the associations of some socio-economic variables (social class, equivalised household income, Health Authority area type) with raised BMI, obesity and WHR are examined. Tables for height, weight and demi-span are appended, but not commented on.

3.5.2 Methods and definitions of measurement

Full details of the protocols for carrying out the measurements are contained in Volume II, Appendix B and are briefly summarised here. Height and weight were measured during the interview visit while waist and hip circumferences and demi-span were measured during the nurse visit.

Height

Height was measured using a portable stadiometer with a sliding head plate, a base plate and three connecting rods marked with a metric measuring scale. Informants were asked to remove shoes. One measurement was taken, with the informant stretching to the maximum height and the head positioned in the Frankfort plane. The reading was recorded to the nearest millimetre.

Weight

Weight was measured using a Soehnle electronic scale with a digital display. Informants were asked to remove shoes and any bulky clothing. A single measurement was recorded to the nearest 100g. Informants who were pregnant, chairbound, or unsteady on their feet were not weighed. Informants who weighed more than 130 kg were asked for their estimated weights because the scales are inaccurate above this level: these estimated weights were included in the analysis.

In the analysis of height and weight, data from those who were considered by the interviewer to have unreliable measurements, for example those who had excessive clothing on, were excluded from the analysis.

Body Mass Index (BMI)

In order to define overweight or obesity, a measurement is required which allows for differences in weight due to height. A widely accepted measure of weight for height, the Body Mass Index (BMI), defined as weight (kg)/height (m^2), has been used for this purpose in the Health Survey series. However BMI does not distinguish between mass due to body fat and mass due to muscular physique. It also does not take account of the distribution of fat.

BMI was calculated for all those informants for whom a valid height and weight measurement was recorded. Adult informants were classified into the following BMI groups:

BMI (kg/m²)	Description
20 or less	Underweight
Over 20-25	Desirable
Over 25-30	Overweight
Over 30	Obese

In the 1998 report the obese category has been split further into 30-40 and 40+; the latter category defined as morbid obesity. Morbid obesity is recognised as a serious illness which is associated with a poor quality of life and with co-morbidities, and has an economic impact on health care. Weight loss treatments such as behavioural, diet, exercise and drug treatments have shown limited success. Surgical methods have been shown to be more effective for reducing weight in those who are morbidly obese.[56,57] Previous Health Surveys have indicated that the prevalence of morbid obesity in England, particularly in women, is increasing.[58]

Waist and hip

Waist was defined as the midpoint between the lower rib and the upper margin of the iliac crest. Waist was measured using a tape with an insertion buckle at one end. Hip was defined as the widest circumference around the buttocks below the iliac crest. Both measurements were taken twice, using the same tape, and were recorded to the nearest even millimetre. Those whose two waist or hip measurements differed by more than 3 cm had a third measurement taken. The mean of the two valid measurements was used in the analysis.

For waist and hip measurements all those who reported that they had a colostomy or ileostomy, or were chairbound or pregnant, were excluded from the measurement. All those with measurements considered unreliable by the nurse, for example due to excessive clothing or movement, were excluded from the analysis.

Waist-hip ratio

Waist-hip ratio (WHR) was defined as the waist circumference divided by the hip circumference, ie waist girth (m)/hip girth (m). WHR is a measure of deposition of abdominal fat, ie central obesity. Unlike BMI there is no consensus about appropriate WHR criterion levels.[59] For consistency, the same cut-off values as in the 1994 report have been used. A raised WHR has been taken to be 0.95 or more in men and 0.85 or more in women.

WHR was calculated for all informants who agreed to a nurse visit and for whom a valid waist and hip circumference measurement was recorded.

Demi-span

Demi-span is defined as the distance between the mid-point of the sternal notch and the finger roots with the arm outstretched laterally. It is an alternative to height as a measure of skeletal size, especially useful in elderly people in whom a certain height loss occurs with age. Measurements were made with the right arm outstretched using a metal retractable tape. Two measurements were taken to the nearest even millimetre with the informant in light clothing and with bulky jewellery removed. If there was a difference between the two measurements of more than 3 cm, a third measurement was taken. The mean of the two valid measurements was used in the analysis.

All informants aged 65 and over were eligible for the measurement. Measurements considered unreliable, for example, due to excessive clothing, or if there was partial response (where only one measurement was obtained or if the difference between the two measurements was greater than 3 cm and a third measurement was not taken) were excluded from the analysis.

Demi-span measurements are not commented on in this chapter.

Response to anthropometric measurements

Valid height (94%) and weight (93%) measurements were obtained from a majority of informants. Weight and height measurements allowed BMI to be computed for 91% of people aged 16 years and over in both sexes (including 37 informants who gave their estimated weights because they weighed more than 130 kg).

Valid WHR measurements were obtained for 99% of informants aged 16 years and over who were visited by a nurse. Valid demi-span measurements were obtained for 96% of informants aged 65 years and over who were visited by a nurse. **Table 3.40**

3.5.3 Trends in body mass over time, by age

Trends over time in BMI

In 1998, mean BMI was 26.5 kg/m^2 in men and 26.4 kg/m^2 in women. Overall, obesity was more prevalent in women (21.2%) than in men (17.3%), and the prevalence of morbid obesity among women (1.9%) was also higher than in men (0.6%). Both mean BMI and the prevalence of obesity increased: up to a maximum of 27.8 kg/m^2 in men aged 55-64 (prevalence of obesity 23.3%) and to 27.8 kg/m^2 (prevalence of obesity 29.0%) in women aged 65-74. BMI and obesity then decreased in older age groups.

During the period 1994-1998 mean BMI gradually increased among men and women in most age groups. The overall age-standardised increase of 0.44 kg/m^2 in men (95% CI 0.31-0.57) and 0.57 kg/m^2 in women (95% CI 0.41-0.72) was statistically significant in both sexes (p<0.001).

The prevalence of obesity also increased gradually in most age groups in both sexes from 1994 to 1998. The increase was greater in women than men and in those aged 45 years and over than those aged 16-44 years. Looking at all ages, the prevalence of obesity in men rose from 13.8% in 1994 to 17.3% in 1998. In women, the increase was more marked, from 17.3% in 1994 to 21.2% in 1998. **Table 3.41, Figure 31**

Trends over time in WHR

In 1998, mean WHR was greater in men than in women, and, in general, tended to increase with age. This pattern was more marked in women than men. For all ages combined, mean WHR was 0.91 in men and 0.80 in women.

In both sexes the changes in mean WHR from 1994 to 1997 and 1998 were very small and no clear pattern emerged. **Table 3.42**

3.5.4 Body mass differences by socioeconomic status

BMI and social class of head of household

Age-standardised mean BMI did not show a clear pattern by social class in men, being highest in Social Class IIIM (26.7 kg/m^2) and lowest in Social Class I (25.9 kg/m^2). In women, there was a steady increase from Social Class I (25.4 kg/m^2) to Social Class V (27.2 kg/m^2).

In men, the age-standardised prevalence of being overweight was highest in Social Class II (46.8%) and was generally higher in non-manual than manual social classes. The reverse was true for the prevalence of obesity and of morbid obesity which was higher in manual than non-manual social classes. Men from Social Class IIIM showed the highest prevalence (19.6%) of obesity while the prevalence of morbid obesity was highest in Social Class V (1.6%).

Figure 3I

Trends in prevalence of obesity and overweight

☐ Overweight (BMI over 25-30 kg/m^2)
■ Obese (BMI over 30 kg/m^2)

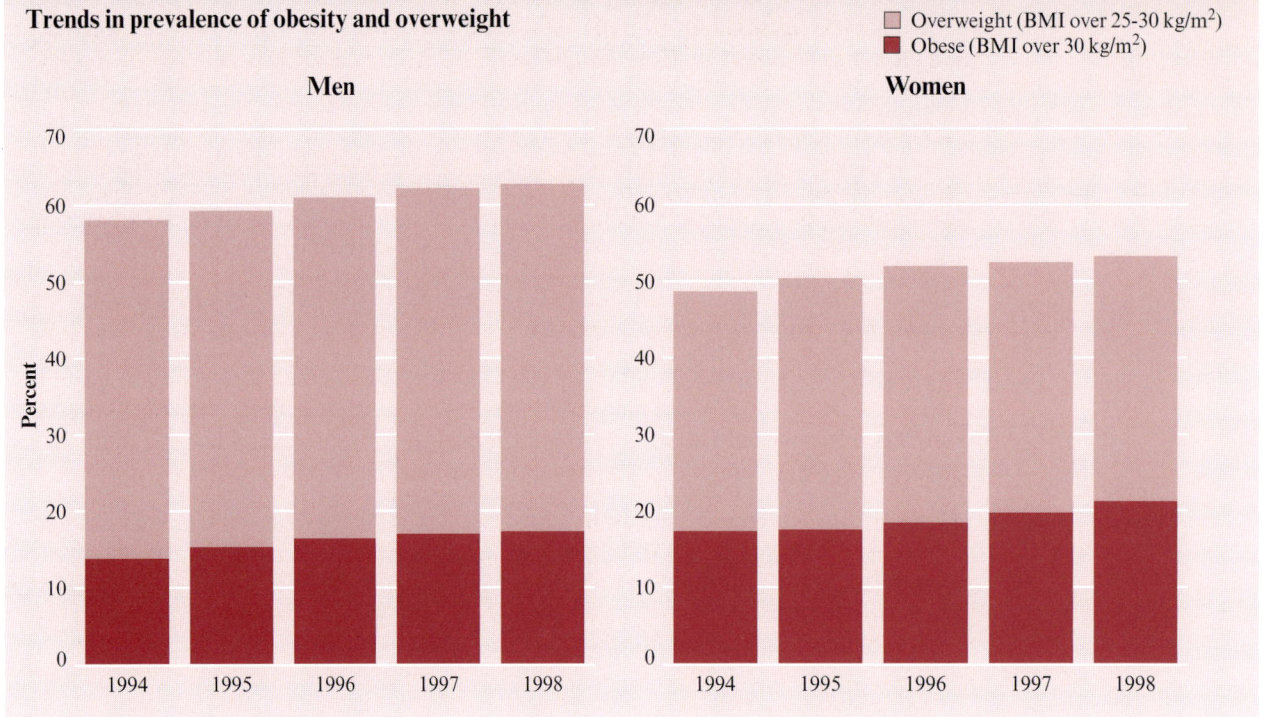

In women, the age-standardised prevalence of being overweight was highest in Social Class II (32.5%). The prevalence of obesity showed a strong social class gradient, increasing progressively from Social Class I (14.4%) to Social Class V, where more than a quarter (28.1%) of women were obese. The prevalence of morbid obesity also increased steadily from Social Class I (0.7%) to Social Class V (3.3%).　　　**Table 3.43, Figure 3J**

WHR and social class of head of household

Mean WHR did not vary consistently from Social Classes I to V in men. The highest mean WHR in men was 0.91 in Social Class IIIM and the lowest was 0.89 in Social Class I and IIINM. In women there was a gradual increase in mean WHR from Social Class I (0.78) to V (0.81).

Figure 3J

Prevalence of obesity and overweight (age-standardised), by social class

☐ Overweight (BMI over 25-30 kg/m^2)
■ Obese (BMI over 30 kg/m^2)

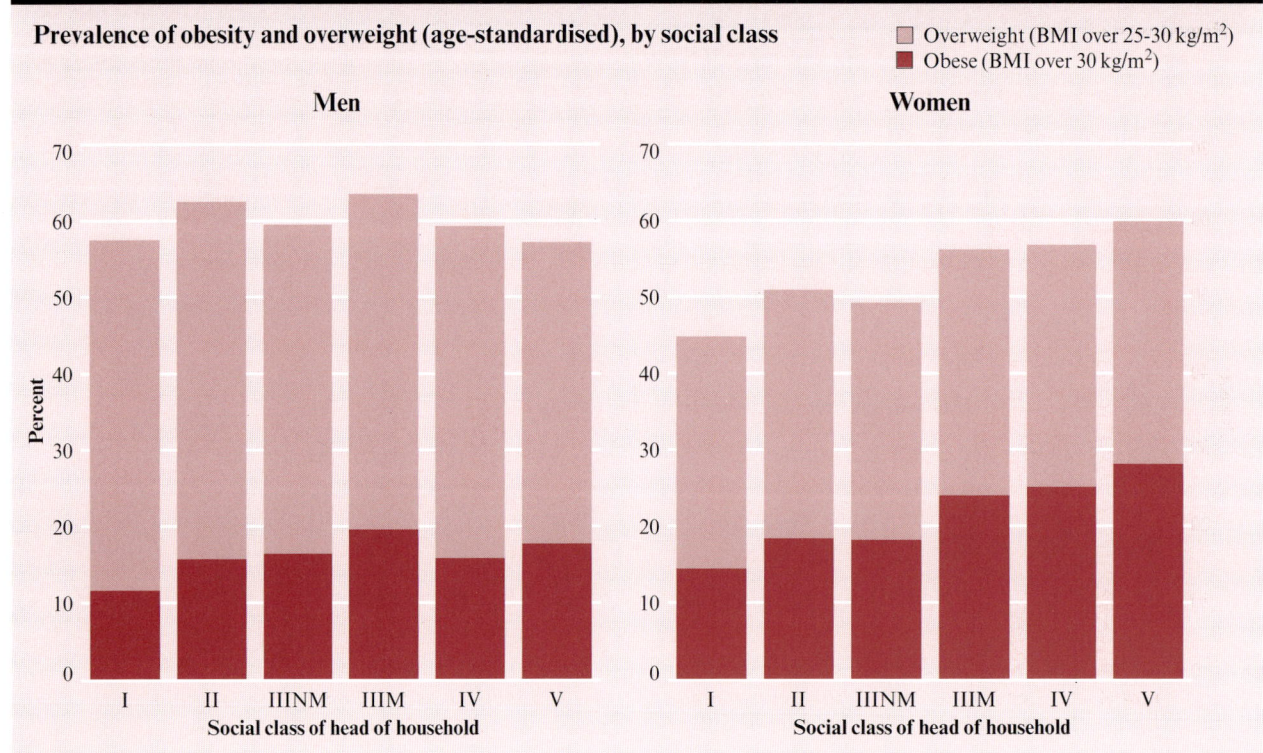

In both sexes, the age-standardised prevalence of raised WHR (≥ 0.95 in men and ≥ 0.85 in women) was higher in informants from manual Social Classes (IIIM, IV, V) than from non-manual Social Classes (I, II, IIINM). Again, the pattern was more evident in women, where the prevalence of raised WHR generally increased from Social Class I (18.0%) to Social Class V (26.6%).

Table 3.44

BMI and equivalised household income

There was no great difference in age-standardised mean BMI in men from the highest to the lowest quintile of equivalised income. In women however, there was a gradual increase in mean BMI from the highest income quintile (25.4 kg/m²) to the lowest income quintile (27.1 kg/m²).

In men, the prevalence of being overweight increased from the lowest income quintile to the highest, where it was 46.8%. No clear pattern emerged in women.

The prevalence of obesity increased from the highest to the lowest income quintile in both men (14.5%, 20.3%) and women (15.9%, 26.3%) respectively.

The prevalence of morbid obesity also showed a strong gradient for equivalised income, increasing for both sexes. In men it increased from 0.6% in the highest income quintile to 1.2% in the lowest income quintile and in women it increased from 0.9% to 3.7% respectively.

Table 3.45, Figure 3K

WHR and equivalised household income

In men, observed mean WHR showed only small differences by income from the highest to lowest quintile. In women, however, there was a stronger gradient for income, increasing from the highest (0.77) to the lowest (0.81) quintile.

In both sexes, the prevalence of age-standardised raised WHR was higher in informants from the lower income quintiles than in those from the higher income quintiles.

Table 3.46

BMI and Health Authority area type

Age-standardised mean BMI was highest in men (26.6 kg/m²) and women (26.7 kg/m²) living in Rural areas. The lowest mean BMI was in men living in Inner London (26.0 kg/m²) and in women living in Prosperous areas (26.0 kg/m²).

In men, no clear pattern of variation in the prevalence of raised BMI was seen by area type. The age-standardised prevalence of being overweight was higher in men in Mature areas

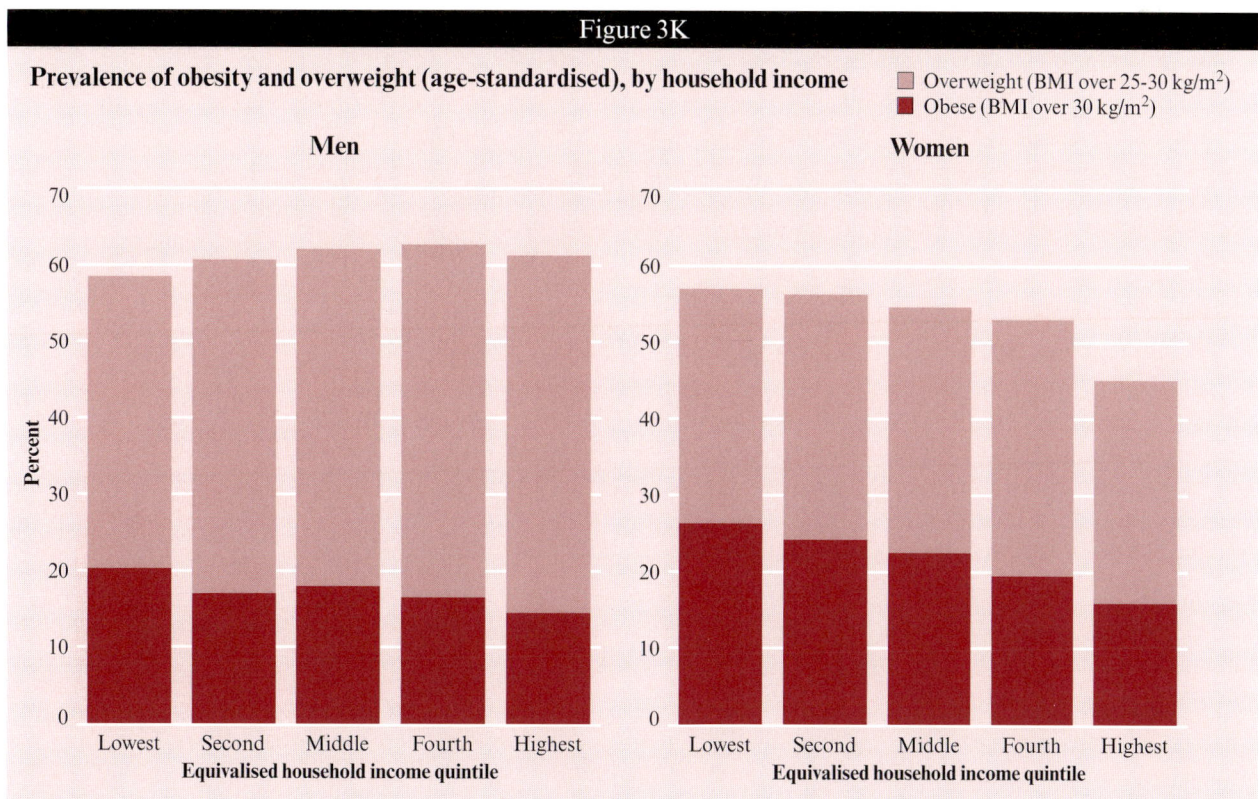

Figure 3K

Prevalence of obesity and overweight (age-standardised), by household income

Legend: Overweight (BMI over 25-30 kg/m²); Obese (BMI over 30 kg/m²)

(46.1%). The prevalence of being obese was higher in Urban areas (19.5%) and the prevalence of being morbidly obese was higher in Inner London (2.2%).

In women, the age-standardised prevalence of being overweight and of being obese was higher in Rural areas (33.3%, 23.0%), however the prevalence of morbid obesity was higher in Mining and Industrial areas (2.1%).   **Table 3.47**

WHR and Health Authority area type

In both sexes, mean WHR showed only small differences between Health Authority area types . In men, mean WHR was highest in Mining and Industrial areas (0.91). In women, mean WHR was highest in Inner London (0.81) and lowest in both Urban and Prosperous areas (0.79).

A similar pattern to mean WHR was seen for the prevalence of age-standardised raised WHR in both sexes. In men, raised WHR was highest in Mining and Industrial areas (30.4%) and for women raised WHR was higher in Inner London (28.8%) than in other areas.   **Table 3.48**

3.6 Blood pressure

3.6.1 Introduction

Observational studies indicate that both systolic (SBP)[60] and diastolic blood pressure (DBP)[61] are positively related to the risk of stroke and of coronary heart disease (CHD) not only among individuals who might be considered 'hypertensive' but also among those who would usually be considered 'normotensive'.[60] In fact, within the wide ranges of BP studied, there was no evidence of any 'threshold' below which lower levels of BP were not associated with lower risks of stroke and of CHD. Studies have also shown that the presence of a wide pulse pressure ($\geq$60 mmHg) has an independent and major impact on coronary disease mortality and is strongly correlated with increased risk for CVD.[62]

Raised blood pressure continues to be a risk factor for subsequent cardiovascular events in patients after myocardial infarction (MI), and approximately 25% of hypertensive patients in the UK have a history of angina pectoris, MI, or both.

Regular blood pressure checks are recommended in 'Our Healthier Nation' as a way of reducing the risk of heart disease and stroke.[63]

Meta-analysis of clinical trials of hypertension management indicates that an average reduction of 5-6 mmHg in DBP is associated with a 12% decrease in mortality from all causes and a highly significant reduction in morbidity and mortality from stroke and CHD.[64]

The main purpose of this section is to present the proportion of adults with high blood pressure and to examine trends in blood pressure over time (Section 3.6.3). Variations in adults' blood pressure are also analysed in relation to socio-economic characteristics, such as social class of the head of household, household income and area of residence (Section 3.6.4).

3.6.2 Content and methods

As in previous rounds of the Health Survey, blood pressure was measured using an automated device, the Dinamap 8100 monitor. Using an appropriately sized cuff, three blood pressure readings were taken on the right arm with the informant in a seated position after five minutes' rest. Systolic, diastolic and mean arterial pressure were displayed on the Dinamap from each measurement. Mean arterial pressure (MAP) was determined by the Dinamap through an indirect measurement: a good approximation of MAP can be obtained by calculating one-third of the difference between DBP and SBP and adding the result to DBP.

The blood pressure variables used in this section are the means of the second and third measurements obtained from the informants in whom three readings were successfully obtained.

Valid blood pressure measurements were obtained from 87.5% of informants who were visited by a nurse. Women who were pregnant were not measured and the remainder was excluded because informants had eaten, drunk alcohol or smoked in the previous half-hour, or because less than three valid readings were obtained, or measurement was refused or not attempted.

Response rates increased with age for both sexes. Women aged 45-64 had a higher response rate (89.7%) than men in the same age group (87.5%), while women aged 16-44 had a lower response rate (mainly because of pregnancy).   **Table 3.56**

In this report, adult informants were classified in one of four groups on the basis of their systolic (SBP) and diastolic (DBP) readings and their current use of anti-hypertensive medication.

Normotensive-untreated	SBP<140 mmHg and DBP<90 mmHg , not currently taking drug prescribed for high blood pressure
Normotensive-treated	SBP<140 mmHg and DBP<90 mmHg, currently taking drug prescribed for high blood pressure
Hypertensive-treated	SBP≥140 mmHg and DBP≥90 mmHg, currently taking drug prescribed for high blood pressure
Hypertensive-untreated	SBP≥140 mmHg and DBP≥90 mmHg, not currently taking drug prescribed for high blood pressure

The three latter categories together are considered as 'hypertensive' for the purpose of this report.

This year the survey's SBP and DBP thresholds for hypertension have been changed from 160/95 to 140/90 mmHg, in accordance with the latest guidelines on hypertension management.[65,66,67] Although the scale of the risk, and hence the potential benefit of drug treatment in patients with blood pressure in the range 140-159 mmHg systolic and 90-99 mmHg diastolic, is questionable, it is clear from prospective observational data that blood pressures in this range are associated with increased risk, particularly among individuals who also have additional cardiovascular risk factors, such as dyslipidaemia or diabetes or target organ damage.[68]

The definition of 'taking antihypertensive drug' in the 1998 survey was the same as in the 1994 Health Survey (in which cardiovascular disease was the principal focus) but different from the 1995, 1996, and 1997 Health Surveys. In 1998 (and in 1994) informants were asked if the medication they took was prescribed to treat their blood pressure, while in 1995-1997 informants were not asked if they were taking the drug specifically to treat their hypertension. In consequence, in 1995-1997 all those who were taking drugs commonly used to treat high blood pressure were classified as 'treated', regardless of whether the drugs were in fact prescribed for that reason.

In the 1998 survey, as in 1994, only those who were taking medication and stated that it was for hypertension were included in the two treatment groups. However, in order to permit comparisons over time, data used in trend analysis have been recomputed for 1994 and 1998 using the same definition as in 1995-1997.

3.6.3   Blood pressure levels in 1998 and trends in blood pressure 1994-1998

In this section mean levels of systolic BP and diastolic BP by age and sex are presented and changes since 1994 in mean SBP and DBP are examined.

Mean systolic blood pressure (SBP), by age

In 1998 men's mean SBP ranged from 128.4 mmHg at age 16-24 to 150.3 mmHg at age 75 and over. Women's SBP ranged from 120.1 mmHg at age 16-24 to 155.4 mmHg at age 75 and over.

There was a general tendency for mean SBP to decrease between 1994 and 1998. This change was greater among women than among men. It was also greater among older than younger age groups. For women aged 75 and over mean SBP fell by 4.6 mmHg, from 159.9 mmHg in 1994 to 155.4 mmHg in 1998. For men in the same age group it fell by 2.0 mmHg, from 152.3 mmHg in 1994 to 150.3 mmHg in 1998. For age groups 55-64 and 65-74 mean SBP fell respectively by 3.1 mmHg and 4.5 mmHg in women and 1.9 mmHg and 2.6 mmHg in men. Falls in mean SBP were also apparent in younger age groups, but to a lesser extent.

Every year mean SBP in the older age groups (those aged 65-74 and those aged 75 and over) was higher among women than men, while the opposite was true in all younger age groups.

Table 3.57

Mean diastolic blood pressure (DBP), by age

In 1998, men's mean DBP ranged from 62.7 mmHg at age 16-24 to 78.7 mmHg at age 75 and over, and women's from 63.6 mmHg to 76.9 mmHg.

DBP showed a slight decrease between 1994 and 1998, mainly in the older age groups (from age 65); there was no evidence of such a trend in young people. As with SBP, the change was greater among older women than older men. For women aged 65-74 mean DBP fell from 79.0 mmHg in 1994 to 76.3 mmHg in 1998. Among women aged 75 and over, it fell from 79.7 mmHg in 1994 to 76.9 mmHg in 1998.

In general, in every survey year, DBP tended to increase with age; in women the upward trend was constant, although it almost flattened out after the mid 50s, while among men there was a decrease from age 55 onwards. This is compatible with other population-based surveys which have shown that, while average SBP rises with age, average DBP peaks in the sixth decade (age 50-59) and then declines.[69] A widening pulse pressure (the difference between SBP and DBP) with age reflects this phenomenon, which is due to pathophysiological changes in the arteries associated with ageing.   **Table 3.58**

Prevalence of high blood pressure -'old' definition

In this section analysis of high blood pressure is presented using the 'old' definition of 'hypertensive' (SBP≥160 mmHg and DBP≥95 mmHg or on medication) in order to permit comparisons with earlier years of the Health Survey.[70] For all subsequent analysis the 'new' definition (SBP≥140 mmHg and DBP≥90 mmHg or on medication) will be used.

Overall, the prevalence of high blood pressure (old definition) in 1998 was 18.4% both in men and in women. Hypertension increased with age in both sexes, rising in men from 1.3% in those aged 16-24 to 44.9% in those aged 75 and over. The corresponding figures for women were 0.4% and 55.2% respectively.

Prevalence was higher in men than in women up to age 55-64, while in the older age groups the opposite was true.   **Table 3.59, Figure 3L**

There was no evidence of a change in the overall prevalence of high blood pressure between 1994 and 1998 but it is worth noting that the prevalence of hypertensive untreated decreased, from 9.5% in 1994 to 8.1% in 1998 for men and from 9.0% in 1994 to 7.1% in 1998 for women.   **Figure 3M**

In 1998, among those with high blood pressure, the treatment rate (defined as the proportion of those with survey defined high blood pressure who were taking anti-hypertensive medication) was 65% (61% in men and 68% in women). Among those who were on treatment, 69% had their blood pressure controlled at the time of measurement. The control rate was defined as the proportion of those taking anti-hypertensive medication who had systolic blood pressure less than 160 mmHg and diastolic blood pressure less than 95 mmHg. The control rate was 71% in men and 67% in women. (Data not shown.)

Prevalence of high blood pressure - 'new' definition

Using the new definition, the prevalence of high blood pressure was 40.8% for men and 32.9% for women. Under this definition, as under the old, the prevalence of high blood pressure was higher in men than in women up to age 55-64, while in the older age groups the opposite was true. In men the prevalence of high blood pressure increased from 16.0% in those aged 16-24 to 72.8% in those aged 75 and over. The corresponding figures for women were 4.2% and 77.6% respectively. Prevalence was higher for men than for women due to the greater number of individuals with levels of DBP between 90 and 95 and of SBP between 140 and 160 among men than among women.

The absolute risk of CHD, and other atherosclerotic diseases, is higher in people aged over 60 than in any other age group. The same proportionate risk reduction will therefore potentially have a much more short-term beneficial impact on those over 60 than on younger age groups. The British Hypertension Society guidelines for the management of hypertension recognise this by recommending that treatment should generally be started at higher levels of BP in younger patients, without other CVD risk factors, than in the elderly.[68]   **Table 3.60, Figure 3L**

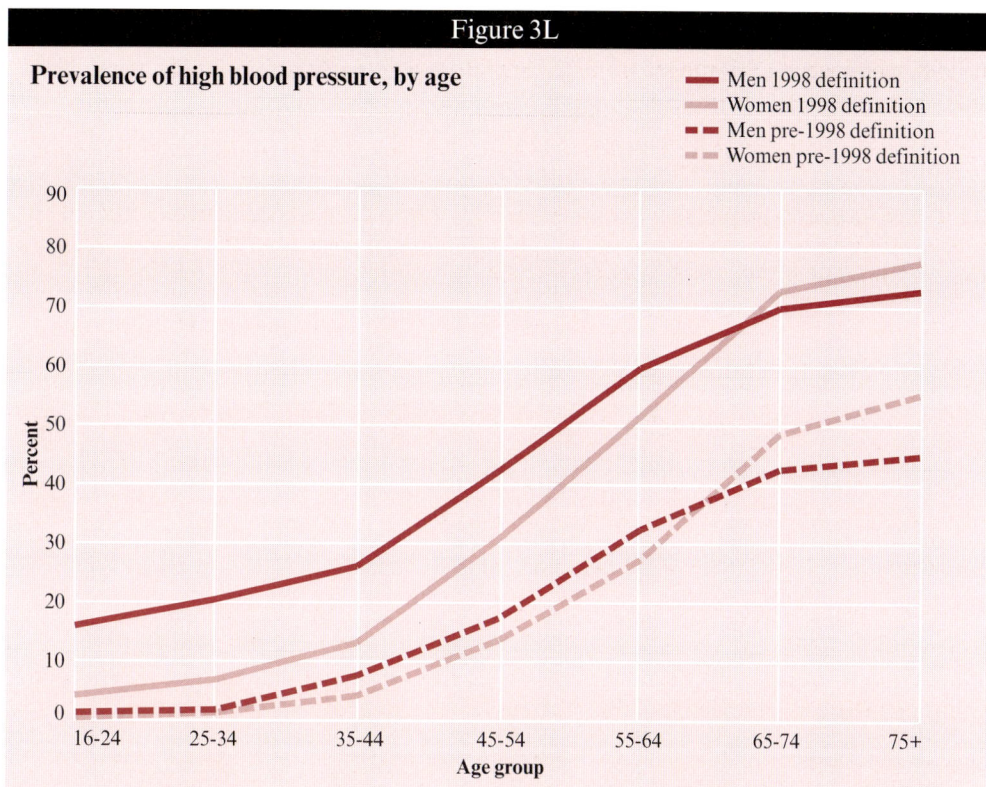

Figure 3L

Prevalence of high blood pressure, by age

Legend:
- Men 1998 definition
- Women 1998 definition
- Men pre-1998 definition
- Women pre-1998 definition

Y-axis: Percent (0–90)
X-axis: Age group (16-24, 25-34, 35-44, 45-54, 55-64, 65-74, 75+)

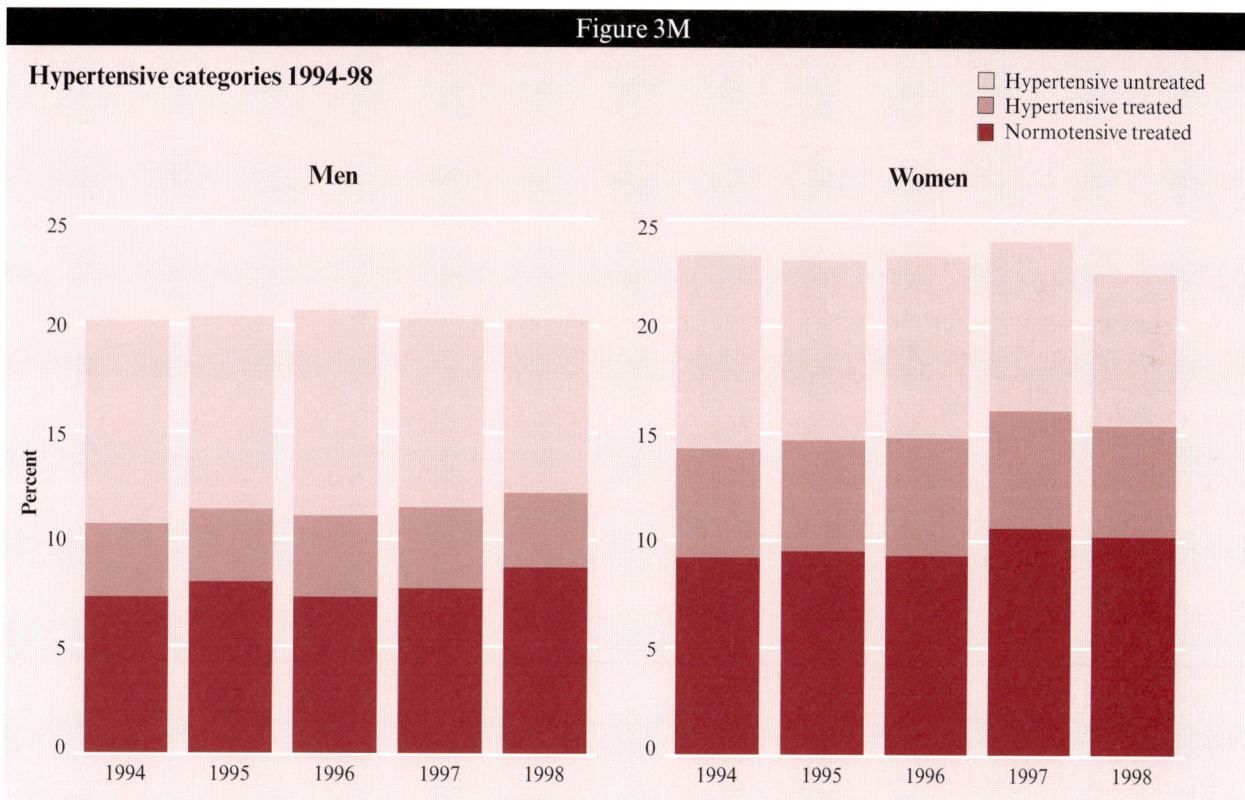

Figure 3M

Hypertensive categories 1994-98

Legend:
- Hypertensive untreated
- Hypertensive treated
- Normotensive treated

Men and **Women**

Y-axis: Percent (0–25)
X-axis: 1994, 1995, 1996, 1997, 1998

3.6.4 Prevalence of high blood pressure (new definition), by socio-economic variables (1998 only)

By social class

Very little variation was found in the prevalence of high blood pressure among social classes, as determined by occupation of head of household. Among women, the age-adjusted prevalence of high blood pressure was slightly lower in Social Classes I and II. No social class gradient was observed among men. The prevalence of high blood pressure was higher in men than in women in all social classes.   **Table 3.61**

By equivalised household income

The prevalence of high blood pressure was examined by quintiles of equivalised household income. Among women, the prevalence of high blood pressure decreased as income increased, from 37.3% in the lowest income quintile to 30.1% in the highest income quintile. No such pattern was found among men. **Table 3.62, Figure 3N**

By Health Authority area type

There was no marked difference in the prevalence of high blood pressure between area types. For men, prevalence was slightly higher in Mining & Industrial (42.2%) and in Prosperous (40.1%) areas than in the other areas. For women, the highest prevalence was again in Mining & Industrial area (36.1%). **Table 3.63**

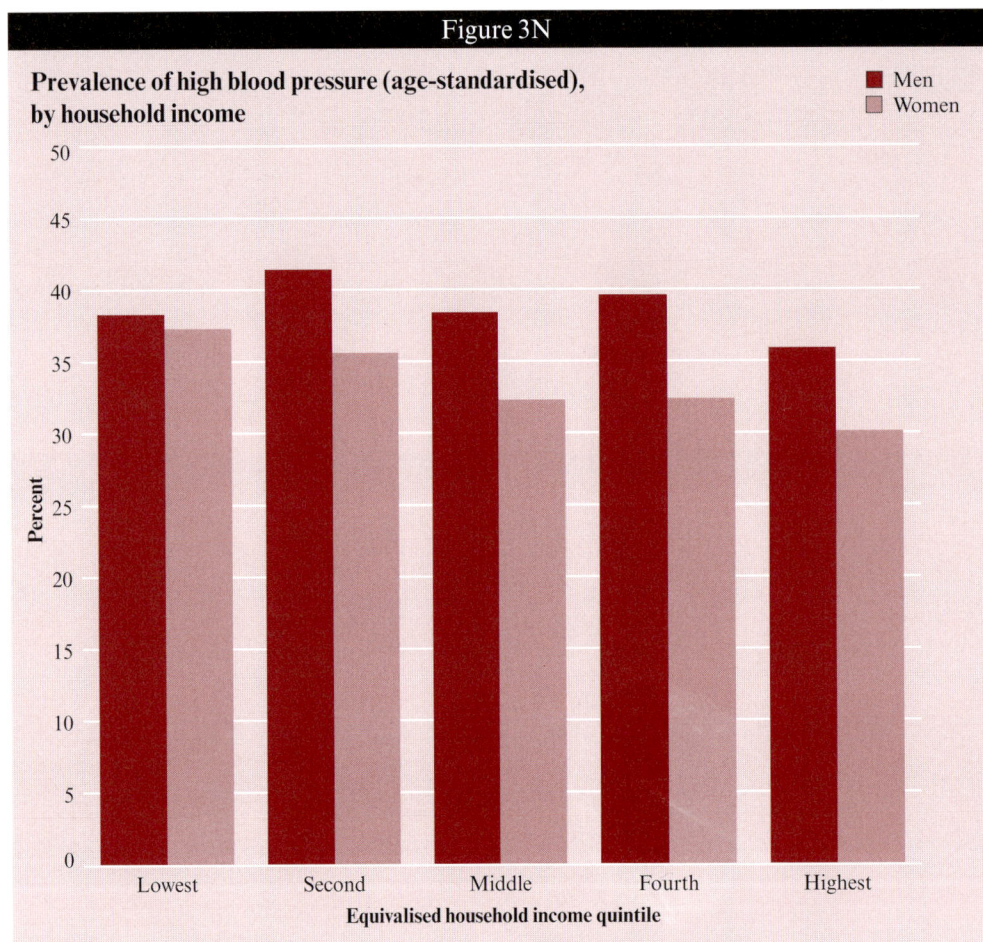

Figure 3N

Prevalence of high blood pressure (age-standardised), by household income

■ Men
■ Women

3.7 Blood analytes

3.7.1 Introduction

This section presents findings on the blood analytes total cholesterol, HDL-cholesterol, C-reactive protein and fibrinogen, which are all independently associated with cardiovascular disease and are therefore important in the determination of cardiovascular risk profile.

A blood sample was obtained from 84% of men and 78% of women who had a nurse visit. The remainder of informants either refused a blood sample or the nurse was unable to obtain a sample from them. The percentage of blood samples obtained was lower in informants aged 16-44, 81% for men and 72% for women. **Table 3.67**

The proportions of informants who had a nurse visit who provided valid measurements were:

	Men	Women
Total cholesterol	79%	74%
HDL-cholesterol	79%	73%
C-reactive protein	80%	74%
Fibrinogen	73%	66%

Table 3.68

3.7.2 Total cholesterol

Meta analyses ,[71,72,73] have confirmed that cholesterol lowering, whether by diet or diet and drugs, decreases coronary heart disease (CHD) risk. Population studies in many countries have repeatedly demonstrated a strong link between mean fat consumption, mean serum cholesterol concentration and the prevalence of CHD.

Joint British recommendations on prevention of coronary heart disease in clinical practice suggest a cholesterol target of less than 5.0 mmol/l for both primary and secondary prevention. The Dutch cholesterol consensus applies the same cut off point for hypercholesterolaemia (total cholesterol 6.5 mmol/l) to men and women.[74]

Several guidelines have been drawn up giving different advice for managing hyperlipidaemia. Unwin et al showed that the application of different cholesterol guidelines leads to considerable variation in decisions to screen and to treat when applied to a population.[75]

It is also important to consider cholesterol in the wider context, together with other risk factors for CHD. The European Atherosclerosis Society and national cholesterol education program guidelines specify two target levels for active intervention: one for drug treatment (if a trial of dietary intervention fails) and the other for intensive dietary intervention only.[76]

The European Atherosclerosis Society considered three categories of people to be treated:

1. People with presence of vascular disease and total cholesterol >5 mmol/l (5<6 mmol/l dietary therapy only);

2. People with coronary heart disease risk >20% over 10 years and total cholesterol >5 mmol/l (5<7 mmol/l dietary therapy only);

3. People with coronary heart disease risk ≥20% and total cholesterol >7 mmol/l (7<8 mmol/l dietary therapy only).

For the purpose of this survey cholesterol was considered to be raised at a level of 6.5 mmol/l or over.

3.7.3 Total cholesterol levels, by age and sex

Cholesterol was approximately normally distributed. Mean cholesterol was 5.5 mmol/l for men and 5.6 mmol/l for women. In women, mean cholesterol increased with age, with a flattening off above the age of 75. In men, starting from a lower level at age 16-24, it increased more rapidly, and from age 25 to about age 50 was higher than in women. After that it levelled off, whereas women's mean cholesterol continued to increase, becoming substantially higher than men's from age 60.

Overall, 18.0% of men and 22.4% of women had a cholesterol level of 6.5 mmol/l or above. The increase in prevalence with age was much greater than the increase in the mean. Among men the prevalence of raised cholesterol increased from 1.9% in those aged 16-24 to 23.8% in those aged 45-54, after which it did not show any further systematic increase. Among women prevalence continued to increase from the youngest age group 16-24 (2.9%) to those aged 65-74 (48.0%), falling slightly to 44.4% among those aged 75 and over. This is consistent with the reported increase in cholesterol after menopause.

The increase in total cholesterol after the menopause may be due to high levels of the HDL fraction of cholesterol (Section 3.7.7). It is therefore important to measure total cholesterol together with its fractions to assess accurately cardiovascular disease risk (see HDL-cholesterol in Section 3.7.6). Actions to lower cholesterol levels should be taken only after HDL-cholesterol has also been measured and found low.   **Table 3.69, Figure 3O**

3.7.4 Change in total cholesterol levels 1994/1998

Mean cholesterol level in 1998 was lower than in 1994 for all age groups in both men and women. Overall it fell from 5.8 mmol/l in 1994 to 5.5 mmol/l in 1998 among men and from 6.0 mmol/l in 1994 to 5.6 mmol/l in 1998 among women.   **Table 3.69**

It should be noted that the laboratory used in 1998 was different from that used in 1994 (see Chapter 8, Sections 8.10.2, 8.10.4). Although they both used the same method, some caution is necessary when interpreting these results.

3.7.5 **Total cholesterol levels, by socio-economic variables**

Social class of head of household

Total cholesterol showed very little social class variation in either sex. To assess the significance of the difference between means an analysis of variance was performed, adjusting for age. To assess the significance of the difference between categorical variables (% of raised total cholesterol) logistic regression was performed.

Among men, age-standardised mean cholesterol varied between 5.3 mmol/l in Social Class IV and 5.5 in Social Class IIINM and V. Among women it was 5.5 mmol/l in Social Class IIINM, compared to 5.6 mmol/l in all other social classes. These differences were not statistically significant.

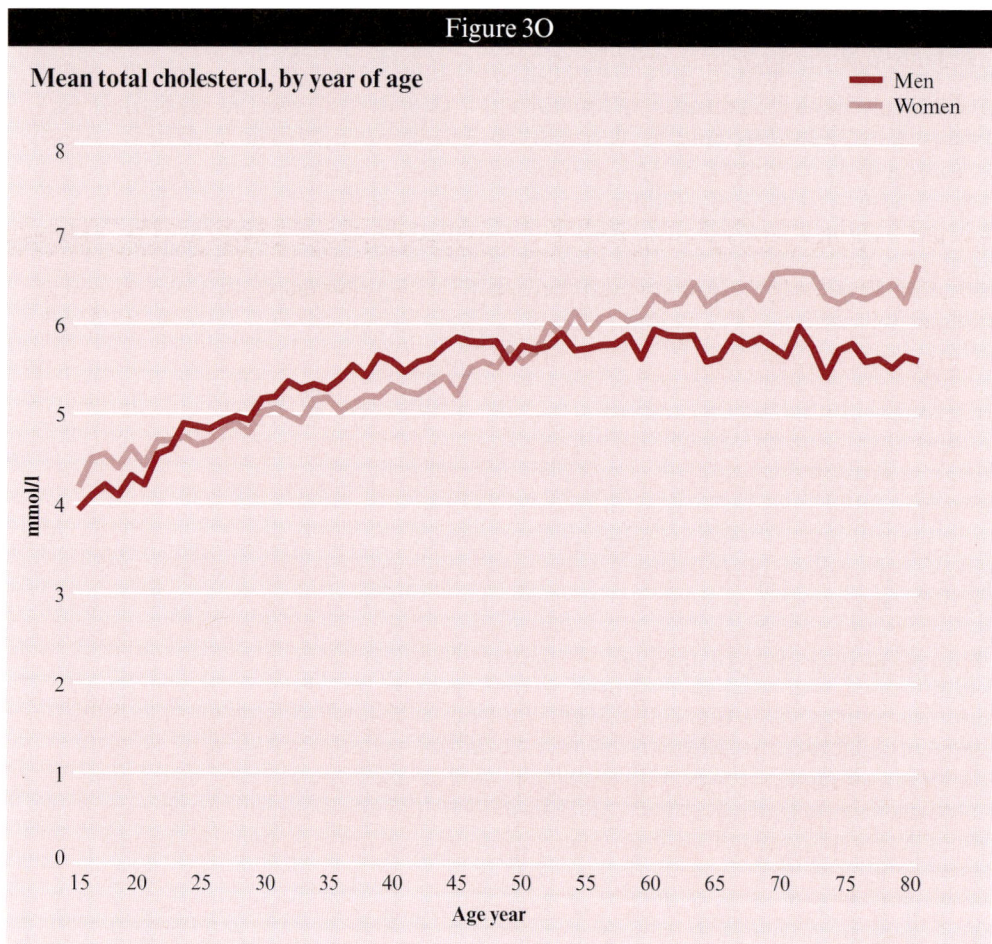

Figure 3O

Mean total cholesterol, by year of age

— Men
— Women

The age-standardised proportion of men with raised cholesterol increased from 14.5% in Social Class I to 21.2% in Social Class IIINM, then decreased to 14.7% in Social Class IV and 19.8% in Social Class V. Among women the prevalence of raised cholesterol was almost the same in each social class, ranging from a minimum of 21.2% in Social Class IIINM to a maximum of 23.7% in Social Class IIIM. **Table 3.70**

Equivalised household income

Small variations in age-adjusted mean total cholesterol by equivalised income quintiles were seen in both sexes.

Among men the age-standardised prevalence of raised cholesterol was higher in the two lowest income quintiles than in the others, while among women there was no clear pattern; no significant differences were found in logistic regression. **Table 3.71, Figure 3P**

Health Authority area type

There were few differences in mean total cholesterol between area types. The proportion of men with raised cholesterol was higher in Urban areas (19.4%) and lower in Rural areas (14.9%) and in Mature areas (15.2%), while women showed a lower prevalence in Inner London (11.3%) than in other area types. These differences were not statistically significant. **Table 3.72**

3.7.6 HDL-cholesterol

High-density lipoprotein cholesterol (HDL-cholesterol) is a fraction of total cholesterol, which constitutes approximately 20% of total cholesterol. Several studies have shown that reduced plasma levels of HDL-cholesterol are associated with increased risk of coronary heart disease.[77,78,79] This effect may be due to the ability of this particle to transport cholesterol from the peripheral tissues to the liver for elimination, thus protecting against atheroma.

The favourable influence of HDL-cholesterol on thrombogenesis has been advocated to explain why low levels of HDL-cholesterol are associated with a worse prognosis after myocardial infarction.[80]

Results from a 21 year follow up of 8,000 men indicated that abnormally low HDL-cholesterol levels carry an excess risk in CHD-free men with total cholesterol <5.2 mmol/l similar to that for their counterparts with higher total cholesterol levels.[81]

Previous studies have demonstrated an association between exercise and elevated HDL-cholesterol. Factors that are known to lower HDL-cholesterol[82] levels are smoking, alcohol consumption, and a raised body mass index and blood pressure.

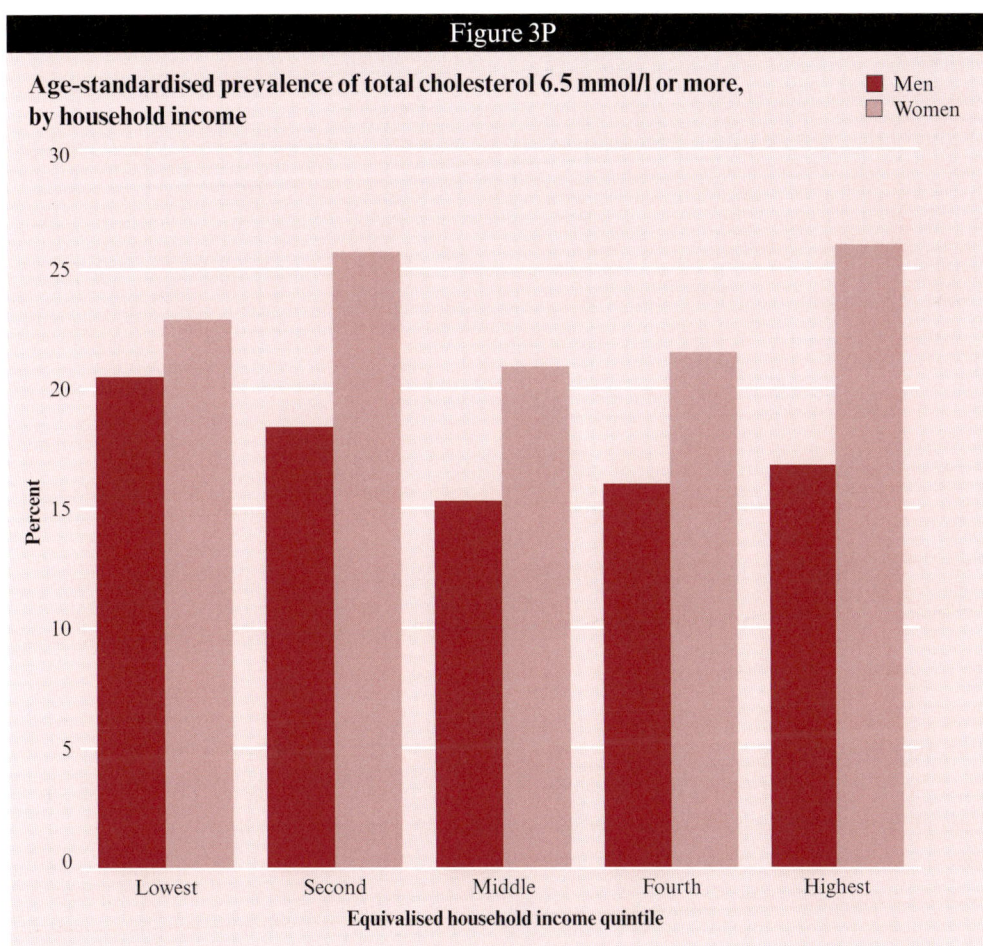

Figure 3P

Age-standardised prevalence of total cholesterol 6.5 mmol/l or more, by household income

Legend: Men, Women

Y-axis: Percent (0–30)
X-axis: Equivalised household income quintile (Lowest, Second, Middle, Fourth, Highest)

A measurement of HDL-cholesterol is essential to assess accurately absolute CHD risk. For example, as low HDL-cholesterol tends to cluster with other risk factors such as diabetes and hypertension reliance on total cholesterol alone in such men or women will often underestimate their risk.

Attention is generally recommended for HDL-cholesterol concentrations ≤0.9 mmol/l. However, the management of low HDL-cholesterol remains an unresolved issue. In particular, isolated low HDL-cholesterol (≤0.9 mmol/l in the absence of total cholesterol >5.2 mmol/l) in CHD-free persons is unlikely to obtain attention.[82]

3.7.7 HDL-cholesterol levels, by age and sex

Women had higher mean HDL-cholesterol than men (1.6 mmol/l versus 1.3 mmol/l). Mean HDL-cholesterol level was the same for all age groups in men, while in women it fluctuated between 1.5 mmol/l and 1.6 mmol/l.

The proportion of informants with an HDL-cholesterol level of 0.9 mmol/l or less was much higher in men (16.9%) than in women (5.4%). Among men it increased from 13% in those aged 16-24 to 19.2% in those aged 65-74, and then decreased to 14.7% in those aged 75 and above. No pattern was observed among women.   **Table 3.73**

3.7.8 HDL-cholesterol levels, by socio-economic variables

Social class of head of household

No difference in age-adjusted mean HDL-cholesterol levels was found between social classes among men (p=0.169 in analysis of variance), while women in manual social classes tended to have a lower mean level than those in non-manual social classes (p<0.001).

The prevalence of HDL-cholesterol levels of 0.9 mmol/l or less in men was slightly lower in Social Classes IV and V. In women prevalence increased from 3.4% in Social Class I to 8.5% in Social Class V. In a logistic regression analysis which adjusted for age the differences were significant for women (p=0.002) but not for men (p=0.09).   **Table 3.74**

Equivalised household income

Mean HDL-cholesterol levels tended to increase as income increased in both sexes.

After adjusting for age, mean HDL-cholesterol variation was statistically significant in both men and women (p<0.001). Differences were significant also for prevalence of HDL-cholesterol levels of 0.9 mmol/l or less (p=0.01 for men and p<0.001 for women).

The prevalence of low HDL-cholesterol among women decreased from 7.9% in the lowest income quintile to 2.9% in the highest income quintile. Among men prevalence was lower in the two highest income quintiles.   **Table 3.75, Figure 3Q**

Health Authority area type

Very small differences were found between areas of residence. Mean HDL-cholesterol was 1.3 mmol/l in all area types for men and fluctuated between 1.5 mmol/l and 1.6 mmol/l for women.

The prevalence of an HDL-cholesterol level of 0.9 mmol/l or less was lowest in Mature areas for both men (14.0%) and women (4.2%).   **Table 3.76**

3.7.9 C-reactive protein (CRP)

C-reactive protein is the major acute phase protein in humans. The measurement of acute phase proteins in blood provides a measurement of inflammation activity. In unchallenged subjects concentrations are usually low, rising several hundredfold in acute illness.

A cross-sectional study showed a relation between C-reactive protein and electrocardiographic abnormalities, symptomatic heart disease, and claudication.[83] C-reactive protein was also associated with cardiovascular risk factors such as raised serum fibrinogen, sialic acid, total cholesterol, triglyceride, glucose, and apolipoprotein B values.

In patients with unstable angina and in chronic coronary heart disease C-reactive protein concentration may be a powerful predictor of subsequent cardiac events.[84]

The follow-up of the Multiple Risk Factor Intervention Trial (MRFIT) has documented a strong relation between levels of C-reactive protein and subsequent risk of CHD deaths among cigarette smokers.[85]

Data from the US Physicians' Health Study demonstrated that CRP is a marker of cardiovascular risk not only among those with stable and unstable angina, the elderly, and selected high-risk patients but also among individuals with no current evidence of cardiovascular disease.[86]

In the literature there is no recommendation for a C-reactive protein threshold. The distribution of C-reactive protein was not normal, being very skewed to the left, so that

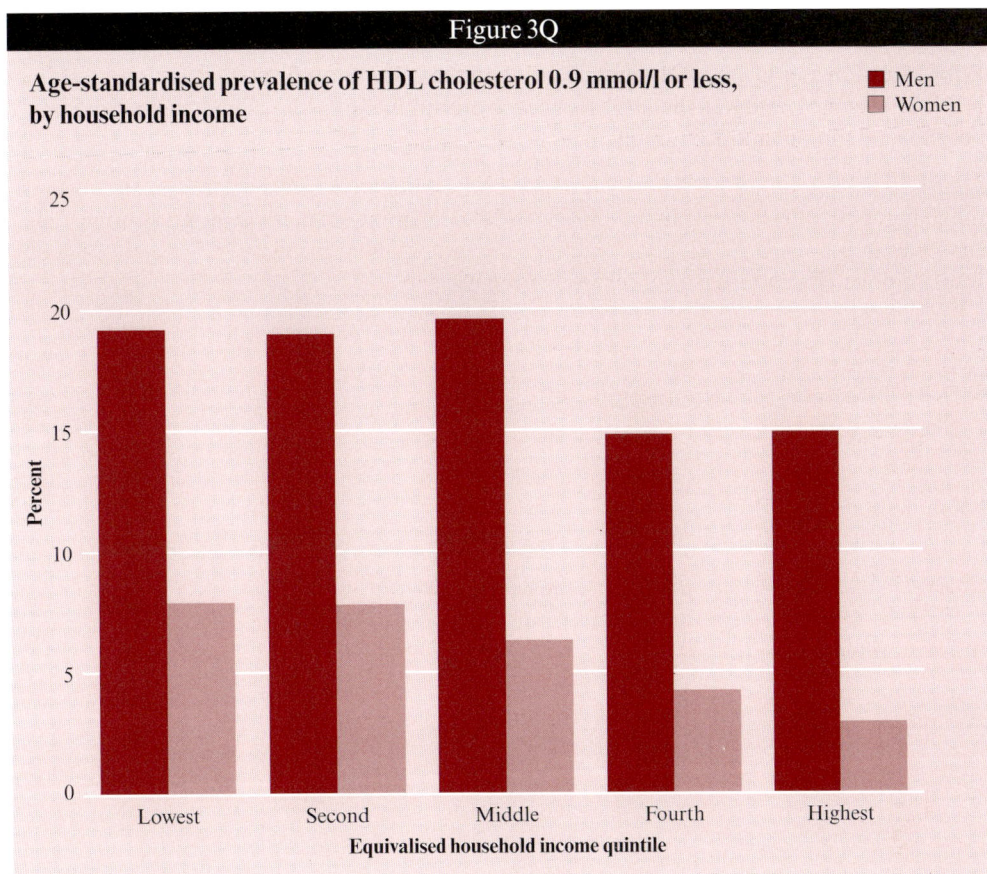

Figure 3Q

Age-standardised prevalence of HDL cholesterol 0.9 mmol/l or less, by household income

Men
Women

Percent (y-axis 0 to 25)

Lowest · Second · Middle · Fourth · Highest

Equivalised household income quintile

even a logarithmic transformation did not normalise it. Quintile distributions are presented in this report. The categories of CRP defined on the basis of the quintile distribution, separately for men and women, are presented below.

mg/l	Men	Women
Bottom quintile	≤0.5	≤0.5
2nd quintile	0.6-1.0	0.6-1.2
3rd quintile	1.1-1.9	1.3-2.4
4th quintile	2.0-3.7	2.5-4.9
Top quintile	>3.7	>4.9

3.7.10 C-reactive protein, by age and sex

C-reactive protein increased with age in both sexes, but this increase was more marked among men. The proportion of men who had a C-reactive protein level in the top quintile increased from 7.6% in those aged 16-24 to 41.9% in those aged 75 and over. In women, the proportion in the top quintile increased from 12.5% in those aged 16-24 to 29.3% in those aged 65-74, then slightly decreased in those aged 75 and above.   Table 3.77

3.7.11 C-reactive protein, by socio-economic variables

Social class of head of household

Among men, the age-standardised proportion in the top quintile of C-reactive protein increased from 14.0% in Social Class I to 21.2% in Social Class IIIM, and then decreased to 19.5% in Social Class V.

A different pattern was found among women. The proportion in the top quintile at first decreased from 19.9% in Social Class I to 16.7% in Social Class II, then increased to 24.2% in Social Class IV and finally decreased slightly in Social Class V.   Table 3.78

Equivalised household income

An income gradient was observed in the proportion in the top quintile of high C-reactive protein. Among men, the proportion decreased from 23.7% in the lowest (equivalised) income quintile and 26.5% in the next lowest to 13.4% in the highest income quintile. Among women, it decreased from 23.3% to 16.5%.   Table 3.79, Figure 3R

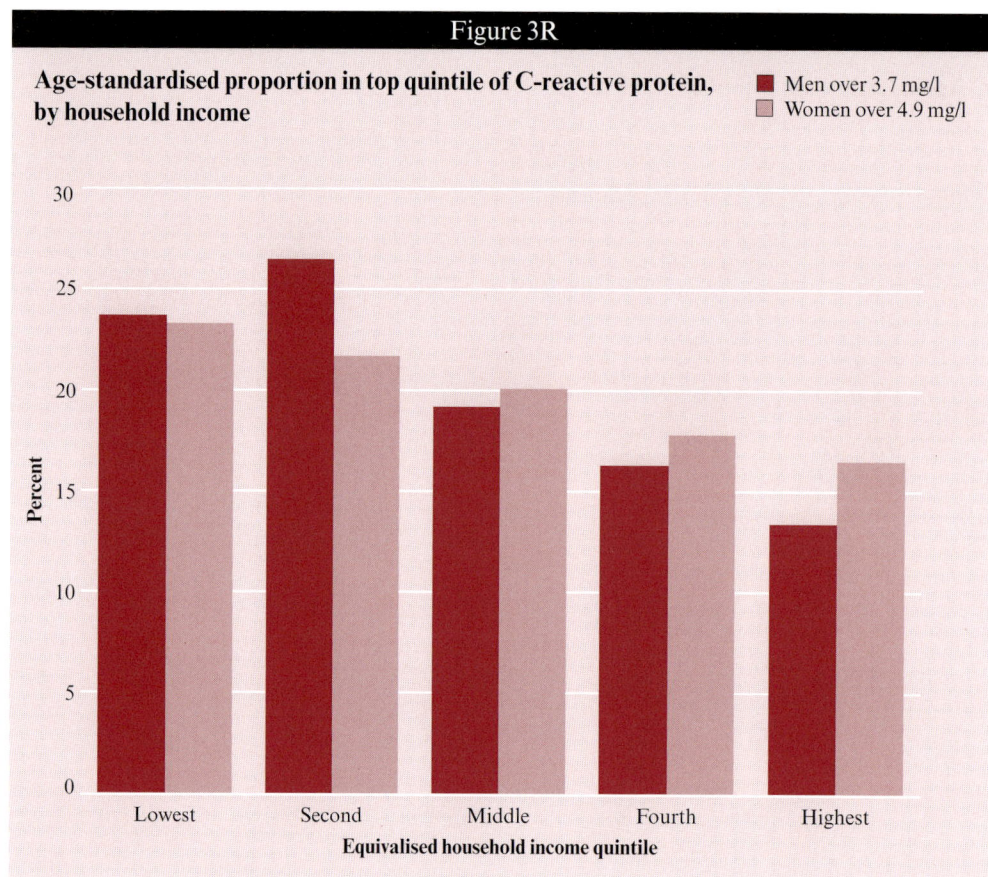

Figure 3R

Age-standardised proportion in top quintile of C-reactive protein, by household income

Legend: ■ Men over 3.7 mg/l ▨ Women over 4.9 mg/l

Equivalised household income quintile

Health Authority area type

There was no marked difference in the prevalence of high C-reactive protein between area types. Among men prevalence was higher in Mining & Industrial areas (21.4%) and lower in Inner London (12.2%), while among women, Inner London (16.7%) and Mature (16.8%) areas had a prevalence slightly lower than others. **Table 3.80**

3.7.12 Fibrinogen

Fibrinogen is a major blood glycoprotein that plays an essential role in haemostasis and the maintenance of blood viscosity. Prospective population studies have established that fibrinogen is an independent predictor for ischaemic heart disease and stroke. These study conclusions have prompted recommendations that fibrinogen determinations be included in the cardiovascular risk profile.

A meta-analysis of studies conducted between 1984 and 1998[87] showed that high plasma fibrinogen levels were associated with an increased risk of cardiovascular disease in healthy as much as in high-risk individuals.

As the laboratory used in 1994 was different comparisons have not been attempted because changes in methodology would affect comparability.

3.7.13 Fibrinogen, by age and sex

Fibrinogen was not normally distributed, hence a log transformation was performed. Although a better approximation to normality was achieved, the log transformation did not normalise the distribution and therefore the arithmetic mean is commented on.

Mean fibrinogen was 2.6 g/l for men and 2.8 g/l for women and increased with age. For men it increased steadily from 2.2 g/l in those aged 16-24 to 3.1 g/l in those aged 75 and above. For women the increase in fibrinogen was more marked after age 45-54, from 2.7 g/l to 3.2 g/l, while it was 2.5g/l and 2.6 g/l in the younger age groups.

Fibrinogen levels were higher in women than in men in all age groups. **Table 3.81, Figure 3S**

Figure 3S

Mean fibrinogen, by age

■ Men
■ Women

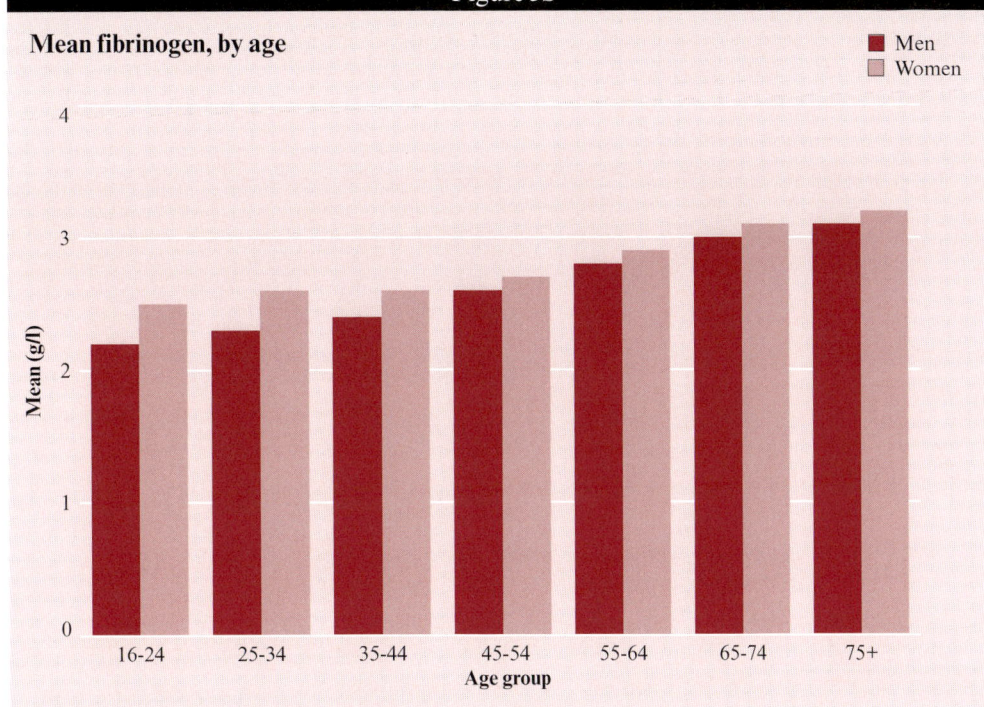

Figure: Bar chart titled "Mean fibrinogen, by age" showing Mean (g/l) on the y-axis (0 to 4) against Age group on the x-axis (16-24, 25-34, 35-44, 45-54, 55-64, 65-74, 75+) for Men and Women.

3.7.14 Fibrinogen, by socio-economic variables

Social class of head of household

A social class gradient was observed: mean fibrinogen value adjusted for age was higher in manual than non-manual social classes in both sexes. **Table 3.82**

Equivalised household income

Mean fibrinogen was negatively associated with income in both men and women. Among men it slightly increased from the lowest income quintile (2.6 g/l) to the next lowest (2.7 g/l), then decreased to 2.4 g/l in the highest income quintile. In women mean fibrinogen showed little changes, from 2.8 g/l in the lowest income quintile to 2.7 g/l in the two highest income quintiles. **Table 3.83**

Health Authority area type

Men showed some differences in mean fibrinogen value (adjusted for age) between area types, while women had similar values. Fibrinogen level was lowest in Inner London for both sexes. **Table 3.84**

References and notes

1 The authors responsible for each section of the chapter were as follows: Section 3.2 (cigarette smoking) Boreham, Section 3.3 (alcohol consumption) Erens, Section 3.4 (eating habits) Hirani and Primatesta, Section 3.5 (body mass) Hirani and Primatesta, Section 3.6 (blood pressure) Falaschetti and Primatesta, Section 3.7 (blood analytes) Falaschetti and Primatesta.

2 Maclure M. *Demonstration of deductive meta-analysis: ethanol intake and risk of myocardial infarction.* Epidemiol Rev 1993; **15**:328-51.

3 Rimm EB, Giovannucci FL, Willett WC, Colditz GA, Ascherio A, Rosner B, Stampfer MJ. *Prospective study of alcohol consumption and risk of coronary heart disease in men.* Lancet 1991; **338**:464-68.

4 *Sensible Drinking: The Report of an Inter-Departmental Working Group*, Department of Health, December 1995.

5 Erens B, Hedges B. *Chapter 7 Alcohol consumption* (Section 7.2.2) in Prescott-Clarke P and Primatesta P (eds) *The Health of Young People '95-'97*, The Stationery Office, London, 1998.

6 Hedges B, di Salvo P. *Chapter 8 Alcohol consumption and smoking in* Prescott-Clarke P and Primatesta P (eds) *The Health Survey for England 1996*, The Stationery Office, London, 1998.

7   In deriving estimates of alcohol consumption, a half pint of normal beer, lager and cider was calculated as one unit, whereas a half pint of strong beer, etc. was 1.5 units.

8   Hedges B. *Chapter 9 Alcohol consumption and smoking* (p.351) in Prescott-Clarke P and Primatesta P (eds) *The Health Survey for England 1995*, The Stationery Office, London, 1997.

9   McKee M, Britton A. *The positive relationship between alcohol and heart disease in Eastern Europe: potential physiological mechanisms*. J Royal Soc Med 1998; **91**:402-7.

10 The percentages in Figure 3A are on different bases, with weekly consumption based on all informants aged 16 and over, and daily consumption based on informants who had drunk alcohol in the past week. However, similar patterns are shown if Figure 3A is redrawn with all percentages calculated on the same base.

11 *Smoking Kills: A White Paper on Tobacco*. The Stationery Office, London, 1998.

12 *Saving Lives: Our Healthier Nation*. The Stationery Office, London, 1999.

13 Korovessis C, Lynn P. *Evaluating the Health Survey for England (HSE) as a vehicle for monitoring trends in smoking*. National Centre for Social Research, London, 1999.

14 A small number of persons aged 18 and over also answered these questions by self-completion rather than by interview, as the interviewer judged that more reliable responses might be obtained by this method.

15 Peto R, Lopez AD, Boreham J et al. *Mortality from smoking in developed countries 1950-2000*. ICRF and WHO, Oxford University Press, 1994.

16 Hedges B, Di Salvo P. *Chapter 8. Alcohol consumption and smoking* in Prescott-Clarke P, Primatesta P. *Health Survey for England '96 Volume 1: Findings*. The Stationery Office, London, 1998.

17 Parish S, Collins R, Peto R et al. *Cigarette smoking, tar yields, and non-fatal myocardial infarction: 14000 cases and 32000 controls in the United Kingdom*. British Medical Journal 1995; **311**(7003):471-477.

18 Benowitz NL, Gourlay SG. *Cardiovascular toxicity of nicotine: implications for nicotine replacement therapy*. JACC June 1997; 29/7:1422-1431.

19 Department of Health, Department of Health and Social Services Northern Ireland, The Scottish Office Department of Health, Welsh Office. *Report of the Scientific Committee on Tobacco and Health*. The Stationery Office, London, 1997.

20 Department of Health 1997 survey of tar, nicotine and carbon monoxide yields of cigarettes.

21 The test cigarettes are conditioned to a standard moisture content by storing them in a standard humidity atmosphere (60+/-2% and temperature 22 +/- 1°C) for at least 48 hours and not more than 10 days. The cigarettes are smoked using a 20 channel Filtrona SM400 automatic smoking machine calibrated to take a puff of 35ml over a period of 2 seconds. Environmental conditions of the room housing the smoking machine must be within the limits of relative humidity 60+/-5% and temperature 22 +/- 2°C while the smoking is in progress The puff is repeated every 60 seconds until the cigarette burns down to a pre-defined butt mark calculated from measurement of the filter and overwrap lengths of the brand. The smoke from each puff is drawn through a 44 mm glass fibre filter trapping the particulate matter of the smoke. Five cigarettes are smoked sequentially through the same filter which is weighed before and after completion of smoking. The filter pad together with the trapped particulate matter are extracted by shaking with an organic solvent (20 mls of propan-2-ol). The solvent is then analysed for nicotine and water content using gas chromatography. 'Tar' is calculated by subtraction of the water and nicotine values from the gain in weight of the filter arising from smoking the cigarettes (all on a 'per cigarette' basis). The vapour phase of the smoke from each set of 5 cigarettes is collected in individual plastic bags before being analysed for carbon monoxide content (%v/v) using a non dispersive infra red technique. For each brand the butt length at which smoking is terminated is calculated from the ISO definition of either filter length + 8 mm or filter overwrap + 3 mm, whichever is the longest. Plain cigarettes are smoked to a butt length of 23 mm.

22 Jarvis MJ, Wardle J. *Social patterning of health behaviours: the case of cigarette smoking*. in: Marmot M, Wilkinson R, eds. Social Determinants of Health. (pp 240-255) Oxford University Press, 1999.

23 A deprivation score was created using social class, tenure, car ownership and employment status as component variables.

24 Department of Health. *Our healthier nation - a contract for health*. The Stationery Office, London, 1998.

25 Graves KL, McGovern PG, Sprafka JM, Folsom AR, Burke GL. *Contribution of dietary lipid change to falling serum cholesterol levels between 1980 to 1982 and 1985 to 1987 in an urban population*. The Minnesota Heart Survey. Ann Epidemiol 1993; **3**:605-13.

26 Rimm EB, Ascherio A, Giovannucci E, Spieglman D, Stampfer MJ, Willett WC. *Vegetable, fruit, and cereal fiber intake and risk of coronary heart disease among men*. JAMA 1996; **275**: 447-51.

27 Law MR, Frost CD, Wald NJ. *Analysis of data from trials of salt reduction*. BMJ 1991; **302**:819-824.

28 World Health Organization. *Diet, nutrition and the prevention of chronic diseases*. WHO Technical Report Series 797, Geneva, Switzerland, 1990;1-203.

29 Dwyer J. *Dietary approaches for reducing cardiovascular disease risks*. J Nutr 1995; **125/3 Suppl**. 656S-665S.

30 Posner BM, Franz MN, Quatromoni PA, Gagnon DR et al. *Secular trends in diet and risk factors for cardiovascular disease: the Framingham Study*. J Am Diet Assoc 1995; **95**:171-9.

31 Golay A, Bobbioni E. *The role of dietary fat in obesity*. Int J Obes Relat Metab Disord 1997; **21 Suppl** 3. S2-11.

32 Kuller LH. *Eating fat or being fat and risk of cardiovascular disease and cancer among women.* Ann Epidemiol 1994; **4**:119-27.

33 Gaziano JM. *Antioxidant vitamins and cardiovascular disease.* Proc Assoc Am Phys 1999; **111/1**:2-9.

34 Gey KF, Moser UK, Jordan P, Stahelin HB, Eichholzer M, Ludin F, Saris WHM, Horrobin DF, Hornstra G. *Increased risk of cardiovascular disease at suboptimal plasma concentrations of essential antioxidants: An epidemiological update with special attention to carotene and vitamin C.* Am J Clin Nutr 1993; **57/5 Suppl.** 787S-797S.

35 INTERSALT Cooperative Research Group. INTERSALT: an international study of electrolyte excretion and blood pressure. Results for 24 hour urinary sodium and potassium excretion. BMJ 1988; **297**:319-28.

36 Appel LJ, Moore TJ, Obarzanek E, Vollmer WM, Svetkey LP, Sacks FM, Bray GA, Vogt TM, Cutler JA, Windhauser MM, Lin PH, Karanja N. *A clinical trial of the effects of dietary patterns on blood pressure.* DASH Collaborative Research Group. N Engl J Med 1997; **336**:1117-1124.

37 The Ministry of Agriculture Fisheries and Food (MAFF). Household food consumption and expenditure. Annual Reports of the National Food Survey Committee. The Stationery Office, London.

38 The Department of Health and MAFF jointly commission the dietary and nutrition surveys throughout England, Wales and Scotland. The most recent report in this series presents the findings of the diet and nutritional status of British adults aged 65 years and over: Finch S, Doyle W, Lowe C, Bates C, Prentice A, Smithers G and Clarke P. *The National Diet and Nutrition Survey: People Aged 65 Years and Over.* The Stationery Office, London, 1998.

39 Roe L, Strong C, Whiteside C, Neil A, Mant D. *Dietary intervention in primary care: Validity of the DINE method for assessment.* Fam Pract 1994; **11**:375-81.

40 Imperial Cancer Research Fund OXCHECK Study Group. *Effectiveness of health checks conducted by nurses in primary care: final results of the OXCHECK study.* BMJ 1995; **310**:1099-1104.

41 Committee on Medical Aspects of Food Policy. *Diet and cardiovascular disease.* HMSO, London, 1984.

42 Roe L. Personal communication.

43 Independent Inquiry into Inequalities in Health Report. The Stationery Office, London, 1998.

44 Pi-Sunyer FX. *The medical hazards of obesity.* Ann Intern Med 1993; **119**:655-660.

45 Franz MJ. *Managing obesity in patients with comorbidities.* J Am Diet Assoc 1998; **98 Suppl 2**:S39-S43.

46 Garrow JS. *Treatment of obesity.* Lancet 1992; **340**:409-413.

47 Effective Health Care. *The prevention and treatment of obesity.* NHS Centre for Reviews and Dissemination, University of York. Churchill Livingstone 1997; **3**:2.

48 Seidell JC. *Obesity in Europe: scaling an epidemic.* Int J Obes 1995; **19 Suppl 3**:S1-S4.

49 Gensini GF, Comeglio M, Colella A. *Classical risk factors and emerging elements in the risk profile for coronary artery disease.* Eur Heart J 1998; **19 Suppl A**:A53-61.

50 Pi-Sunyer FX. *Health implications of obesity.* Am J Clin Nutr 1991; **53 Suppl 6**: 1595S-1603S.

51 Bost L, Primatesta P, Dong W. *Anthropometric measures and children's iron status (Chapter 7)* in Prescott-Clarke P and Primatesta P (eds) Health Survey for England 1996, The Stationery Office, London, 1998.

52 Bost L, Primatesta P, Dong W. *Anthropometric measures and children's iron status (Chapter 8)* in Prescott-Clarke P and Primatesta P (eds) Health Survey for England 1995, The Stationery Office, London, 1997.

53 Colhoun H, Lampe F, Dong W. *Obesity (Chapter 8)* in Colhoun H and Prescott-Clarke P (eds) Health Survey for England 1994, HMSO, London, 1996.

54 Sjostrom L. *Obesity and its relationship to other diseases (Chapter 11.4)* pp 235-239. in Shetty PS, McPherson K (eds). Diet, nutrition and chronic disease: lessons from contrasting worlds 1996. London School of Hygiene and Tropical Medicine Sixth Annual Public Health Forum, 1997, Wiley, London, UK.

55 Kannel WB, Cupples LA, Ramaswami R, Stokes J, Kregor BE, Higgins M. *Regional obesity and risk of cardiovascular disease; the Framingham Study.* J Clin Epidemiol 1991; **44**:183-190.

56 Karlsson J, Sjostrom L, Sullivan M. Swedish obese subjects (SOS) - an intervention study of obesity. Two year follow-up of health related quality of life (HRQL) and eating behaviour after gastric surgery for severe obesity. Int J Obes Relat Metab Disord 1998; **22**:113-26.

57 NHS CRD. *The prevention and treatment of obesity.* Effective healthcare. University of York, 1997; **3**:2-12.

58 Prescott-Clarke P and Primatesta P (eds) *Health Survey for England : Adult Reference Tables 1997* (unpublished).

59 Molarius A, Seidell JC. *Selection of anthropometric indicators for classification of abdominal fatness - a critical review.* Int J Obes 1998; **22**:719-727.

60 Stamler J, Stamler R, Neaton JD. *Blood pressure, systolic and diastolic, and cardiovascular risks.* Arch Intern Med 1993; **153**:598-615.

61 MacMahon S, Peto R, Cutler J, Collins R, Sorlie P, Neaton J, Abbott R, Godwin J, Dyer A, Stomeer J. *Blood pressure, stroke, and coronary heart disease. Part 1. Prolonged differences in blood pressure: prospective observational studies corrected for the regression dilution bias.* Lancet 1990; **335**:765-774.

62 Millar JA, Liver AF, Burke V. *Pulse pressure as risk factor for cardiovascular events in the MRC mild hypertension trial.* J Hypertens 1999; **17**:1065-1072.

63 Saving Lives: *Our Healthier Nation. Cm 4386.*The Stationery Office. London, July 1999.

64 Collins R, MacMahon S. *Blood pressure, antihypertensive drug treatment and the risks of stroke and of coronary heart disease.* Br Med Bull 1994; **50**:272-298.

65 Joint National Committee on Prevention, Detection, Evaluation and Treatment of High Blood Pressure and the National High Blood Pressure Education Program Coordinating Committee. *The sixth report of the Joint National Committee on prevention, detection, evaluation, and treatment of high blood pressure.* Arch Intern Med 1997; **157**:2413-2446.

66 1999 World Health Organization – International Society of Hypertension Guidelines for the Management of Hypertension. J Hypertens 1999; **17**:151-183.

67 Ramsay LE, Williams B, Johnston GD, MacGregor GA, Poston L, Potter JF, Poulter NR, Russell G. British *Hypertension Society guidelines for hypertension management 1999: Summary.* BMJ 1999; **319**:630-635.

68 Ramsay LE, Williams B, Johnston GD, MacGregor GA, Poston L, Potter JF, Poulter NR, Russell G. *Guidelines for management of hypertension: Report of the third working party of the British Hypertension Society, 1999.* J Human Hypertens 1999; **13**:569-592.

69 Burt VL, Whelton P, Roccella EJ. Prevalence of hypertension in the US adult population. *Results from the Third National Health Nutrition Examination Survey, 1988-1991.* Hypertension 1995; **25**:305-313.

70 Colhoun HM, Dong W, Poulter NR. *Blood pressure screening, management and control in England; results from the Health Survey for England 1994.* J Hypertens 1998; **16**:747-753.

71 Law MR, Wald NJ, Thompson SG. By how much and how quickly does reduction in serum cholesterol concentration lower risk of ischaemic heart disease? BMJ 1994; **308**:367-73.

72 Law MR, Thompson SG, Wald NJ. Assessing possible hazards of reducing serum cholesterol. BMJ 1994; **308**:373-9.

73 Gould AL, Rossouw JE, Santanello NC, et al. *Cholesterol reduction yields clinical benefit. A new look at old data.* Circulation 1995; **91**:2274-82.

74 Anonymous. *Netherlands cholesterol consensus update.* Heart Bulletin 1990; **23** (suppl):9-21.

75 Unwin N, Thomson R, O'Byrne AM, Laker M, Armstrong H. *Implications of applying widely accepted cholesterol screening and management guidelines to a British adult population: cross sectional study of cardiovascular disease and risk factors.* BMJ 1998; **317**:1125-1129.

76 Walker ARP. *Cholesterol: how low is low enough?* BMJ 1999; **318**:538.

77 Miller NE, Thelle DS, Forde OH, Mjos OD. *The Tromso Heart Study: high-density lipoprotein and coronary heart disease: a prospective case-control study.* Lancet 1977; **2**:965-968.

78 Castelli WP, Garrison RJ, Wilson PWF, Abbott RD, Kalousdian S, Kannel WB. *Incidence of coronary heart disease and lipoprotein cholesterol levels: the Framingham Study.* JAMA 1986; **256**:2835-2838.

79 Gordon DJ, Probstfield JL, Garrison RJ, Neaton JD, Castelli WP, Knoke JD, Jacobs DR Jr, Bangdiwala S, Tyroler A. *High-density lipoprotein cholesterol and cardiovascular disease: four prospective American studies.* Circulation 1989; **79**:8-15.

80 Berge KG, Canner PL, Hainline A Jr. *High-density lipoprotein cholesterol and prognosis after myocardial infarction.* Circulation 1982; **66**:1176-1178.

81 Goldbourt U; Yaari S; Medalie JH. *Isolated low HDL Cholesterol as a risk factor for coronary heart disease mortality. A 21 year follow-up of 8000 men.* Arterioscler Thromb Vasc Biol 1997; **17**:107-13.

82 Gibbons LW, Blair SN, Cooper KH, Smith M. *Association between coronary heart disease risk factors and physical fitness in healthy adult women.* Circulation 1983; **67**:977-983.

83 Mendall MA, Patel P, Ballam L, Strachan D, Northfield TC. *C-reactive protein and its relation to cardiovascular risk factors: a population based cross sectional study.* BMJ 1996; **312**:1061-5.

84 Liuzzo G, Biasucci LM, Gallimore JR, et al. *The prognostic value of C-reactive protein and serum amyloid a protein in severe unstable angina.* N Engl J Med 1994; **331**:417-24.

85 Lewis H. Kuller, Russel P. Tracy et al. *Relation of C-reactive protein and coronary heart disease in the MRFIT nested case-control study.* Am J Epidemiol 1996; **144**:537-47.

86 Ridker PM, Glynn RJ, Hennekens CH. *C-reactive protein adds to the predictive value of total and HDL cholesterol in determining risk of first myocardial infarction.* Circulation 1998; **97**:2007-2011.

87 Maresca G, Di Blasio A. Marchioli R, Di Minno G. *Measuring plasma fibrinogen to predict stroke and myocardial infarction.* Arterioscler Thromb Vasc Biol 1999; **19**:1368-1377.

Tables

Table 3.1

Estimated usual weekly alcohol consumption level, by age and sex

Aged 16 and over   *1998*

Alcohol consumption level (units per week)	Age							Total
	16-24	25-34	35-44	45-54	55-64	65-74	75 +	
	%	%	%	%	%	%	%	%
Men								
Have never drunk alcohol	7	5	3	2	3	4	4	4
Ex-drinker	1	2	3	3	5	6	11	4
Under 1	6	5	5	7	9	11	16	7
1-10	26	31	32	29	35	38	39	32
Over 10-21	18	25	23	22	20	21	17	22
Over 21-35	18	17	17	17	17	13	8	16
Over 35-50	11	7	9	10	7	5	3	8
Over 50	13	8	8	9	5	3	2	7
Mean units	23.9	19.0	19.8	20.6	16.2	12.2	9.0	18.0
Standard error of the mean	1.04	0.62	0.67	0.74	0.63	0.53	0.54	0.28
Women								
Have never drunk alcohol	10	6	5	5	8	11	16	8
Ex-drinker	2	3	3	4	5	9	10	5
Under 1	9	14	15	17	21	27	28	18
1-7	35	37	39	36	39	31	29	36
Over 7-14	17	20	18	18	14	12	10	16
Over 14-21	11	10	10	10	7	6	4	9
Over 21-35	10	8	7	7	5	3	3	6
Over 35	7	3	3	3	1	1	0	3
Mean units	10.8	8.4	8.1	7.9	5.5	4.5	3.4	7.2
Standard error of the mean	0.52	0.31	0.30	0.27	0.24	0.25	0.21	0.12
Bases								
Men	*831*	*1330*	*1302*	*1287*	*985*	*834*	*560*	*7129*
Women	*970*	*1630*	*1570*	*1480*	*1147*	*966*	*903*	*8666*

Table 3.2

Estimated usual weekly alcohol consumption level (observed and age standardised), by social class of head of household and sex

Aged 16 and over   *1998*

Estimated units of alcohol per week	Social class of head of household						Social class of head of household					
	I	II	IIINM	IIIM	IV	V	I	II	IIINM	IIIM	IV	V
	Men						**Women**					
Observed												
% consuming more than 21/14[a] units of alcohol per week	28	34	31	29	30	29	21	23	19	15	12	11
Estimated mean weekly units	15.5	19.1	18.6	17.1	18.0	19.9	8.0	8.7	7.2	6.4	6.1	5.7
Standard error of the mean	0.72	0.46	0.87	0.46	0.85	2.06	0.43	0.23	0.29	0.21	0.35	0.55
Standardised												
% consuming more than 21/14[a] units of alcohol per week	28	35	32	30	31	29	20	22	20	15	13	12
Estimated mean weekly units	15.8	19.4	19.0	17.5	18.7	19.9	7.7	8.6	7.6	6.2	6.2	6.3
Standard error of the mean	0.74	0.46	0.88	0.47	0.87	2.04	0.42	0.23	0.29	0.21	0.36	0.59
Bases	*501*	*2162*	*710*	*2249*	*1027*	*332*	*512*	*2488*	*1340*	*2196*	*1364*	*493*

[a] 21 for men, 14 for women.

Table 3.3

Estimated usual weekly alcohol consumption level (observed and age standardised), by equivalised household income and sex

Aged 16 and over   *1998*

Estimated units of alcohol per week	Equivalised annual household income quintile				
	Up to £7,186	Over £7,186 to £10,834	Over £10,834 to £17,890	Over £17,890 to £27,705	Over £27,705
Men					
Observed					
% consuming more than 21 units of alcohol per week	24	23	29	36	39
Estimated mean weekly units	15.2	15.1	17.0	20.5	21.3
Standard error of the mean	0.80	0.86	0.56	0.63	0.56
Standardised					
% consuming more than 21 units of alcohol per week	26	26	28	36	38
Estimated mean weekly units	16.5	17.3	17.1	20.3	21.1
Standard error of the mean	0.85	0.99	0.57	0.63	0.57
Women					
Observed					
% consuming more than 14 units of alcohol per week	13	11	17	19	28
Estimated mean weekly units	5.7	4.9	7.1	8.0	10.4
Standard error of the mean	0.32	0.25	0.29	0.27	0.31
Standardised					
% consuming more than 14 units of alcohol per week	13	13	17	19	26
Estimated mean weekly units	5.7	5.7	7.0	7.8	9.8
Standard error of the mean	0.31	0.28	0.29	0.27	0.30
Bases					
Men	*988*	*991*	*1434*	*1386*	*1355*
Women	*1398*	*1479*	*1647*	*1490*	*1383*

Table 3.4

Estimated usual weekly alcohol consumption level (observed and age standardised), by Health Authority area type and sex

Aged 16 and over   *1998*

Estimated units of alcohol per week	Health Authority area type					
	Inner London	Mining & Industrial	Urban	Mature	Prosperous	Rural
Men						
Observed						
% consuming more than 21 units of alcohol per week	27	34	34	30	31	29
Estimated mean weekly units	14.9	19.4	19.4	17.6	17.9	17.1
Standard error of the mean	1.22	0.74	0.74	0.69	0.51	0.58
Standardised						
% consuming more than 21 units of alcohol per week	26	34	35	30	31	29
Estimated mean weekly units	14.2	19.7	19.7	18.0	18.4	17.6
Standard error of the mean	1.21	0.75	0.75	0.70	0.51	0.59
Women						
Observed						
% consuming more than 14 units of alcohol per week	21	18	18	17	18	17
Estimated mean weekly units	8.1	7.7	7.8	7.0	7.1	6.6
Standard error of the mean	0.78	0.33	0.39	0.28	0.22	0.21
Standardised						
% consuming more than 14 units of alcohol per week	20	19	18	18	17	17
Estimated mean weekly units	7.6	7.8	7.9	7.1	7.1	6.6
Standard error of the mean	0.74	0.33	0.39	0.28	0.22	0.21
Bases						
Men	*237*	*1096*	*1043*	*1092*	*1931*	*1730*
Women	*306*	*1285*	*1333*	*1302*	*2378*	*2062*

Table 3.5

Estimated usual weekly alcohol consumption level (observed and age standardised), by region and sex

Aged 16 and over   *1998*

Estimated units of alcohol per week	Region							
	Northern & Yorkshire	North West	Trent	West Midlands	Anglia & Oxford	North Thames	South Thames	South & West
Men								
Observed								
% consuming more than 21 units of alcohol per week	36	33	32	30	28	25	30	31
Estimated mean weekly units	21.1	19.3	18.3	17.4	16.2	15.4	17.5	18.3
Standard error of the mean	0.90	0.77	0.80	0.78	0.71	0.72	0.69	0.74
Standardised								
% consuming more than 21 units of alcohol per week	37	33	32	31	28	26	31	32
Estimated mean weekly units	21.6	19.4	18.5	17.9	16.3	15.9	17.7	19.0
Standard error of the mean	0.91	0.77	0.81	0.81	0.71	0.74	0.70	0.76
Women								
Observed								
% consuming more than 14 units of alcohol per week	19	20	16	15	17	14	19	18
Estimated mean weekly units	7.6	8.3	6.7	6.5	7.0	6.4	7.6	7.1
Standard error of the mean	0.31	0.36	0.33	0.39	0.34	0.36	0.37	0.28
Standardised								
% consuming more than 14 units of alcohol per week	20	20	16	16	17	14	19	19
Estimated mean weekly units	7.9	8.2	6.8	6.5	6.8	6.4	7.5	7.3
Standard error of the mean	0.32	0.36	0.34	0.39	0.34	0.38	0.37	0.28
Bases								
Men	*1023*	*967*	*791*	*734*	*805*	*909*	*887*	*1013*
Women	*1242*	*1126*	*935*	*911*	*956*	*1110*	*1175*	*1211*

Table 3.6

Estimated usual weekly alcohol consumption level, by survey year

Aged 16 and over   *1994-98*

Alcohol consumption level (units per week)[a]	Survey year						Survey year				
	1994	1995	1996	1997	1998		1994	1995	1996	1997	1998
	%	%	%	%	%		%	%	%	%	%
	Men						**Women**				
Have never drunk alcohol	4	4	4	4	4		8	8	7	8	8
Ex-drinker	3	3	3	3	4		4	4	4	5	5
Under 1	8	9	8	8	7		20	22	20	18	18
1-10 (1-7)	33	34	33	33	32		38	37	37	36	36
Over 10-21 (7-14)	22	22	22	23	22		16	16	17	17	16
Over 21-35 (14-21)	15	14	15	16	16		9	7	8	8	9
Over 35-50 (21-35)	7	8	8	7	8		3	5	5	6	6
Over 50 (35)	8	7	7	7	7		2	2	2	2	3
Mean units	17.8	16.9	17.5	16.9	18.0		6.3	6.2	6.6	6.7	7.2
Standard error of the mean	0.27	0.25	0.27	0.32	0.28		0.11	0.10	0.11	0.15	0.12
Bases	*7172*	*7314*	*7473*	*3836*	*7129*		*8620*	*8694*	*8934*	*4637*	*8666*

[a] Unbracketed figures refer to men, bracketed to women.

Table 3.7

Number of days on which alcohol consumed in past week, by age and sex

Aged 16 and over drinking alcohol in past 7 days   *1998*

Number of days	Age							Total
	16-24	25-34	35-44	45-54	55-64	65-74	75 +	
	%	%	%	%	%	%	%	%
Men								
1	25	22	20	17	21	24	26	21
2	22	24	22	18	19	17	16	20
3	18	18	15	14	13	10	9	15
4	12	12	11	10	10	7	5	10
5	8	7	8	8	6	5	2	7
6	7	5	6	7	5	5	4	6
7	9	12	18	26	25	32	38	21
Women								
1	36	35	32	30	34	34	32	33
2	25	25	23	19	20	17	20	22
3	17	15	13	14	12	11	6	13
4	9	9	10	9	7	5	4	8
5	6	5	7	6	4	2	3	5
6	3	3	5	4	3	3	2	4
7	4	8	10	18	20	27	32	15
Bases								
Men	*646*	*1039*	*1041*	*1033*	*753*	*591*	*345*	*5448*
Women	*621*	*1055*	*1063*	*1002*	*690*	*478*	*386*	*5295*

Table 3.8

Estimated alcohol consumption on heaviest drinking day in last week, by age and sex

Aged 16 and over drinking alcohol in past 7 days   1998

Alcohol consumption (units per day)	Age 16-24	25-34	35-44	45-54	55-64	65-74	75 +	Total
	%	%	%	%	%	%	%	%
Men								
Under 2 units	11	11	13	14	20	29	44	17
2, under 3 units	13	14	15	15	19	23	22	16
3, under 4 units	4	7	8	8	9	8	7	7
4, under 5 units	5	9	14	14	13	14	11	12
5, under 6 units	3	4	3	3	4	3	2	3
6, under 8 units	6	10	10	14	14	11	7	11
8 or more units	58	46	37	32	23	12	6	33
Women								
Under 2 units	19	20	26	26	40	53	68	32
2, under 3 units	16	20	23	25	28	26	19	23
3, under 4 units	9	12	13	16	13	9	8	12
4, under 5 units	11	10	11	11	10	6	3	10
5, under 6 units	7	7	6	6	3	3	0	5
6, under 8 units	14	13	11	9	4	3	1	9
8 or more units	24	17	9	6	3	2	1	10
Bases								
Men	*514*	*1038*	*1039*	*1032*	*752*	*592*	*345*	*5312*
Women	*545*	*1055*	*1062*	*1002*	*690*	*477*	*386*	*5217*

Table 3.9

Estimated alcohol consumption on heaviest drinking day in last week (observed and age standardised), by social class of head of household and sex

Aged 16 and over drinking alcohol in past 7 days   1998

Alcohol consumption (units per day)	Social class of head of household I	II	IIINM	IIIM	IV	V	Social class of head of household I	II	IIINM	IIIM	IV	V
	%	%	%	%	%	%	%	%	%	%	%	%
	Men						**Women**					
Observed												
Under 2 units	21	17	18	17	15	18	38	30	32	32	30	33
2, under 3 units	21	17	16	16	16	15	21	23	24	23	23	23
3, under 4 units	11	8	8	6	6	3	12	15	11	10	11	8
4, under 5 units	12	11	11	14	11	9	11	10	8	10	10	9
5, under 6 units	5	4	3	3	3	2	6	5	5	5	5	6
6, under 8 units	9	11	10	10	12	11	7	8	10	10	10	11
8 or more units	21	30	35	34	37	42	5	9	10	10	11	10
Standardised												
Under 2 units	20	17	18	16	15	17	43	33	31	35	31	32
2, under 3 units	20	17	16	16	16	14	20	22	24	22	24	23
3, under 4 units	11	8	7	6	6	3	11	14	11	10	11	8
4, under 5 units	11	10	10	13	11	9	11	9	9	9	9	9
5, under 6 units	5	4	3	3	3	2	5	5	5	5	5	6
6, under 8 units	9	11	10	10	12	11	6	8	10	9	9	12
8 or more units	24	33	35	36	38	44	5	9	10	9	11	11
Bases	*379*	*1742*	*544*	*1631*	*708*	*211*	*354*	*1765*	*810*	*1248*	*691*	*233*

Table 3.10

Estimated alcohol consumption on heaviest drinking day in last week (observed and age standardised), by equivalised household income and sex

Aged 16 and over drinking alcohol in past 7 days   *1998*

Alcohol consumption (units per day)	Equivalised annual household income quintile				
	Up to £7,186	Over £7,186 to £10,834	Over £10,834 to £17,890	Over £17,890 to £27,705	Over £27,705
	%	%	%	%	%
Men					
Observed					
Under 2 units	18	24	19	17	12
2, under 3 units	17	16	18	17	14
3, under 4 units	4	5	7	8	10
4, under 5 units	14	13	13	11	11
5, under 6 units	3	3	3	3	5
6, under 8 units	12	11	10	10	12
8 or more units	32	28	31	35	36
Standardised					
Under 2 units	16	19	18	18	14
2, under 3 units	15	14	17	17	15
3, under 4 units	4	5	7	8	10
4, under 5 units	14	13	12	10	10
5, under 6 units	3	3	3	3	5
6, under 8 units	12	11	10	9	11
8 or more units	36	34	33	34	35
Women					
Observed					
Under 2 units	30	41	33	28	23
2, under 3 units	21	24	21	24	23
3, under 4 units	10	8	11	14	16
4, under 5 units	11	9	10	9	10
5, under 6 units	5	5	5	5	7
6, under 8 units	9	9	9	9	10
8 or more units	14	5	10	10	11
Standardised					
Under 2 units	31	35	36	33	29
2, under 3 units	21	23	21	23	24
3, under 4 units	10	8	11	14	14
4, under 5 units	11	11	10	9	11
5, under 6 units	5	5	5	5	5
6, under 8 units	9	11	9	8	8
8 or more units	13	6	10	9	9
Bases					
Men	*598*	*639*	*1070*	*1127*	*1169*
Women	*672*	*702*	*989*	*1017*	*1081*

Table 3.11

Estimated alcohol consumption on heaviest drinking day in last week (observed and age standardised), by Health Authority area type and sex

Aged 16 and over drinking alcohol in past 7 days   *1998*

Alcohol consumption (units per day)	Health Authority area type					
	Inner London	Mining & Industrial	Urban	Mature	Prosperous	Rural
	%	%	%	%	%	%
Men						
Observed						
Under 2 units	17	13	15	18	20	18
2, under 3 units	15	14	12	19	18	18
3, under 4 units	10	6	7	7	9	7
4, under 5 units	14	11	13	11	10	14
5, under 6 units	6	4	3	3	4	3
6, under 8 units	10	12	11	11	11	10
8 or more units	29	40	40	31	28	31
Standardised						
Under 2 units	19	13	15	17	20	18
2, under 3 units	18	14	12	19	17	18
3, under 4 units	9	6	6	7	8	7
4, under 5 units	14	11	12	10	10	13
5, under 6 units	8	3	3	3	4	3
6, under 8 units	10	11	11	10	11	9
8 or more units	23	42	41	33	30	32
Women						
Observed						
Under 2 units	26	27	27	35	34	33
2, under 3 units	23	23	23	22	22	24
3, under 4 units	14	10	13	12	13	12
4, under 5 units	6	12	10	9	9	10
5, under 6 units	11	5	5	5	5	4
6, under 8 units	11	11	11	9	8	8
8 or more units	9	12	10	9	9	8
Standardised						
Under 2 units	32	30	29	36	36	34
2, under 3 units	21	22	23	22	22	23
3, under 4 units	13	10	13	12	12	12
4, under 5 units	5	11	10	9	8	10
5, under 6 units	10	5	5	5	5	4
6, under 8 units	10	10	11	9	7	8
8 or more units	9	12	10	9	9	9
Bases						
Men	*143*	*829*	*746*	*807*	*1494*	*1293*
Women	*159*	*754*	*774*	*784*	*1516*	*1230*

Table 3.12

Estimated alcohol consumption on heaviest drinking day in last week (observed and age standardised), by region and sex

Aged 16 and over drinking alcohol in past 7 days   *1998*

Alcohol consumption (units per day)	Region							
	Northern & Yorkshire	North West	Trent	West Midlands	Anglia & Oxford	North Thames	South Thames	South & West
	%	%	%	%	%	%	%	%
Men								
Observed								
Under 2 units	13	15	17	17	18	21	19	19
2, under 3 units	13	12	14	18	19	21	16	19
3, under 4 units	5	7	8	5	7	8	9	9
4, under 5 units	11	11	12	16	11	9	13	12
5, under 6 units	4	3	3	3	4	4	3	4
6, under 8 units	12	10	10	11	10	12	10	11
8 or more units	41	41	36	31	31	25	30	27
Standardised								
Under 2 units	12	15	16	16	18	20	18	18
2, under 3 units	13	12	14	17	18	21	16	18
3, under 4 units	5	7	8	5	7	8	9	9
4, under 5 units	11	11	12	15	11	9	13	12
5, under 6 units	4	3	3	3	4	4	4	4
6, under 8 units	12	10	10	10	10	12	10	11
8 or more units	43	42	37	33	31	27	31	29
Women								
Observed								
Under 2 units	28	26	34	30	34	31	35	34
2, under 3 units	22	21	21	30	21	25	23	22
3, under 4 units	10	12	12	13	11	12	14	13
4, under 5 units	12	11	10	9	9	10	6	10
5, under 6 units	5	5	5	5	6	5	4	6
6, under 8 units	9	14	11	6	9	9	8	7
8 or more units	13	11	8	8	10	8	9	9
Standardised								
Under 2 units	27	26	34	29	35	32	36	34
2, under 3 units	21	21	21	30	21	24	23	21
3, under 4 units	10	12	12	13	11	12	14	13
4, under 5 units	12	11	9	9	9	9	6	10
5, under 6 units	5	5	5	5	6	5	4	6
6, under 8 units	10	14	11	6	9	9	7	7
8 or more units	14	11	8	9	9	9	9	9
Bases								
Men	*1030*	*979*	*797*	*746*	*812*	*915*	*893*	*1021*
Women	*1249*	*1135*	*941*	*913*	*961*	*1118*	*1183*	*1215*

Table 3.13

Self-reported cigarette smoking status, by age and sex

Aged 16 and over   *1998*

Self-reported cigarette smoking status	Age							Total
	16-24	25-34	35-44	45-54	55-64	65-74	75 +	
	%	%	%	%	%	%	%	%
Men								
Current cigarette smoker	41	36	31	28	23	18	9	28
Ex-regular cigarette smoker	6	13	23	35	47	54	62	31
Never regular cigarette smoker	53	50	46	37	29	28	28	40
Women								
Current cigarette smoker	38	34	30	26	25	19	10	27
Ex-regular cigarette smoker	8	14	18	24	25	33	33	21
Never regular cigarette smoker	54	53	52	50	50	48	57	52
Bases								
Men	823	1335	1304	1285	985	836	561	7129
Women	964	1629	1571	1483	1147	967	906	8667

Table 3.14

Self-reported cigarette smoking status (observed and age standardised), by social class of head of household and sex

Aged 16 and over   *1998*

Self-reported cigarette smoking status	Social class of head of household							Social class of head of household					
	I	II	IIINM	IIIM	IV	V		I	II	IIINM	IIIM	IV	V
	%	%	%	%	%	%		%	%	%	%	%	%
	Men							**Women**					
Observed													
Current cigarette smoker	14	20	27	33	36	41		15	21	28	29	35	34
Ex-regular cigarette smoker	28	34	30	32	31	25		16	23	21	21	20	25
Never regular cigarette smoker	58	45	42	35	33	34		69	56	51	50	45	41
Standardised													
Current cigarette smoker	15	22	28	34	38	42		14	21	29	28	36	37
Ex-regular cigarette smoker	25	32	30	29	29	23		18	23	20	21	20	23
Never regular cigarette smoker	60	46	43	37	34	35		68	56	51	51	44	40
Bases	499	2166	707	2246	1031	334		511	2488	1340	2200	1366	492

Table 3.15

**Self-reported cigarette smoking status (observed and age standardised),
by equivalised household income and sex**

Aged 16 and over   *1998*

Self-reported cigarette smoking status	Equivalised annual household income quintile				
	Up to £7,186	Over £7,186 to £10,834	Over £10,834 to £17,890	Over £17,890 to £27,705	Over £27,705
	%	%	%	%	%
Men					
Observed					
Current cigarette smoker	37	33	27	27	22
Ex-regular cigarette smoker	30	33	34	30	29
Never regular cigarette smoker	32	34	39	43	49
Standardised					
Current cigarette smoker	42	37	28	26	21
Ex-regular cigarette smoker	25	25	32	31	31
Never regular cigarette smoker	33	38	41	43	49
Women					
Observed					
Current cigarette smoker	37	27	28	24	21
Ex-regular cigarette smoker	20	25	21	20	21
Never regular cigarette smoker	43	48	51	56	59
Standardised					
Current cigarette smoker	37	32	28	23	18
Ex-regular cigarette smoker	20	20	21	21	24
Never regular cigarette smoker	42	48	51	56	58
Bases					
Men	*992*	*997*	*1430*	*1384*	*1353*
Women	*1403*	*1480*	*1643*	*1488*	*1382*

Table 3.16

**Self-reported cigarette smoking status (observed and age standardised),
by Health Authority area type and sex**

Aged 16 and over   *1998*

Self-reported cigarette smoking status	Health Authority area type					
	Inner London	Mining & Industrial	Urban	Mature	Prosperous	Rural
	%	%	%	%	%	%
Men						
Observed						
Current cigarette smoker	34	31	29	28	27	26
Ex-regular cigarette smoker	25	30	32	32	33	31
Never regular cigarette smoker	41	39	39	40	40	43
Standardised						
Current cigarette smoker	33	32	29	29	29	27
Ex-regular cigarette smoker	27	27	31	29	30	29
Never regular cigarette smoker	40	41	40	41	41	44
Women						
Observed						
Current cigarette smoker	31	31	30	25	25	25
Ex-regular cigarette smoker	17	19	22	21	23	22
Never regular cigarette smoker	51	50	48	54	53	53
Standardised						
Current cigarette smoker	31	31	30	26	25	26
Ex-regular cigarette smoker	20	18	22	20	23	22
Never regular cigarette smoker	49	51	48	54	53	53
Bases						
Men	*236*	*1098*	*1041*	*1092*	*1932*	*1730*
Women	*306*	*1288*	*1332*	*1299*	*2378*	*2064*

Table 3.17

Self-reported cigarette smoking status (observed and age standardised), by region and sex

Aged 16 and over   *1998*

Self-reported cigarette smoking status	Region							
	Northern & Yorkshire	North West	Trent	West Midlands	Anglia & Oxford	North Thames	South Thames	South & West
	%	%	%	%	%	%	%	%
Men								
Observed								
Current cigarette smoker	28	30	31	26	29	29	28	26
Ex-regular cigarette smoker	30	31	31	31	31	30	34	34
Never regular cigarette smoker	42	40	38	43	40	41	38	40
Standardised								
Current cigarette smoker	29	30	32	27	29	30	29	28
Ex-regular cigarette smoker	28	29	28	28	30	28	32	31
Never regular cigarette smoker	43	41	40	45	41	42	39	41
Women								
Observed								
Current cigarette smoker	31	29	27	27	26	23	27	25
Ex-regular cigarette smoker	21	18	24	19	22	23	21	22
Never regular cigarette smoker	48	53	48	54	52	54	52	52
Standardised								
Current cigarette smoker	32	28	28	27	25	23	26	26
Ex-regular cigarette smoker	20	18	24	19	23	23	21	21
Never regular cigarette smoker	48	53	49	54	52	54	52	52
Bases								
Men	*1023*	*969*	*792*	*734*	*808*	*911*	*881*	*1011*
Women	*1245*	*1130*	*938*	*909*	*956*	*1114*	*1169*	*1206*

Table 3.18

Self-reported cigarette smoking status, by survey year, age and sex

Aged 16 and over   *1994-98*

Self-reported cigarette smoking status	Age							Total
	16-24	25-34	35-44	45-54	55-64	65-74	75 +	
	%	%	%	%	%	%	%	%

Men

Current cigarette smoker

1994	35	36	31	30	22	21	12	28
1995	36	39	31	30	24	18	11	29
1996	38	39	34	30	23	19	14	30
1997	36	39	31	27	25	20	12	29
1998	41	36	31	28	23	18	9	28

Ex-regular cigarette smoker

1994	8	17	29	41	48	60	65	34
1995	7	13	23	37	44	61	58	31
1996	5	13	22	35	43	53	63	30
1997	5	11	22	36	46	55	69	31
1998	6	13	23	35	47	54	62	31

Never regular cigarette smoker

1994	58	47	40	29	30	20	23	37
1995	57	48	45	34	32	22	30	40
1996	57	48	44	34	34	28	23	40
1997	58	49	46	37	29	25	20	40
1998	53	50	46	37	29	28	28	40

Women

Current cigarette smoker

1994	34	33	28	29	24	19	11	27
1995	37	32	27	30	24	19	10	27
1996	35	34	30	29	24	20	10	27
1997	38	33	28	27	23	18	11	27
1998	38	34	30	26	25	19	10	27

Ex-regular cigarette smoker

1994	9	14	20	25	25	36	31	22
1995	8	14	20	24	25	33	28	21
1996	8	14	18	25	25	33	32	21
1997	9	14	18	24	27	34	29	21
1998	8	14	18	24	25	33	33	21

Never regular cigarette smoker

1994	57	53	51	46	51	45	58	51
1995	56	54	52	46	50	48	62	52
1996	57	52	53	47	51	48	57	52
1997	53	53	53	48	50	48	60	52
1998	54	53	52	50	50	48	57	52

Bases

Men

1994	*955*	*1433*	*1329*	*1126*	*1000*	*876*	*440*	*7159*
1995	*918*	*1395*	*1386*	*1183*	*1000*	*920*	*519*	*7321*
1996	*938*	*1363*	*1410*	*1323*	*996*	*895*	*554*	*7479*
1997	*464*	*739*	*739*	*694*	*535*	*455*	*243*	*3869*
1998	*823*	*1335*	*1304*	*1285*	*985*	*836*	*561*	*7129*

Women

1994	*1071*	*1723*	*1520*	*1295*	*1056*	*1119*	*825*	*8609*
1995	*1074*	*1737*	*1502*	*1378*	*1120*	*1059*	*836*	*8706*
1996	*1101*	*1675*	*1603*	*1492*	*1087*	*1100*	*881*	*8939*
1997	*538*	*916*	*832*	*806*	*585*	*545*	*438*	*4660*
1998	*964*	*1629*	*1571*	*1483*	*1147*	*967*	*906*	*8667*

Table 3.19

Estimated odds ratios for prevalence of cigarette smoking

Aged 16 and over *1998*

Independent variables	Men			Women		
	N	Odds ratio[a]	95% CI	N	Odds ratio[a]	95% CI
Age		p=0.0000			p=0.0000	
16-24	678	2.07	1.77 - 2.41	790	2.14	1.85 - 2.47
25-34	1148	2.08	1.82 - 2.37	1444	1.95	1.73 - 2.20
35-44	1174	1.59	1.40 - 1.82	1387	1.56	1.38 - 1.76
45-54	1105	1.27	1.11 - 1.46	1261	1.21	1.07 - 1.38
55-64	829	0.88	0.75 - 1.03	926	0.97	0.84 - 1.12
65-74	696	0.56	0.46 - 0.67	761	0.55	0.47 - 0.66
75 and over	444	0.23	0.18 - 0.31	645	0.24	0.19 - 0.30
Social class of head of household		p=0.0000			p=0.0000	
I	433	0.60	0.47 - 0.78	441	0.60	0.47 - 0.76
II	1868	0.78	0.68 - 0.89	2127	0.90	0.80 - 1.02
IINM	614	0.93	0.79 - 1.10	1153	1.13	0.99 - 1.29
IIM	1962	1.20	1.07 - 1.34	1891	0.98	0.88 - 1.10
IV	889	1.30	1.13 - 1.50	1168	1.28	1.13 - 1.45
V	308	1.46	1.18 - 1.81	434	1.30	1.08 - 1.57
Equivalised household income quintile		p=0.0000			p=0.0000	
Bottom quintile	957	1.25	1.09 - 1.42	1322	1.27	1.14 - 1.43
Second quintile	982	1.28	1.12 - 1.46	1419	1.14	1.02 - 1.28
Middle quintile	1418	0.88	0.78 - 0.98	1629	1.01	0.91 - 1.12
Fourth quintile	1371	0.91	0.81 - 1.02	1470	0.85	0.76 - 0.95
Top quintile	1346	0.79	0.69 - 0.90	1374	0.80	0.70 - 0.92
Health Authority area type		p=0.0838			p=0.2417	
Inner London	177	1.32	1.00 - 1.74	254	1.09	0.86 - 1.39
Mining & Industrial	961	0.98	0.86 - 1.13	1099	1.06	0.93 - 1.20
Urban Centres	898	0.88	0.76 - 1.02	1112	1.05	0.92 - 1.19
Mature	888	0.99	0.85 - 1.14	1022	0.97	0.85 - 1.11
Prospering	1653	1.03	0.91 - 1.16	1999	0.97	0.87 - 1.08
Rural	1497	0.86	0.76 - 0.97	1728	0.88	0.78 - 0.98
Level of educational qualification		p=0.0000			p=0.0000	
Degree/NVQ 4,5	950	0.67	0.57 - 0.78	796	0.60	0.51 - 0.70
A level/NVQ 3	1481	1.00	0.90 - 1.11	1336	0.89	0.79 - 1.00
O level/NVQ 1,2	1960	1.01	0.91 - 1.11	2614	1.14	1.04 - 1.25
No qualifications	1683	1.49	1.32 - 1.68	2468	1.64	1.47 - 1.84

[a] Odds ratios are relative to average, not to a designated reference category.

Table 3.20

Saliva cotinine levels, by age and sex

Aged 16 and over with a valid saliva cotinine measurement   *1998*

Saliva cotinine levels (ng/ml)	Age							Total
	16-24	25-34	35-44	45-54	55-64	65-74	75+	
Men								
75th percentile	190	182	185	191	151	6	2	149
90th percentile	316	367	423	435	412	353	130	379
95th percentile	382	443	521	521	506	457	253	474
Mean	101	104	110	110	102	76	35	97
Standard error of the mean	5.9	5.5	6.0	6.1	7.2	6.6	5.7	2.4
% 15 ng/ml and over	46	37	34	33	30	23	16	32
Women								
75th percentile	103	117	128	11	4	2	1	47
90th percentile	246	330	381	323	329	240	42	309
95th percentile	323	425	469	447	434	369	231	416
Mean	70	86	93	74	70	51	24	72
Standard error of the mean	4.8	4.7	5.2	4.8	5.4	5.2	3.7	2.0
% 15 ng/ml and over	38	34	31	24	23	18	11	27
Bases								
Men	*577*	*952*	*957*	*947*	*672*	*585*	*364*	*5054*
Women	*635*	*1049*	*1059*	*994*	*716*	*565*	*460*	*5478*

Table 3.21

Estimated odds ratios for prevalence of saliva cotinine 15 ng/ml or over

Aged 16 and over with valid saliva cotinine measurement   *1998*

Independent variables	Men			Women		
	N	Odds ratio[a]	95% CI	N	Odds ratio[a]	95% CI
Age		p=0.0000			p=0.0000	
16-24	472	1.99	1.67 - 2.39	513	2.24	1.87 - 2.69
25-34	830	1.62	1.39 - 1.89	939	1.98	1.70 - 2.31
35-44	864	1.45	1.25 - 1.68	950	1.63	1.40 - 1.89
45-54	827	1.18	1.01 - 1.37	863	1.11	0.95 - 1.30
55-64	581	0.93	0.78 - 1.10	602	0.89	0.74 - 1.07
65-74	498	0.60	0.49 - 0.73	459	0.52	0.41 - 0.65
75 and over	300	0.33	0.24 - 0.43	343	0.27	0.20 - 0.37
Social class of head of household		p=0.0000			p=0.0002	
I	308	0.55	0.41 - 0.73	301	0.69	0.52 - 0.91
II	1408	0.90	0.78 - 1.03	1400	0.82	0.71 - 0.95
IINM	418	0.90	0.74 - 1.10	759	1.01	0.86 - 1.18
IIM	1388	1.34	1.18 - 1.53	1225	0.99	0.87 - 1.13
IV	629	1.23	1.04 - 1.45	719	1.33	1.14 - 1.56
V	221	1.37	1.07 - 1.75	265	1.33	1.05 - 1.68
Equivalised household income quintile		p=0.0088			p=0.0018	
Bottom quintile	630	1.22	1.04 - 1.42	783	1.20	1.03 - 1.38
Second quintile	675	1.17	1.01 - 1.36	856	1.22	1.05 - 1.41
Middle quintile	1021	0.88	0.77 - 1.00	1089	1.00	0.89 - 1.14
Fourth quintile	1038	0.93	0.82 - 1.06	1013	0.81	0.71 - 0.93
Top quintile	1008	0.86	0.74 - 1.00	928	0.84	0.72 - 0.99
Health Authority area type		p=0.6425			p=0.0143	
Inner London	113	1.18	0.84 - 1.66	167	1.09	0.81 - 1.47
Mining & Industrial	698	1.05	0.90 - 1.24	705	1.12	0.96 - 1.31
Urban Centres	585	0.91	0.76 - 1.08	642	1.13	0.96 - 1.33
Mature	613	0.94	0.79 - 1.11	628	0.92	0.77 - 1.09
Prospering	1259	1.01	0.89 - 1.16	1378	0.98	0.86 - 1.12
Rural	1104	0.93	0.81 - 1.07	1149	0.80	0.69 - 0.92
Level of educational qualification		p=0.0000			p=0.0000	
Degree/NVQ 4,5	703	0.68	0.57 - 0.80	542	0.55	0.45 - 0.67
A level/NVQ 3	1088	0.91	0.81 - 1.03	904	0.92	0.80 - 1.06
O level/NVQ 1,2	1438	1.08	0.97 - 1.21	1781	1.18	1.05 - 1.32
No qualifications	1143	1.49	1.30 - 1.71	1442	1.69	1.46 - 1.95

[a] Odds ratios are relative to average, not to a designated reference category.

Table 3.22

Number of cigarettes smoked per smoker, by age and sex

Aged 16 and over currently smoking cigarettes   *1998*

Cigarettes smoked per day	Age							Total
	16-24	25-34	35-44	45-54	55-64	65-74	75 +	
	%	%	%	%	%	%	%	%
Men								
Under 10 cigarettes	34	30	17	19	18	22	48	25
10 to under 20 cigarettes	44	41	39	30	37	44	29	39
20 and over	23	29	44	50	45	34	23	37
Mean	12.7	13.9	17.3	18.2	18.2	14.8	12.2	15.7
Standard error of the mean	0.42	0.40	0.50	0.58	0.75	0.70	1.65	0.22
Women								
Under 10 cigarettes	43	31	25	18	25	32	46	30
10 to under 20 cigarettes	40	41	40	42	43	46	34	41
20 and over	16	28	35	39	32	22	21	29
Mean	11.0	13.1	14.9	16.0	14.3	12.3	11.1	13.6
Standard error of the mean	0.37	0.33	0.40	0.44	0.50	0.50	0.83	0.17
Bases								
Men	*332*	*484*	*400*	*361*	*231*	*148*	*52*	*2008*
Women	*361*	*546*	*467*	*390*	*289*	*183*	*92*	*2328*

Table 3.23

Number of cigarettes smoked per smoker (observed and age standardised), by social class of head of household and sex

Aged 16 and over currently smoking cigarettes   *1998*

Cigarettes smoked per day	Social class of head of household			
	I & II	IIINM	IIIM	IV & V
	%	%	%	%
Men				
Observed				
Under 10 cigarettes	32	28	20	22
10 to under 20 cigarettes	37	38	40	39
20 and over	31	34	40	39
Mean	14.3	15.1	16.4	16.1
Standard error of the mean	0.45	0.70	0.34	0.46
Standardised				
Under 10 cigarettes	33	29	21	22
10 to under 20 cigarettes	35	36	41	38
20 and over	32	35	38	40
Mean	14.5	15.2	16.1	16.2
Standard error of the mean	0.46	0.73	0.34	0.47
Women				
Observed				
Under 10 cigarettes	36	29	27	26
10 to under 20 cigarettes	38	45	43	42
20 and over	26	27	31	32
Mean	12.5	13.8	14.0	14.2
Standard error of the mean	0.34	0.42	0.32	0.32
Standardised				
Under 10 cigarettes	36	30	27	27
10 to under 20 cigarettes	38	43	41	42
20 and over	26	26	32	31
Mean	12.5	13.6	13.8	14.0
Standard error of the mean	0.34	0.42	0.32	0.32
Bases				
Men	*514*	*193*	*729*	*509*
Women	*601*	*373*	*639*	*640*

Table 3.24

Number of cigarettes smoked per smoker (observed and age standardised), by equivalised household income and sex

Aged 16 and over currently smoking cigarettes   *1998*

Cigarettes smoked per day	Equivalised annual household income quintile				
	Up to £7,186	Over £7,186 to £10,834	Over £10,834 to £17,890	Over £17,890 to £27,705	Over £27,705
	%	%	%	%	%
Men					
Observed					
Under 10 cigarettes	21	18	24	22	33
10 to under 20 cigarettes	39	42	39	37	36
20 and over	39	39	36	40	31
Mean	16.4	16.6	15.3	16.4	14.1
Standard error of the mean	0.54	0.58	0.48	0.49	0.58
Standardised					
Under 10 cigarettes	22	18	28	23	35
10 to under 20 cigarettes	38	42	39	36	32
20 and over	40	40	33	41	33
Mean	16.5	16.8	14.5	16.5	14.3
Standard error of the mean	0.55	0.60	0.48	0.51	0.62
Women					
Observed					
Under 10 cigarettes	25	24	28	36	38
10 to under 20 cigarettes	39	44	44	41	41
20 and over	36	32	28	23	21
Mean	14.7	14.3	13.7	12.3	11.9
Standard error of the mean	0.37	0.41	0.36	0.42	0.46
Standardised					
Under 10 cigarettes	29	25	27	37	41
10 to under 20 cigarettes	36	43	45	41	37
20 and over	35	32	28	21	22
Mean	14.2	14.3	13.7	12.2	11.6
Standard error of the mean	0.37	0.42	0.35	0.42	0.46
Bases					
Men	*368*	*328*	*384*	*373*	*291*
Women	*519*	*396*	*466*	*356*	*285*

Table 3.25

Number of cigarettes smoked per smoker (observed and age standardised), by Health Authority area type and sex

Aged 16 and over currently smoking cigarettes   *1998*

Cigarettes smoked per day	Health Authority area type					
	Inner London	Mining & Industrial	Urban	Mature	Prosperous	Rural
	%	%	%	%	%	%
Men						
Observed						
Under 10 cigarettes	42	15	24	26	29	23
10 to under 20 cigarettes	35	43	36	38	39	37
20 and over	23	41	40	36	32	40
Mean	11.9	16.9	16.0	15.5	14.8	16.3
Standard error of the mean	1.00	0.52	0.56	0.57	0.43	0.49
Standardised						
Under 10 cigarettes	36	16	25	26	29	24
10 to under 20 cigarettes	33	44	36	37	39	37
20 and over	31	40	40	37	32	38
Mean	13.7	16.6	15.9	15.9	14.7	16.0
Standard error of the mean	1.08	0.51	0.56	0.64	0.43	0.48
Women						
Observed						
Under 10 cigarettes	36	22	27	36	30	31
10 to under 20 cigarettes	39	44	39	36	44	42
20 and over	25	34	34	28	26	27
Mean	13.1	14.8	14.5	13.1	13.0	13.2
Standard error of the mean	0.86	0.42	0.43	0.48	0.32	0.34
Standardised						
Under 10 cigarettes	33	24	29	36	31	32
10 to under 20 cigarettes	43	43	37	36	44	42
20 and over	24	33	33	28	25	26
Mean	13.3	14.5	14.3	13.1	12.7	13.0
Standard error of the mean	0.83	0.42	0.43	0.47	0.32	0.34
Bases						
Men	*81*	*344*	*298*	*308*	*527*	*450*
Women	*96*	*400*	*397*	*330*	*583*	*522*

Table 3.26

Number of cigarettes smoked per smoker (observed and age standardised), by region and sex

Aged 16 and over currently smoking cigarettes   1998

Cigarettes smoked per day	Region							
	Northern & Yorkshire	North West	Trent	West Midlands	Anglia & Oxford	North Thames	South Thames	South & West
	%	%	%	%	%	%	%	%
Men								
Observed								
Under 10 cigarettes	18	18	23	24	24	29	31	31
10 to under 20 cigarettes	41	40	39	35	41	40	41	33
20 and over	41	42	39	41	35	31	28	37
Mean	16.8	16.8	16.2	16.0	15.3	14.9	13.8	15.2
Standard error of the mean	0.58	0.57	0.66	0.75	0.62	0.65	0.57	0.62
Standardised								
Under 10 cigarettes	19	20	24	26	24	29	34	33
10 to under 20 cigarettes	42	38	38	35	41	39	38	31
20 and over	40	42	39	39	35	32	28	36
Mean	16.6	17.1	16.1	15.5	15.1	15.2	13.5	15.0
Standard error of the mean	0.58	0.66	0.66	0.73	0.62	0.66	0.57	0.62
Women								
Observed								
Under 10 cigarettes	26	22	33	25	30	30	37	34
10 to under 20 cigarettes	42	41	44	39	44	38	39	42
20 and over	32	37	23	36	25	32	24	24
Mean	14.1	15.5	12.7	14.6	13.2	13.9	12.5	12.4
Standard error of the mean	0.42	0.47	0.49	0.53	0.51	0.53	0.48	0.40
Standardised								
Under 10 cigarettes	28	22	34	31	29	33	36	33
10 to under 20 cigarettes	41	41	43	35	45	36	42	44
20 and over	32	37	23	34	26	31	22	23
Mean	13.9	15.6	12.5	14.0	13.2	13.4	12.5	12.3
Standard error of the mean	0.43	0.47	0.48	0.55	0.48	0.51	0.48	0.40
Bases								
Men	*285*	*287*	*244*	*188*	*232*	*262*	*248*	*262*
Women	*386*	*323*	*256*	*245*	*246*	*257*	*310*	*305*

Table 3.27

Estimated odds ratios for proportion of current smokers who smoke 20 or more cigarettes per day

Aged 16 and over currently smoking cigarettes *1998*

Independent variables	Men			Women		
	N	Odds ratio[a]	95% CI	N	Odds ratio[a]	95% CI
Age		p=0.0000			p=0.0000	
16-24	264	0.54	0.40 - 0.72	295	0.59	0.43 - 0.79
25-34	415	0.96	0.76 - 1.22	485	1.14	0.90 - 1.43
35-44	362	1.51	1.20 - 1.89	410	1.64	1.31 - 2.05
45-54	296	2.06	1.61 - 2.63	332	1.76	1.39 - 2.23
55-64	197	1.38	1.05 - 1.83	238	1.21	0.93 - 1.59
65-74	126	0.85	0.60 - 1.20	145	0.64	0.45 - 0.93
75 and over	43	0.53	0.29 - 0.98	66	0.67	0.40 - 1.12
Social class of head of household		p=0.6895			p=0.9070	
I	61	0.74	0.44 - 1.24	65	1.03	0.61 - 1.75
II	376	0.97	0.77 - 1.24	460	1.00	0.79 - 1.26
IINM	168	0.94	0.69 - 1.28	328	1.01	0.79 - 1.30
IIM	648	1.14	0.93 - 1.39	556	0.98	0.80 - 1.21
IV	322	1.14	0.89 - 1.45	408	0.88	0.70 - 1.11
V	128	1.14	0.81 - 1.62	154	1.11	0.80 - 1.53
Equivalised household income quintile		p=0.0967			p=0.0021	
Bottom quintile	343	1.04	0.84 - 1.29	484	1.41	1.16 - 1.73
Second quintile	321	1.03	0.83 - 1.28	388	1.23	1.00 - 1.52
Middle quintile	384	0.87	0.71 - 1.06	464	1.01	0.83 - 1.23
Fourth quintile	368	1.27	1.03 - 1.55	354	0.77	0.61 - 0.96
Top quintile	287	0.85	0.66 - 1.08	281	0.74	0.56 - 0.97
Health Authority area type		p=0.2509			p=0.5151	
Inner London	65	0.63	0.39 - 1.03	81	0.92	0.59 - 1.42
Mining & Industrial	300	1.07	0.84 - 1.36	337	1.11	0.88 - 1.40
Urban Centres	254	1.14	0.89 - 1.46	337	1.18	0.94 - 1.48
Mature	241	1.18	0.91 - 1.53	267	1.00	0.77 - 1.29
Prosperous	446	0.93	0.75 - 1.15	504	0.90	0.73 - 1.11
Rural	397	1.18	0.95 - 1.46	445	0.93	0.75 - 1.15
Level of educational qualification		p=0.0154			p=0.0410	
Degree/NVQ 4,5	158	0.87	0.65 - 1.17	127	0.75	0.52 - 1.09
A level/NVQ 3	410	0.88	0.72 - 1.07	323	0.87	0.68 - 1.11
O level/NVQ 1,2	583	0.96	0.80 - 1.14	786	1.14	0.95 - 1.38
No qualifications	552	1.37	1.12 - 1.67	735	1.34	1.08 - 1.65

[a] Odds ratios are relative to average, not to a designated reference category.

Table 3.28

Estimated odds ratios for the proportion of current cigarette smokers who have saliva cotinine levels at or above the 75th percentile[b]

Aged 16 and over currently smoking cigarettes   *1998*

Independent variables	Men			Women		
	N	Odds ratio[a]	95% CI	N	Odds ratio[a]	95% CI
Age		p=0.0000			p=0.0000	
16-24	177	0.43	0.27 - 0.68	198	0.37	0.24 - 0.58
25-34	291	0.72	0.52 - 0.98	311	0.89	0.67 - 1.19
35-44	248	1.53	1.15 - 2.02	284	1.58	1.21 - 2.06
45-54	213	1.63	1.22 - 2.18	208	1.33	0.99 - 1.81
55 and over	242	1.32	0.98 - 1.77	254	1.42	1.05 - 1.92
Social class of head of household		p=0.9317			p=0.5819	
I	39	0.79	0.33 - 1.86	48	0.86	0.40 - 1.85
II	274	1.05	0.73 - 1.50	283	0.84	0.60 - 1.20
IINM	102	1.27	0.78 - 2.06	207	1.08	0.77 - 1.53
IIM	441	1.05	0.78 - 1.40	358	1.06	0.79 - 1.42
IV	221	0.92	0.64 - 1.33	262	1.30	0.94 - 1.79
V	94	0.99	0.61 - 1.59	97	0.92	0.58 - 1.47
Equivalised household income quintile		p=0.2685			p=0.2500	
Bottom quintile	224	1.12	0.82 - 1.52	283	1.28	0.96 - 1.72
Second quintile	195	1.33	0.99 - 1.80	233	0.86	0.64 - 1.15
Middle quintile	278	0.91	0.69 - 1.20	314	0.83	0.64 - 1.09
Fourth quintile	268	0.80	0.59 - 1.07	239	1.03	0.75 - 1.41
Top quintile	206	0.93	0.65 - 1.32	186	1.06	0.72 - 1.56
Health Authority area type		p=0.7244			p=0.3560	
Inner London	39	0.69	0.29 - 1.61	55	1.34	0.75 - 2.39
Mining & Industrial	213	0.92	0.65 - 1.31	218	0.98	0.72 - 1.35
Urban Centres	151	1.02	0.68 - 1.51	199	0.71	0.51 - 1.00
Mature	158	1.16	0.79 - 1.72	158	0.89	0.60 - 1.31
Prosperous	328	1.06	0.77 - 1.46	343	1.16	0.88 - 1.53
Rural	282	1.26	0.91 - 1.73	282	1.03	0.77 - 1.39
Level of educational qualification		p=0.2651			p=0.0136	
Degree/NVQ 4,5	115	0.77	0.49 - 1.22	88	0.55	0.29 - 1.01
A level/NVQ 3	283	0.91	0.67 - 1.24	212	0.86	0.59 - 1.25
O level/NVQ 1,2	419	1.07	0.82 - 1.38	522	1.56	1.17 - 2.08
No qualifications	354	1.33	1.00 - 1.78	433	1.36	0.99 - 1.88
Number of cigarettes smoked per day		p=0.0000			p=0.0000	
Less than 10	277	0.31	0.21 - 0.45	371	0.31	0.24 - 0.42
10 up to less than 20	445	1.25	0.98 - 1.60	532	1.20	0.98 - 1.47
20 or more	449	2.59	2.04 - 3.29	352	2.66	2.15 - 3.28
Type of cigarettes smoked		p=0.0201			p=0.0069	
Roll-ups	294	1.48	1.13 - 1.92	77	1.24	0.81 - 1.89
10+ mg/cigarette tar	550	0.91	0.72 - 1.16	570	1.34	1.05 - 1.70
<10 mg/cigarette tar	233	0.79	0.57 - 1.10	477	0.79	0.61 - 1.03
Unknown[c]	94	0.94	0.62 - 1.42	131	0.76	0.52 - 1.11

[a] Odds ratios are relative to average, not to a designated reference category.

[b] 75th percentile saliva cotinine levels for cigarette smokers were 431.5 ng/ml for men and 369.0 ng/ml for women.

[c] Unknown includes cigarettes where the informant did not know the brand name, where there was not enough information given to determine the brand of cigarette, imported brands, or where the brand was not analysed by the Laboratory of Government Chemists.

Table 3.29

Type of cigarette smoked, by age and sex

Aged 16 and over currently smoking cigarettes   *1998*

Type of cigarette smoked	Age					Total
	16-24	25-34	35-44	45-54	55+	
	%	%	%	%	%	%
Men						
Roll-ups	15	23	28	31	31	26
Branded cigarette						
Tar yield 10 mg/cigarette or more	54	46	48	44	41	46
Tar yield under 10 mg/cigarette	22	25	18	18	16	20
Unknown[a]	9	7	6	7	12	8
Women						
Roll-ups	5	8	7	8	5	7
Branded cigarette						
Tar yield 10 mg/cigarette or more	52	48	50	42	33	44
Tar yield under 10 mg/cigarette	30	36	32	36	48	37
Unknown[a]	13	9	10	14	13	12
Bases						
Men	*345*	*484*	*400*	*362*	*432*	*2023*
Women	*372*	*546*	*467*	*389*	*564*	*2338*

[a] Unknown includes cigarettes where the informant did not know the brand name, where there
was not enough information given to determine the brand of cigarette, imported brands,
or where the brand was not analysed by the Laboratory of Government Chemists.

HSE '98 / 3 RISK FACTORS FOR CADIOVASCULAR DISEASE

Table 3.30

Type of cigarette smoked (observed and age standardised), by social class of head of household and sex

Aged 16 and over currently smoking cigarettes   *1998*

Type of cigarette smoked	Social class of head of household			
	I & II	IIINM	IIIM	IV & V
	%	%	%	%
Men				
Observed				
Roll-ups	16	15	30	34
Branded cigarette				
Tar yield 10 mg/cigarette or more	44	52	47	46
Tar yield under 10 mg/cigarette	33	24	14	12
Unknown[a]	7	9	8	8
Standardised				
Roll-ups	16	15	30	35
Branded cigarette				
Tar yield 10 mg/cigarette or more	45	51	48	45
Tar yield under 10 mg/cigarette	32	25	14	12
Unknown[a]	8	9	9	8
Women				
Observed				
Roll-ups	4	7	8	8
Branded cigarette				
Tar yield 10 mg/cigarette or more	34	43	49	50
Tar yield under 10 mg/cigarette	50	38	33	28
Unknown[a]	11	12	11	14
Standardised				
Roll-ups	3	7	8	8
Branded cigarette				
Tar yield 10 mg/cigarette or more	33	42	48	48
Tar yield under 10 mg/cigarette	53	39	33	30
Unknown[a]	11	13	11	14
Bases				
Men	*516*	*196*	*733*	*513*
Women	*604*	*373*	*641*	*643*

[a] Unknown includes cigarettes where the informant did not know the brand name, where there was not enough information given to determine the brand of cigarette, imported brands, or where the brand was not analysed by the Laboratory of Government Chemists.

Table 3.31

Type of cigarette smoked (observed and age standardised), by equivalised household income and sex

Aged 16 and over currently smoking cigarettes   *1998*

Type of cigarette smoked	Equivalised annual household income quintile				
	Up to £7,186	Over £7,186 to £10,834	Over £10,834 to £17,890	Over £17,890 to £27,705	Over £27,705
	%	%	%	%	%
Men					
Observed					
Roll-ups	32	32	28	22	13
Branded cigarette					
Tar yield 10 mg/cigarette or more	43	47	48	51	41
Tar yield under 10 mg/cigarette	14	14	17	20	38
Unknown[a]	11	7	6	8	7
Standardised					
Roll-ups	34	31	28	21	12
Branded cigarette					
Tar yield 10 mg/cigarette or more	42	48	50	50	44
Tar yield under 10 mg/cigarette	13	14	16	21	38
Unknown[a]	10	7	6	8	7
Women					
Observed					
Roll-ups	10	9	8	2	4
Branded cigarette					
Tar yield 10 mg/cigarette or more	55	47	47	42	28
Tar yield under 10 mg/cigarette	24	33	35	44	57
Unknown[a]	11	12	9	11	12
Standardised					
Roll-ups	9	9	8	2	3
Branded cigarette					
Tar yield 10 mg/cigarette or more	51	47	46	37	28
Tar yield under 10 mg/cigarette	28	32	37	49	60
Unknown[a]	12	12	9	12	9
Bases					
Men	*372*	*332*	*386*	*375*	*292*
Women	*519*	*400*	*468*	*358*	*285*

[a] Unknown includes cigarettes where the informant did not know the brand name, where there was not enough information given to determine the brand of cigarette, imported brands, or where the brand was not analysed by the Laboratory of Government Chemists.

Table 3.32

Type of cigarette smoked (observed and age standardised), by Health Authority area type and sex

Aged 16 and over currently smoking cigarettes   *1998*

Type of cigarette smoked	Health Authority area type					
	Inner London	Mining & Industrial	Urban	Mature	Prosperous	Rural
	%	%	%	%	%	%
Men						
Observed						
Roll-ups	16	28	25	24	24	29
Branded cigarette						
Tar yield 10 mg/cigarette or more	46	54	49	44	45	42
Tar yield under 10 mg/cigarette	31	12	21	25	23	17
Unknown[a]	7	6	6	7	8	12
Standardised						
Roll-ups	24	27	24	26	26	31
Branded cigarette						
Tar yield 10 mg/cigarette or more	43	54	50	43	45	41
Tar yield under 10 mg/cigarette	24	12	21	24	21	16
Unknown[a]	10	6	6	8	7	12
Women						
Observed						
Roll-ups	3	6	6	8	6	9
Branded cigarette						
Tar yield 10 mg/cigarette or more	48	48	52	38	40	44
Tar yield under 10 mg/cigarette	41	36	33	41	43	33
Unknown[a]	8	10	9	14	11	14
Standardised						
Roll-ups	5	5	5	8	6	8
Branded cigarette						
Tar yield 10 mg/cigarette or more	47	47	51	38	39	42
Tar yield under 10 mg/cigarette	39	37	33	40	44	37
Unknown[a]	9	11	10	14	11	13
Bases						
Men	*81*	*345*	*298*	*311*	*532*	*456*
Women	*96*	*401*	*399*	*333*	*586*	*523*

[a] Unknown includes cigarettes where the informant did not know the brand name, where there was not enough information given to determine the brand of cigarette, imported brands, or where the brand was not analysed by the Laboratory of Government Chemists.

Table 3.33

Type of cigarette smoked (observed and age standardised), by region and sex

Aged 16 and over currently smoking cigarettes 1998

Type of cigarette smoked	Region							
	Northern & Yorkshire	North West	Trent	West Midlands	Anglia & Oxford	North Thames	South Thames	South & West
	%	%	%	%	%	%	%	%
Men								
Observed								
Roll-ups	26	25	27	27	28	27	22	27
Branded cigarette								
Tar yield 10 mg/cigarette or more	53	49	44	46	46	45	42	43
Tar yield under 10 mg/cigarette	15	20	18	16	20	23	24	23
Unknown[a]	6	7	11	11	6	5	13	8
Standardised								
Roll-ups	25	25	26	27	30	28	22	27
Branded cigarette								
Tar yield 10 mg/cigarette or more	54	47	45	47	45	45	44	44
Tar yield under 10 mg/cigarette	16	20	18	15	20	22	22	22
Unknown[a]	6	7	11	11	5	5	12	7
Women								
Observed								
Roll-ups	7	3	8	4	9	5	6	10
Branded cigarette								
Tar yield 10 mg/cigarette or more	48	43	49	52	42	43	39	40
Tar yield under 10 mg/cigarette	34	45	29	34	35	44	40	36
Unknown[a]	10	9	14	9	14	8	15	15
Standardised								
Roll-ups	7	4	8	4	7	5	7	8
Branded cigarette								
Tar yield 10 mg/cigarette or more	46	41	50	52	42	42	37	38
Tar yield under 10 mg/cigarette	36	46	30	35	34	45	41	38
Unknown[a]	12	9	13	9	17	8	16	16
Bases								
Men	*286*	*288*	*244*	*190*	*236*	*262*	*251*	*266*
Women	*387*	*325*	*256*	*246*	*246*	*259*	*311*	*308*

[a] Unknown includes cigarettes where the informant did not know the brand name, where there was not enough information given to determine the brand of cigarette, imported brands, or where the brand was not analysed by the Laboratory of Government Chemists.

Table 3.34

Fat and fibre, by age and sex

Aged 16 and over with valid scores   *1998*

Fat/fibre consumption	Age							Total
	16-24	25-34	35-44	45-54	55-64	65-74	75 +	
	%	%	%	%	%	%	%	%
Men								
Fat consumption								
Low (under 30)	27	41	44	44	46	39	34	40
Medium (30-40)	35	35	33	32	32	34	38	34
High (over 40)	38	24	24	23	22	27	28	26
Mean fat score	38.7	33.7	33.1	32.9	32.3	34.2	34.9	34.0
Standard error of the mean	0.51	0.37	0.38	0.38	0.42	0.47	0.51	0.16
Fibre consumption								
Low (under 30)	65	58	58	52	48	42	39	53
Medium (30-40)	29	29	29	31	35	35	37	31
High (over 40)	7	13	13	17	17	23	24	16
Mean fibre score	26.3	28.3	28.4	30.2	30.7	32.8	32.8	29.6
Standard error of the mean	0.34	0.32	0.32	0.33	0.35	0.40	0.49	0.14
Women								
Fat consumption								
Low (under 30)	55	64	62	68	65	54	48	61
Medium (30-40)	29	26	28	24	26	33	34	28
High (over 40)	16	9	10	8	9	14	18	11
Mean fat score	29.9	27.1	27.9	26.9	26.9	29.5	31.8	28.3
Standard error of the mean	0.39	0.26	0.28	0.42	0.31	0.36	0.58	0.14
Fibre consumption								
Low (under 30)	72	71	64	57	52	44	49	60
Medium (30-40)	22	22	25	31	31	37	33	28
High (over 40)	6	7	11	12	17	19	18	12
Mean fibre score	24.6	25.4	26.8	28.3	30.0	31.7	30.8	27.9
Standard error of the mean	0.33	0.26	0.28	0.29	0.34	0.37	0.38	0.12
Bases								
Men								
Fat	*766*	*1168*	*1159*	*1151*	*881*	*764*	*515*	*6404*
Fibre	*725*	*1097*	*1056*	*1072*	*821*	*706*	*472*	*5949*
Women								
Fat	*880*	*1433*	*1352*	*1259*	*994*	*879*	*829*	*7626*
Fibre	*846*	*1370*	*1303*	*1225*	*961*	*812*	*768*	*7285*

Table 3.35

Adds salt to food at the table, by age and sex

Aged 16 and over   1998

Adds salt at the table	Age							Total
	16-24	25-34	35-44	45-54	55-64	65-74	75 +	
	%	%	%	%	%	%	%	%
Men								
Adds salt without tasting food	34	31	36	34	36	36	39	35
Tastes the food, then generally adds salt	10	9	9	11	10	12	9	10
Tastes the food, only occasionally adds salt	17	17	16	16	15	16	18	16
Rarely, or never, adds salt at the table	39	43	39	39	39	36	34	39
Women								
Adds salt without tasting food	26	26	27	23	22	20	22	24
Tastes the food, then generally adds salt	8	9	10	10	12	12	12	10
Tastes the food, only occasionally adds salt	19	16	17	18	19	19	19	18
Rarely, or never, adds salt at the table	46	49	46	49	48	49	47	48
Bases								
Men	873	1336	1304	1287	986	836	562	7184
Women	1005	1630	1570	1483	1147	967	907	8709

Table 3.36

Fat and fibre (observed and age-standardised), by social class of head of household and sex

Aged 16 and over with valid scores   1998

Fat/fibre consumption	Social class of head of household						Social class of head of household					
	I	II	IIINM	IIIM	IV	V	I	II	IIINM	IIIM	IV	V
	% %		%	%	%	%	%	%	%	%	%	%
	Men						**Women**					
Observed												
Fat consumption												
Low (under 30)	45	46	47	36	35	33	63	65	60	61	56	53
Medium (30-40)	36	33	30	34	35	30	30	27	27	28	29	30
High (over 40)	19	21	23	29	29	37	7	8	13	11	15	16
Fibre consumption												
Low (under 30)	44	49	51	56	57	58	50	54	58	63	65	65
Medium (30-40)	34	33	31	32	29	29	32	31	30	27	24	23
High (over 40)	21	18	19	12	13	13	18	14	12	10	11	12
Standardised												
Fat consumption												
Low (under 30)	45	45	47	36	35	33	60	64	61	60	57	54
Medium (30-40)	36	34	30	34	35	30	33	28	27	28	28	30
High (over 40)	19	21	23	30	29	38	7	8	12	12	15	17
Fibre consumption												
Low (under 30)	45	49	50	57	58	59	47	54	59	63	66	68
Medium (30-40)	34	33	31	31	29	29	33	31	29	27	23	21
High (over 40)	21	18	19	12	13	12	20	14	12	10	11	11
Bases												
Fat	435	1951	631	2050	924	296	441	2169	1179	1957	1217	432
Fibre	392	1809	580	1880	873	295	410	2089	1119	1832	1177	437

Table 3.37

Fat and fibre (observed and age-standardised), by equivalised household income and sex

Aged 16 and over with valid scores   *1998*

Fat/fibre consumption	Equivalised annual household income quintile				
	Up to £7,186	Over £7,186 to £10,834	Over £10,834 to £17,890	Over £17,890 to £27,705	Over £27,705
	%	%	%	%	%
Men					
Observed					
Fat consumption					
Low (under 30)	34	37	35	41	51
Medium (30-40)	33	33	34	36	31
High (over 40)	32	29	30	23	19
Fibre consumption					
Low (under 30)	58	53	51	51	52
Medium (30-40)	30	32	32	33	31
High (over 40)	12	14	17	16	17
Standardised					
Fat consumption					
Low (under 30)	34	37	35	40	50
Medium (30-40)	33	33	34	37	31
High (over 40)	33	30	31	23	19
Fibre consumption					
Low (under 30)	59	55	52	51	53
Medium (30-40)	29	31	32	33	31
High (over 40)	12	14	17	16	16
Women					
Observed					
Fat consumption					
Low (under 30)	52	57	59	65	71
Medium (30-40)	30	29	30	27	23
High (over 40)	18	14	11	8	6
Fibre consumption					
Low (under 30)	66	57	60	57	58
Medium (30-40)	24	29	28	31	29
High (over 40)	10	13	13	12	13
Standardised					
Fat consumption					
Low (under 30)	51	57	59	64	71
Medium (30-40)	31	29	30	28	23
High (over 40)	18	14	11	8	6
Fibre consumption					
Low (under 30)	67	58	59	57	58
Medium (30-40)	24	30	28	30	29
High (over 40)	10	13	13	12	13
Bases					
Men					
Fat	*883*	*905*	*1296*	*1261*	*1196*
Fibre	*826*	*873*	*1188*	*1162*	*1112*
Women					
Fat	*1249*	*1344*	*1470*	*1306*	*1171*
Fibre	*1203*	*1265*	*1417*	*1229*	*1120*

Table 3.38

Fat and fibre (observed and age-standardised), by Health Authority area type and sex

Aged 16 and over with valid scores   *1998*

Fat/fibre consumption	Health Authority area type					
	Inner London	Mining & Industrial	Urban	Mature	Prosperous	Rural
	%	%	%	%	%	%
Men						
Observed						
Fat consumption						
Low (under 30)	50	38	45	42	43	35
Medium (30-40)	31	36	31	33	33	36
High (over 40)	19	26	24	25	24	30
Fibre consumption						
Low (under 30)	62	53	57	53	52	51
Medium (30-40)	27	31	30	31	31	34
High (over 40)	11	16	13	16	17	15
Standardised						
Fat consumption						
Low (under 30)	50	37	45	42	42	34
Medium (30-40)	30	36	31	32	34	35
High (over 40)	19	27	24	26	24	30
Fibre consumption						
Low (under 30)	63	54	57	54	53	52
Medium (30-40)	27	30	29	30	31	34
High (over 40)	10	16	13	16	16	15
Women						
Observed						
Fat consumption						
Low (under 30)	59	59	61	63	63	57
Medium (30-40)	28	28	27	28	27	29
High (over 40)	14	13	11	9	10	13
Fibre consumption						
Low (under 30)	70	59	64	57	58	58
Medium (30-40)	22	27	25	29	30	30
High (over 40)	8	13	11	14	12	12
Standardised						
Fat consumption						
Low (under 30)	58	59	61	63	63	57
Medium (30-40)	28	28	27	28	28	30
High (over 40)	14	13	12	10	10	13
Fibre consumption						
Low (under 30)	71	60	64	58	58	59
Medium (30-40)	22	27	24	29	30	29
High (over 40)	7	13	12	14	12	12
Bases						
Men						
Fat	*191*	*987*	*934*	*963*	*1747*	*1582*
Fibre	*175*	*958*	*870*	*879*	*1611*	*1456*
Women						
Fat	*242*	*1138*	*1173*	*1125*	*2089*	*1859*
Fibre	*242*	*1092*	*1123*	*1077*	*1996*	*1755*

Table 3.39

Fat and fibre (observed and age-standardised), by region and sex

Aged 16 and over with valid scores   *1998*

Fat/fibre consumption	Region							
	Northern & Yorkshire	North West	Trent	West Midlands	Anglia & Oxford	North Thames	South Thames	South & West
	%	%	%	%	%	%	%	%
Men								
Observed								
Fat consumption								
Low (under 30)	40	38	37	40	37	46	46	40
Medium (30-40)	33	33	37	34	35	31	33	35
High (over 40)	27	29	27	26	27	23	22	25
Fibre consumption								
Low (under 30)	52	55	52	56	55	55	51	50
Medium (30-40)	31	29	35	30	30	32	34	31
High (over 40)	17	16	13	14	15	14	16	19
Standardised								
Fat consumption								
Low (under 30)	39	37	37	39	37	45	46	40
Medium (30-40)	33	34	36	34	35	32	32	35
High (over 40)	28	30	27	27	28	23	21	24
Fibre consumption								
Low (under 30)	53	56	52	56	56	55	51	51
Medium (30-40)	31	29	35	30	29	31	34	30
High (over 40)	16	15	13	14	14	13	15	19
Women								
Observed								
Fat consumption								
Low (under 30)	57	59	57	64	61	64	64	60
Medium (30-40)	29	29	31	26	28	26	26	30
High (over 40)	14	12	12	10	11	10	10	10
Fibre consumption								
Low (under 30)	60	60	58	63	60	61	58	56
Medium (30-40)	28	26	29	27	27	28	30	31
High (over 40)	13	14	13	10	13	11	12	13
Standardised								
Fat consumption								
Low (under 30)	57	58	57	63	60	64	64	59
Medium (30-40)	29	30	31	26	28	26	26	30
High (over 40)	14	13	12	11	11	10	10	10
Fibre consumption								
Low (under 30)	60	60	58	63	61	61	58	57
Medium (30-40)	27	27	28	27	26	28	30	30
High (over 40)	13	14	13	10	13	11	12	13
Bases								
Men								
Fat	*928*	*872*	*720*	*658*	*747*	*788*	*781*	*910*
Fibre	*886*	*796*	*663*	*640*	*681*	*774*	*685*	*824*
Women								
Fat	*1107*	*988*	*843*	*803*	*842*	*954*	*1026*	*1063*
Fibre	*1079*	*936*	*795*	*779*	*811*	*963*	*944*	*978*

Table 3.40

Response to anthropometric measurements, by age and sex

Aged 16 and over who were interviewed/had a nurse visit   *1998*

Response to anthropometric measurements	Age							Total
	16-24	25-34	35-44	45-54	55-64	65-74	75 +	
	%	%	%	%	%	%	%	%
Men								
Height	96	97	97	96	95	92	81	95
Weight	95	94	94	93	93	92	86	93
BMI	94	94	94	93	92	89	77	91
Waist-hip	99	99	99	99	99	99	96	99
Demi-span	a	a	a	a	a	98	96	97
Women								
Height	97	97	98	96	94	92	77	94
Weight	95	94	93	93	92	90	85	92
BMI	94	94	93	92	91	88	75	90
Waist-hip	99	100	99	99	98	97	95	98
Demi-span	a	a	a	a	a	98	92	95
Bases								
Men								
Height, weight, BMI (interviewed)	875	1338	1305	1289	987	837	562	7193
Waist-hip (saw nurse)	698	1132	1128	1138	858	730	480	6164
Demi-span[a] (saw nurse)	a	a	a	a	a	725	467	1192
Women								
Height (interviewed)	1006	1630	1573	1484	1148	967	907	8715
Weight, BMI (interviewed, not pregnant)	960	1530	1551	1484	1148	967	907	8547
Waist-hip (saw nurse)	788	1297	1334	1297	999	818	723	7256
Demi-span[a] (saw nurse)	a	a	a	a	a	812	715	1527

[a] Measured only in those aged 65 and over.

Table 3.41

Body mass index (BMI), 1994-98, by age and sex

Aged 16 and over with both valid height and weight measurements   *1994-98*

BMI (kg/m^2)	Age							Total
	16-24	25-34	35-44	45-54	55-64	65-74	75 +	
	%	%	%	%	%	%	%	%
Men								
1994								
20 or under	16.0	4.8	1.9	1.8	1.4	2.9	2.6	4.5
Over 20-25	53.4	45.6	36.4	30.3	29.4	26.1	34.6	37.3
Over 25-30	24.9	39.8	46.2	50.7	51.4	53.1	48.2	44.3
Over 30-40	5.5	9.5	15.1	16.7	17.4	17.6	13.9	13.4
Over 40	0.2	0.4	0.4	0.5	0.4	0.2	0.8	0.4
All over 30 (obese)	*5.7*	*9.8*	*15.5*	*17.2*	*17.8*	*17.9*	*14.7*	*13.8*
Mean	23.5	25.3	26.4	26.8	27.0	27.0	26.5	26.0
Standard error of the mean	0.12	0.10	0.11	0.11	0.12	0.13	0.21	0.05
1995								
20 or under	16.2	3.7	2.9	1.4	1.5	2.7	3.1	4.4
Over 20-25	54.0	44.9	34.3	30.0	25.7	29.3	33.9	36.4
Over 25-30	24.1	39.6	46.8	49.3	51.3	50.2	48.8	44.0
Over 30-40	5.8	11.4	15.6	18.8	21.5	17.3	14.2	15.0
Over 40	-	0.4	0.4	0.6	-	0.5	-	0.3
All over 30 (obese)	*5.8*	*11.8*	*16.0*	*19.4*	*21.5*	*17.8*	*14.2*	*15.3*
Mean	23.5	25.6	26.5	27.1	27.2	26.8	26.1	26.1
Standard error of the mean	0.13	0.10	0.11	0.12	0.12	0.13	0.18	0.05
1996								
20 or under	16.4	4.1	1.6	2.2	1.2	2.6	2.8	4.2
Over 20-25	55.4	40.7	34.5	27.3	24.5	26.2	33.8	34.7
Over 25-30	22.1	42.7	47.8	49.4	50.7	51.5	47.4	44.6
Over 30-40	5.8	12.2	15.6	20.5	23.2	19.4	16.1	16.1
Over 40	0.2	0.3	0.5	0.6	0.3	0.2	-	0.4
All over 30 (obese)	*6.1*	*12.5*	*16.1*	*21.1*	*23.6*	*19.6*	*16.1*	*16.4*
Mean	23.4	25.8	26.7	27.2	27.6	27.0	26.3	26.3
Standard error of the mean	0.12	0.11	0.10	0.11	0.13	0.13	0.17	0.05
1997								
20 or under	17.0	4.1	2.0	1.0	0.6	1.0	4.1	4.0
Over 20-25	56.3	40.3	32.4	25.3	24.9	24.9	34.2	33.9
Over 25-30	21.6	42.5	48.2	52.0	47.2	55.8	49.7	45.2
Over 30-40	4.6	12.3	16.7	20.2	26.6	17.9	11.9	16.2
Over 40	0.4	0.8	0.8	1.3	0.8	0.5	-	0.8
All over 30 (obese)	*5.0*	*13.1*	*17.5*	*21.6*	*27.4*	*18.4*	*11.9*	*17.0*
Mean	23.2	25.9	26.9	27.4	27.8	27.3	26.1	26.5
Standard error of the mean	0.17	0.15	0.15	0.16	0.19	0.18	0.25	0.07
1998								
20 or under	13.5	3.1	2.4	1.9	0.9	1.7	3.9	3.6
Over 20-25	58.7	40.6	32.9	24.8	23.6	21.7	32.1	33.5
Over 25-30	22.7	40.4	47.9	52.0	52.2	55.3	48.0	45.5
Over 30-40	5.1	15.3	16.4	20.1	22.4	20.4	15.7	16.7
Over 40	0.1	0.6	0.5	1.1	0.9	0.8	0.2	0.6
All over 30 (obese)	*5.2*	*15.9*	*16.8*	*21.2*	*23.3*	*21.2*	*15.9*	*17.3*
Mean	23.5	26.1	26.7	27.4	27.8	27.5	26.4	26.5
Standard error of the mean	0.13	0.12	0.11	0.12	0.13	0.14	0.19	0.05

continued...

Table 3.41 *continued*

BMI (kg/m²)	Age							Total
	16-24	25-34	35-44	45-54	55-64	65-74	75 +	
	%	%	%	%	%	%	%	%
Women								
1994								
20 or under	19.6	9.5	4.9	3.8	2.4	4.9	8.0	7.4
Over 20-25	52.2	52.9	50.3	42.0	33.4	29.1	39.6	43.9
Over 25-30	20.3	24.7	27.9	36.4	38.7	40.7	36.1	31.4
Over 30-40	7.1	11.6	15.0	16.5	23.2	23.0	15.4	15.7
Over 40	0.8	1.3	1.8	1.3	2.3	2.3	0.9	1.6
All over 30 (obese)	*7.9*	*12.9*	*16.9*	*17.8*	*25.5*	*25.3*	*16.3*	*17.3*
Mean	23.5	24.8	25.7	26.3	27.5	27.3	25.7	25.8
Standard error of the mean	0.14	0.12	0.13	0.14	0.16	0.15	0.18	0.06
1995								
20 or under	17.2	9.0	5.6	3.9	2.2	4.4	8.6	7.1
Over 20-25	56.4	53.1	46.8	38.2	32.9	26.4	33.6	42.5
Over 25-30	18.5	24.7	31.0	36.3	41.6	45.1	40.8	32.9
Over 30-40	7.6	11.8	15.1	19.7	21.0	23.1	16.6	16.1
Over 40	*0.4*	*1.5*	*1.4*	*1.8*	*2.2*	*1.1*	*0.3*	*1.4*
All over 30 (obese)	*8.0*	*13.3*	*16.6*	*21.5*	*23.2*	*24.1*	*17.0*	*17.5*
Mean	23.4	24.9	25.8	26.8	27.3	27.2	26.1	25.9
Standard error of the mean	0.13	0.12	0.13	0.14	0.15	0.15	0.18	0.06
1996								
20 or under	17.3	7.9	5.8	3.2	3.5	5.2	6.4	6.9
Over 20-25	56.2	49.3	47.1	38.2	28.2	27.2	33.4	41.2
Over 25-30	18.6	27.9	29.7	39.4	40.8	43.1	40.3	33.6
Over 30-40	7.0	13.4	16.0	17.5	25.7	23.1	19.2	17.0
Over 40	0.9	1.5	1.5	1.7	1.8	1.4	0.7	1.4
All over 30 (obese)	*7.9*	*14.9*	*17.5*	*19.2*	*27.5*	*24.5*	*19.9*	*18.4*
Mean	23.5	25.2	25.8	26.6	27.7	27.3	26.4	26.0
Standard error of the mean	0.14	0.12	0.13	0.13	0.15	0.15	0.18	0.05
1997								
20 or under	16.5	8.2	6.7	3.8	4.0	4.4	7.7	7.1
Over 20-25	56.1	50.5	43.6	37.5	29.2	27.1	29.6	40.4
Over 25-30	18.8	26.8	31.5	36.3	36.8	43.6	40.7	32.8
Over 30-40	7.8	12.3	15.4	19.6	26.1	23.0	21.7	17.4
Over 40	0.8	2.2	2.8	2.9	4.0	1.9	0.3	2.3
All over 30 (obese)	*8.6*	*14.5*	*18.2*	*22.5*	*30.1*	*24.8*	*21.9*	*19.7*
Mean	23.6	25.2	26.1	26.9	28.0	27.5	26.5	26.2
Standard error of the mean	0.19	0.18	0.20	0.19	0.25	0.23	0.24	0.08
1998								
20 or under	18.6	7.7	4.3	3.7	3.0	4.5	7.2	6.6
Over 20-25	54.0	48.8	45.1	36.3	29.2	25.3	34.6	40.0
Over 25-30	16.6	27.1	30.1	36.1	39.2	41.3	37.4	32.1
Over 30-40	9.5	14.7	17.5	21.9	26.3	27.2	20.0	19.3
Over 40	1.2	1.6	3.0	2.0	2.3	1.8	0.7	1.9
All over 30 (obese)	*10.7*	*16.3*	*20.5*	*23.9*	*28.6*	*29.0*	*20.7*	*21.2*
Mean	23.8	25.5	26.4	27.0	27.6	27.8	26.4	26.4
Standard error of the mean	0.16	0.13	0.14	0.14	0.16	0.17	0.18	0.06

continued...

Table 3.41 *continued*

BMI (kg/m²)	Age							Total
	16-24	25-34	35-44	45-54	55-64	65-74	75 +	
Bases								
Men								
1994	*935*	*1373*	*1288*	*1076*	*925*	*816*	*382*	*6795*
1995	*869*	*1309*	*1296*	*1078*	*919*	*820*	*416*	*6707*
1996	*908*	*1290*	*1348*	*1247*	*938*	*831*	*435*	*6997*
1997	*476*	*710*	*714*	*667*	*511*	*414*	*193*	*3685*
1998	*825*	*1261*	*1229*	*1197*	*910*	*745*	*433*	*6600*
Women								
1994	*990*	*1524*	*1418*	*1227*	*988*	*1048*	*689*	*7884*
1995	*979*	*1521*	*1394*	*1258*	*1028*	*936*	*613*	*7729*
1996	*1016*	*1500*	*1493*	*1385*	*1007*	*986*	*677*	*8064*
1997	*510*	*816*	*780*	*766*	*552*	*479*	*351*	*4254*
1998	*903*	*1433*	*1449*	*1373*	*1043*	*853*	*676*	*7730*

Table 3.42

Waist-hip ratio (WHR), 1994, 1997, 1998, by age and sex

Aged 16 and over with both valid waist and hip measurements   *1994, 1997, 1998*

WHR	Age							Total
	16-24	25-34	35-44	45-54	55-64	65-74	75 +	
Men								
1994								
Mean	0.83	0.87	0.90	0.92	0.94	0.94	0.94	0.90
Standard error of the mean	0.002	0.002	0.002	0.002	0.002	0.002	0.003	0.001
1997								
Mean	0.82	0.88	0.91	0.93	0.95	0.95	0.94	0.91
Standard error of the mean	0.003	0.002	0.002	0.002	0.003	0.003	0.004	0.001
1998								
Mean	0.82	0.87	0.90	0.93	0.94	0.95	0.94	0.91
Standard error of the mean	0.002	0.002	0.002	0.002	0.002	0.002	0.003	0.001
Women								
1994								
Mean	0.75	0.77	0.78	0.79	0.81	0.83	0.85	0.79
Standard error of the mean	0.002	0.001	0.002	0.002	0.002	0.002	0.002	0.001
1997								
Mean	0.75	0.77	0.78	0.81	0.82	0.83	0.85	0.80
Standard error of the mean	0.003	0.002	0.002	0.002	0.003	0.003	0.004	0.001
1998								
Mean	0.75	0.77	0.79	0.80	0.81	0.83	0.84	0.80
Standard error of the mean	0.002	0.002	0.002	0.002	0.002	0.002	0.002	0.001
Bases								
Men								
1994	*968*	*1434*	*1329*	*1127*	*1001*	*877*	*442*	*7178*
1997	*492*	*739*	*740*	*694*	*535*	*455*	*243*	*3898*
1998	*875*	*1338*	*1305*	*1289*	*987*	*837*	*562*	*7193*
Women								
1994	*1080*	*1723*	*1520*	*1300*	*1059*	*1120*	*829*	*8631*
1997	*560*	*916*	*833*	*806*	*585*	*545*	*439*	*4684*
1998	*1006*	*1630*	*1573*	*1484*	*1148*	*967*	*907*	*8715*

Table 3.43

Raised and mean body mass index (observed and age-standardised), by social class of head of household and sex

Aged 16 and over with both valid height and weight measurements   *1998*

BMI (kg/m²)	Social class of head of household						Social class of head of household					
	I	II	IIINM	IIIM	IV	V	I	II	IIINM	IIIM	IV	V
	%	%	%	%	%	%	%	%	%	%	%	%
	Men						**Women**					
Observed												
Over 25-30 (overweight)	47.5	48.8	42.6	44.9	43.9	39.9	30.4	32.8	31.7	32.5	31.7	34.0
Over 30 (obese)	11.9	16.5	16.5	20.5	16.1	17.9	15.1	18.4	18.9	24.4	24.9	27.5
Over 40 (morbid obesity)	*0.4*	*0.6*	*0.2*	*0.8*	*0.5*	*1.7*	*0.8*	*1.5*	*1.1*	*2.5*	*2.7*	*2.8*
Mean	26.1	26.7	26.2	26.8	26.2	26.3	25.4	26.1	26.0	26.8	26.9	27.2
Standard error of the mean	0.17	0.09	0.16	0.09	0.14	0.27	0.22	0.10	0.14	0.12	0.16	0.27
Standardised												
Over 25-30 (overweight)	45.9	46.8	43.1	43.9	43.5	39.5	30.4	32.5	31.0	32.2	31.7	31.8
Over 30 (obese)	11.6	15.7	16.4	19.6	15.8	17.7	14.4	18.4	18.2	24.0	25.1	28.1
Over 40 (morbid obesity)	*0.4*	*0.5*	*0.2*	*0.8*	*0.5*	*1.6*	*0.7*	*1.5*	*1.1*	*2.4*	*2.8*	*3.3*
Mean	25.9	26.5	26.2	26.7	26.2	26.2	25.4	26.0	25.9	26.7	26.9	27.2
Standard error of the mean	0.17	0.09	0.16	0.10	0.14	0.26	0.21	0.10	0.14	0.12	0.16	0.28
Bases	*461*	*2031*	*662*	*2072*	*938*	*301*	*471*	*2231*	*1193*	*1983*	*1201*	*429*

Table 3.44

Waist-hip ratio (observed and age-standardised), by social class of head of household and sex

Aged 16 and over with both valid waist and hip measurements   *1998*

WHR	Social class of head of household						Social class of head of household					
	I	II	IIINM	IIIM	IV	V	I	II	IIINM	IIIM	IV	V
	Men						**Women**					
Observed												
Mean	0.90	0.91	0.90	0.92	0.91	0.91	0.78	0.79	0.79	0.80	0.80	0.81
Standard error of the mean	0.003	0.002	0.003	0.002	0.003	0.005	0.003	0.001	0.002	0.002	0.002	0.003
% with waist-hip ratio 0.95 (0.85) and over[a]	23.2	26.2	23.0	35.0	30.1	31.4	15.7	17.5	20.0	21.3	25.0	28.7
Standardised												
Mean	0.89	0.90	0.90	0.91	0.90	0.90	0.78	0.79	0.79	0.80	0.80	0.81
Standard error of the mean	0.003	0.002	0.003	0.002	0.003	0.005	0.003	0.001	0.002	0.002	0.002	0.003
% with waist-hip ratio 0.95 (0.85) and over[a]	20.1	23.6	22.6	31.4	28.3	28.7	18.0	18.4	18.0	21.9	24.3	26.6
Bases	*418*	*1896*	*601*	*1926*	*863*	*273*	*432*	*2062*	*1098*	*1836*	*1117*	*390*

[a] Unbracketed figure refers to men, bracketed figure to women.

Table 3.45

**Raised and mean body mass index (observed and age-standardised),
by equivalised household income and sex**

Aged 16 and over with both valid height and weight measurements   *1998*

BMI (kg/m²)	Equivalised annual household income quintile				
	Up to £7,186	Over £7,186 to £10,834	Over £10,834 to £17,890	Over £17,890 to £27,705	Over £27,705
	%	%	%	%	%
Men					
Observed					
Over 25-30 (overweight)	38.9	46.1	45.4	46.5	48.6
Over 30 (obese)	20.1	18.1	18.7	17.6	14.8
Over 40 (morbid obesity)	*1.1*	*0.8*	*0.8*	*0.5*	*0.4*
Mean	26.4	26.7	26.6	26.6	26.5
Standard error of the mean	0.15	0.14	0.12	0.11	0.10
Standardised					
Over 25-30 (overweight)	38.2	43.7	44.1	46.2	46.8
Over 30 (obese)	20.3	17.0	18.0	16.5	14.5
Over 40 (morbid obesity)	*1.2*	*0.8*	*0.8*	*0.4*	*0.6*
Mean	26.4	26.4	26.5	26.4	26.4
Standard error of the mean	0.15	0.14	0.12	0.11	0.11
Women					
Observed					
Over 25-30 (overweight)	30.1	34.4	32.4	32.8	30.1
Over 30 (obese)	26.0	24.3	22.7	19.2	15.2
Over 40 (morbid obesity)	*3.8*	*2.1*	*1.7*	*1.6*	*1.2*
Mean	27.0	26.8	26.5	26.2	25.5
Standard error of the mean	0.17	0.15	0.13	0.13	0.13
Standardised					
Over 25-30 (overweight)	30.7	32.1	32.1	33.5	29.2
Over 30 (obese)	26.3	24.2	22.5	19.5	15.9
Over 40 (morbid obesity)	*3.7*	*2.3*	*1.5*	*1.4*	*0.9*
Mean	27.1	26.7	26.4	26.2	25.4
Standard error of the mean	0.17	0.15	0.13	0.13	0.13
Bases					
Men	*885*	*907*	*1344*	*1324*	*1288*
Women	*1248*	*1305*	*1501*	*1362*	*1256*

Table 3.46

**Waist-hip ratio (observed and age-standardised),
by equivalised household income and sex**

Aged 16 and over with both valid waist and hip measurements   *1998*

WHR	Equivalised annual household income quintile				
	Up to £7,186	Over £7,186 to £10,834	Over £10,834 to £17,890	Over £17,890 to £27,705	Over £27,705
Men					
Observed					
Mean	0.92	0.92	0.91	0.90	0.90
Standard error of the mean	0.003	0.003	0.002	0.002	0.002
% with waist-hip ratio 0.95 and over	37.4	38.0	31.0	25.8	19.2
Standardised					
Mean	0.91	0.91	0.91	0.90	0.90
Standard error of the mean	0.003	0.003	0.002	0.002	0.002
% with waist-hip ratio 0.95 and over	34.1	29.7	28.0	25.3	20.2
Women					
Observed					
Mean	0.81	0.81	0.79	0.78	0.77
Standard error of the mean	0.002	0.002	0.002	0.002	0.002
% with waist-hip ratio 0.85 and over	27.1	29.5	19.1	14.1	11.1
Standardised					
Mean	0.81	0.80	0.80	0.79	0.78
Standard error of the mean	0.002	0.002	0.002	0.002	0.002
% with waist-hip ratio 0.85 and over	27.3	23.8	19.6	17.4	16.3
Bases					
Men	*824*	*839*	*1257*	*1232*	*1197*
Women	*1121*	*1216*	*1421*	*1284*	*1153*

Table 3.47

Raised and mean body mass index (observed and age-standardised), by Health Authority area type and sex

Aged 16 and over with both valid height and weight measurements   *1998*

BMI (kg/m²)	Health Authority area type					
	Inner London	Mining & Industrial	Urban	Mature	Prosperous	Rural
	%	%	%	%	%	%
Men						
Observed						
Over 25-30 (overweight)	36.5	46.4	43.4	46.8	45.8	46.4
Over 30 (obese)	15.3	17.6	19.8	14.7	16.3	18.8
Over 40 (morbid obesity)	*1.8*	*0.6*	*0.5*	*0.3*	*0.6*	*0.9*
Mean	25.8	26.6	26.6	26.3	26.4	26.8
Standard error of the mean	0.29	0.13	0.14	0.12	0.09	0.11
Standardised						
Over 25-30 (overweight)	38.9	45.3	42.7	46.1	44.6	44.9
Over 30 (obese)	16.5	16.6	19.5	14.3	15.9	18.1
Over 40 (morbid obesity)	*2.2*	*0.6*	*0.5*	*0.3*	*0.6*	*0.8*
Mean	26.0	26.4	26.5	26.2	26.3	26.6
Standard error of the mean	0.30	0.13	0.14	0.12	0.09	0.11
Women						
Observed						
Over 25-30 (overweight)	21.8	32.0	31.6	33.5	31.8	33.6
Over 30 (obese)	21.4	22.0	22.5	19.5	19.3	23.2
Over 40 (morbid obesity)	*1.5*	*2.1*	*1.5*	*1.9*	*2.0*	*2.0*
Mean	25.7	26.5	26.4	26.2	26.1	26.7
Standard error of the mean	0.35	0.15	0.15	0.15	0.11	0.12
Standardised						
Over 25-30 (overweight)	22.7	31.7	31.6	33.2	31.2	33.3
Over 30 (obese)	22.9	21.5	22.5	19.1	19.0	23.0
Over 40 (morbid obesity)	*2.0*	*2.1*	*1.5*	*1.8*	*2.0*	*2.0*
Mean	26.1	26.4	26.4	26.2	26.0	26.7
Standard error of the mean	0.36	0.15	0.15	0.15	0.11	0.12
Bases						
Men	*222*	*1029*	*959*	*1019*	*1809*	*1562*
Women	*266*	*1180*	*1160*	*1178*	*2132*	*1814*

Table 3.48

Waist-hip ratio (observed and age-standardised), by Health Authority area type and sex

Aged 16 and over with both valid waist and hip measurements   *1998*

WHR	Health Authority area type					
	Inner London	Mining & Industrial	Urban	Mature	Prosperous	Rural
Men						
Observed						
Mean	0.90	0.92	0.91	0.91	0.91	0.91
Standard error of the mean	0.006	0.002	0.003	0.002	0.002	0.002
% with waist-hip ratio 0.95 and over	25.2	33.8	29.6	26.4	27.6	29.4
Standardised						
Mean	0.90	0.91	0.90	0.90	0.90	0.90
Standard error of the mean	0.006	0.002	0.003	0.002	0.002	0.002
% with waist-hip ratio 0.95 and over	27.3	30.4	27.8	24.8	25.0	26.6
Women						
Observed						
Mean	0.81	0.80	0.79	0.80	0.79	0.80
Standard error of the mean	0.005	0.002	0.002	0.002	0.001	0.002
% with waist-hip ratio 0.85 and over	25.6	21.2	20.9	20.6	18.5	22.2
Standardised						
Mean	0.81	0.80	0.79	0.80	0.79	0.80
Standard error of the mean	0.005	0.002	0.002	0.002	0.001	0.002
% with waist-hip ratio 0.85 and over	28.8	20.5	21.3	19.9	18.9	22.1
Bases						
Men	*162*	*953*	*883*	*915*	*1685*	*1497*
Women	*230*	*1076*	*1074*	*1051*	*1993*	*1716*

Table 3.49

Raised and mean body mass index (observed and age-standardised), by region and sex

Aged 16 and over with both valid height and weight measurements   *1998*

BMI (kg/m²)	Region							
	Northern & Yorkshire	North West	Trent	West Midlands	Anglia & Oxford	North Thames	South Thames	South & West
	%	%	%	%	%	%	%	%
Men								
Observed								
Over 25-30 (overweight)	46.3	45.5	47.7	43.4	43.6	47.6	43.0	46.4
Over 30 (obese)	17.4	15.5	17.6	22.9	16.9	14.5	19.6	15.8
Over 40 (morbid obesity)	*0.4*	*0.6*	*0.6*	*1.2*	*0.5*	*0.6*	*0.6*	*0.7*
Mean	26.4	26.4	26.5	27.0	26.4	26.3	26.7	26.5
Standard error of the mean	0.13	0.14	0.16	0.18	0.15	0.13	0.14	0.13
Standardised								
Over 25-30 (overweight)	45.6	44.4	47.2	42.1	42.9	46.7	42.0	44.9
Over 30 (obese)	16.8	15.1	16.7	22.4	16.7	14.0	19.1	15.4
Over 40 (morbid obesity)	*0.4*	*0.5*	*0.6*	*1.1*	*0.5*	*0.5*	*0.6*	*0.8*
Mean	26.3	26.3	26.4	26.9	26.3	26.2	26.5	26.4
Standard error of the mean	0.13	0.14	0.16	0.18	0.15	0.13	0.14	0.13
Women								
Observed								
Over 25-30 (overweight)	31.0	32.9	29.6	34.7	34.4	29.7	30.6	34.6
Over 30 (obese)	23.5	20.6	24.4	22.3	19.4	21.4	18.6	20.1
Over 40 (morbid obesity)	*2.4*	*1.6*	*2.2*	*2.2*	*1.7*	*1.6*	*1.8*	*1.7*
Mean	26.6	26.3	26.7	26.7	26.2	26.3	25.8	26.5
Standard error of the mean	0.16	0.16	0.19	0.19	0.17	0.17	0.16	0.15
Standardised								
Over 25-30 (overweight)	30.3	32.8	29.0	34.0	34.9	29.8	30.6	33.9
Over 30 (obese)	23.0	20.3	24.4	22.2	19.4	20.9	18.6	19.6
Over 40 (morbid obesity)	*2.5*	*1.6*	*2.2*	*2.3*	*1.7*	*1.6*	*1.8*	*1.7*
Mean	26.5	26.2	26.6	26.6	26.2	26.2	25.8	26.4
Standard error of the mean	0.16	0.16	0.19	0.19	0.17	0.17	0.16	0.15
Bases								
Men	*966*	*907*	*698*	*645*	*757*	*853*	*812*	*962*
Women	*1120*	*1043*	*807*	*770*	*861*	*995*	*1047*	*1087*

Table 3.50

Waist-hip ratio (observed and age-standardised), by region and sex

Aged 16 and over with both valid waist and hip measurements   *1998*

WHR	Region							
	Northern & Yorkshire	North West	Trent	West Midlands	Anglia & Oxford	North Thames	South Thames	South & West
Men								
Observed								
Mean	0.90	0.91	0.91	0.92	0.90	0.92	0.91	0.90
Standard error of the mean	0.002	0.002	0.003	0.003	0.003	0.003	0.003	0.002
% with waist-hip ratio 0.95 and over	27.5	28.5	35.1	34.3	23.9	31.3	29.5	25.2
Standardised								
Mean	0.90	0.91	0.91	0.91	0.90	0.91	0.90	0.90
Standard error of the mean	0.002	0.002	0.003	0.003	0.003	0.003	0.003	0.002
% with waist-hip ratio 0.95 and over	24.8	27.0	31.9	31.8	23.1	27.9	27.2	22.4
Women								
Observed								
Mean	0.79	0.80	0.81	0.79	0.79	0.80	0.79	0.80
Standard error of the mean	0.002	0.002	0.003	0.002	0.002	0.002	0.002	0.002
% with waist-hip ratio 0.85 and over	20.7	17.7	25.7	19.0	18.5	22.3	21.2	20.9
Standardised								
Mean	0.79	0.80	0.81	0.79	0.80	0.80	0.79	0.79
Standard error of the mean	0.002	0.002	0.003	0.002	0.002	0.002	0.002	0.002
% with waist-hip ratio 0.85 and over	19.7	18.0	26.0	19.2	20.0	21.7	21.5	20.5
Bases								
Men	*911*	*813*	*682*	*613*	*719*	*705*	*742*	*910*
Women	*1053*	*944*	*762*	*740*	*779*	*836*	*993*	*1033*

Table 3.51

Height, by age and sex

Aged 16 and over with a valid measurement   *1998*

Height (cm)	Age							Total
	16-24	25-34	35-44	45-54	55-64	65-74	75 +	
Men								
Mean	176.6	176.6	175.6	174.8	173.1	171.2	168.4	174.4
Standard error of the mean	0.24	0.19	0.19	0.19	0.22	0.24	0.31	0.09
5th percentile	165.4	165.5	164.8	163.9	161.4	160.3	156.9	162.5
10th percentile	168.0	167.9	167.1	166.1	164.1	162.8	158.8	165.3
Median	176.9	176.3	175.1	174.7	173.1	171.2	168.6	174.4
90th percentile	184.8	185.3	184.6	183.2	182.0	179.9	176.6	183.6
95th percentile	187.3	188.0	187.9	186.3	184.3	181.6	178.4	186.4
Women								
Mean	163.4	163.0	162.5	161.4	160.2	157.8	154.7	161.0
Standard error of the mean	0.21	0.16	0.16	0.16	0.19	0.20	0.25	0.07
5th percentile	152.6	152.6	152.5	151.6	150.5	147.8	143.5	149.9
10th percentile	155.0	155.1	154.6	153.7	152.2	150.2	145.8	152.4
Median	163.5	162.8	162.3	161.4	160.1	157.6	154.9	161.0
90th percentile	171.7	171.2	170.5	169.3	167.9	165.9	163.3	169.5
95th percentile	174.2	174.1	173.2	171.6	170.4	167.6	165.2	172.2
Bases								
Men	*841*	*1298*	*1267*	*1236*	*935*	*771*	*453*	*6801*
Women	*980*	*1587*	*1540*	*1430*	*1083*	*887*	*697*	*8204*

Table 3.52

Weight, by age and sex

Aged 16 and over with a valid measurement　　　　　　　　　　　　　　　*1998*

Weight (kg)	Age							Total
	16-24	25-34	35-44	45-54	55-64	65-74	75 +	
Men								
Mean	73.3	81.6	82.3	83.9	83.3	80.8	74.8	80.8
Standard error of the mean	0.44	0.40	0.39	0.39	0.46	0.47	0.58	0.17
5th percentile	55.9	60.9	62.7	63.8	62.8	61.2	55.0	60.1
10th percentile	58.7	65.0	66.3	68.0	67.7	65.7	58.8	64.1
Median	71.8	80.0	80.7	83.2	82.2	79.9	74.1	79.6
90th percentile	89.5	100.0	98.8	100.5	100.1	96.7	91.9	98.4
95th percentile	97.6	107.5	107.2	106.3	107.2	104.1	98.4	105.2
Women								
Mean	63.6	67.8	69.8	70.4	70.9	69.2	63.4	68.3
Standard error of the mean	0.45	0.38	0.39	0.37	0.42	0.44	0.45	0.16
5th percentile	47.8	49.8	51.7	51.3	52.6	48.9	43.6	49.5
10th percentile	49.7	52.8	54.2	54.4	55.9	54.0	47.3	52.7
Median	60.8	64.8	66.8	68.3	69.1	68.1	62.6	65.9
90th percentile	82.1	87.8	89.0	88.6	87.5	86.4	80.4	86.6
95th percentile	92.5	95.7	99.2	96.5	95.4	90.2	85.0	94.5
Bases								
Men	*827*	*1265*	*1235*	*1206*	*919*	*772*	*485*	*6709*
Women	*909*	*1441*	*1451*	*1385*	*1057*	*875*	*769*	*7887*

Table 3.53

Demi-span, by age and sex

Aged 65 and over with a valid measurement　　　　　　　*1998*

Demi-span (cm)	Age			Total
	65-74	75-84	85 +	
Men				
Mean	81.2	79.8	78.9	80.6
Standard error of the mean	0.15	0.20	0.41	0.12
5th percentile	74.8	73.7	72.9	74.4
10th percentile	76.5	74.8	74.7	75.6
Median	81.5	80.0	79.0	80.8
90th percentile	85.9	84.8	83.4	85.4
95th percentile	87.4	86.3	84.5	86.8
Women				
Mean	73.9	72.6	71.4	73.2
Standard error of the mean	0.13	0.16	0.42	0.10
5th percentile	68.3	66.4	64.2	67.2
10th percentile	69.6	68.1	65.4	68.5
Median	73.8	72.6	71.7	73.2
90th percentile	78.2	77.3	76.1	77.7
95th percentile	79.8	78.7	77.5	79.1
Bases				
Men	*713*	*376*	*70*	*1159*
Women	*796*	*545*	*114*	*1455*

Table 3.54

Height, 1994-98, by age and sex

Aged 16 and over with a valid measurement — *1994-98*

Height (cm)	Age							Total
	16-24	25-34	35-44	45-54	55-64	65-74	75 +	
Men								
1994								
Mean	176.6	176.7	176.2	174.8	173.1	170.9	168.7	174.6
Standard error of the mean	0.23	0.18	0.20	0.21	0.22	0.24	0.39	0.09
1995								
Mean	176.8	176.6	175.8	174.7	173.2	170.9	168.2	174.5
Standard error of the mean	0.23	0.19	0.18	0.20	0.22	0.22	0.31	0.09
1996								
Mean	176.3	176.6	175.7	174.4	173.2	170.9	168.0	174.4
Standard error of the mean	0.23	0.19	0.19	0.19	0.22	0.22	0.30	0.09
1997								
Mean	176.7	176.4	175.8	174.7	172.9	170.9	168.5	174.5
Standard error of the mean	0.32	0.26	0.25	0.26	0.29	0.33	0.46	0.12
1998								
Mean	176.6	176.6	175.6	174.8	173.1	171.2	168.4	174.4
Standard error of the mean	0.24	0.19	0.19	0.19	0.22	0.24	0.31	0.09
Women								
1994								
Mean	163.0	163.3	162.3	161.9	160.4	158.4	154.6	161.1
Standard error of the mean	0.21	0.16	0.17	0.18	0.19	0.19	0.23	0.08
1995								
Mean	163.1	162.8	162.1	161.3	159.9	158.1	154.6	160.9
Standard error of the mean	0.19	0.16	0.17	0.17	0.18	0.20	0.25	0.07
1996								
Mean	163.1	163.2	162.2	161.4	159.9	157.8	154.7	161.0
Standard error of the mean	0.19	0.15	0.16	0.17	0.19	0.19	0.23	0.07
1997								
Mean	162.9	163.1	162.4	161.4	159.4	158.2	154.3	160.9
Standard error of the mean	0.27	0.21	0.23	0.22	0.26	0.28	0.30	0.10
1998								
Mean	163.4	163.0	162.5	161.4	160.2	157.8	154.7	161.0
Standard error of the mean	0.21	0.16	0.16	0.16	0.19	0.20	0.25	0.07
Bases								
Men								
1994	*949*	*1394*	*1299*	*1093*	*948*	*826*	*390*	*6899*
1995	*892*	*1352*	*1331*	*1121*	*944*	*847*	*435*	*6922*
1996	*927*	*1330*	*1378*	*1280*	*955*	*848*	*444*	*7162*
1997	*483*	*722*	*727*	*680*	*516*	*420*	*196*	*3744*
1998	*841*	*1298*	*1267*	*1236*	*935*	*771*	*453*	*6801*
Women								
1994	*1059*	*1678*	*1471*	*1259*	*1011*	*1063*	*706*	*8247*
1995	*1050*	*1686*	*1456*	*1317*	*1067*	*975*	*640*	*8191*
1996	*1093*	*1642*	*1576*	*1436*	*1043*	*1011*	*698*	*8499*
1997	*549*	*900*	*820*	*784*	*562*	*493*	*354*	*4462*
1998	*980*	*1587*	*1540*	*1430*	*1083*	*887*	*697*	*8204*

Table 3.55

Weight, 1994-98, by age and sex

Aged 16 and over with a valid measurement   *1994-98*

Weight (kg)	Age							Total
	16-24	25-34	35-44	45-54	55-64	65-74	75 +	
Men								
1994								
Mean	73.5	79.2	82.0	82.1	81.2	79.0	75.3	79.4
Standard error of the mean	0.43	0.34	0.38	0.39	0.42	0.44	0.61	0.16
1995								
Mean	73.6	79.8	81.9	82.6	81.7	78.2	74.0	79.5
Standard error of the mean	0.44	0.36	0.36	0.38	0.41	0.43	0.54	0.16
1996								
Mean	72.8	80.7	82.4	82.7	82.8	78.9	74.1	80.0
Standard error of the mean	0.43	0.38	0.36	0.37	0.43	0.43	0.51	0.16
1997								
Mean	72.7	80.8	83.3	83.9	83.1	79.8	74.3	80.6
Standard error of the mean	0.61	0.52	0.51	0.54	0.58	0.62	0.75	0.23
1998								
Mean	73.3	81.6	82.3	83.9	83.3	80.8	74.8	80.8
Standard error of the mean	0.44	0.40	0.39	0.39	0.46	0.47	0.58	0.17
Women								
1994								
Mean	62.6	66.1	67.6	68.8	70.7	68.6	61.7	66.9
Standard error of the mean	0.38	0.34	0.36	0.37	0.42	0.40	0.45	0.15
1995								
Mean	62.2	65.9	67.8	69.7	69.8	68.3	62.5	66.9
Standard error of the mean	0.37	0.33	0.36	0.37	0.40	0.40	0.45	0.15
1996								
Mean	62.7	67.0	67.8	69.3	70.7	68.2	63.4	67.3
Standard error of the mean	0.38	0.34	0.35	0.35	0.40	0.40	0.42	0.14
1997								
Mean	62.6	67.2	68.8	70.2	71.1	69.0	62.7	67.8
Standard error of the mean	0.52	0.50	0.54	0.51	0.63	0.59	0.58	0.21
1998								
Mean	63.6	67.8	69.8	70.4	70.9	69.2	63.4	68.3
Standard error of the mean	0.45	0.38	0.39	0.37	0.42	0.44	0.45	0.16
Bases								
Men								
1994	*943*	*1388*	*1295*	*1082*	*939*	*829*	*392*	*6868*
1995	*868*	*1313*	*1300*	*1091*	*930*	*847*	*459*	*6808*
1996	*909*	*1296*	*1353*	*1254*	*945*	*847*	*489*	*7093*
1997	*476*	*713*	*715*	*669*	*514*	*430*	*221*	*3738*
1998	*827*	*1265*	*1235*	*1206*	*919*	*772*	*485*	*6709*
Women								
1994	*998*	*1533*	*1434*	*1239*	*997*	*1061*	*719*	*7981*
1995	*982*	*1530*	*1394*	*1269*	*1036*	*964*	*700*	*7875*
1996	*1024*	*1504*	*1501*	*1399*	*1017*	*1023*	*771*	*8239*
1997	*511*	*816*	*782*	*770*	*561*	*497*	*395*	*4332*
1998	*909*	*1441*	*1451*	*1385*	*1057*	*875*	*769*	*7887*

Table 3.56

Response to blood pressure measurement, by age and sex

Aged 16 and over who had a nurse visit   *1998*

Response to blood pressure measurement	Men			Total	Women			Total
	16-44	45-64	65 +		16-44	45-64	65 +	
	%	%	%	%	%	%	%	%
Valid BP measurement	86.5	87.5	90.5	87.6	84.4	89.7	90.8	87.4
Ate, drank alcohol, or smoked in previous half hour	12.7	11.1	5.5	10.8	9.9	8.4	4.6	8.4
Three valid readings not obtained	0.7	1.2	3.6	1.4	0.9	1.7	3.9	1.8
Pregnant	-	-	-	-	4.6	-	-	2.2
Refused, not obtained, not attempted	0.1	0.2	0.3	0.2	0.2	0.2	0.7	0.3
Bases	*2959*	*1996*	*1210*	*6165*	*3584*	*2296*	*1541*	*7421*

Table 3.57

Systolic blood pressure, 1994-98, by age and sex

Aged 16 and over with valid blood pressure readings   *1994-98*

Systolic blood pressure (mmHg)	Age							Total
	16-24	25-34	35-44	45-54	55-64	65-74	75 +	
Men								
1994								
Mean	130.1	131.2	132.4	136.1	144.0	150.4	152.3	137.6
Standard error of the mean	0.44	0.33	0.40	0.54	0.66	0.78	1.20	0.23
Median	130.0	130.0	131.0	134.0	142.0	149.0	151.0	135.0
1995								
Mean	131.1	132.0	132.7	136.6	143.8	149.6	151.1	138.1
Standard error of the mean	0.43	0.36	0.38	0.53	0.67	0.74	1.11	0.23
Median	131.0	132.0	132.0	135.0	141.0	148.0	148.0	135.5
1996								
Mean	130.4	132.5	132.3	137.4	144.4	151.7	154.2	138.6
Standard error of the mean	0.42	0.35	0.39	0.48	0.64	0.79	1.13	0.23
Median	129.0	131.5	131.0	135.5	142.5	150.5	153.0	135.5
1997								
Mean	128.9	131.2	132.7	135.4	143.7	148.5	153.6	137.3
Standard error of the mean	0.60	0.49	0.53	0.63	0.94	1.04	1.52	0.31
Median	128.5	130.0	131.5	134.0	142.0	146.0	151.5	135.0
1998								
Mean	128.4	130.4	131.2	136.2	142.1	147.7	150.3	136.8
Standard error of the mean	0.47	0.37	0.41	0.49	0.71	0.80	1.03	0.24
Median	127.5	130.0	130.5	135.0	140.5	147.0	149.0	134.0
Women								
1994								
Mean	121.4	121.8	124.7	132.2	143.2	153.7	159.9	134.3
Standard error of the mean	0.38	0.32	0.39	0.53	0.68	0.75	0.99	0.27
Median	121.0	120.0	123.0	129.0	140.0	151.0	159.0	129.0
1995								
Mean	121.7	121.8	124.3	132.5	142.3	153.5	159.1	134.0
Standard error of the mean	0.39	0.31	0.39	0.51	0.67	0.80	1.06	0.27
Median	121.0	121.0	123.0	130.0	140.0	151.0	156.0	129.0
1996								
Mean	121.4	122.4	124.4	132.4	144.8	151.9	159.7	134.2
Standard error of the mean	0.35	0.32	0.38	0.51	0.71	0.76	0.96	0.26
Median	120.5	121.5	122.5	130.0	142.8	149.5	157.5	129.5
1997								
Mean	121.2	121.1	124.6	130.7	141.6	151.9	158.1	133.2
Standard error of the mean	0.53	0.42	0.55	0.66	0.86	1.01	1.30	0.35
Median	120.5	120.5	122.5	128.0	139.0	150.5	156.5	128.5
1998								
Mean	120.1	120.5	123.5	131.7	140.1	149.2	155.4	132.5
Standard error of the mean	0.41	0.34	0.38	0.53	0.67	0.80	0.95	0.26
Median	120.0	119.5	122.0	129.0	138.0	147.5	153.5	128.0

continued...

Table 3.57 *continued*

Systolic blood pressure (mmHg)	Age							Total
	16-24	25-34	35-44	45-54	55-64	65-74	75 +	
Bases								
Men								
1994	*710*	*1167*	*1110*	*922*	*817*	*727*	*347*	*5800*
1995	*699*	*1076*	*1112*	*939*	*803*	*749*	*420*	*5798*
1996	*741*	*1069*	*1143*	*1056*	*817*	*761*	*425*	*6012*
1997	*373*	*577*	*603*	*584*	*443*	*384*	*199*	*3163*
1998	*594*	*984*	*981*	*981*	*766*	*665*	*430*	*5401*
Women								
1994	*806*	*1278*	*1247*	*1070*	*861*	*884*	*609*	*6755*
1995	*780*	*1308*	*1224*	*1080*	*915*	*825*	*608*	*6740*
1996	*849*	*1289*	*1336*	*1224*	*900*	*879*	*642*	*7119*
1997	*405*	*683*	*682*	*659*	*484*	*446*	*333*	*3692*
1998	*692*	*1142*	*1190*	*1164*	*896*	*751*	*648*	*6483*

Table 3.58

Diastolic blood pressure, 1994-98, by age and sex

Aged 16 and over with valid blood pressure readings   *1994-98*

Diastolic blood pressure (mmHg)	Age							Total
	16-24	25-34	35-44	45-54	55-64	65-74	75 +	
Men								
1994								
Mean	63.5	70.5	76.4	80.8	83.4	82.1	80.7	76.3
Standard error of the mean	0.39	0.28	0.32	0.37	0.39	0.45	0.71	0.17
Median	63.0	70.0	76.0	80.0	83.0	81.0	80.0	76.0
1995								
Mean	63.8	71.1	76.6	81.3	83.1	82.0	79.0	76.6
Standard error of the mean	0.38	0.31	0.30	0.37	0.39	0.46	0.66	0.17
Median	63.0	71.0	77.0	81.0	83.0	81.0	78.0	76.0
1996								
Mean	63.8	71.4	76.9	81.4	83.0	82.6	80.1	76.9
Standard error of the mean	0.36	0.30	0.30	0.33	0.37	0.44	0.66	0.16
Median	63.5	71.0	76.5	81.0	82.5	82.0	79.0	76.5
1997								
Mean	63.2	71.4	76.9	79.9	82.7	81.3	78.9	76.3
Standard error of the mean	0.46	0.42	0.43	0.44	0.57	0.57	0.89	0.22
Median	63.0	71.5	76.5	79.5	82.0	80.5	78.5	76.0
1998								
Mean	62.7	70.5	76.5	80.8	82.0	81.0	78.7	76.2
Standard error of the mean	0.42	0.31	0.34	0.36	0.44	0.47	0.62	0.17
Median	62.0	70.0	76.0	80.5	81.0	80.5	78.0	76.0
Women								
1994								
Mean	64.0	68.4	71.3	74.5	76.9	79.0	79.7	72.8
Standard error of the mean	0.32	0.27	0.29	0.35	0.39	0.45	0.63	0.15
Median	63.0	68.0	71.0	74.0	77.0	78.0	78.0	72.0
1995								
Mean	63.8	67.8	71.2	74.5	76.7	78.7	79.4	72.6
Standard error of the mean	0.32	0.26	0.30	0.33	0.42	0.45	0.60	0.15
Median	63.0	68.0	71.0	74.0	76.0	78.0	78.0	72.0
1996								
Mean	64.3	68.8	71.5	74.8	78.0	78.0	78.6	73.0
Standard error of the mean	0.31	0.26	0.29	0.33	0.40	0.44	0.59	0.15
Median	64.0	68.0	71.0	74.5	77.5	77.5	77.5	72.0
1997								
Mean	63.6	68.0	71.9	73.6	76.0	77.4	78.6	72.4
Standard error of the mean	0.45	0.35	0.41	0.42	0.52	0.56	0.82	0.20
Median	63.0	67.5	71.0	72.5	75.5	77.5	76.5	71.5
1998								
Mean	63.6	68.6	71.6	74.0	75.4	76.3	76.9	72.3
Standard error of the mean	0.34	0.27	0.30	0.34	0.40	0.45	0.56	0.15
Median	63.5	68.5	71.5	73.5	74.5	76.5	75.5	71.5

continued...

Table 3.58 *continued*

Systolic blood pressure (mmHg)	Age							Total
	16-24	25-34	35-44	45-54	55-64	65-74	75 +	
Bases								
Men								
1994	*710*	*1167*	*1110*	*922*	*817*	*727*	*347*	*5800*
1995	*699*	*1076*	*1112*	*939*	*803*	*749*	*420*	*5798*
1996	*741*	*1069*	*1143*	*1056*	*817*	*761*	*425*	*6012*
1997	*373*	*577*	*603*	*584*	*443*	*384*	*199*	*3163*
1998	*594*	*984*	*981*	*981*	*766*	*665*	*430*	*5401*
Women								
1994	*806*	*1278*	*1247*	*1070*	*861*	*884*	*609*	*6755*
1995	*780*	*1308*	*1224*	*1080*	*915*	*825*	*608*	*6740*
1996	*849*	*1289*	*1336*	*1224*	*900*	*879*	*642*	*7119*
1997	*405*	*683*	*682*	*659*	*484*	*446*	*333*	*3692*
1998	*692*	*1142*	*1190*	*1164*	*896*	*751*	*648*	*6483*

Table 3.59

Blood pressure level using pre-1998 definition,[a] by age and sex

Blood pressure level	Age							Total
	16-24	25-34	35-44	45-54	55-64	65-74	75 +	
	%	%	%	%	%	%	%	%
Men								
Normotensive untreated	98.7	98.2	92.4	82.6	67.6	57.4	55.1	81.6
Normotensive treated	-	0.3	1.8	5.4	11.4	13.4	13.0	5.7
Hypertensive treated	-	-	0.5	1.5	6.0	7.2	9.5	2.9
Hypertensive untreated	1.3	1.5	5.3	10.5	15.0	22.0	22.3	9.9
All with high blood pressure	*1.3*	*1.8*	*7.6*	*17.4*	*32.4*	*42.6*	*44.9*	*18.4*
Women								
Normotensive untreated	99.6	98.7	95.8	86.3	72.7	51.4	44.8	81.6
Normotensive treated	0.1	0.5	1.8	4.6	10.8	18.2	15.0	6.4
Hypertensive treated	-	-	0.6	1.6	4.7	11.7	16.8	4.1
Hypertensive untreated	0.3	0.8	1.8	7.6	11.8	18.6	23.5	8.0
All with high blood pressure	*0.4*	*1.3*	*4.2*	*13.7*	*27.3*	*48.6*	*55.2*	*18.4*
Bases								
Men	*594*	*984*	*981*	*981*	*766*	*665*	*430*	*5401*
Women	*692*	*1142*	*1190*	*1164*	*896*	*751*	*648*	*6483*

[a] Pre 1998 informants were considered hypertensive if their systolic blood pressure was 160 mmHg or over or their diastolic blood pressure was 95 mmHg or over or they were taking medicine affecting blood pressure. The definition of hypertension was changed in 1998, but this table presents 1998 data using the pre-1998 definition for comparability purposes. The new definition is presented in Table 3.60. 'Treated' means taking medication prescribed for high blood pressure.

Table 3.60

Blood pressure level using 1998 definition,[a] by age and sex

Aged 16 and over with valid blood pressure readings and data on medication — *1998*

Blood pressure level	Age							Total
	16-24	25-34	35-44	45-54	55-64	65-74	75 +	
	%	%	%	%	%	%	%	%
Men								
Normotensive untreated	84.0	79.5	73.9	57.7	40.2	30.1	27.2	59.2
Normotensive treated	-	0.1	1.2	2.8	5.1	5.4	4.9	2.5
Hypertensive treated	-	0.2	1.1	4.2	12.3	15.2	17.7	6.0
Hypertensive untreated	16.0	20.2	23.8	35.4	42.4	49.3	50.2	32.3
All with high blood pressure	*16.0*	*20.5*	*26.1*	*42.3*	*59.8*	*69.9*	*72.8*	*40.8*
Women								
Normotensive untreated	95.8	93.1	86.8	69.2	48.4	27.2	22.4	67.1
Normotensive treated	0.1	0.4	1.2	2.6	5.0	8.0	4.8	2.9
Hypertensive treated	-	0.1	1.2	3.6	10.5	22.0	27.0	7.6
Hypertensive untreated	4.0	6.4	10.8	24.6	36.0	42.9	45.8	22.5
All with high blood pressure	*4.2*	*6.9*	*13.2*	*30.8*	*51.6*	*72.8*	*77.6*	*32.9*
Bases								
Men	*594*	*984*	*981*	*981*	*766*	*665*	*430*	*5401*
Women	*692*	*1142*	*1190*	*1164*	*896*	*751*	*648*	*6483*

[a] In 1998 informants were considered hypertensive if their systolic blood pressure was 140 mmHg or over or their diastolic blood pressure was 90 mmHg or over or they were taking medicine affecting blood pressure. See Table 3.59 for the definition in use prior to 1998. 'Treated' means taking medication prescribed for high blood pressure.

Table 3.61

Blood pressure level using 1998 definition[a] (observed and age-standardised), by social class of head of household and sex

Aged 16 and over with valid blood pressure readings and data on medication — *1998*

Blood pressure level	Social class of head of household						Social class of head of household					
	I	II	IIINM	IIIM	IV	V	I	II	IIINM	IIIM	IV	V
	%	%	%	%	%	%	%	%	%	%	%	%
	Men						**Women**					
Observed												
Normotensive untreated	63.1	60.1	62.6	54.8	62.2	56.3	75.4	70.9	62.0	67.6	63.9	58.5
Normotensive treated	2.1	2.4	2.1	3.0	2.6	2.5	2.5	2.5	3.1	2.8	3.4	3.2
Hypertensive treated	5.5	5.3	5.4	7.3	5.8	6.3	4.2	5.8	10.2	7.5	8.8	8.6
Hypertensive untreated	29.4	32.3	29.9	34.9	29.4	35.0	18.0	20.9	24.8	22.1	23.9	29.7
All with high blood pressure	*36.9*	*39.9*	*37.4*	*45.2*	*37.8*	*43.8*	*24.6*	*29.1*	*38.0*	*32.4*	*36.1*	*41.5*
Standardised												
Normotensive untreated	65.7	62.0	62.8	58.2	64.8	59.8	68.6	68.7	65.6	65.8	65.6	64.1
Normotensive treated	1.9	2.1	2.1	2.7	2.2	2.1	2.7	2.7	2.7	2.8	3.2	2.7
Hypertensive treated	4.9	4.8	5.2	6.3	5.0	5.3	5.7	6.7	8.7	8.6	8.1	7.0
Hypertensive untreated	27.5	31.1	29.9	32.9	28.0	32.8	23.0	21.9	22.9	22.8	23.1	26.2
All with high blood pressure	*34.3*	*38.0*	*37.2*	*41.8*	*35.2*	*40.2*	*31.4*	*31.3*	*34.4*	*34.2*	*34.4*	*35.9*
Bases	*385*	*1686*	*522*	*1694*	*770*	*240*	*406*	*1875*	*981*	*1684*	*1008*	*347*

[a] In 1998 informants were considered hypertensive if their systolic blood pressure was 140 mmHg or over or their diastolic blood pressure was 90 mmHg or over or they were taking medicine affecting blood pressure. See Table 3.59 for the definition in use prior to 1998. 'Treated' means taking medication prescribed for high blood pressure.

Table 3.62

Blood pressure level using 1998 definition[a] (observed and age-standardised), by equivalised household income and sex

Aged 16 and over with valid blood pressure readings and data on medication
1998

Blood pressure level	Equivalised annual household income quintile				
	Up to £7,186	Over £7,186 to £10,834	Over £10,834 to £17,890	Over £17,890 to £27,705	Over £27,705
	%	%	%	%	%
Men					
Observed					
Normotensive untreated	56.1	48.5	58.7	62.9	66.6
Normotensive treated	2.3	3.5	3.1	2.7	1.5
Hypertensive treated	7.3	9.6	6.2	4.8	3.2
Hypertensive untreated	34.4	38.4	32.0	29.6	28.8
All with high blood pressure	*43.9*	*51.5*	*41.3*	*37.1*	*33.4*
Standardised					
Normotensive untreated	61.7	58.6	61.6	60.4	64.1
Normotensive treated	1.8	2.3	2.7	2.7	1.8
Hypertensive treated	5.8	6.3	5.5	5.9	4.1
Hypertensive untreated	30.6	32.7	30.2	31.0	30.0
All with high blood pressure	*38.3*	*41.4*	*38.4*	*39.6*	*35.9*
Women					
Observed					
Normotensive untreated	62.9	50.7	70.4	75.5	79.7
Normotensive treated	2.7	4.1	3.1	1.8	1.8
Hypertensive treated	8.5	14.1	7.0	5.1	2.8
Hypertensive untreated	25.9	31.1	19.5	17.7	15.7
All with high blood pressure	*37.1*	*49.3*	*29.6*	*24.5*	*20.3*
Standardised					
Normotensive untreated	62.7	64.4	67.7	67.6	69.9
Normotensive treated	2.7	3.1	3.3	2.0	3.2
Hypertensive treated	8.4	8.8	8.1	9.3	5.3
Hypertensive untreated	26.1	23.7	20.8	21.0	21.6
All with high blood pressure	*37.3*	*35.6*	*32.3*	*32.4*	*30.1*
Bases					
Men	*710*	*747*	*1129*	*1094*	*1071*
Women	*1000*	*1103*	*1308*	*1188*	*1039*

[a] In 1998 informants were considered hypertensive if their systolic blood pressure was 140 mmHg or over or their diastolic blood pressure was 90 mmHg or over or they were taking medicine affecting blood pressure. See Table 3.59 for the definition in use prior to 1998. 'Treated' means taking medication prescribed for high blood pressure.

Table 3.63

Blood pressure level using 1998 definition[a] (observed and age-standardised), by Health Authority area type and sex

Aged 16 and over with valid blood pressure readings and data on medication   *1998*

Blood pressure level	Health Authority area type					
	Inner London	Mining & Industrial	Urban	Mature	Prosperous	Rural
	%	%	%	%	%	%
Men						
Observed						
Normotensive untreated	67.4	55.1	60.3	62.4	57.3	60.4
Normotensive treated	2.1	2.4	2.3	2.8	2.8	2.2
Hypertensive treated	3.5	7.4	5.4	5.8	6.7	5.1
Hypertensive untreated	27.0	35.1	32.0	29.0	33.2	32.2
All with high blood pressure	*32.6*	*44.9*	*39.7*	*37.6*	*42.7*	*39.6*
Standardised						
Normotensive untreated	63.7	57.8	61.9	64.5	59.9	62.8
Normotensive treated	2.4	2.2	2.2	2.6	2.5	2.0
Hypertensive treated	4.4	6.5	5.0	5.1	5.9	4.5
Hypertensive untreated	29.5	33.6	30.9	27.8	31.7	30.7
All with high blood pressure	*36.3*	*42.2*	*38.1*	*35.5*	*40.1*	*37.2*
Women						
Observed						
Normotensive untreated	74.5	62.7	67.4	67.4	68.2	67.2
Normotensive treated	4.1	2.3	3.6	3.3	2.6	2.7
Hypertensive treated	5.1	8.7	6.3	8.5	7.0	8.1
Hypertensive untreated	16.3	26.3	22.7	20.7	22.2	22.1
All with high blood pressure	*25.5*	*37.3*	*32.6*	*32.6*	*31.8*	*32.8*
Standardised						
Normotensive untreated	68.1	63.9	67.6	68.1	67.6	67.2
Normotensive treated	4.5	2.2	3.5	3.3	2.6	2.7
Hypertensive treated	7.0	8.5	6.3	8.5	7.5	8.2
Hypertensive untreated	20.4	25.4	22.6	20.1	22.3	21.8
All with high blood pressure	*31.9*	*36.1*	*32.4*	*31.9*	*32.4*	*32.8*
Bases						
Men	*141*	*828*	*773*	*808*	*1501*	*1350*
Women	*196*	*972*	*981*	*960*	*1812*	*1562*

[a] In 1998 informants were considered hypertensive if their systolic blood pressure was 140 mmHg or over or their diastolic blood pressure was 90 mmHg or over or they were taking medicine affecting blood pressure. See Table 3.59 for the definition in use prior to 1998. 'Treated' means taking medication prescribed for high blood pressure.

Table 3.64

Mean arterial pressure (MAP), by age and sex

Aged 16 and over with valid blood pressure readings   *1998*

Mean arterial pressure (mmHg)	Age							Total
	16-24	25-34	35-44	45-54	55-64	65-74	75 +	
Men								
Mean	87.5	92.3	96.4	101.3	105.4	107.0	106.1	98.9
Standard error of the mean	0.39	0.31	0.36	0.42	0.54	0.57	0.71	0.19
5th percentile	72.9	77.5	80.0	82.0	83.0	83.0	82.5	78.5
10th percentile	76.0	80.0	83.0	85.5	86.0	87.5	87.1	82.5
Median	87.0	92.0	95.0	100.5	105.0	107.0	105.3	97.5
90th percentile	99.5	104.0	110.9	118.5	124.5	125.5	126.0	118.0
95th percentile	104.0	109.0	117.0	124.0	131.5	130.4	130.0	124.5
Women								
Mean	84.9	87.8	91.6	96.8	101.2	104.6	106.1	95.4
Standard error of the mean	0.33	0.29	0.33	0.40	0.48	0.53	0.66	0.18
5th percentile	71.0	73.0	74.5	76.5	79.9	81.0	81.0	75.0
10th percentile	73.5	76.0	77.5	80.5	83.5	86.1	86.0	78.5
Median	84.5	87.0	91.0	95.3	100.5	104.5	105.3	93.5
90th percentile	96.9	100.5	106.0	115.0	118.0	123.4	128.5	115.0
95th percentile	100.0	105.0	112.7	122.0	128.0	129.0	135.0	121.9
Bases								
Men	*594*	*984*	*981*	*981*	*766*	*665*	*430*	*5401*
Women	*692*	*1142*	*1190*	*1164*	*896*	*751*	*648*	*6483*

Table 3.65

Pulse pressure, by age and sex

Aged 16 and over with valid blood pressure readings   *1998*

Pulse pressure (mmHg)	Age							Total
	16-24	25-34	35-44	45-54	55-64	65-74	75 +	
Men								
Mean	65.7	59.9	54.7	55.4	60.1	66.7	71.6	60.6
Standard error of the mean	0.41	0.31	0.30	0.31	0.48	0.57	0.78	0.17
5th percentile	48.9	44.5	40.5	39.6	40.5	44.5	45.5	42.0
10th percentile	53.0	47.5	43.0	43.5	44.5	49.0	52.0	45.6
Median	65.5	59.5	54.0	54.5	59.5	65.5	71.8	59.5
90th percentile	79.0	73.0	67.5	68.5	77.2	85.5	91.5	77.0
95th percentile	83.1	77.5	71.0	72.5	83.3	92.9	101.0	83.0
Women								
Mean	56.4	51.9	51.8	57.7	64.7	72.8	78.5	60.3
Standard error of the mean	0.35	0.26	0.27	0.36	0.48	0.58	0.69	0.19
5th percentile	42.5	38.0	38.5	40.0	43.5	48.5	51.0	40.0
10th percentile	45.0	41.0	40.5	43.0	47.0	54.0	58.0	43.5
Median	56.0	51.5	50.5	57.0	64.0	71.0	77.0	58.0
90th percentile	68.0	63.0	63.5	73.0	82.5	94.0	102.1	80.5
95th percentile	71.7	66.0	68.5	79.4	90.5	101.0	109.5	90.5
Bases								
Men	*594*	*984*	*981*	*981*	*766*	*665*	*430*	*5401*
Women	*692*	*1142*	*1190*	*1164*	*896*	*751*	*648*	*6483*

Table 3.66

Blood pressure level using 1998 definition[a] (observed and age-standardised), by region and sex

Aged 16 and over with valid blood pressure readings and data on medication — 1998

Blood pressure level	Region							
	Northern & Yorkshire	North West	Trent	West Midlands	Anglia & Oxford	North Thames	South Thames	South & West
	%	%	%	%	%	%	%	%
Men								
Observed								
Normotensive untreated	54.5	63.7	58.8	58.0	61.2	60.6	59.8	57.8
Normotensive treated	2.4	2.4	1.9	2.4	3.8	2.8	2.4	2.1
Hypertensive treated	6.3	6.6	5.5	6.9	4.2	6.4	7.2	5.3
Hypertensive untreated	36.8	27.3	33.8	32.7	30.8	30.2	30.6	34.8
All with high blood pressure	*45.5*	*36.3*	*41.2*	*42.0*	*38.8*	*39.4*	*40.2*	*42.2*
Standardised								
Normotensive untreated	57.0	64.9	61.6	60.8	61.7	63.5	61.5	61.0
Normotensive treated	2.2	2.3	1.7	2.1	3.8	2.6	2.2	1.9
Hypertensive treated	5.5	6.2	4.8	5.9	4.1	5.5	6.7	4.5
Hypertensive untreated	35.3	26.6	31.9	31.2	30.4	28.4	29.6	32.7
All with high blood pressure	*43.0*	*35.1*	*38.4*	*39.2*	*38.3*	*36.5*	*38.5*	*39.0*
Women								
Observed								
Normotensive untreated	61.8	70.1	66.9	67.2	68.8	69.7	68.8	64.7
Normotensive treated	2.6	2.5	2.9	3.6	1.9	3.5	3.3	2.8
Hypertensive treated	8.4	7.1	7.0	6.2	8.0	8.7	7.4	7.6
Hypertensive untreated	27.2	20.3	23.3	23.0	21.4	18.1	20.5	24.9
All with high blood pressure	*38.2*	*29.9*	*33.1*	*32.8*	*31.2*	*30.3*	*31.2*	*35.3*
Standardised								
Normotensive untreated	64.0	69.4	67.1	67.6	66.2	68.8	67.6	65.8
Normotensive treated	2.4	2.5	2.9	3.4	2.1	3.4	3.4	2.7
Hypertensive treated	7.7	7.3	7.0	6.2	9.2	9.2	8.0	7.4
Hypertensive untreated	25.9	20.8	23.0	22.7	22.6	18.5	21.0	24.1
All with high blood pressure	*36.0*	*30.6*	*32.9*	*32.4*	*33.8*	*31.2*	*32.4*	*34.2*
Bases								
Men	*783*	*700*	*622*	*548*	*624*	*597*	*679*	*848*
Women	*944*	*847*	*718*	*647*	*701*	*745*	*917*	*964*

[a] In 1998 informants were considered hypertensive if their systolic blood pressure was 140 mmHg or over or their diastolic blood pressure was 90 mmHg or over or they were taking medicine affecting blood pressure. See Table 3.59 for the definition in use prior to 1998. 'Treated' means taking medication prescribed for high blood pressure.

Table 3.67

Response to blood sample, by age and sex

Aged 16 and over who had a nurse visit   1998

Response to blood sample	Men			Total	Women			Total
	16-44	45-64	65 +		16-44	45-64	65 +	
	%	%	%	%	%	%	%	%
Blood obtained	81	87	85	84	72	85	80	78
Consent given, no blood obtained	4	3	5	4	7	5	5	6
Ineligible[a]	5	4	6	5	10	3	6	7
Refused	10	6	5	8	11	7	10	10
Bases	*2959*	*1996*	*1210*	*6165*	*3584*	*2296*	*1541*	*7421*

[a] Pregnant or on anticoagulant drugs.

Table 3.68

Percentages providing valid samples for each analyte, by age and sex

Aged 16 and over who had a nurse visit   1998

Blood analytes	Men			Total	Women			Total
	16-44	45-64	65 +		16-44	45-64	65 +	
	%	%	%	%	%	%	%	%
Total cholesterol	77	81	80	79	69	80	73	74
HDL-cholesterol	77	80	80	79	69	80	73	73
C-reactive protein	77	84	83	80	69	82	76	74
Fibrinogen	74	74	68	73	65	73	61	66
Bases	*2959*	*1996*	*1210*	*6165*	*3584*	*2296*	*1541*	*7421*

Table 3.69

Total cholesterol, 1994 and 1998, by age and sex

Aged 16 and over with a valid sample   *1994,1998*

Total cholesterol (mmol/l)	Age							Total
	16-24	25-34	35-44	45-54	55-64	65-74	75 +	
Men								
1994								
Mean	4.7	5.3	6.0	6.3	6.2	6.2	5.9	5.8
Standard error of the mean	0.04	0.03	0.03	0.04	0.04	0.05	0.07	0.02
5th percentile	3.4	3.7	4.3	4.5	4.5	4.4	4.1	3.9
10th percentile	3.6	4.1	4.6	4.8	4.9	4.8	4.4	4.3
Median	4.6	5.3	5.9	6.2	6.2	6.1	5.9	5.7
90th percentile	5.9	6.8	7.5	7.8	7.7	7.8	7.4	7.4
95th percentile	6.3	7.3	8.0	8.4	8.1	8.2	8.1	8.0
% ≥6.5 mmol/l	3.6	14.7	30.9	39.3	40.7	38.3	30.1	27.9
1998								
Mean	4.4	5.1	5.5	5.8	5.8	5.8	5.5	5.5
Standard error of the mean	0.04	0.03	0.03	0.03	0.04	0.05	0.05	0.02
5th percentile	3.2	3.6	3.9	4.2	4.3	4.1	3.9	3.7
10th percentile	3.4	3.9	4.3	4.5	4.6	4.4	4.2	4.1
Median	4.3	5.0	5.4	5.7	5.8	5.8	5.5	5.4
90th percentile	5.5	6.5	6.9	7.2	7.1	7.2	6.9	6.9
95th percentile	5.8	7.0	7.3	7.6	7.6	7.6	7.3	7.3
% ≥6.5 mmol/l	1.9	10.8	16.9	23.8	22.9	26.4	20.2	18.0
Women								
1994								
Mean	4.9	5.2	5.5	6.1	6.8	7.0	6.8	6.0
Standard error of the mean	0.04	0.03	0.03	0.04	0.04	0.04	0.06	0.02
5th percentile	3.6	3.8	3.9	4.4	4.9	5.1	4.8	4.0
10th percentile	3.8	4.0	4.4	4.7	5.4	5.5	5.1	4.4
Median	4.8	5.1	5.4	6.0	6.7	7.0	6.7	5.8
90th percentile	6.1	6.4	6.7	7.5	8.5	8.5	8.5	7.8
95th percentile	6.4	7.0	7.2	8.0	9.0	9.1	9.0	8.4
% ≥6.5 mmol/l	4.8	9.8	13.4	32.2	57.4	67.4	57.6	31.9
1998								
Mean	4.6	4.9	5.2	5.7	6.2	6.5	6.3	5.6
Standard error of the mean	0.04	0.03	0.03	0.03	0.04	0.05	0.05	0.02
5th percentile	3.4	3.6	3.9	4.1	4.5	4.6	4.5	3.9
10th percentile	3.6	3.9	4.1	4.5	4.9	5.0	4.9	4.1
Median	4.5	4.8	5.1	5.5	6.1	6.4	6.3	5.5
90th percentile	5.7	6.2	6.4	7.1	7.6	8.0	7.8	7.2
95th percentile	6.0	6.6	6.8	7.5	8.0	8.6	8.2	7.7
% ≥6.5 mmol/l	2.9	6.7	8.8	22.2	37.4	48.0	44.4	22.4
Bases								
Men								
1994	*635*	*1090*	*1069*	*856*	*755*	*634*	*306*	*5345*
1998	*423*	*910*	*960*	*937*	*673*	*584*	*387*	*4874*
Women								
1994	*588*	*1097*	*1104*	*967*	*765*	*786*	*510*	*5817*
1998	*450*	*967*	*1067*	*1080*	*764*	*594*	*536*	*5458*

Table 3.70

Total cholesterol (observed and age-standardised), by social class of head of household and sex

Aged 16 and over with a valid sample

1998

Total cholesterol (mmol/l)	Social class of head of household							Social class of head of household					
	I	II	IIINM	IIIM	IV	V		I	II	IIINM	IIIM	IV	V
	Men							**Women**					
Observed													
Mean	5.5	5.5	5.4	5.5	5.4	5.5		5.4	5.6	5.6	5.6	5.6	5.7
Standard error of the mean	0.06	0.03	0.05	0.03	0.04	0.08		0.07	0.03	0.04	0.03	0.04	0.07
5th percentile	4.0	3.8	3.6	3.7	3.7	3.8		3.8	3.9	3.9	3.8	3.9	3.9
10th percentile	4.2	4.1	3.9	4.1	4.0	4.0		4.0	4.2	4.2	4.1	4.1	4.2
Median	5.4	5.5	5.3	5.5	5.3	5.4		5.3	5.4	5.5	5.4	5.5	5.5
90th percentile	6.9	6.9	7.0	6.9	6.8	6.8		6.9	7.1	7.3	7.1	7.2	7.4
95th percentile	7.4	7.4	7.4	7.3	7.2	7.4		7.6	7.6	7.9	7.6	7.8	7.8
% ≥6.5 mmol/l	15.7	17.9	21.1	19.0	15.1	19.5		5.6	5.6	5.5	5.6	5.6	5.6
Standardised													
Mean	5.4	5.4	5.5	5.4	5.3	5.5		16.7	21.2	23.2	22.9	24.2	25.6
Standard error of the mean	0.06	0.03	0.05	0.03	0.04	0.09		0.07	0.03	0.04	0.03	0.04	0.07
% ≥6.5 mmol/l	14.5	16.6	21.2	17.9	14.7	19.8		22.2	22.6	21.2	23.7	23.3	22.6
Bases	*338*	*1539*	*470*	*1540*	*694*	*210*		*323*	*1610*	*836*	*1420*	*831*	*293*

Table 3.71

**Total cholesterol (observed and age-standardised),
by equivalised household income and sex**

Aged 16 and over with a valid sample   *1998*

Total cholesterol (mmol/l)	Equivalised annual household income quintile				
	Up to £7,186	Over £7,186 to £10,834	Over £10,834 to £17,890	Over £17,890 to £27,705	Over £27,705
Men					
Observed					
Mean	5.5	5.5	5.4	5.5	5.5
Standard error of the mean	0.05	0.04	0.03	0.04	0.03
5th percentile	3.6	3.7	3.8	3.7	3.9
10th percentile	4.0	4.1	4.1	4.1	4.2
Median	5.4	5.5	5.4	5.4	5.4
90th percentile	7.0	6.9	6.8	6.9	6.9
95th percentile	7.5	7.4	7.2	7.3	7.4
% ≥6.5 mmol/l	20.9	20.6	16.7	16.4	17.5
Standardised					
Mean	5.5	5.4	5.4	5.4	5.4
Standard error of the mean	0.05	0.04	0.04	0.04	0.04
% ≥6.5 mmol/l	20.5	18.4	15.3	16.0	16.8
Women					
Observed					
Mean	5.6	5.9	5.5	5.4	5.4
Standard error of the mean	0.04	0.04	0.03	0.04	0.04
5th percentile	3.8	3.9	3.8	3.8	3.8
10th percentile	4.1	4.3	4.1	4.1	4.1
Median	5.5	5.9	5.4	5.2	5.3
90th percentile	7.2	7.6	7.0	6.9	6.9
95th percentile	7.5	8.1	7.6	7.5	7.4
% ≥6.5 mmol/l	22.5	33.1	20.0	17.7	15.9
Standardised					
Mean	5.6	5.7	5.5	5.5	5.7
Standard error of the mean	0.04	0.04	0.04	0.04	0.04
% ≥6.5 mmol/l	22.9	25.7	20.9	21.5	26.0
Bases					
Men	*611*	*666*	*1023*	*992*	*1002*
Women	*819*	*912*	*1118*	*997*	*920*

Table 3.72

Total cholesterol (observed and age-standardised), by Health Authority area type and sex

Aged 16 and over with a valid sample   *1998*

Total cholesterol (mmol/l)	Health Authority area type					
	Inner London	Mining & Industrial	Urban	Mature	Prosperous	Rural
Men						
Observed						
Mean	5.4	5.5	5.5	5.4	5.5	5.4
Standard error of the mean	0.11	0.04	0.04	0.04	0.03	0.03
5th percentile	3.3	3.8	3.8	3.7	3.8	3.8
10th percentile	3.8	4.1	4.1	4.0	4.1	4.1
Median	5.3	5.5	5.5	5.3	5.4	5.4
90th percentile	7.0	6.9	7.0	6.8	7.0	6.8
95th percentile	7.3	7.5	7.4	7.2	7.4	7.2
% ≥6.5 mmol/l	17.7	19.5	20.4	16.3	18.6	16.1
Standardised						
Mean	5.3	5.5	5.5	5.3	5.4	5.4
Standard error of the mean	0.11	0.04	0.04	0.04	0.03	0.03
% ≥6.5 mmol/l	16.8	18.5	19.4	15.2	17.3	14.9
Women						
Observed						
Mean	5.3	5.6	5.5	5.6	5.5	5.6
Standard error of the mean	0.10	0.04	0.04	0.04	0.03	0.03
5th percentile	3.6	3.9	3.8	3.9	3.8	3.9
10th percentile	4.0	4.1	4.1	4.1	4.1	4.2
Median	5.1	5.5	5.5	5.5	5.4	5.5
90th percentile	7.1	7.2	7.2	7.2	7.0	7.3
95th percentile	7.6	7.7	7.6	7.8	7.6	7.7
% ≥6.5 mmol/l	12.3	25.3	21.6	22.5	21.6	23.0
Standardised						
Mean	5.2	5.6	5.5	5.6	5.5	5.6
Standard error of the mean	0.09	0.04	0.04	0.04	0.03	0.03
% ≥6.5 mmol/l	11.3	24.9	21.4	23.2	21.9	24.2
Bases						
Men	*124*	*755*	*697*	*712*	*1396*	*1190*
Women	*154*	*826*	*801*	*791*	*1567*	*1319*

Table 3.73

HDL-cholesterol, by age and sex

Aged 16 and over with a valid sample   1998

HDL-cholesterol (mmol/l)	Age							Total
	16-24	25-34	35-44	45-54	55-64	65-74	75 +	
Men								
Mean	1.3	1.3	1.3	1.3	1.3	1.3	1.3	1.3
Standard error of the mean	0.02	0.01	0.01	0.01	0.01	0.02	0.02	0.01
5th percentile	0.8	0.8	0.8	0.8	0.8	0.7	0.8	0.8
10th percentile	0.9	0.9	0.9	0.9	0.9	0.9	0.9	0.9
Median	1.3	1.3	1.3	1.2	1.2	1.2	1.3	1.3
90th percentile	1.7	1.7	1.8	1.8	1.8	1.7	1.8	1.8
95th percentile	1.9	1.9	1.9	2.0	1.9	1.9	2.1	1.9
% ≤0.9 mmol/l	13.0	16.8	16.2	17.3	19.0	19.2	14.7	16.9
Women								
Mean	1.5	1.5	1.5	1.6	1.6	1.5	1.6	1.6
Standard error of the mean	0.03	0.01	0.01	0.01	0.02	0.02	0.02	0.01
5th percentile	1.0	0.9	0.9	0.9	0.9	0.9	1.0	0.9
10th percentile	1.1	1.1	1.1	1.1	1.1	1.0	1.1	1.1
Median	1.5	1.5	1.5	1.5	1.5	1.5	1.5	1.5
90th percentile	2.0	2.0	2.1	2.2	2.1	2.1	2.2	2.1
95th percentile	2.1	2.2	2.2	2.4	2.3	2.3	2.3	2.3
% ≤0.9 mmol/l	4.2	6.1	5.5	5.4	5.2	6.9	3.5	5.4
Bases								
Men	*422*	*907*	*958*	*935*	*670*	*583*	*387*	*4862*
Women	*450*	*963*	*1063*	*1077*	*762*	*591*	*536*	*5442*

Table 3.74

HDL-cholesterol (observed and age-standardised), by social class of head of household and sex

Aged 16 and over with a valid sample   1998

HDL-cholesterol (mmol/l)	Social class of head of household							Social class of head of household					
	I	II	IIINM	IIIM	IV	V		I	II	IIINM	IIIM	IV	V
	Men							**Women**					
Observed													
Mean	1.3	1.3	1.3	1.3	1.3	1.3		1.6	1.6	1.6	1.5	1.5	1.5
Standard error of the mean	0.02	0.01	0.02	0.01	0.01	0.03		0.03	0.01	0.02	0.01	0.01	0.02
5th percentile	0.7	0.8	0.8	0.8	0.8	0.8		1.0	1.0	1.0	0.9	0.9	0.9
10th percentile	0.8	0.9	0.9	0.9	0.9	0.9		1.2	1.1	1.1	1.1	1.0	1.0
Median	1.3	1.3	1.3	1.2	1.3	1.2		1.6	1.6	1.5	1.5	1.5	1.4
90th percentile	1.9	1.8	1.7	1.7	1.8	1.9		2.2	2.1	2.1	2.1	2.0	2.0
95th percentile	2.1	1.9	1.9	1.9	1.9	2.1		2.5	2.3	2.3	2.2	2.3	2.2
% ≤0.9 mmol/l	16.9	15.5	18.2	19.0	15.2	14.4		3.4	3.9	4.9	6.4	6.3	8.2
Standardised													
Mean	1.3	1.3	1.3	1.3	1.3	1.3		1.7	1.6	1.6	1.5	1.5	1.5
Standard error of the mean	0.02	0.01	0.02	0.01	0.01	0.03		0.03	0.01	0.02	0.01	0.01	0.02
% ≤0.9 mmol/l	16.3	15.4	18.1	18.8	15.2	14.1		3.4	4.0	4.9	6.4	6.2	8.5
Bases	*338*	*1535*	*467*	*1539*	*691*	*209*		*323*	*1606*	*831*	*1416*	*830*	*292*

Table 3.75

HDL-cholesterol (observed and age-standardised), by equivalised household income and sex

Aged 16 and over with a valid sample   *1998*

HDL-cholesterol (mmol/l)	Equivalised annual household income quintile				
	Up to £7,186	Over £7,186 to £10,834	Over £10,834 to £17,890	Over £17,890 to £27,705	Over £27,705
Men					
Observed					
Mean	1.2	1.3	1.3	1.3	1.3
Standard error of the mean	0.01	0.01	0.01	0.01	0.01
5th percentile	0.7	0.8	0.8	0.8	0.8
10th percentile	0.8	0.8	0.9	0.9	0.9
Median	1.2	1.2	1.2	1.3	1.3
90th percentile	1.7	1.7	1.8	1.8	1.8
95th percentile	1.9	1.9	1.9	2.0	2.0
% ≤0.9 mmol/l	18.7	18.8	19.6	15.2	14.6
Standardised					
Mean	1.2	1.3	1.3	1.3	1.3
Standard error of the mean	0.01	0.01	0.01	0.01	0.01
% ≤0.9 mmol/l	19.2	19.0	19.6	14.8	14.9
Women					
Observed					
Mean	1.5	1.5	1.5	1.6	1.7
Standard error of the mean	0.01	0.01	0.02	0.01	0.01
5th percentile	0.9	0.9	0.9	1.0	1.1
10th percentile	1.0	1.0	1.0	1.1	1.2
Median	1.4	1.5	1.5	1.5	1.6
90th percentile	2.0	2.1	2.1	2.1	2.2
95th percentile	2.2	2.3	2.2	2.3	2.4
% ≤0.9 mmol/l	8.0	6.8	6.6	3.9	2.4
Standardised					
Mean	1.5	1.5	1.6	1.6	1.7
Standard error of the mean	0.01	0.01	0.02	0.01	0.01
% ≤0.9 mmol/l	7.9	7.8	6.3	4.2	2.9
Bases					
Men	*610*	*664*	*1018*	*993*	*999*
Women	*816*	*910*	*1113*	*993*	*919*

Table 3.76

HDL-cholesterol (observed and age-standardised), by Health Authority area type and sex

Aged 16 and over with a valid sample   *1998*

HDL-cholesterol (mmol/l)	Health Authority area type					
	Inner London	Mining & Industrial	Urban	Mature	Prosperous	Rural
Men						
Observed						
Mean	1.3	1.3	1.3	1.3	1.3	1.3
Standard error of the mean	0.04	0.01	0.01	0.01	0.01	0.01
5th percentile	0.7	0.8	0.8	0.8	0.8	0.8
10th percentile	0.9	0.9	0.8	0.9	0.8	0.9
Median	1.2	1.2	1.2	1.3	1.3	1.2
90th percentile	1.9	1.8	1.8	1.8	1.8	1.7
95th percentile	2.3	2.0	2.0	1.9	2.0	1.9
% ≤0.9 mmol/l	17.1	18.0	18.7	13.9	17.8	15.7
Standardised						
Mean	1.3	1.3	1.3	1.3	1.3	1.3
Standard error of the mean	0.04	0.01	0.01	0.01	0.01	0.01
% ≤0.9 mmol/l	16.1	17.8	18.1	14.0	17.7	15.4
Women						
Observed						
Mean	1.6	1.5	1.5	1.6	1.6	1.6
Standard error of the mean	0.04	0.01	0.02	0.01	0.01	0.01
5th percentile	0.9	0.9	0.9	1.0	1.0	0.9
10th percentile	1.1	1.1	1.1	1.1	1.1	1.1
Median	1.6	1.5	1.5	1.5	1.5	1.5
90th percentile	2.2	2.1	2.1	2.1	2.1	2.1
95th percentile	2.3	2.2	2.3	2.3	2.3	2.3
% ≤0.9 mmol/l	6.5	6.2	7.0	4.3	4.8	5.2
Standardised						
Mean	1.6	1.5	1.5	1.6	1.6	1.6
Standard error of the mean	0.03	0.01	0.01	0.01	0.01	0.01
% ≤0.9 mmol/ll	7.2	5.9	6.7	4.2	5.0	5.5
Bases						
Men	*123*	*750*	*696*	*711*	*1396*	*1186*
Women	*153*	*824*	*799*	*788*	*1562*	*1316*

Table 3.77

C-reactive protein, by age and sex

Aged 16 and over with a valid sample | | | | | | | *1998*

C-reactive protein (mg/l)	Age							Total
	16-24	25-34	35-44	45-54	55-64	65-74	75 +	
Men								
Mean	1.3	2.1	1.9	2.6	3.6	5.0	6.7	3.0
Standard error of the mean	0.13	0.17	0.09	0.13	0.22	0.38	0.53	0.09
≤0.5[a]	46.6	34.7	29.4	21.1	11.9	7.9	5.4	23.1
0.6-1.0	21.1	21.0	22.4	19.2	17.7	13.9	13.1	19.0
1.1-1.9	14.5	20.8	21.0	20.4	21.2	20.0	16.2	19.8
2.0-3.7	10.3	12.6	15.3	20.6	23.3	22.3	23.4	18.1
>3.7	7.6	10.9	11.9	18.8	25.9	35.9	41.9	20.0
Women								
Mean	2.6	3.1	2.8	3.3	4.0	4.8	5.3	3.6
Standard error of the mean	0.26	0.16	0.17	0.18	0.22	0.26	0.40	0.08
≤0.5[a]	31.5	27.6	28.7	19.9	13.9	6.7	8.5	20.4
0.6-1.2	22.6	20.1	25.7	23.5	19.3	15.8	17.2	21.2
1.3-2.4	17.4	17.7	16.5	21.2	22.2	22.0	20.1	19.5
2.5-4.9	15.9	18.0	13.7	19.2	20.2	26.2	26.8	19.4
>4.9	12.5	16.6	15.3	16.3	24.2	29.3	27.5	19.6
Bases								
Men	*408*	*902*	*959*	*953*	*717*	*610*	*389*	*4938*
Women	*447*	*950*	*1062*	*1078*	*796*	*627*	*542*	*5502*

[a] These values correspond to the quintiles, specific for men and women.

Table 3.78

C-reactive protein (observed and age-standardised), by social class of head of household and sex

Aged 16 and over with a valid sample   *1998*

C-reactive protein (mg/l)	Social class of head of household						Social class of head of household					
	I	II	IIINM	IIIM	IV	V	I	II	IIINM	IIIM	IV	V
	Men						**Women**					
Observed												
Mean	2.4	2.8	3.1	3.4	3.3	2.4	3.7	3.4	3.4	3.4	4.1	4.1
Standard error of the mean	0.24	0.14	0.28	0.17	0.25	0.24	0.42	0.17	0.19	0.13	0.21	0.44
≤0.5 (≤0.5)[a]	25.8	24.4	27.0	20.8	22.5	20.3	28.7	22.7	19.4	19.0	16.7	18.9
0.6-1.0 (0.6-1.2)	21.2	18.4	16.9	18.9	19.0	22.6	20.8	21.4	24.1	21.3	19.3	16.9
1.1-1.9 (1.3-1.4)	20.6	21.0	17.7	19.2	19.5	18.9	16.2	20.7	18.1	19.9	18.8	22.3
2.0-3.7 (2.5-4.9)	17.4	18.1	19.2	18.3	17.0	17.5	15.3	19.3	19.7	19.1	20.7	20.3
>3.7 (>4.9)	15.1	18.1	19.2	22.7	22.0	20.8	19.0	15.9	18.6	20.8	24.5	21.6
Standardised												
Mean	2.3	2.7	3.0	3.1	3.0	2.3	4.0	3.5	3.3	3.5	4.1	3.9
Standard error of the mean	0.23	0.14	0.26	0.16	0.23	0.22	0.45	0.18	0.18	0.13	0.21	0.43
≤0.5 (≤0.5)[a]	26.6	25.8	26.9	22.9	24.0	21.7	26.8	21.7	20.4	18.6	17.1	20.0
0.6-1.0 (0.6-1.2)	21.3	18.3	17.2	19.4	19.5	23.4	19.7	20.8	24.8	21.0	19.4	18.5
1.1-1.9 (1.3-1.4)	20.9	20.9	17.7	19.1	19.4	18.8	18.1	20.5	18.1	20.0	18.7	21.2
2.0-3.7 (2.5-4.9)	17.1	17.6	19.5	17.4	16.8	16.7	15.5	20.3	18.5	19.1	20.6	19.6
>3.7 (>4.9)	14.0	17.3	18.8	21.2	20.3	19.5	19.9	16.7	18.2	21.3	24.2	20.8
Bases	*345*	*1554*	*474*	*1570*	*699*	*212*	*327*	*1611*	*849*	*1435*	*836*	*301*

[a] These values correspond to the quintiles, specific for men (unbracketed) and women (bracketed).

Table 3.79

C-reactive protein (observed and age-standardised),
by equivalised household income and sex

Aged 16 and over with a valid sample   *1998*

C-reactive protein (mg/l)	Equivalised annual household income quintile				
	Up to £7,186	Over £7,186 to £10,834	Over £10,834 to £17,890	Over £17,890 to £27,705	Over £27,705
Men					
Observed					
Mean	3.5	4.3	3.3	2.6	2.0
Standard error of the mean	0.26	0.27	0.24	0.14	0.12
≤0.5[a]	19.1	14.5	22.9	25.7	30.9
0.6-1.0	17.6	16.8	18.1	18.6	21.1
1.1-1.9	17.6	17.2	20.9	21.7	19.3
2.0-3.7	19.6	19.7	17.9	18.2	16.0
>3.7	26.1	31.8	20.2	15.8	12.7
Standardised					
Mean	3.2	3.6	3.1	2.6	2.1
Standard error of the mean	0.22	0.24	0.23	0.14	0.12
≤0.5[a]	21.9	19.1	24.7	25.1	29.8
0.6-1.0	18.9	18.1	18.4	18.3	21.3
1.1-1.9	17.2	17.0	20.6	22.1	19.7
2.0-3.7	18.2	19.3	17.2	18.2	15.8
>3.7	23.7	26.5	19.2	16.3	13.4
Women					
Observed					
Mean	3.7	4.2	3.5	3.2	2.9
Standard error of the mean	0.19	0.22	0.18	0.18	0.19
≤0.5[a]	17.0	15.2	21.9	22.4	26.3
0.6-1.2	21.2	19.5	19.7	23.3	23.3
1.3-2.4	18.1	20.9	19.6	19.0	19.5
2.5-4.9	20.9	19.7	19.3	18.4	16.8
>4.9	22.9	24.7	19.5	16.7	14.1
Standardised					
Mean	3.8	3.9	3.7	3.6	3.5
Standard error of the mean	0.19	0.22	0.20	0.21	0.23
≤0.5[a]	16.9	18.5	21.7	20.1	23.0
0.6-1.2	20.9	20.7	19.3	23.0	22.8
1.3-2.4	18.4	19.9	19.1	19.3	18.6
2.5-4.9	20.5	19.1	19.8	19.9	19.1
>4.9	23.3	21.7	20.1	17.8	16.5
Bases					
Men	*624*	*674*	*1036*	*1000*	*1010*
Women	*831*	*928*	*1128*	*1003*	*913*

[a] These values correspond to the quintiles, specific for men and women.

Table 3.80

C-reactive protein (observed and age-standardised), by Health Authority area type and sex

Aged 16 and over with a valid sample *1998*

C-reactive protein (mg/l)	Health Authority area type					
	Inner London	Mining & Industrial	Urban	Mature	Prosperous	Rural
Men						
Observed						
Mean	2.1	3.1	3.3	2.9	2.8	3.2
Standard error of the mean	0.34	0.19	0.26	0.23	0.15	0.19
≤0.5[a]	29.0	19.7	22.0	24.7	24.9	22.2
0.6-1.0	28.2	16.8	18.7	18.9	19.5	18.8
1.1-1.9	12.9	21.1	21.1	20.2	19.3	19.3
2.0-3.7	16.1	19.6	16.1	17.8	17.4	19.5
>3.7	13.7	22.8	22.1	18.4	18.9	20.1
Standardised						
Mean	2.0	2.9	3.1	2.8	2.6	3.0
Standard error of the mean	0.31	0.18	0.25	0.22	0.14	0.18
≤0.5[a]	30.5	21.0	23.9	26.2	26.8	24.2
0.6-1.0	28.8	17.3	19.3	19.4	19.3	19.1
1.1-1.9	13.4	21.0	20.6	19.6	19.4	19.1
2.0-3.7	15.0	19.3	15.9	17.1	16.8	18.8
>3.7	12.2	21.4	20.4	17.7	17.7	18.7
Women						
Observed						
Mean	3.0	3.8	3.7	3.1	3.8	3.5
Standard error of the mean	0.36	0.22	0.23	0.18	0.17	0.16
≤0.5[a]	24.0	19.7	20.1	19.2	20.6	21.0
0.6-1.2	24.7	20.9	20.2	22.2	22.2	19.6
1.3-2.4	17.5	17.5	20.0	20.5	19.5	20.1
2.5-4.9	16.9	21.2	18.6	21.6	17.2	20.2
>4.9	16.9	20.7	21.1	16.5	20.5	19.2
Standardised						
Mean	3.0	3.7	3.7	3.2	3.9	3.6
Standard error of the mean	0.35	0.22	0.23	0.19	0.18	0.17
≤0.5[a]	23.8	19.5	19.9	19.0	20.3	20.7
0.6-1.2	24.8	20.6	20.8	22.3	22.2	19.4
1.3-2.4	17.3	18.3	19.8	20.1	19.2	19.9
2.5-4.9	17.4	21.2	18.2	21.9	17.2	20.3
>4.9	16.7	20.4	21.3	16.8	21.1	19.6
Bases						
Men	*124*	*762*	*706*	*718*	*1423*	*1205*
Women	*154*	*832*	*811*	*790*	*1584*	*1331*

[a] These values correspond to the quintiles, specific for men and women.

Table 3.81

Fibrinogen, by age and sex

Aged 16 and over with a valid sample   *1998*

Fibrinogen (g/l)	Age							Total
	16-24	25-34	35-44	45-54	55-64	65-74	75 +	
Men								
Mean	2.2	2.3	2.4	2.6	2.8	3.0	3.1	2.6
Standard error of the mean	0.02	0.02	0.02	0.02	0.03	0.03	0.04	0.01
Geometric mean	2.1	2.2	2.4	2.5	2.7	3.0	3.1	2.5
5th percentile	1.5	1.5	1.6	1.7	1.9	2.0	2.1	1.7
10th percentile	1.6	1.7	1.8	1.9	2.0	2.2	2.3	1.8
Median	2.1	2.2	2.4	2.5	2.7	3.0	3.1	2.5
90th percentile	2.8	3.1	3.2	3.4	3.7	4.0	4.1	3.5
95th percentile	3.0	3.3	3.6	3.7	4.0	4.3	4.5	3.8
Women								
Mean	2.5	2.6	2.6	2.7	2.9	3.1	3.2	2.8
Standard error of the mean	0.03	0.02	0.02	0.02	0.03	0.04	0.04	0.01
Geometric mean	2.5	2.5	2.5	2.7	2.9	3.0	3.1	2.7
5th percentile	1.7	1.7	1.8	1.8	2.0	2.1	2.0	1.8
10th percentile	1.8	1.8	1.9	2.0	2.1	2.3	2.3	2.0
Median	2.5	2.5	2.5	2.6	2.9	3.1	3.1	2.7
90th percentile	3.3	3.5	3.4	3.5	3.8	4.0	4.0	3.7
95th percentile	3.8	3.8	3.9	3.9	4.2	4.6	4.4	4.0
Bases								
Men	*386*	*869*	*927*	*868*	*603*	*495*	*332*	*4480*
Women	*411*	*914*	*994*	*985*	*685*	*509*	*428*	*4926*

Table 3.82

Fibrinogen (observed and age-standardised), by social class of head of household and sex

Aged 16 and over with a valid sample   *1998*

Fibrinogen (g/l)	Social class of head of household						Social class of head of household					
	I	II	IIINM	IIIM	IV	V	I	II	IIINM	IIIM	IV	V
	Men						**Women**					
Observed												
Mean	2.5	2.5	2.5	2.6	2.6	2.6	2.7	2.7	2.8	2.8	2.8	2.9
Standard error of the mean	0.04	0.02	0.03	0.02	0.03	0.04	0.04	0.02	0.03	0.02	0.02	0.05
Geometric mean	2.4	2.5	2.4	2.5	2.5	2.6	2.6	2.6	2.7	2.7	2.7	2.8
5th percentile	1.6	1.6	1.6	1.7	1.7	1.8	1.8	1.8	1.8	1.8	1.9	1.8
10th percentile	1.8	1.8	1.8	1.8	1.9	1.9	1.9	2.0	2.0	2.0	2.0	2.0
Median	2.4	2.4	2.4	2.6	2.5	2.6	2.6	2.6	2.7	2.7	2.7	2.8
90th percentile	3.4	3.4	3.4	3.5	3.5	3.6	3.6	3.6	3.7	3.7	3.7	3.9
95th percentile	3.8	3.8	3.8	4.0	3.9	3.7	4.0	3.9	4.1	4.1	4.1	4.1
Standardised												
Mean	2.5	2.5	2.5	2.6	2.6	2.6	2.7	2.7	2.8	2.8	2.8	2.8
Standard error of the mean	0.04	0.02	0.03	0.02	0.03	0.04	0.04	0.02	0.03	0.02	0.02	0.04
Geometric mean	2.4	2.4	2.4	2.5	2.5	2.5	2.6	2.6	2.7	2.7	2.7	2.8
Bases	*317*	*1389*	*438*	*1419*	*644*	*195*	*288*	*1469*	*743*	*1294*	*747*	*262*

Table 3.83

Fibrinogen (observed and age-standardised), by equivalised household income and sex

Aged 16 and over with a valid sample   *1998*

Fibrinogen (g/l)	Equivalised annual household income quintile				
	Up to £7,186	Over £7,186 to £10,834	Over £10,834 to £17,890	Over £17,890 to £27,705	Over £27,705
Men					
Observed					
Mean	2.7	2.8	2.6	2.5	2.4
Standard error of the mean	0.03	0.03	0.02	0.02	0.02
Geometric mean	2.6	2.7	2.5	2.4	2.3
5th percentile	1.7	1.7	1.7	1.6	1.6
10th percentile	1.9	1.9	1.8	1.8	1.7
Median	2.6	2.7	2.5	2.4	2.3
90th percentile	3.7	3.8	3.5	3.3	3.2
95th percentile	4.1	4.1	3.9	3.6	3.5
Standardised					
Mean	2.6	2.7	2.5	2.5	2.4
Standard error of the mean	0.03	0.03	0.02	0.02	0.02
Geometric mean	2.5	2.6	2.5	2.4	2.4
Women					
Observed					
Mean	2.8	2.9	2.7	2.7	2.6
Standard error of the mean	0.03	0.03	0.02	0.02	0.02
Geometric mean	2.7	2.8	2.7	2.6	2.5
5th percentile	1.8	1.9	1.8	1.8	1.7
10th percentile	2.0	2.1	1.9	1.9	1.9
Median	2.8	2.9	2.7	2.6	2.5
90th percentile	3.8	3.8	3.7	3.5	3.4
95th percentile	4.1	4.2	4.0	3.9	3.8
Standardised					
Mean	2.8	2.8	2.8	2.7	2.7
Standard error of the mean	0.03	0.03	0.02	0.02	0.03
Geometric mean	2.8	2.7	2.7	2.7	2.6
Bases					
Men	*544*	*606*	*947*	*926*	*933*
Women	*725*	*808*	*1010*	*921*	*837*

Table 3.84

Fibrinogen (observed and age-standardised), by Health Authority area type and sex

Aged 16 and over with a valid sample   *1998*

Fibrinogen (g/l)	Health Authority area type					
	Inner London	Mining & Industrial	Urban	Mature	Prosperous	Rural
Men						
Observed						
Mean	2.4	2.7	2.6	2.5	2.6	2.6
Standard error of the mean	0.06	0.03	0.03	0.03	0.02	0.02
Geometric mean	2.3	2.6	2.5	2.5	2.5	2.5
5th percentile	1.4	1.7	1.6	1.6	1.7	1.7
10th percentile	1.6	1.9	1.8	1.8	1.8	1.8
Median	2.4	2.6	2.5	2.4	2.4	2.5
90th percentile	3.3	3.7	3.5	3.4	3.4	3.5
95th percentile	3.5	4.0	4.0	3.7	3.8	3.8
Standardised						
Mean	2.4	2.6	2.5	2.5	2.5	2.6
Standard error of the mean	0.05	0.03	0.03	0.02	0.02	0.02
Geometric mean	2.3	2.5	2.5	2.4	2.4	2.5
Women						
Observed						
Mean	2.7	2.8	2.8	2.8	2.8	2.8
Standard error of the mean	0.06	0.03	0.03	0.03	0.02	0.02
Geometric mean	2.6	2.7	2.7	2.7	2.7	2.7
5th percentile	1.7	1.8	1.8	1.8	1.8	1.8
10th percentile	2.0	2.0	2.0	2.0	2.0	2.0
Median	2.7	2.7	2.7	2.7	2.7	2.7
90th percentile	3.5	3.8	3.7	3.6	3.6	3.7
95th percentile	4.2	4.1	4.0	4.0	4.0	4.1
Standardised						
Mean	2.7	2.8	2.8	2.8	2.8	2.8
Standard error of the mean	0.06	0.03	0.03	0.03	0.02	0.02
Geometric mean	2.6	2.7	2.7	2.7	2.7	2.7
Bases						
Men	*114*	*697*	*631*	*653*	*1295*	*1090*
Women	*140*	*734*	*702*	*707*	*1426*	*1217*

Table 3.85

Total cholesterol (observed and age-standardised), by region and sex

Aged 16 and over with a valid sample   *1998*

| Total cholesterol (mmol/l) | Region | | | | | | | |
	Northern & Yorkshire	North West	Trent	West Midlands	Anglia & Oxford	North Thames	South Thames	South & West
Men								
Observed								
Mean	5.6	5.4	5.4	5.6	5.5	5.5	5.4	5.4
Standard error of the mean	0.04	0.04	0.05	0.05	0.05	0.05	0.04	0.04
5th percentile	3.9	3.7	3.6	3.9	3.8	3.8	3.7	3.7
10th percentile	4.2	4.0	4.0	4.2	4.1	4.2	4.0	4.1
Median	5.6	5.4	5.4	5.5	5.4	5.5	5.4	5.3
90th percentile	7.0	6.8	6.8	7.0	7.0	7.0	6.8	6.9
95th percentile	7.5	7.3	7.2	7.4	7.4	7.3	7.3	7.2
%≥6.5 mmol/l	21.7	16.5	15.8	20.1	17.3	18.6	16.9	16.9
Standardised								
Mean	5.5	5.4	5.3	5.5	5.4	5.4	5.4	5.3
Standard error of the mean	0.04	0.04	0.05	0.05	0.05	0.05	0.04	0.04
%≥6.5 mmol/l	20.3	15.8	14.6	19.2	16.6	17.1	16.1	15.7
Women								
Observed								
Mean	5.7	5.6	5.6	5.6	5.5	5.5	5.5	5.6
Standard error of the mean	0.04	0.05	0.05	0.05	0.05	0.05	0.04	0.04
5th percentile	3.9	3.9	3.9	3.9	3.9	3.8	3.7	3.8
10th percentile	4.2	4.2	4.2	4.1	4.1	4.0	4.1	4.1
Median	5.6	5.5	5.5	5.5	5.3	5.4	5.4	5.6
90th percentile	7.3	7.1	7.4	7.2	7.1	7.1	7.1	7.2
95th percentile	7.8	7.6	7.9	7.6	7.5	7.6	7.7	7.7
%≥6.5 mmol/l	25.4	20.2	22.7	23.9	21.1	21.5	21.7	22.2
Standardised								
Mean	5.6	5.6	5.6	5.5	5.5	5.5	5.5	5.6
Standard error of the mean	0.04	0.05	0.05	0.05	0.05	0.05	0.04	0.04
%≥6.5 mmol/l	23.7	20.4	22.6	23.4	22.3	21.6	22.5	21.7
Bases								
Men	*701*	*647*	*532*	*497*	*595*	*553*	*622*	*727*
Women	*796*	*699*	*576*	*593*	*598*	*606*	*819*	*771*

Table 3.86

HDL-cholesterol (observed and age-standardised), by region and sex

Aged 16 and over with a valid sample   *1998*

HDL-cholesterol (mmol/l)	Region							
	Northern & Yorkshire	North West	Trent	West Midlands	Anglia & Oxford	North Thames	South Thames	South & West
Men								
Observed								
Mean	1.3	1.3	1.3	1.3	1.3	1.3	1.3	1.3
Standard error of the mean	0.01	0.01	0.02	0.02	0.01	0.02	0.01	0.01
5th percentile	0.8	0.8	0.8	0.8	0.7	0.8	0.8	0.8
10th percentile	0.9	0.9	0.9	0.9	0.8	0.9	0.9	0.9
Median	1.2	1.2	1.2	1.3	1.2	1.2	1.3	1.3
90th percentile	1.8	1.7	1.7	1.8	1.7	1.8	1.8	1.8
95th percentile	2.0	2.0	1.9	1.9	1.9	1.9	2.0	1.9
% ≤0.9 mmol/l	17.2	16.9	18.0	16.9	19.4	16.5	15.5	15.2
Standardised								
Mean	1.3	1.3	1.3	1.3	1.3	1.3	1.3	1.3
Standard error of the mean	0.01	0.01	0.02	0.02	0.01	0.02	0.01	0.01
% ≤0.9 mmol/l	16.6	16.9	17.7	17.0	19.1	16.7	15.3	14.8
Women								
Observed								
Mean	1.5	1.6	1.5	1.6	1.6	1.6	1.6	1.6
Standard error of the mean	0.01	0.02	0.02	0.02	0.03	0.02	0.01	0.02
5th percentile	0.9	0.9	1.0	1.0	0.9	0.9	1.0	0.9
10th percentile	1.0	1.1	1.1	1.1	1.1	1.1	1.1	1.1
Median	1.5	1.5	1.5	1.5	1.5	1.5	1.6	1.5
90th percentile	2.1	2.1	2.1	2.1	2.1	2.1	2.2	2.1
95th percentile	2.3	2.3	2.3	2.3	2.3	2.3	2.3	2.3
% ≤0.9 mmol/l	7.7	5.2	4.9	4.4	5.4	6.6	3.1	6.0
Standardised								
Mean	1.5	1.6	1.5	1.6	1.6	1.6	1.6	1.6
Standard error of the mean	0.01	0.02	0.02	0.02	0.03	0.02	0.01	0.02
% ≤0.9 mmol/l	7.5	5.0	4.8	4.5	5.4	6.6	3.0	5.9
Bases								
Men	*699*	*646*	*528*	*497*	*593*	*552*	*621*	*726*
Women	*793*	*698*	*576*	*592*	*596*	*603*	*815*	*769*

Table 3.87

C-reactive protein (observed and age-standardised), by region and sex

Aged 16 and over with a valid sample   *1998*

C-reactive protein (mg/l)	Region							
	Northern & Yorkshire	North West	Trent	West Midlands	Anglia & Oxford	North Thames	South Thames	South & West
Men								
Observed								
Mean	3.2	3.0	3.4	3.3	2.6	3.1	2.8	2.8
Standard error of the mean	0.24	0.22	0.29	0.30	0.20	0.32	0.19	0.21
≤0.5[a]	22.1	21.8	19.9	20.5	26.2	22.7	26.2	24.4
0.6-1.0	17.8	19.9	18.4	15.9	20.2	20.4	19.3	19.3
1.1-1.9	19.8	20.1	20.6	22.5	18.4	21.3	16.1	20.4
2.0-3.7	18.4	17.2	18.2	20.2	17.4	17.9	18.2	17.6
>3.7	21.8	21.0	23.0	20.9	17.7	17.6	20.2	18.3
Standardised								
Mean	3.0	2.9	3.3	3.1	2.6	2.9	2.7	2.6
Standard error of the mean	0.24	0.22	0.28	0.28	0.19	0.29	0.18	0.19
≤0.5[a]	24.1	23.0	21.9	22.5	27.0	24.7	27.6	27.0
0.6-1.0	18.8	19.9	18.3	16.2	20.4	21.0	19.2	19.5
1.1-1.9	19.3	20.2	20.4	22.5	18.4	20.8	16.0	20.3
2.0-3.7	17.8	16.8	17.5	19.3	17.1	17.3	17.7	16.8
>3.7	20.1	20.2	21.8	19.5	17.1	16.2	19.4	16.4
Women								
Observed								
Mean	4.0	3.2	3.7	3.9	3.3	3.4	3.3	3.8
Standard error of the mean	0.26	0.17	0.24	0.30	0.21	0.22	0.22	0.25
≤0.5[a]	18.2	23.0	19.8	20.9	22.7	22.1	19.4	18.1
0.6-1.2	20.8	20.9	18.2	19.4	21.9	20.8	22.4	23.6
1.3-2.4	18.8	19.3	19.1	18.9	20.1	19.6	21.7	18.3
2.5-4.9	20.3	19.2	20.7	21.6	15.6	16.5	18.5	21.8
>4.9	21.8	17.6	22.2	19.2	19.7	20.9	17.9	18.1
Standardised								
Mean	3.9	3.2	3.7	3.9	3.4	3.5	3.4	3.8
Standard error of the mean	0.26	0.17	0.24	0.30	0.22	0.23	0.22	0.25
≤0.5[a]	19.0	22.8	20.0	21.1	21.9	22.0	19.0	18.3
0.6-1.2	21.1	20.7	17.9	19.2	21.4	20.9	22.1	23.8
1.3-2.4	18.5	19.4	18.8	18.9	20.1	19.8	21.6	18.2
2.5-4.9	20.0	19.4	20.7	21.7	16.2	16.4	19.1	21.7
>4.9	21.4	17.7	22.6	19.1	20.4	20.9	18.2	18.0
Bases:								
Men	*701*	*657*	*539*	*511*	*603*	*563*	*633*	*731*
Women	*797*	*709*	*581*	*598*	*603*	*611*	*820*	*783*

[a] These values correspond to the quintiles, specific for men and women.

Table 3.88

Fibrinogen (observed and age-standardised), by region and sex

Aged 16 and over with a valid sample   *1998*

Fibrinogen (g/l)	Region							
	Northern & Yorkshire	North West	Trent	West Midlands	Anglia & Oxford	North Thames	South Thames	South & West
Men								
Observed								
Mean	2.6	2.6	2.6	2.7	2.6	2.5	2.5	2.6
Standard error of the mean	0.03	0.03	0.03	0.03	0.03	0.03	0.03	0.03
Geometric mean	2.5	2.5	2.5	2.6	2.5	2.4	2.5	2.5
5th percentile	1.7	1.7	1.6	1.7	1.7	1.6	1.6	1.7
10th percentile	1.8	1.8	1.8	1.9	1.8	1.8	1.8	1.8
Median	2.5	2.5	2.4	2.6	2.5	2.4	2.4	2.5
90th percentile	3.5	3.5	3.5	3.5	3.4	3.4	3.5	3.5
95th percentile	3.9	3.9	3.9	3.9	3.8	3.7	3.8	3.8
Standardised								
Mean	2.6	2.6	2.5	2.6	2.5	2.5	2.5	2.5
Standard error of the mean	0.03	0.03	0.03	0.03	0.03	0.03	0.03	0.03
Geometric mean	2.5	2.5	2.4	2.5	2.5	2.4	2.4	2.4
Women								
Observed								
Mean	2.8	2.7	2.7	2.9	2.8	2.7	2.7	2.8
Standard error of the mean	0.03	0.03	0.03	0.03	0.03	0.03	0.02	0.03
Geometric mean	2.7	2.6	2.7	2.8	2.7	2.7	2.6	2.7
5th percentile	1.8	1.8	1.8	1.8	1.8	1.8	1.8	1.9
10th percentile	2.0	1.9	2.0	2.0	2.0	2.0	2.0	2.0
Median	2.7	2.6	2.7	2.8	2.7	2.7	2.6	2.7
90th percentile	3.8	3.6	3.7	3.9	3.7	3.6	3.5	3.7
95th percentile	4.3	4.0	4.0	4.3	4.0	4.1	3.9	4.0
Standardised								
Mean	2.8	2.7	2.7	2.9	2.8	2.7	2.7	2.8
Standard error of the mean	0.03	0.03	0.03	0.03	0.03	0.03	0.02	0.03
Geometric mean	2.7	2.6	2.7	2.8	2.7	2.7	2.6	2.7
Bases								
Men	*642*	*599*	*464*	*471*	*559*	*505*	*576*	*664*
Women	*705*	*642*	*494*	*550*	*551*	*532*	*747*	*705*

Relationship of CVD to risk factors and socio-demographic factors

Paola Primatesta

SUMMARY

- In both men and women, the mean age of those with CVD was 60.4. The mean age of those without CVD was 43.8 in men and 45.2 in women.

- After age standardisation, the prevalence of the main CVD risk factors was as follows: 49% of men with CVD had high blood pressure compared with 39% of those without CVD; 25% were physically inactive vs 17%; and 23% had low HDL-cholesterol vs 16% respectively. Current smoking prevalence was not higher in those with CVD than in those without; this was true in both sexes. In women 44% of those with CVD had high blood pressure compared with 33% of those without CVD; 33% were physically inactive vs 22%; 8% had low HDL-cholesterol vs 5%.

- Hypertension is a major risk factor for CVD. On the whole, a higher proportion of informants with high blood pressure were physically inactive, were overweight or obese, had high total cholesterol and low HDL-cholesterol than of those without high blood pressure.

- Further analyses were carried out on informants aged 35 and over with IHD or stroke. The contribution of each risk factor once the others were simultaneously taken into account was assessed by multiple regression models. In men, high blood pressure, high levels of fibrinogen and high GHQ12 scores (indicative of possible psychiatric morbidity) remained independently associated with IHD or stroke, while the relation between social class and IHD or stroke was eliminated by simultaneous adjustment for age and biological, behavioural and psychological risk factors. For women, low physical activity and high GHQ12 scores, in addition to manual social class, remained associated with the disease.

4.1 Introduction

CVD continues to be the leading cause of death and disability in all industrialised nations, in spite of a steady decline during the last decades. Together with many other contributing factors, plasma cholesterol, cigarette smoking and hypertension are established as major risk factors for CVD.[1] The decline in CVD mortality observed in most western countries has been attributed to some extent to a decline in these risk factors.[2]

However, there may be socio-economic differences in this downward trend.[3] Those in low socio-economic status groups tend to exhibit smaller reductions or a delayed onset of decline in rates of CVD and cerebrovascular mortality.[4] The disparity in CVD risk between social classes may be explained by differences in health behaviour (smoking, diet, physical activity), biological factors (blood pressure, adiposity, diabetes mellitus and lipid profile), psychosocial variables (social support and hostility), or the environment (living conditions and access to and use of health services). Several studies have shown an association, in both men and women, between low socio-economic status and smoking, obesity, sedentary lifestyle, high blood pressure, poor lipid profile, poor haemostatic profile and psychosocial factors.[5] The mechanisms underlying this social gradient are still not entirely understood. A better understanding of these mechanisms would enable the development of better-targeted strategies to reduce socio-economic inequalities in cardiovascular health.

Changes in CVD prevalence between 1994 and 1998 are reported in Chapter 2, and CVD risk factor profiles and trends in Chapter 3. In the present chapter the associations between disease and a variety of risk factors and socio-economic characteristics are considered.

4.2 Methods and definitions

The measurement of the various risk factors is described in detail in Chapter 3. Briefly, for the purpose of this chapter, risk factors were defined as follows.

Current cigarette smokers were those who reported that they regularly smoked cigarettes at the time of the survey. Alcohol consumption above 21 units per week for men or above 14 units per week for women is presented. Physically inactive informants were those who reported less than one occasion of 15 minutes activity over the 4 weeks prior to the interview. In surveys before 1998 high blood pressure was defined as taking medication affecting blood pressure or having a systolic blood pressure of 160 mmHg or over or a diastolic blood pressure of 95 mmHg or over. In 1998 levels were changed from 160 to 140 mmHg and from 95 to 90 mmHg respectively. Both definitions are presented in this chapter. Being overweight or obese was defined as a body mass index above 25 kg/m^2. A raised waist-hip ratio was taken to be 0.95 or more in men and 0.85 or more in women. Raised total cholesterol was defined as total cholesterol of 6.5 mmol/l or above, and low HDL-cholesterol as HDL-cholesterol of 0.9 mmol/l or below. C-reactive protein and fibrinogen were divided into sex-specific quintiles and the prevalence of the highest quintile is presented here. Family history of CVD was defined as a premature parental death, ie the death of either parent before the age of 65 from a cardiovascular cause. Psychological risk factors were measured by the General Health Questionnaire (GHQ12). The GHQ12 (self-administered) was based on twelve questions, which asked informants about their general level of happiness, depression, anxiety and sleep disturbance over the past four weeks. A threshold score of 4 or more was used to identify possible psychiatric disorder. Manual social class (belonging to Social Classes IIIM, IV or V) and the lowest equivalised household income quintile were the chosen indicators of low socio-economic status.

4.3 Prevalence of risk factors, by age, separately for those with and without a CVD condition

In both men and women, the mean age of those with CVD was 60.4. The mean age of those without CVD was 43.8 in men and 45.2 in women (data not shown).

Smoking and drinking were not more prevalent among informants with CVD than among those without. This was not unexpected as many people would have decreased their consumption of cigarettes and alcohol after having been diagnosed. In fact current smoking prevalence was lower among men with CVD in all age groups (except for those aged 45-64 where the prevalence was the same, at 26%). In women the overall prevalence was also lower in those with CVD (23%) than in those without (28%), but in the younger age groups a higher proportion of women with CVD smoked than of those without. The prevalence of estimated weekly alcohol consumption above 21 units in men (14 in women) was also lower in those with a reported diagnosis of CVD, from age 45 onwards. It is nevertheless worth noting that between a fifth and a quarter (21% of men and 23% of women overall) of informants with CVD were still smoking, and 23% of men and 12% of women were still drinking more than 21 (14) units of alcohol per week.

In the younger age group, the proportion physically inactive was not very different between those with and without CVD, but the difference increased with age, so that overall twice as many informants with CVD were inactive compared with those without the diagnosis. As noted for the other behavioural characteristics, the direction of the relationship between the two variables cannot be assessed in a cross-sectional study: it is possible that informants reduced their activity after CVD was diagnosed.

The prevalence of high blood pressure was higher in those with CVD than in those without, in all age groups and in both sexes. With the new definition the prevalence was 31%, 70% and 85% in men aged 16-44, 45-64 and 65 and above with CVD, and 21%, 49% and 75% respectively in those without CVD. Changing the levels from the old to the new definition meant a two-fold increase in the prevalence of high blood pressure in those without CVD, while the increase was smaller, of about 25%, in those with CVD. In men mean SBP was 141 mmHg in those with CVD and 136 mmHg in those without CVD, and in women it was 142 and 131 respectively (data not shown).

Overall, 71% of men with CVD had a BMI >25 kg/m², compared to 61% of those without CVD, although no differences were observed among those aged 65 and above. In women the differences in the different age groups were less marked. Similarly, the prevalence of obesity (i.e. BMI >30 kg/m²) was higher in men and women of all age groups with CVD than in those without CVD; overall, 23% of men with CVD were obese compared to 16% of those without CVD. The corresponding figures in women were 27% and 20% (data not shown). In both sexes more marked differences were seen in the prevalence of raised waist-hip ratio than in the prevalence of overweight and obesity; overall, the prevalence of raised waist-hip ratio was more than 60% higher in those with CVD than in those without CVD (42% vs. 25% in men and 33% vs. 18% in women).

Serum lipids measured in the 1998 Health Survey were total cholesterol and HDL-cholesterol. A less favourable profile (with raised total cholesterol and low HDL-cholesterol) was shown among informants with CVD, with larger differences for HDL-cholesterol in all age groups in both sexes. Mean total and HDL-cholesterol were also higher in informants with CVD than in those without (data not shown).

Other blood analytes reported in several studies as positively associated with CVD are C-reactive protein and fibrinogen: the Health Survey data also showed levels of these analytes to be higher in informants with CVD than in those without CVD. Table 4.1 shows the proportion of informants in the highest quintile for C-reactive protein, and mean fibrinogen levels: in both sexes and in all age groups, these measures were higher among those with CVD than those without CVD, .

A family history of CVD showed a higher prevalence in informants with CVD, especially among the younger age groups in both sexes. This may be due to the fact that younger informants may be more likely to recall the cause of parental death than older informants.

54% of men with CVD were from manual social classes, a proportion similar to that of men without CVD (51%), while 22% of men with CVD were in the lowest equivalised household income quintile compared with 15% of those without CVD. Among women 53% of those with self-reported CVD belonged to manual social classes compared to 48% of women without CVD, and the difference in the proportions in the lowest equivalent income quintile was of about the same magnitude. **Table 4.1**

After age standardisation, the prevalences of risk factors among those with CVD appeared to be reduced, but the differences between those with and without CVD still remained; hence the differences observed were mainly attributable to reasons other than the age difference between the two groups. Not all the factors shown in Table 4.1 were significantly associated with CVD in both sexes. In men, a significantly larger proportion of informants with CVD than of those without CVD were physically inactive, were hypertensive (according to the new definition), had a raised waist-hip ratio, had low HDL-cholesterol, were in the highest C-reactive protein quintile, had a family history of CVD and scored high on GHQ12, as shown in the following table:

Age-adjusted prevalence of CVD risk factors in men with and without CVD

	With CVD (%)	Without CVD (%)	p
High blood pressure	49	39	<.001
Physically inactive	25	17	<.001
Low HDL-cholesterol	23	16	<.001
Family history of CVD	19	12	<.001
GHQ12≥4	20	11	<.01
Highest CRP quintile	23	18	<.01
Raised WHR	28	25	<.01

In women the same risk factors as in men showed significant differences between those with and without CVD, and manual social class showed a significant positive association with CVD.

Age-adjusted prevalence of CVD risk factors in women with and without CVD

	With CVD (%)	Without CVD (%)	p
High blood pressure	44	33	<.001
Physically inactive	33	22	<.001
Low HDL-cholesterol	8	5	<.001
Family history of CVD	17	14	<.001
GHQ12≥4	28	17	<.001
Highest CRP quintile	23	19	<.001
Raised WHR	24	19	<.001
Manual social class	52	48	<.01

4.4 Prevalence of risk factors, by age, separately for those with and without high BP

Hypertension is a major risk factor for CVD. Several studies found a high prevalence of CVD risk factors in those with high blood pressure, including an altered lipid profile and a high prevalence of obesity.[6] These factors are known further to increase the risk of CVD in people with high blood pressure.

On the whole, a larger proportion of informants with high blood pressure were physically inactive, were overweight or obese, had a raised waist-hip ratio, had high total and low HDL-cholesterol, were in the highest C-reactive protein quintile, had higher mean fibrinogen levels (significant in women only), had a family history of CVD than those without high blood pressure. This was true in both sexes and most age groups. In addition, men with high blood pressure had a higher prevalence of alcohol consumption above 21 units per week. Women in manual social classes and in households in the lowest income quintile were also more likely to have high blood pressure.   **Table 4.2**

After age was adjusted for, the differences for most risk factors were still appreciable and those that were statistically significant in men are shown in the table opposite.

As already pointed out in Chapter 3, high blood pressure in men did not show a significant association with social class or equivalised income once age was adjusted for.

In women, the age-adjusted prevalence of risk factors showing statistically significant differences between those with and without high blood pressure is shown opposite.

Age-adjusted prevalence of risk factors in men with and without high blood pressure

	With high blood pressure	Without high blood pressure	p
	(%)	(%)	
Physically inactive	21	15	<.001
Raised WHR	32	20	<.001
Raised total cholesterol	19	16	<.05
Low HDL cholesterol	18	16	<.05
Highest CRP quintile	20	17	<.01
Family history of CVD	15	12	<.001

Age-adjusted prevalence of risk factors in women with and without high blood pressure

	With high blood pressure	Without high blood pressure	p
	(%)	(%)	
Physically inactive	25	20	<.001
Raised WHR	28	15	<.001
Raised total cholesterol	26	20	<.001
Low HDL cholesterol	7	4	<.001
Fibrinogen top quintile	21	15	<.001
Highest CRP quintile	24	16	<.001
Family history of CVD	17	13	<.001
Lowest income quintile	22	17	<.001
Manual social class	51	47	<.001

4.5 Prevalence of risk factors, by age, separately for those with and without IHD or stroke

IHD and stroke are severe manifestations of CVD. As already noted in Chapter 2, the prevalence of these conditions was higher in men than in women, although the sex differential tended to narrow with advancing age. This sex differential may result from a combination of genetic and life-style factors, including smoking and drinking, that can determine the disease through risk factors such as hypertension, hypercholesterolaemia, abdominal fat distribution and haemostatic factors.[7]

The prevalence of various risk factors in men and women by age is shown in Table 4.3. This table includes informants aged 16-44, among whom coronary and cerebrovascular events are relatively rare, for completeness.

As well as current smokers, 'ever' smokers were also examined. As pointed out above, the prevalence of some risk factors, mainly behavioural ones, should be interpreted with caution given that the disease is likely to have induced some modification in the lifestyle of many individuals affected. Moreover, people with these risk factors may have been more at risk of dying of CVD than those without the risk factors, leaving a population with CVD with lower than average prevalence of risk factors.

For those aged 16-44 and those aged 65 and over, the prevalence of current cigarette smoking was lower in those with IHD or stroke than in those without, while among both men and women aged 45-64 with IHD or stroke the prevalence of smoking was higher (among women) or the same (in men) as in those without IHD or stroke. The proportion who had ever smoked (either currently or in the past) was higher in those with IHD or stroke than in those without, in all age groups and in both sexes. As noted in Chapter 3, the prevalence of current cigarette smoking was slightly higher in men (28%) than women (27%). The proportion of men who had ever smoked (currently or in the past) was appreciably higher (59%) than the corresponding proportion of women (48%).

The prevalence of estimated weekly alcohol consumption above 21 units in men (14 in women) was higher in those without IHD or stroke, possibly mainly due to changes in habits after the event.

Women tended to be more physically inactive than men, and those who had a diagnosis of IHD or stroke were less active than those without the diagnosis.

Chapter 3 shows that mean SBP was higher in men than in women in young and middle age groups, although after the menopausal age the situation was reversed. This was also true for the prevalence of hypertension, and is confirmed looking at the prevalence in those with and without IHD or stroke. Using both definitions, the prevalence of high blood pressure was higher in those with than in those without IHD or stroke.

Being overweight or obese, and having a raised waist-hip ratio, were both more prevalent in informants with IHD or stroke. Among women with IHD or stroke the prevalence of raised waist-hip ratio was 42% (highest in those aged 45-64, at 46%) and in men with IHD or stroke it was 50%. It was pointed out in Chapter 3 that men have more abdominal fat than women, and this has been shown to be a risk factor for coronary artery disease in both men and women. Similar sex differences were observed in those without IHD or stroke (where the prevalence was 25% in men, 18% in women).

Raised total cholesterol showed only small differences in men and women between those with and without IHD or stroke, although women tended to have higher prevalence than men. This may be due partly to the fact that women, throughout adult life, tend to have greater mean HDL-cholesterol levels.[8] The prevalence of low HDL-cholesterol was in fact higher in men than in women, both among those with and without IHD or stroke. The high level of HDL-cholesterol in women may contribute to the coronary disease sex differential, although it has been shown that for any given HDL-cholesterol level, women still have considerably less risk of disease than men.[9]

The proportion of both men and women in the highest quintile of fibrinogen and C-reactive protein was higher in men and women with IHD or stroke than in their counterparts without the condition. Some studies have shown that both the relative risk of coronary artery disease and the absolute increase in risk of disease, in the highest tertile of plasma fibrinogen compared with the lowest, was higher in men than in women, although a substantial difference in risk of disease persisted within each tertile.[10] In keeping with the higher rates of CVD it might be expected that men have higher levels of fibrinogen than women do, but the data show that women have slightly higher mean fibrinogen than men at all ages. This has been confirmed in other studies.[11] The information on the relation between haemostatic factors and CVD in women remains sparse.   **Table 4.3**

In summary, most of the risk factors considered showed a higher prevalence in informants with IHD or stroke than without, in most age groups and both sexes.

Potential causes for the sex differential in coronary and cerebrovascular conditions may lie partly in differences between men and women in their susceptibility to these and other less well-established risk factors.[7]

After age standardisation, the prevalence of risk factors remained higher among those with IHD or stroke than in those without, as shown in the following tables (confined to those aged 35 and over):

Men aged 35 and over

	With IHD or stroke (%)	Without IHD or stroke (%)	p
Ever smoked	74	68	<.001
High blood pressure (1998)	76	50	<.001
Physically inactive	44	23	<.001
Raised WHR	47	35	<.001
Low HDL-cholesterol	21	17	<.001
Highest CRP quintile	27	22	<.001
Fibrinogen highest quintile	27	22	<.01
Family history of CVD	24	18	<.01
GHQ12≥4	28	12	<.001
Lowest income quintile	23	14	<.001
Manual social class	59	50	<.01

Women aged 35 and over

	With IHD or stroke (%)	Without IHD or stroke (%)	p
Ever smoked	66	55	<.001
High blood pressure (1998)	60	46	<.001
Physically inactive	53	28	<.001
Raised WHR	42	25	<.001
Low HDL-cholesterol	10	5	<.001
Highest CRP quintile	37	21	<.001
Family history of CVD	27	18	<.001
GHQ12≥4	38	16	<.001
Lowest income quintile	27	18	<.01
Manual social class	59	47	<.001

4.6 Factors associated with CVD

Section 4.5 looked at the association between each individual risk factor with IHD or stroke. This section examines the contribution of each risk factor once the others have simultaneously been taken into account.

The data reported in Chapter 3 provide evidence of an inverse association between socio-economic status and CVD risk factors. Manual social class was associated with smoking, high body mass and raised waist-hip ratio in both sexes, and high blood pressure and low HDL-cholesterol in women (see Chapter 3, Sections 3.3, 3.5, 3.6, 3.7).

Equivalised household income was inversely associated with smoking prevalence, obesity and raised waist-hip ratio in both sexes; and total cholesterol and high blood pressure in women. Income level was positively associated with HDL-cholesterol in both sexes (see Chapter 3, Sections 3.3, 3.5, 3.6, 3.7).

Further analyses were done to assess the contribution of these and other risk factors to the social class and income gradient in IHD and stroke. This was done in two stages. The first phase was to examine the relation between socio-economic status and IHD/stroke with separate adjustment for each group of explanatory risk factors and age. The various risk factors were grouped into six sets:

● Unhealthy lifestyle patterns (smoking, high waist-hip ratio, lack of physical activity)

● High blood pressure

● Serum lipids (total and HDL-cholesterol)

● Haemostatic factors (fibrinogen and CRP)

● Family history of CVD

● Psychological factors (GHQ12).

To assess the impact of risk factor adjustment on the odds of having IHD, percentage reductions were calculated by taking each set of risk factors at a time in the baseline logistic regression model, according to the formula:[12]

$$\left(\frac{OR\ (unadjusted) - OR\ (adjusted)}{OR\ (unadjusted) - 1} \right) \times 100$$

In the second stage, the relation between socio-economic status and IHD/stroke was adjusted by all these risk factors simultaneously.

Age was adjusted for in all analyses. These analyses were restricted to informants aged 35 and over, given the low prevalence of the outcome of interest in the younger age groups.

The percentage reductions in the odds of IHD or stroke associated with manual social class in men, after adjustment for the different sets of risk factors, are shown in the following table:

Logistic regression model	Adjusted for	OR (95% CI)	% reduction
I	Age	1.31 (1.00, 1.74)	-
II	Age + high blood pressure	1.31 (1.00, 1.74)	0
III	Age + family history of CVD	1.31 (1.00, 1.73)	0
IV	Age + haemostatic factors	1.31 (0.98, 1.92)	0
V	Age + serum lipids	1.29 (0.98, 1.71)	-6
VI	Age + lifestyle factors	1.25 (0.94, 1.68)	-19
VII	Age + GHQ12	1.20 (0.90, 1.60)	-35
VIII	Age + all factors	1.21 (0.85, 1.72)	-32

There was no reduction in the odds after separate adjustment for high blood pressure, family history and haemostatic factors, whereas adjusting for lifestyle factors reduced the odds by 19%, and the association between manual social class and IHD or stroke was no longer significant (p=0.12). Adjusting for GHQ12 scores (an indicator of psychiatric morbidity) resulted in the largest reduction in the odds (35%). After further adjustment for all the risk factors, the excess odds for IHD or stroke in men were reduced by 32% to 1.21 (95% CI 0.85, 1.72).

Similar models were run for women. The percentage reductions in the odds of IHD or stroke, after adjustment for the different sets of risk factors, are shown in the following table:

Logistic regression model	Adjusted for	OR (95% CI)	% reduction
I	Age	1.86 (1.34, 2.59)	-
II	Age + high blood pressure	1.86 (1.33, 2.58)	0
III	Age + family history of CVD	1.85 (1.32, 2.56)	-1
IV	Age + GHQ12	1.82 (1.30, 2.53)	-5
V	Age + serum lipids	1.82 (1.30, 2.53)	-5
VI	Age + lifestyle factors	1.80 (1.29, 2.53)	-7
VII	Age + haemostatic factors	1.72 (1.16, 2.54)	-16
VIII	Age + all factors	1.59 (1.06, 2.38)	-31

The percentage reduction in the odds after separate adjustment for GHQ12 and lipids was 5%, and after adjusting separately for haemostatic factors the largest reduction in the odds was achieved (16%). After further adjustment for all these factors the excess odds of IHD or stroke associated with manual social class in women was reduced by 31%, but remained statistically significant (p=.02), which suggests that the observed association between IHD or stroke and social class was not entirely explained by the risk factors considered in these analyses. These findings confirm that the association between socio-economic status and IHD or stroke in women was accounted for by a large number of known factors. However, even though the risk factors examined were strongly associated with the outcome, the adjustments failed to account completely for the elevated risk associated with low socio-economic status.

Table 4.4 presents the results of regression model VIII, applied to both men and women, which simultaneously adjusted for all risk factors. Among men, high blood pressure, high levels of fibrinogen, and high GHQ12 scores (of 4 or more, indicative of possible psychiatric morbidity) remained independently associated with IHD or stroke, while the relation between social class and IHD or stroke was eliminated by simultaneous adjustment for age and biological, behavioural and psychological risk factors. For women, low physical activity and high GHQ12 scores, in addition to manual social class, remained associated with the disease.

Table 4.4

Similar results were seen when the analyses were repeated with equivalised household income instead of social class as an indicator of socio-economic status (data not shown).

These multivariate analyses can be interpreted as controlling for variables that have an intermediate role in the chain of causation between manual social class and IHD or stroke. If their role is stronger in men than in women this could explain why the association becomes statistically non-significant after multivariate control in men but not in women. Caution is necessary when interpreting these results: whether these factors are causal or simple mediators cannot be determined in a cross-sectional study. Detection of causal mechanisms requires longitudinal studies.

References and notes

1   Gordon T, Kannel WB. *Multiple risk function for predicting coronary artery disease: the concept, accuracy, and application*. Am Heart J 1982; **103**:1031-39.

2   Dobson A, Evans A, Ferrario M, Kuulasmaa K, Moltchanov V, Sans S, Tunstall-Pedoe H, Tuomilehto J, Wedel H, Yarnell J for the WHO MONICA Project. *Changes in estimated coronary risk in the 1980s: data from 38 populations in the WHO MONICA project*. Ann Med 1998; **30**:199-205.

3   Marmot MG, McDowall ME. *Mortality decline and widening social inequalities*. Lancet 1986; **2**:274-76.

4   Wing S, Barnett E, Casper M, Tyroler HA. *Geographic and socioeconomic variations in the onset of decline of coronary heart disease mortality in white women*. Am J Public Health 1992; **82**:204-9.

5   Kaplan GA, Keil JE. *Socioeconomic factors and cardiovascular disease: a review of the literature*. Circulation 1993; **88**:1973-98.

6   Stamler J, Stamler R, Neaton JD. *Blood pressure, systolic and diastolic, and cardiovascular risk: US population data*. Arch Intern Med 1993; **153**:598-615.

7   Price JF, Fowkes FGR. *Risk factors and the sex differential in coronary artery disease*. Epidemiology 1997; **8**:584-91.

8   Kannel WB. *Metabolic risk factors for coronary heart disease in women: perspectives from the Framingham Study*. Am Heart J 1987; **114**:413-19.

9   Stensvold I, Urdal P, Thurmer H, Tverdal A, Lund-Larsen PG, Foss OP. *High-density lipoprotein cholesterol and coronary, cardiovascular and all cause mortality among middle-aged Norwegian men and women*. Eur Heart J 1992; **13**:1155-63.

10 Kannel WB, Wolf PA, Castelli WP, D'Agostino RB. *Fibrinogen and risk of cardiovascular disease: the Framingham Study*. JAMA 1987; **258**:1183-86.

11 Meade TW, Vickers MW, Thompson SG, Stirling Y, Haines AP, Miller GJ. *Epidemiological characteristics of platelet aggregability*. BMJ 1985; **290**:428-32.

12 Lynch JW, Kaplan GA, Cohen RD, Tuomilehto J, Salonen JT. *Do cardiovascular risk factors explain the relation between socioeconomic status, risk of all-cause mortality, cardiovascular mortality, and acute miocardial infarction?* Am J Epidemiol 1996; **144**:934-42.

Tables

Table 4.1

Prevalence of risk factors amongst those with and without CVD conditions, by age and sex

Aged 16 and over   *1998*

Risk factors	With CVD			Total	Without CVD			Total
	16-44	45-64	65 +		16-44	45-64	65 +	
	%	%	%	%	%	%	%	%
Men								
Current cigarette smoker	34	26	13	21	35	26	15	30
Alcohol >21 units/week	37	27	15	23	35	34	19	32
Physically inactive	11	41	54	42	10	20	34	16
High blood pressure (old definition)[a]	14	55	72	56	4	22	46	16
High blood pressure (1998 definition)[a]	31	70	85	71	21	49	75	38
BMI >25 kg/m^2 (overweight or obese)	57	78	72	71	52	73	72	61
Waist-hip ratio >0.95	14	46	49	42	12	38	46	25
Cholesterol ≥6.5 mmol/l	15	20	22	20	11	24	25	18
HDL-cholesterol ≤0.9 mmol/l	23	22	22	22	15	17	15	16
Highest C-reactive protein quintile	13	27	44	32	11	21	35	18
Mean fibrinogen (g/l)	2.37	2.74	3.13	2.84	2.33	2.66	3.06	2.54
Family has history of CVD	16	28	22	23	7	19	18	12
Manual social class	49	54	55	54	51	51	54	51
Lowest equivalised household income quintile	17	19	27	22	15	12	23	15
Women								
Current cigarette smoker	38	30	12	23	33	25	16	28
Alcohol >14 units/week	24	11	7	12	21	18	10	18
Physically inactive	14	37	67	47	12	17	49	20
High blood pressure (old definition)[a]	6	45	80	54	2	20	55	17
High blood pressure (1998 definition)[a]	14	59	92	65	9	39	76	30
BMI >25 kg/m^2 (overweight or obese)	45	67	66	61	42	63	65	52
Waist-hip ratio >0.85	12	34	43	33	9	21	37	18
Cholesterol ≥6.5 mmol/l	10	27	45	32	7	29	47	21
HDL-cholesterol ≤0.9 mmol/l	5	12	8	9	6	4	4	5
Highest C-reactive protein quintile	18	27	32	28	15	19	27	18
Mean fibrinogen (g/l)	2.68	2.96	3.24	3.00	2.59	2.80	3.10	2.74
Family has history of CVD	12	24	25	22	8	19	22	14
Manual social class	49	54	54	53	48	47	49	48
Lowest equivalised household income quintile	24	21	24	23	20	13	23	18
Bases								
Men								
Whole sample[b]	204	406	520	1130	3314	1870	879	6063
All who had a nurse visit[c]	177	367	456	1000	2782	1629	754	5165
All who gave a blood sample[d]	140	305	360	805	2212	1440	665	4317
Women								
Whole sample[b]	278	352	598	1228	3931	2280	1276	7487
All who had a nurse visit[c]	243	313	518	1074	3341	1983	1023	6347
All who gave a blood sample[d]	173	250	385	808	2380	1698	843	4921

[a] In surveys before 1998 ('old definition'), informants were considered hypertensive if their systolic blood pressure pressure was 160 mmHg or over or their diastolic blood pressure was 95 mmHg or over or they were taking medicine affecting blood pressure. In 1998 levels were changed from 160 and 95 to 140 and 90 ('1998 definition'). Figures using both definitions are presented in the table.

[b] Bases vary: those shown are for the whole sample and apply to current cigarette smoking, alcohol consumption, physical activity, BMI, house hold income, family history of CVD, and social class.

[c] Bases vary: those shown are for informants who had a nurse visit and apply to blood pressure readings and waist-hip measurements.

[d] Bases vary: those shown are for informants who gave a blood sample and apply to total cholesterol, HDL-cholesterol, C-reactive protein and fibrinogen.

Table 4.2

Prevalence of risk factors amongst those with and without high blood pressure, by age and sex

Aged 16 and over | | | | | | | | *1998*

Risk factors	With high blood pressure[a]			Total	Without high blood pressure[a]			Total
	16-44	45-64	65 +		16-44	45-64	65 +	
	%	%	%	%	%	%	%	%
Men								
Current cigarette smoker	28	22	11	19	32	23	13	28
Alcohol >21 units/week	43	34	18	30	33	29	15	30
Physically inactive	12	29	40	29	9	18	31	13
BMI >25 kg/m² (overweight or obese)	69	82	76	77	48	67	67	55
Waist-hip ratio >0.95	22	48	50	42	9	29	39	17
Cholesterol ≥6.5 mmol/l	16	25	24	22	11	22	23	15
HDL-cholesterol ≤0.9 mmol/l	18	21	18	19	16	16	17	16
Highest C-reactive protein quintile	13	23	40	27	10	20	28	14
Mean fibrinogen (g/l)	2.37	2.70	3.10	2.76	2.31	2.62	2.96	2.45
Family has history of CVD	11	23	21	20	7	18	17	11
Manual social class	50	55	54	53	50	47	51	49
Lowest equivalised household income quintile	13	14	24	17	13	11	23	13
Women								
Current cigarette smoker	26	24	11	18	31	23	15	28
Alcohol >14 units/week	23	17	8	13	22	16	15	20
Physically inactive	11	25	56	38	12	16	37	14
BMI >25 kg/m² (overweight or obese)	68	75	69	71	39	56	50	45
Waist-hip ratio >0.85	22	34	39	35	8	16	31	12
Cholesterol ≥6.5 mmol/l	14	35	48	39	6	24	42	14
HDL-cholesterol ≤0.9 mmol/l	9	8	6	7	5	3	4	5
Highest C-reactive protein quintile	19	28	30	28	15	13	22	15
Mean fibrinogen (g/l)	2.72	2.93	3.19	3.03	2.57	2.73	2.93	2.65
Family has history of CVD	12	24	24	23	8	17	22	11
Manual social class	50	53	49	51	48	44	49	47
Lowest equivalised household income quintile	22	18	22	21	18	11	18	16
Bases								
Men								
All who had a nurse visit[b]	560	922	866	2348	1999	825	229	3053
All who gave a blood sample[c]	461	791	734	1986	1585	741	198	2524
Women								
All who had a nurse visit[b]	276	862	1139	2277	2748	1198	260	4206
All who gave a blood sample[c]	215	723	911	1849	2049	1039	219	3307

[a] The 1998 definition of high blood pressure was used. See footnote to Table 4.1.

[b] Bases vary: those shown are for informants who had a nurse visit and a valid blood pressure measurement.

[c] Bases vary: those shown are for informants who gave a blood sample and apply to total cholesterol, HDL-cholesterol, C-reactive protein and fibrinogen.

Table 4.3

Prevalence of risk factors amongst those with and without IHD or stroke, by age and sex

Aged 16 and over *1998*

Risk factors	With IHD or stroke			Total	Without IHD or stroke			Total
	16-44	45-64	65 +		16-44	45-64	65 +	
	%	%	%	%	%	%	%	%
Men								
Current cigarette smoker	[13]	26	13	18	35	26	15	29
Ever smoked	[58]	82	81	80	55	70	75	63
Alcohol >21 units/week	[35]	23	14	18	35	34	19	32
Physically inactive	[29]	52	55	53	10	21	36	17
High blood pressure (old definition)[a]	[44]	69	78	73	4	23	48	17
High blood pressure (1998 definition)[a]	[50]	79	87	83	22	50	76	39
BMI >25 kg/m^2 (overweight or obese)	[70]	81	75	77	52	74	71	62
Waist-hip ratio >0.95	[29]	52	51	50	12	38	46	25
Cholesterol ≥6.5 mmol/l	[29]	21	22	22	12	24	24	18
HDL-cholesterol ≤0.9 mmol/l	[21]	20	21	21	16	18	16	17
Highest C-reactive protein quintile	[18]	29	46	39	11	21	36	18
Highest fibrinogen quintile	[17]	36	49	44	8	21	39	17
Family has history of CVD	[21]	30	19	23	8	19	19	13
Manual social class	[67]	58	58	58	51	50	53	51
Lowest equivalised household income quintile	[32]	25	28	27	15	12	24	15
Women								
Current cigarette smoker	[41]	33	13	19	33	25	15	27
Ever smoked	[65]	67	58	61	53	55	55	54
Alcohol >14 units/week	[32]	8	7	9	21	17	9	18
Physically inactive	[21]	56	69	63	12	18	51	21
High blood pressure (old definition)[a]	[-]	64	84	74	3	21	58	19
High blood pressure (1998 definition)[a]	[4]	74	92	83	9	40	79	32
BMI >25 kg/m^2 (overweight or obese)	[34]	74	64	65	42	63	65	53
Waist-hip ratio >0.85	[32]	46	42	42	9	22	38	18
Cholesterol ≥6.5 mmol/l	[21]	30	45	41	7	28	47	21
HDL-cholesterol ≤0.9 mmol/l	[7]	17	9	10	5	5	4	5
Highest C-reactive protein quintile	[43]	29	34	33	15	19	27	19
Highest fibrinogen quintile	[14]	33	36	34	11	18	31	17
Family has history of CVD	[12]	31	26	26	8	19	22	14
Manual social class	[45]	66	55	57	48	47	50	48
Lowest equivalised household income quintile	[34]	30	24	26	20	14	23	19
Bases								
Men								
All who had a nurse visit[b]	*24*	*218*	*370*	*612*	*3493*	*2057*	*1027*	*6577*
All who gave a blood sample[c]	*17*	*161*	*261*	*439*	*2334*	*1584*	*763*	*4681*
Women								
All who had a nurse visit[b]	*34*	*131*	*375*	*540*	*4175*	*2500*	*1499*	*8174*
All who gave a blood sample[c]	*14*	*82*	*248*	*344*	*2539*	*1865*	*980*	*5384*

[a] See footnote to Table 4.1.

[b] Bases vary: those shown are for informants who had a nurse visit and apply to blood pressure readings and waist-hip measurements.

[c] Bases vary: those shown are for informants who gave a blood sample and apply to total cholesterol, HDL-cholesterol, C-reactive protein and fibrinogen.

Table 4.4

Odds ratios and 95% confidence intervals for the age-adjusted[a] associations between social class and IHD or stroke, adjusted for all risk factors

Aged 35 and over with valid measurments *1998*

Variable	N	Odds ratio	95% CI[b]	Variable	N	Odds ratio	95% CI[b]
Men *Base 2349*				**Women** *Base 2585*			
Social class of head of household (p=0.3656)				**Social class of head of household (p=0.0268)**			
Non manual[c]	1174	1.00		Non manual[c]	1378	1.00	
Manual	1175	1.18	0.83,1.68	Manual	1207	1.58	1.05,2.38
C-reactive protein (p=0.1399)				**C-reactive protein (p=0.2413)**			
Lowest quintile[c]	464	1.00		Lowest quintile[c]	491	1.00	
2nd quintile	441	1.51	0.66,3.45	2nd quintile	590	1.30	0.56,3.02
3rd quintile	474	1.83	0.83,4.05	3rd quintile	525	1.07	0.45,2.52
4th quintile	455	1.07	0.46,2.45	4th quintile	477	1.05	0.44,2.48
Highest quintile	515	1.88	0.84,4.24	Highest quintile	502	1.84	0.80,4.25
Fibrinogen level (p=0.1335)				**Fibrinogen level (p=0.2414)**			
Lowest quintile[c]	400	1.00		Lowest quintile[c]	551	1.00	
2nd quintile	423	3.22	1.05,9.86	2nd quintile	463	1.31	0.54,3.20
3rd quintile	468	4.18	1.42,12.32	3rd quintile	628	1.22	0.54,2.75
4th quintile	530	3.30	1.13,9.69	4th quintile	476	2.12	0.97,4.64
Highest quintile	528	3.72	1.25,11.06	Highest quintile	467	1.55	0.69,3.49
Total cholesterol level (p=0.9681)				**Total cholesterol level (p=0.9210)**			
6.5 mmol/l[c]	1834	1.00		6.5 mmol/l[c]	1900	1.00	
6.5 mmol/l	515	0.99	0.66,1.49	6.5 mmol/l	685	1.02	0.67,1.55
HDL-cholesterol level (p=0.8523)				**HDL-cholesterol level (p=0.3236)**			
>0.9 mmol/l[c]	1946	1.00		>0.9 mmol/l[c]	2458	1.00	
≤0.9 mmol/l	403	1.04	0.67,1.63	≤0.9 mmol/l	127	1.46	0.69,3.12
Family has history of CVD (p=0.3061)				**Family has history of CVD (p=0.2011)**			
No[c]	1915	1.00		No[c]	2114	1.00	
Yes	434	1.24	0.82,1.86	Yes	471	1.34	0.85,2.11
Ever smoked (p=0.1645)				**Ever smoked (p=0.9729)**			
Never smoked[c]	776	1.00		Never smoked[c]	1155	1.00	
Has smoked	1573	1.36	0.88,2.11	Has smoked	1430	0.99	0.66,1.49
Physical activity (p=0.1359)				**Physical activity (p=0.0032)**			
Active[c]	1878	1.00		Active[c]	2026	1.00	
Inactive	471	1.33	0.91,1.94	Inactive	559	1.93	1.25,2.98
Waist-hip ratio (p=0.9925)				**Waist-hip ratio (p=0.9963)**			
0.95[c]	1556	1.00		0.85[c]	2030	1.00	
0.95 and over	793	1.00	0.70,1.43	0.85 and over	555	1.00	0.64,1.55
High blood pressure (1998 definition) (p=0.0480)				**High blood pressure (1998 definition) (p=0.1412)**			
No high blood pressure[c]	1222	1.00		No high blood pressure[c]	1598	1.00	
Has high blood pressure	1127	1.52	1.00,2.32	Has high blood pressure	987	1.45	0.88,2.36
GHQ12 (p<0.0001)				**GHQ12 (p=0.0067)**			
Score 0[c]	1576	1.00		Score 0[c]	1487	1.00	
Score 1-3	506	2.14	1.42,3.21	Score 1-3	655	1.66	1.05,2.64
Score 4+	267	3.67	2.29,5.88	Score 4+	443	2.19	1.31,3.67

[a] Adjusted for age using linear regression.

[b] Confidence interval.

[c] Reference category.

Physical activity

5

Gillian Prior

SUMMARY

- Men were more likely than women to have participated in all activity types except heavy housework.

- The activity type most commonly reported by men was sports and exercise: 42% of men had participated in some sports and exercise (of at least 15 minutes' duration) in the past four weeks. Participation by women in sports was lower at 36%. The proportion of men and women participating in sports and exercise decreased rapidly with age.

- The most common activity type for women was heavy housework; 58% of women had participated in this, compared with 38% of men. Participation in heavy housework was lowest in those aged 16-24 and those aged 75 and over.

- 22% of men were classified as at least moderately active at work (on the basis of their occupation and their own rating of their physical activity at work), compared with 12% of women.

- Combining all activity types, 80% of men and 76% of women reported at least one occasion of physical activity (of at least 15 minutes' duration) in the last four weeks. This proportion tended to fall with age, particularly after age 35.

- Participation in physical activities was summarised into activity groups; Group 3 is the level that fulfils the current activity guidelines, which are that adults should take part in physical activities of at least moderate intensity and of at least 30 minutes' duration, on most days (at least five days a week). Men overall were far more likely to be classified in Group 3 (37%) than were women (25%).

- Among men, the proportion in Group 3 fell steadily with age from 58% of those aged 16-24 to 7% of those aged 75 and over.

- Among women, the proportion in Group 3 was fairly level at 30%-32% in women aged 16-54, before falling with age to just 4% among women aged 75 and over.

- Among men, there was no change since 1994 in the proportion in Group 3. Among women, there was a small increase, from 22% in 1994 to 25% in 1998.

- Participation in physical activities overall tended to increase with increasing household income, particularly among men. Participation in sports and exercise and walking was strongly related to household income, with men and women in higher income quintiles being more likely to take part in these activities.

- Contrarily, because of the greater contribution of occupational activity in the manual social classes, the proportion of men in activity Group 3 was highest in Social Class V, and lower in the non-manual social classes. Similarly the proportion of men in Group 3 was lower in the lowest and highest income quintiles than in the middle incomes. Among women there was no clear pattern according to income or social class in the proportions in Group 3. These findings were confirmed by logistic regression.

5.1 Introduction

5.1.1 Background

Increasing physical activity among adults has long been the subject of public health promotion policies, and the White Paper *Saving Lives: Our Healthier Nation* emphasises the importance of physical activity as one of the key determinants of good health.[1] The health benefits of a physically-active lifestyle are well documented. Physical activity is one of the major risk factors for coronary heart disease which has been targeted by government health strategies since the early 1990s.[2,3] Lack of physical activity has been shown to contribute to a range of other health conditions such as non-insulin dependent diabetes and osteoporosis, while participation in physical activity promotes good mental health.[4] In addition there have been for many years internationally-accepted recommendations about the amount and type of physical activity among adults that is beneficial for health.[5]

Physical activity questions have been included regularly in the Health Survey since it began in 1991. When the Health Survey adult physical activity module was first developed the recommended level of physical activity for adults was that they should take part in at least three occasions a week of vigorous activity lasting 20 minutes or more.[6] By the mid-1990s however the emphasis shifted towards encouraging people to take part in regular activity at a moderate level. Although regular vigorous activity has been shown to produce maximum cardiac benefit for an individual, for the majority of the population this may have been an unrealistic target. It was felt that the greatest health gain for the population as a whole would be achieved by encouraging the least active to become a little more active, and so moderate activity became more important for health promotion. The recommended guidelines were revised to say that adults should take part in at least 30 minutes of moderate activity, ideally on a daily basis (at least five days a week).[7]

Recently the emphasis has shifted further, towards encouraging the accumulation of shorter bouts of activity (of as little as 10 minutes) in order to reach the daily target of 30 minutes.[8,9,10]

The Health Survey physical activity questions were revised for the 1997 and 1998 surveys to address the issue of accumulation, and to allow better estimation of the amount of time spent participating in different activities.

5.1.2 Methodology

The Health Survey adult physical activity module was developed for the 1991 Health Survey, and the questions were repeated in the 1992-1994 surveys with minor changes in 1993-1994. The questions were included again in the 1997 and 1998 surveys, with further revisions.[11,12]

The original Health Survey questions were based on those used in the Allied Dunbar National Fitness Survey (ADNFS), which was carried out in 1989.[13] The level of physical activity has been measured by the time spent being active, the intensity of the activity (in terms of energy expenditure) and the frequency with which it is done.

Types of activity

Four main types of activity were asked about in the questionnaire:

- Occupational activity (activity at work)

- Activity at home (housework, gardening, DIY)

- Walks of 15 minutes or more

- Sports and exercise activities.

For each activity type informants were asked on how many days in the last four weeks they had participated in the activity for at least 15 minutes a time. They were then asked how long they had usually spent participating in the activity.

For occupational activity, the concept of an 'occasion' was not applicable, so no data on frequency or duration was collected. In summary variables, occupational activity was counted as 20 days in the last four weeks for full-time workers and 12 days in the last four weeks for part-time workers.

For walking, informants were asked on how many days they had taken more than one walk of at least 15 minutes. If they had taken more than one walk a day, the total time spent walking on that day was calculated as twice the average time per walk. Informants were also asked to assess their usual walking pace as 'fast (at least 4 miles per hour)', 'brisk', 'steady average' or 'slow'.

For sports and exercise activities, informants were asked whether the effort of the activity was usually enough to make them out of breath or sweaty.

Intensity level

In order to create a summary classification for this chapter, activities have been classified into intensity levels, based on an estimate of the energy cost of the activities. The levels are:

Vigorous   Activities with an energy cost of at least 7.5 kcal/min

Moderate   Activities with an energy cost of at least 5 kcal/min but less than 7.5 kcal/min

Light   Activities with an energy cost of at least 2 kcal/min but less than 5 kcal/min

Inactive   Activities with an energy cost of less than 2 kcal/min.

For sports and exercise, activities were classified according to the nature of the activity, and the informant's assessment of the amount of effort involved. For example, 'swimming' was counted as 'vigorous' if the effort was usually enough to make the informant out of breath or sweaty, otherwise as 'moderate'.[14]

For walking, walks of 15 minutes or more at a 'brisk' or 'fast' pace were classified as 'moderate'. Walks at a 'slow' or 'steady average' pace were classified as 'light'.

For home activity, informants were given examples of types of housework/gardening and DIY that counted as 'heavy' and 'light'. Heavy housework and heavy gardening/DIY were classified as 'moderate', other gardening/DIY as 'light' and light housework only as 'inactive'.[15]

For occupational activity (activity at work), a combination of factors was used for classification. The level of activity was assigned by combining the Standard Occupational Classification (SOC) code of the informant's job with the answer to a question about how physically active informants felt themselves to be in their jobs. For example, informants who said that they were very physically active in their jobs were only classified as doing 'vigorous' activity at work if their job was one of a short list of occupations; otherwise they were classified as 'moderately active' at work.[16]

5.2 Components of activity

5.2.1 Number of days' participation in different activities

Table 5.1 shows the number of days' participation in the last four weeks in heavy housework, heavy manual/DIY, walking, sports and exercise and occupational activity (for at least 15 minutes a time), together with the mean number of days based on all informants (so that non-participation is counted as zero days).

In addition the table shows a summary classification of the number of days' participation in any physical activity for at least 15 minutes a time. It should be noted that overall this classification probably over-estimates the number of active days, as it assumes that each type of activity was done on a different day. So, for example, if an informant had participated in heavy housework and walking on the same day, it would be counted as two days of activity in the summary classification.

The activity type most commonly reported by men was sports and exercise. 42% of men reported having participated in some sports and exercise (of at least 15 minutes' duration) in the last four weeks. Participation in sports and exercise among women was lower at 36%; however this was still the second-most common activity type among women.

Among both men and women the proportion participating in sports decreased rapidly with age. Nearly 8 out of 10 men aged 16-24 (77%) had done some sports, and 29% had participated on 20 days or more in the last four weeks. By age 45-54 just over a third of men (36%) had participated in sports and exercise, and only 6% had done so on 20 days or more.

By age 75 and over only 7% of men had done any sports and exercise. The mean number of days' sports and exercise peaked at 11.4 among men aged 16-24, falling to 3.4 among men aged 45-54.

In younger age groups (up to age 35-44) men were significantly more likely than women to have done any sports; in the older age groups (age 45 and over) the proportions of men and women reporting any participation in sports were roughly the same. 57% of women aged 16-24 had participated in sports, and 11% had done so on 20 days or more. By age 45-54, 36% of women reported any sports participation, the same proportion as among men. The mean number of days' participation in sports fell from 5.9 among women aged 16-24 to 3.2 among those aged 45-54 and 0.3 among those aged 75 and over. **Table 5.1, Figure 5A**

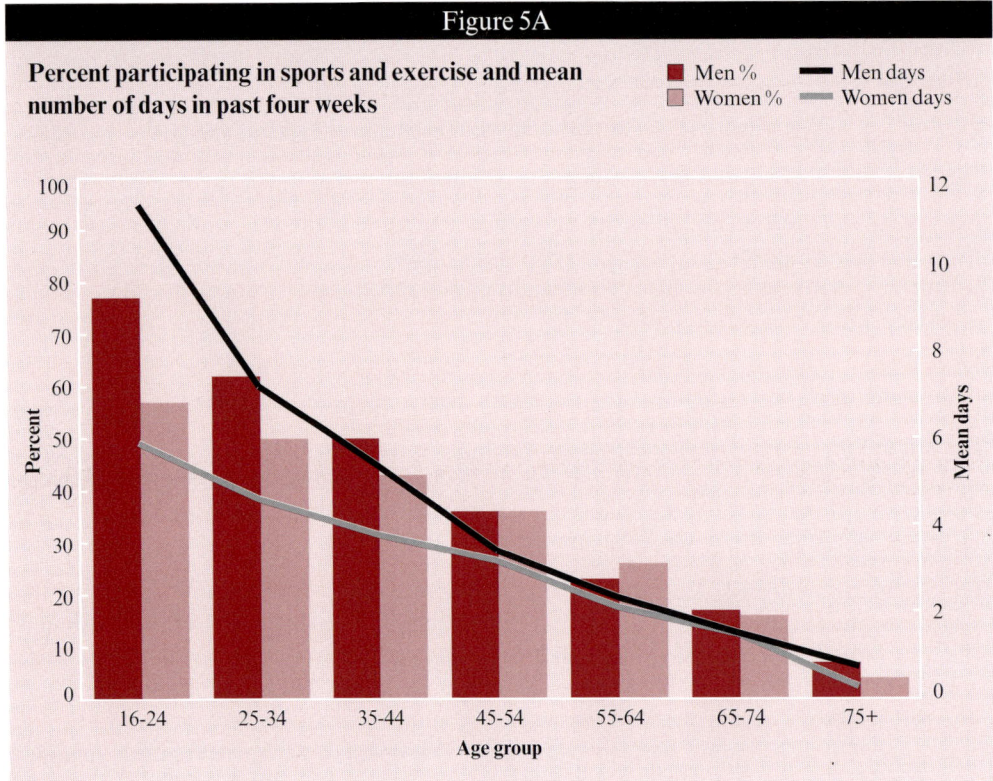

Figure 5A

Percent participating in sports and exercise and mean number of days in past four weeks

Among women the most common type of activity was heavy housework; 58% of women had participated in this in the last four weeks. Participation in housework was lower among men at 38% overall, although it was the second most common activity type for men. In all except the oldest age group the proportion of women who had participated in heavy housework was higher than of men.

Among women, participation in housework initially increased with age from around a half of those aged 16-24, to around 7 in 10 of those aged 25-44, before falling to around 6 in 10 among those aged 45-64, and just over a quarter of women aged 75 and over. The mean number of days' housework peaked at 4.6 among women aged 35-44.

Among men, participation in heavy housework was lowest in those aged 16-24 (28%), rising to 45% among those aged 25-34, falling again to 31% in men aged 55-64. There was a second smaller peak in participation in housework among men of retirement age – 40% of men aged 65-74 reported having done some heavy housework. The proportion fell again among those aged 75 and over. The number of days' housework reported by men was significantly lower than for women overall, with a peak of 2.5 days among men aged 65-74. **Table 5.1, Figure 5B**

The third major component of activity was walking; 32% of men and 24% of women had participated in walking (at a fast or brisk pace) in the last four weeks. Among men there was a steady decline with age in the proportion reporting any walking, from 53% of men aged 16-24 to 32% of those aged 45-54 and 9% of those aged 75 and over. The mean number of days similarly fell from 8.9 in men aged 16-24 to 1.4 in those aged 75 and over.

Among women, although the proportion reporting any walking fell with age the decline was less marked than among men. 35% of women aged 16-24 had participated in walking,

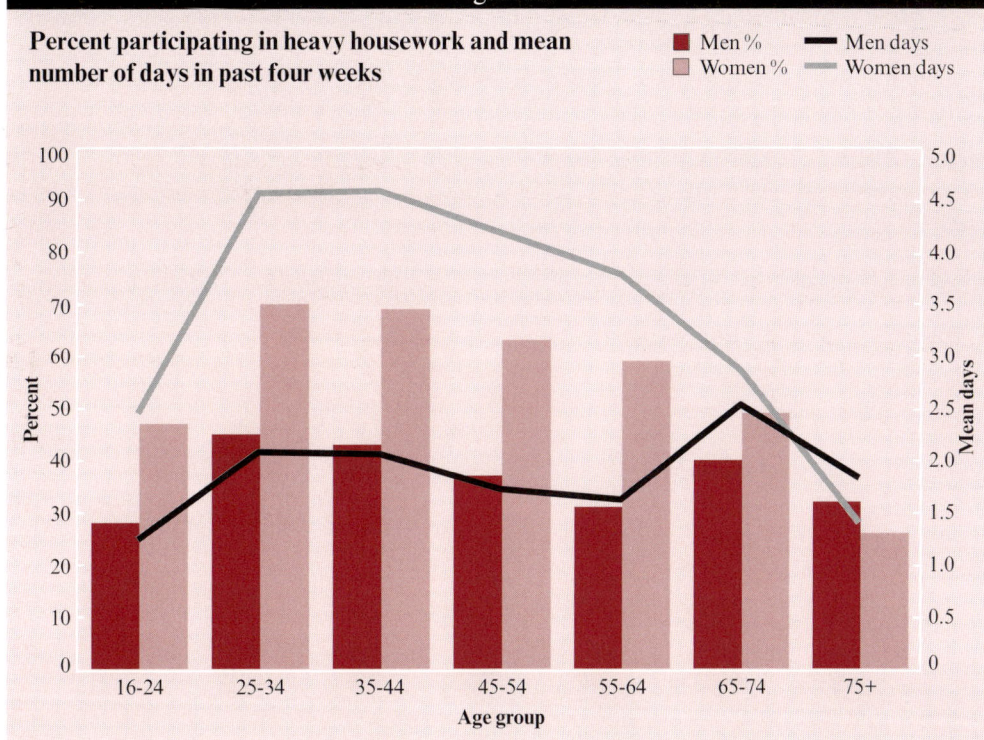

Figure 5B

Percent participating in heavy housework and mean number of days in past four weeks

Men %   Men days
Women %   Women days

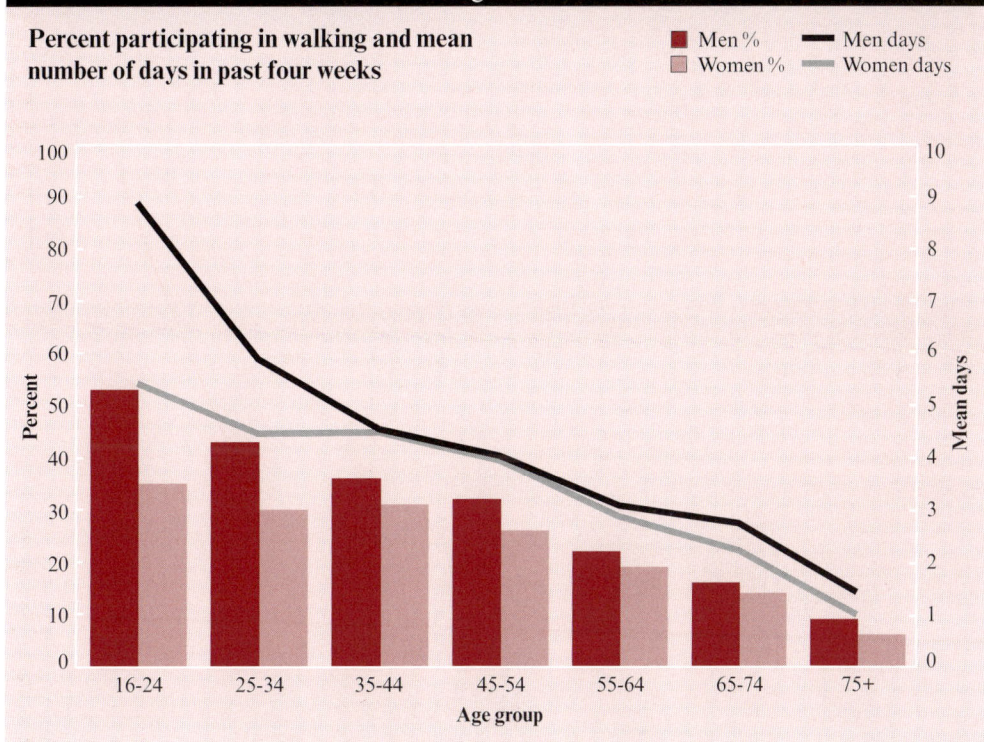

Figure 5C

Percent participating in walking and mean number of days in past four weeks

Men %   Men days
Women %   Women days

falling to 26% of those aged 45-54 and 6% of those aged 75 and over. The mean number of days' walking among women similarly fell from 5.4 in women aged 16-24, to 3.9 in those aged 45-54 and 1.0 in those aged 75 and over.   **Table 5.1, Figure 5C**

Heavy manual work/DIY was a significant part of men's overall physical activity; 31% of men overall reported at least one occasion of this activity. Participation in this type of activity was lowest at the ends of the age range – 16% of men aged 16-24 and 17% of those aged 75 and over reported any manual work/DIY. Among men aged 25-74 the proportion who had done any manual work was fairly steady at around 35%. Women were much less likely to report having done any heavy manual work/DIY – only 12% overall; again lowest in the youngest and oldest age groups.

There was a similar difference between men and women in the proportions reporting occupational activity. 22% of men overall were at least moderately active at work, compared with 12% of women. Among both men and women the proportion reporting occupational activity was fairly steady in those aged 16-54, falling slightly in those aged 55-64 and virtually disappearing in those aged 65 and over.

Figure 5D shows the mean number of days' participation in the main activity categories (heavy housework, sports and exercise and walking) by men and women in the past four weeks.

Figure 5D

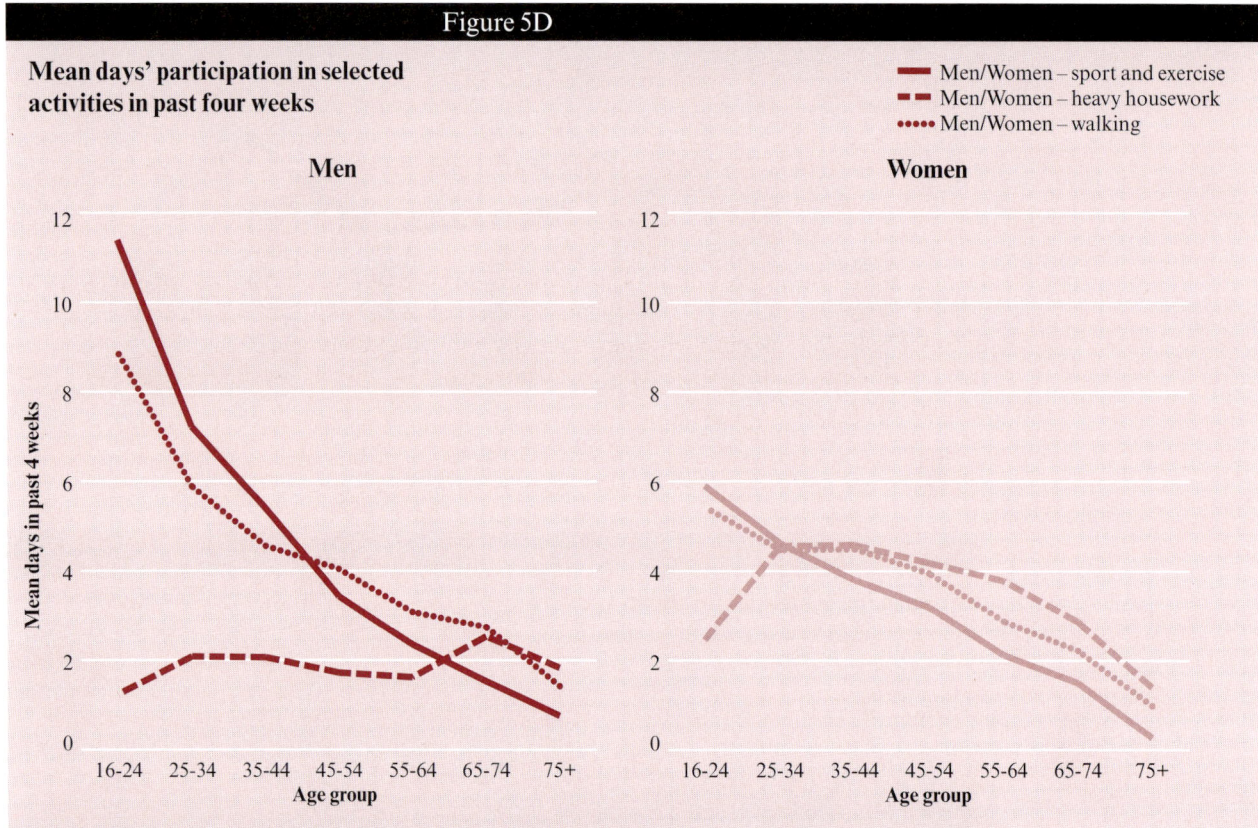

Figure 5D

Mean days' participation in selected activities in past four weeks

— Men/Women – sport and exercise
--- Men/Women – heavy housework
••••• Men/Women – walking

Men

Women

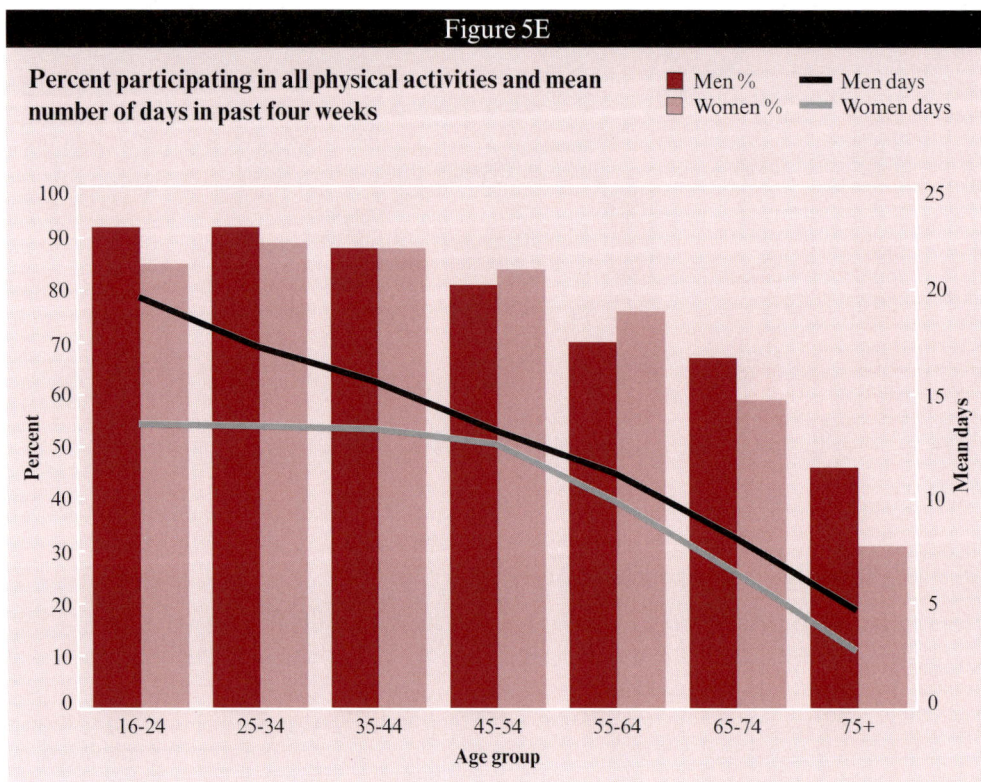

Figure 5E

Percent participating in all physical activities and mean number of days in past four weeks

Men % — Men days
Women % — Women days

Looking at the summary classification of participation in all types of activity, men overall were slightly more likely to have participated in physical activities than women (80% vs. 76%), and to have participated for a larger number of days (mean 13.7 among men, 11.0 among women). However this was not the case in all age groups.

Among men, participation in physical activity was highest at 92% in those aged 16-34. Participation rates then fell steadily with age to 67% among men aged 65-74, with a sharp drop to 46% among men aged 75 and over. The mean number of days' participation similarly fell steadily from 19.7 days by men aged 16-24 to 8.2 days by those aged 65-74, with a sharper drop to 4.7 days in men aged 75 and over.

Among women, participation in physical activity initially increased from 85% of women aged 16-24 to 89% of those aged 25-34. Participation then fell steadily to 76% among women aged 55-64, falling further to 31% in women aged 75 and over. The mean number of days' participation remained fairly steady at around 13.5 in women aged 16-44, falling to 2.7 days in those aged 75 and over.

Table 5.1, Figure 5E

5.2.2 Time spent participating in different activities

In addition to the number of days participating in each type of activity, informants were asked how long they had spent participating on each occasion. Table 5.2 shows the number of hours' participation in each type of activity per week, calculated by multiplying the number of days on which the activity was carried out by the average time per occasion, and converting to a weekly figure.

Figures are shown separately for each activity type, and for the summary classification of all physical activities. For the summary classification, occupational activity is counted as 10 hours per week for full-time workers, 6 hours per week for part-time workers.

Overall, 38% of men and 25% of women took part in physical activities for 7 hours or more per week, that is, at least one hour a day on average. Among men, the mean number of hours fell steadily with age, from 9.6 hours in men aged 16-24 to 6.5 in men aged 55-64 and 1.9 in those aged 75 and over.

Among women the mean number of hours per week spent in physical activities initially increased from 5.4 among those aged 16-24 to 6.2 among those aged 35-44, before falling again to 4.4 among women aged 55-64 and 1.0 among those aged 75 and over. As with

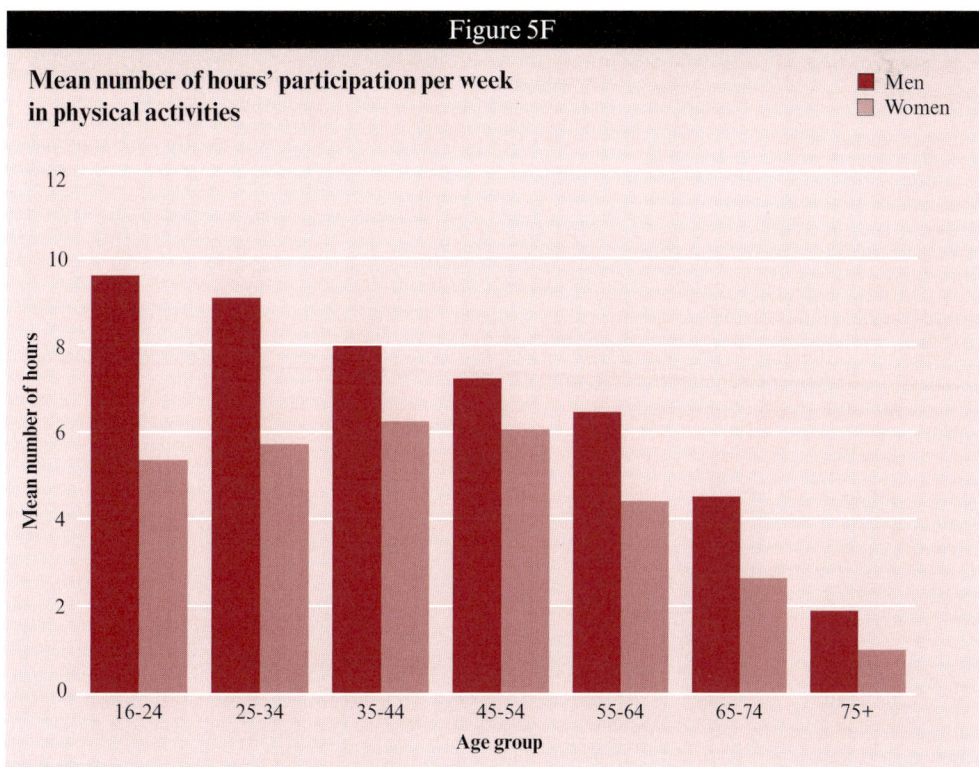

Figure 5F

Mean number of hours' participation per week in physical activities

■ Men
■ Women

participation in activities overall, the differential between men and women in the number of hours' participation in physical activities grew less with increasing age.   **Table 5.2, Figure 5F**

5.2.3 Maximum intensity level attained

Table 5.3 shows the maximum intensity level attained, by age and sex. This summary measure classifies informants according to the maximum intensity level reached in any type of activity in the four weeks prior to interview. In this measure, no account is taken of the frequency of the activity or of the duration, so that the overall proportions of men and women classified as active at a moderate level or higher are slightly higher than in the previous tables.

In the last four weeks, the majority of men (81%) and women (78%) had participated in at least one occasion of moderate/vigorous activity (including some who had done so for less than 15 minutes only).

Nearly a third of men (32%) and 22% of women had participated in activity at a vigorous level. For 12% of men and women the maximum intensity of activity reported was light activity; 10% of women and 7% of men reported no occasions of physical activity of at least light intensity.

Among both men and women the proportion who had participated in vigorous activity fell steadily with age, from 67% (men) and 41% (women) among those aged 16-24, to 13% of men and women aged 55-64. The proportion of people aged 65 and over who had done any vigorous activity was very small.

The proportion of men and women who were wholly inactive remained at 5% or less in all age groups up to age 54, before increasing rapidly with age: by age 75 and over a quarter of men and 39% of women reported no occasions of activity of at least light intensity. However at the other end of the activity scale significant proportions of those aged 75 and over were physically active: over a third of women (35%) and nearly half of men (48%) in this age group had been active at a moderate (or vigorous) level.   **Table 5.3**

5.2.4 Physical activity at work

All adults who were in paid employment or self-employed in the four weeks prior to interview were asked whether at work they were mainly sitting down, standing up or walking about; whether they did any climbing in the course of their work (excluding climbing stairs), and whether they had to lift or carry things at work that they found heavy. Answers to these questions are summarised in Table 5.4.

Similar proportions of men (44%) and women (41%) said that when at work they were mainly walking about. Nearly half of men (49%) said that their work involved lifting and/or carrying heavy loads, as did 41% of women. Men were far more likely than women to say their work involved climbing (30% compared with 8%).

Overall only 32% of men said that their work involved none of these physical activities; 40% that it involved at least two of these. Fewer women reported physical activities at work overall: 40% said that their work involved none of these activities, and around a quarter that it involved at least two. There was no consistent variation with age in participation in these activities at work, except for lifting and/or carrying heavy loads, which was most frequently reported by men and women aged 16-24.   **Table 5.4**

5.3 Overall levels of physical activity

5.3.1 Definitions of summary measures

Frequency-intensity level of activity

The frequency-intensity classification uses information available on the frequency and duration of activities as well as on the intensity of activity. This scale is similar to that used in the 1994 Health Survey report. The scale is intended to measure activity levels compared with the 'old' physical activity guidelines, which were that adults should take part in vigorous physical activities of 20 minutes' duration, three times a week. For this reason, only activities of a minimum duration of 20 minutes are included in this scale.

For occupational activity, full-time workers are counted as 20 days in four weeks of activity, part-time workers as 12 days in four weeks.

The classification is as follows:

Level 0 No occasions of moderate activity of at least 20 minutes' duration

Level 1 One to four occasions of at least moderate activity (once a week or less)

Level 2 Five to 11 occasions of at least moderate activity (more than once, less than three times a week)

Level 3 12 or more occasions of moderate activity (three times a week or more)

Level 4 12 or more occasions of a mixture of moderate and vigorous activity (three times a week or more)

Level 5 12 or more occasions of vigorous activity (three times a week or more).

Summary activity level

Most analyses in this chapter use a revised summary activity level, which classifies informants according to the revised physical activity guidelines (which are that adults should take part in five or more occasions a week of activity of at least moderate intensity, of 30 minutes' or more duration).

For the revised summary activity level, the minimum duration for all activities is 30 minutes. As before, full-time workers who were at least moderately active in their work are counted as 20 days' activity in the last four weeks, part-time workers as 12 days' activity.

The summary activity level classification is as follows:

Group 1 – low activity	Up to three occasions of moderate or vigorous activity of at least 30 minutes' duration in the last four weeks (less than once a week)
Group 2 – medium activity	Four to 19 occasions of moderate or vigorous activity of at least 30 minutes' duration in the last four weeks (at least once, less than five days a week)
Group 3 – high activity	20 or more occasions of moderate or vigorous activity of at least 30 minutes' duration in the last four weeks (at least five days a week).

5.3.2 **Participation in physical activities**

Frequency-intensity level of activity

Table 5.5 shows the distributions for the 'old' frequency-intensity summary measure for men and women in different age groups.

Perhaps the most striking finding here is the low proportion of adults who were active at Level 5, the level consistent with maximum cardiac benefit. Only in younger men did significant proportions report this level of activity. Overall 11% of men and 5% of women were active at Level 5. There was a steep decline with age in the proportions active at Level 5; among men this fell from 30% of men aged 16-24 to 8% of men aged 45-54. The decline among women with age was less steep, albeit from a lower peak: from 10% of women aged 16-24 to 4% of women aged 45-54. In both men and women aged 55 and over the proportions active at Level 5 were negligible.

As seen in previous sections in this chapter, overall activity levels tended to decline with age, particularly among men. At age 16-24, 70% of men were active at Level 3 and above (that is, at least 3 occasions a week of moderate or vigorous activity of 20 minutes or more). This proportion fell steadily to 40% among men aged 55-64, falling further to 15% of men aged 75 and over.

Among women aged 16-24 the proportion active at Level 3 and above was much lower than for men in the same age group, at 46%. However this proportion remained fairly level through to age 45-54 (45%), falling to 34% among women aged 55-64, down to 8% among women aged 75 and over. Thus the differential in activity levels between men and women was much less marked from age 45 than for younger age groups.   **Table 5.5**

Summary activity level

Table 5.7 shows the average number of days per week of participation in 30 minutes or more moderate or vigorous activity by men and women, and the summary activity level, by age group. Figure 5G shows proportions of men and women in Group 1, Group 2 and Group 3 by age.

Figure 5G

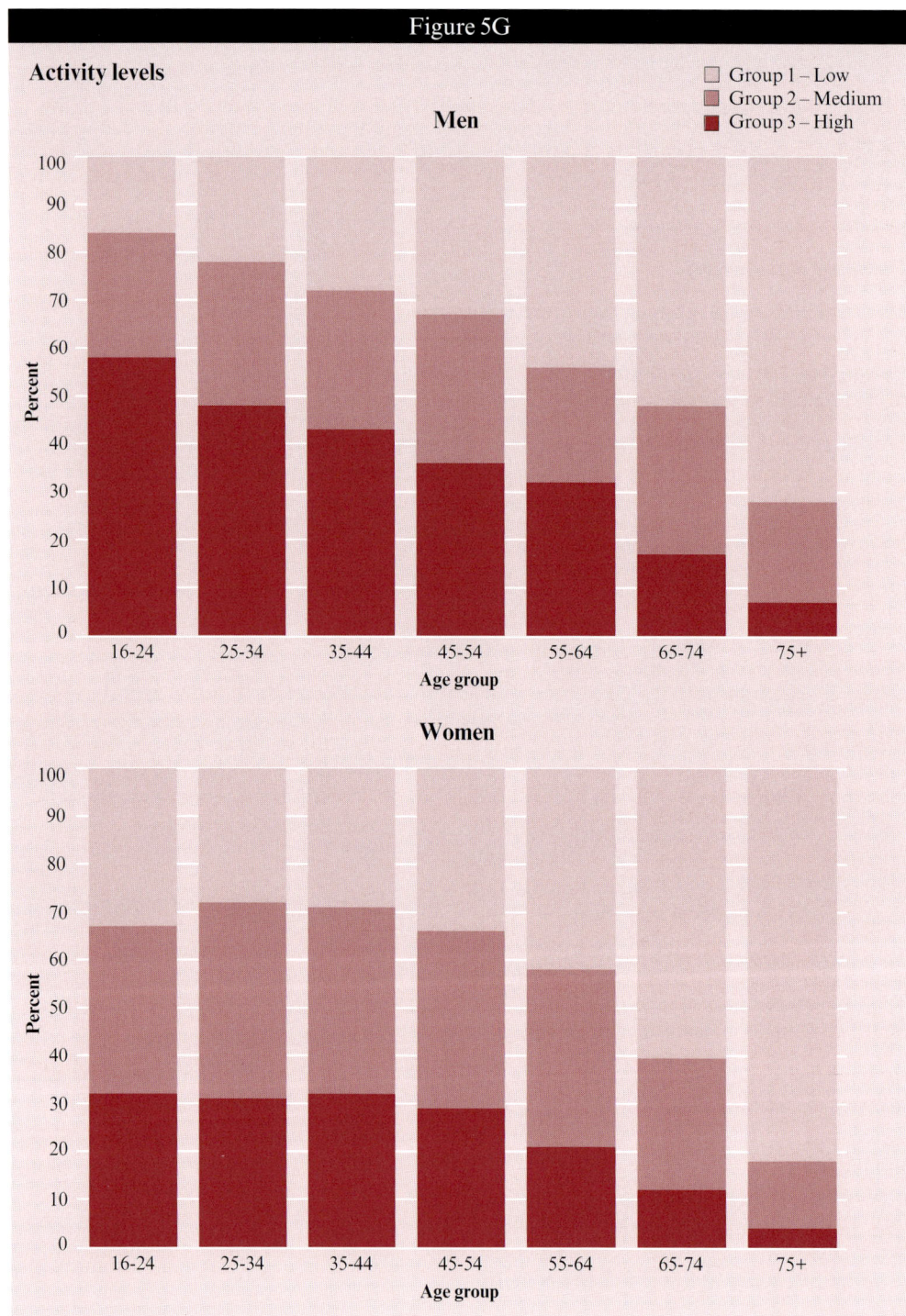

Figure 5G

Among men, over a third overall (37%) were classified in Group 3 (high activity). As seen for the other activity measures, this proportion fell steadily with age, from 58% of men aged 16-24 to 7% of those aged 75 and over.

Among women, a quarter overall were classified in Group 3. As before this proportion was fairly level at 30-32% in women aged 16-54, before falling with age to 4% among women aged 75 and over.

Group 3 is the level of activity that fulfils the current physical activity recommendations; Figure 5H illustrates the proportions of men and women achieving this level of activity.

Figure 5H

Proportion reaching 5 x 30 minutes guideline (Group 3)

■ Men
□ Women

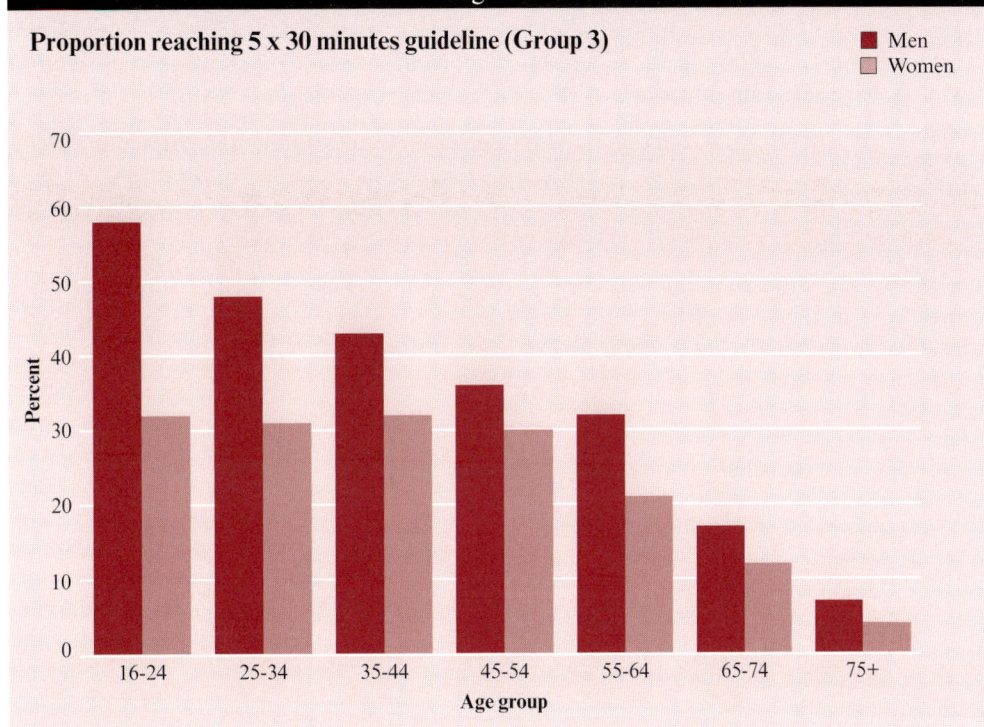

As the chart shows, up to age 44 men were more likely than women to be classified in Group 3, that is, to meet the target activity level. From age 45 and above the difference between men and women was much less marked, as activity levels in both sexes declined rapidly with advancing years.

Table 5.7, Figure 5H

Combined activity classification

As the two recommended guideline levels for physical activity are different, an informant who met one of the guideline levels would not necessarily meet the other. For example, someone who did only three bouts of vigorous activity of 20 minutes' duration per week would meet the 'old' guideline level (and indeed would be obtaining cardiac benefit from the activity), but would not meet the revised guideline level.

Table 5.9 presents figures for the two classifications combined, that is, the proportions of people active at either, both or neither of the guideline levels.

Overall far more men and women reached the revised guideline activity level (ie 5 x 30 minutes moderate activity per week) than the old level (ie 3 x 20 minutes vigorous activity per week). Most people who were active at the old guideline level also met the revised guideline activity level. Overall 40% of men and 26% of women met either or both of the guideline activity levels.

Table 5.9

5.3.3 Trends since 1994

Tables 5.6 and 5.8 show trends in the 'old' frequency-intensity activity classification, and in the 'new' summary activity level, since 1994.

There were some differences in questions between the 1994 and 1998 surveys that affect the comparability of both these classifications. In the 1994 survey, information on the duration of home activities (ie housework and manual work/DIY) was not collected. Instead information was collected on the number of days' participation in these activities, lasting at least 15 minutes. In the summary classifications for 1994, all reported occurrences of housework and manual work/DIY are counted towards the total. This means that, for example, some occurrences of housework that lasted only 15 minutes will be included towards the total count, presented as activities lasting at least 20 minutes.

In the 1998 survey, information on the duration of all activities was collected, so the summary classifications impose cut-offs on the duration of activities of 20 or 30 minutes. So some occurrences of housework or manual work/DIY that would have been counted in the summary variables in 1994 would not be counted in 1998. This means that the total number of occasions of reported moderate activity would be expected to be slightly higher in 1994 than in 1998. The number of occasions of vigorous activity are not affected, as home activities would never be counted as vigorous.

Trends in frequency-intensity level

There was no significant difference in the proportion of males and females active at Level 3 and above (that is, active at least three times a week). 49% of men in 1994 and 48% in 1998 were active at this level, as were 38% of women in both years. There were no significant differences in these proportions over time in the different age groups.

The proportions of men and women in the lowest activity category, Level 0 (i.e. no reported occasions of activity of at least 20 minutes' duration) did appear to increase between 1994 and 1998 in both men (17% in 1994, 23% in 1998) and women (19% in 1994, 26% in 1998). However this is likely to be an artefactual consequence of the change in the classification, noted above. That is to say, a proportion of those who in 1994 were coded as activity Level 1 or 2 as a consequence of doing 15 minutes of housework or manual work/DIY, were coded as Level 0 in 1998.

Table 5.6

Trends in summary activity level

Table 5.8 shows proportions of men and women in the summary activity level groups in 1994 and 1998. Group 3 on the summary activity level identifies those informants who met the current activity level, that is, took part in moderate or vigorous activities of at least 30 minutes' duration, on at least five days a week.

The proportion of men in activity Group 3 was 37% in 1994, and remained at exactly this proportion in 1998. There were no significant differences in any age groups among men, except among the 16-24 group, where the proportion in Group 3 increased from 50% in 1994 to 58% in 1998.

Among women the proportion meeting the guideline activity levels increased slightly, from 22% in 1994 to 25% in 1998. There were small increases in the proportion in Group 3 in all age groups up to age 54.

As with the frequency-intensity scale, the proportion of men and women in the lowest activity group (Group 1) appeared to increase between 1994 and 1998 (among men, from 30% to 35%; among women, from 35% to 41%). However it is likely that this increase was due to the changes in the questionnaire in 1998.

Table 5.8

5.4 Physical activity levels by socio-economic indicators

5.4.1 Components of activity and summary of activity levels by socio-economic indicators

Social class and equivalised household income

Participation in physical activities overall tended to increase with increasing household income, particularly among men. The age-standardised proportion of men who participated in any physical activities increased from 70% in the lowest income quintile to 86% and 85% in the two highest quintiles. Among women the age-standardised proportion who participated in any physical activity was 78% or 79% in the three higher income quintiles, but only 70% in the lowest quintile. The pattern according to social class was similar: among men, the age-standardised proportion participating was higher in Social Classes I and II; among women it was higher in Social Classes I, II and IIINM.

Looking at participation in the different components of activity by income and social class, clearer patterns emerge. Among both men and women, participation in sports and exercise increased rapidly with increasing household income. The age-standardised proportion of men who took part in sports increased from 31% in the lowest household income quintile to 55% in the highest quintile; equivalent figures for women were 24% and 45%. A similar pattern was apparent in participation by social class; that is, rates of participation in sports and exercise tended to be higher in Social Classes I and II.

Participation in walking was also strongly related to household income and social class, with men and women in higher income quintiles more likely to have participated in walking. Age-standardised proportions of men increased from 27% in the lowest income quintile to 41% in the highest; equivalent percentages for women were 19% and 30%.

Similarly, proportions walking tended to be non-manual in the non-manual social classes.

Participation in physical activity at work was, as might be expected, strongly related to social class, particularly for men. In the manual social classes around a third of men (age-standardised) participated in occupational activity, more than twice the proportion in the non-manual classes. Among women participation in occupational activity was particularly high in Social Class V. In terms of household income, participation in physical activity at work was highest in the middle income quintiles.   **Table 5.14, 5.15, Figure 5I**

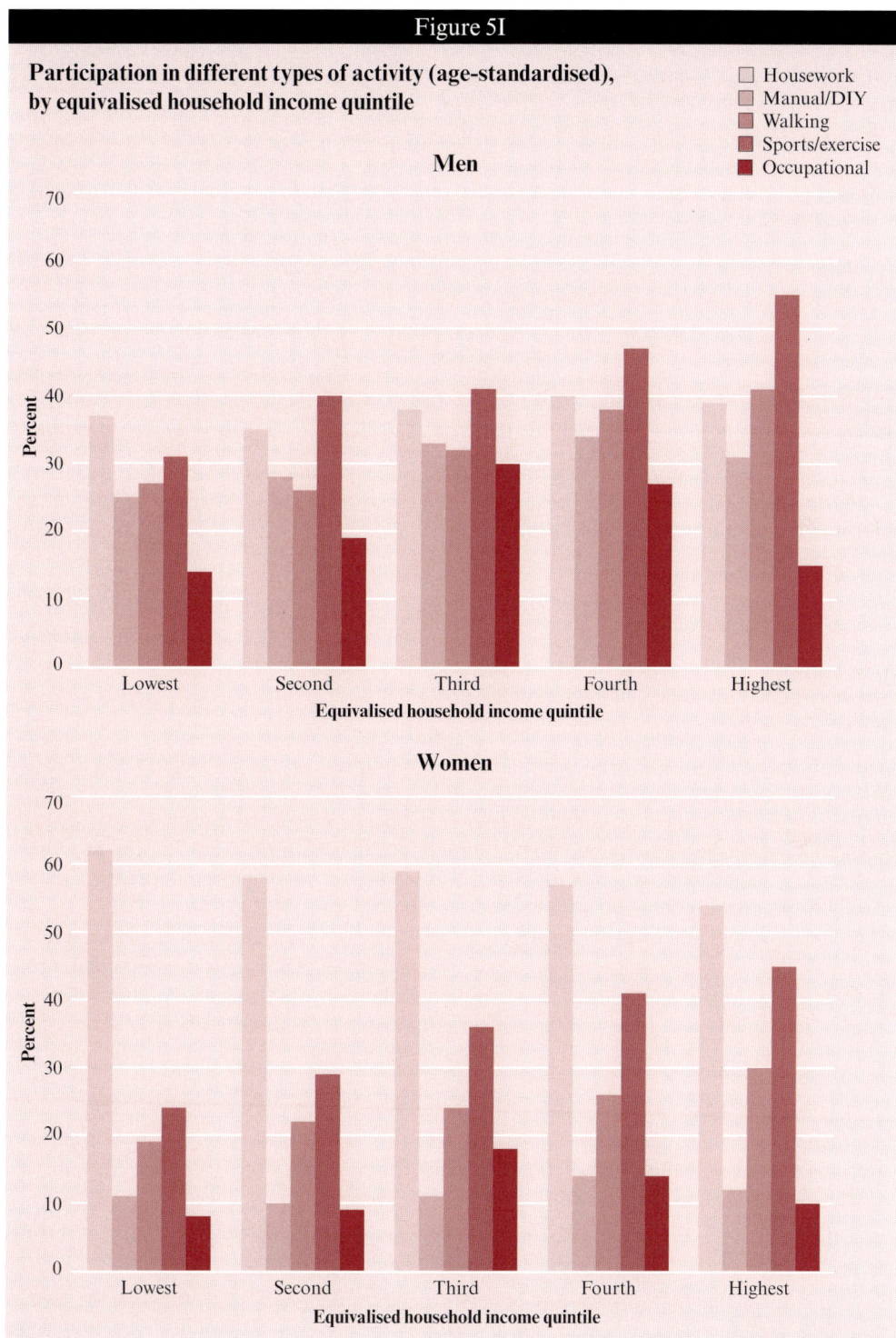

Figure 5I

Participation in different types of activity (age-standardised), by equivalised household income quintile

Legend: Housework, Manual/DIY, Walking, Sports/exercise, Occupational

Men

X-axis: Equivalised household income quintile (Lowest, Second, Third, Fourth, Highest)

Women

X-axis: Equivalised household income quintile (Lowest, Second, Third, Fourth, Highest)

Looking at the proportions of men and women in Group 3 of the summary activity level (that is, meeting the current physical activity guidelines), the pattern according to social class and income is less clear. Among men the age-standardised proportion in Group 3 was highest in Social Class V (50%), and lower in the non-manual social classes (31%-33% in Social Classes I, II and IIINM); the opposite pattern to that seen for participation in physical activities overall. This apparent discrepancy is due to the greater importance of occupational activity in the manual social classes, since informants who were physically active at work are automatically coded into the highest activity group. Similarly the age-standardised proportion of men in Group 3 was lower in the lowest (32%) and highest (34%) income quintiles than it was in the middle quintiles (40%-44%).

Among women there was no clear pattern according to household income or social class in the proportion in Group 3. **Table 5.10, 5.11**

Health Authority area type

The overall rate of participation in physical activities was lowest in Inner London for both men and women, and tended to be lower in the more urban area types (Inner London, Mining and Industrial, Urban) than in the less urban areas (Mature, Prosperous and Rural), particularly for men. The age-standardised proportion of men participating in physical activity was 68% in Inner London, compared with 76%-78% in the other urban areas and 82% to 85% in the suburban/rural areas. Among women the lowest participation rate was in Inner London (70%), the highest in Rural areas (78%), but the gradient across area types was less clear.

Looking at the types of activity, participation in housework was particularly low among men in Inner London (32% compared with 37%-39% in the other area types); among women participation in housework was lowest in Inner London (53%) and Mature and Prosperous area types (54%), and highest in Rural areas (62%).

Participation in heavy manual work/DIY was also particularly low in Inner London (9% for men, compared with 35% in Rural areas).

Participation in walking was lowest for both men and women in the Mining and Industrial and Urban areas, and highest in Prosperous areas. Participation in sports and exercise was highest in the Prosperous and Mature area types. **Table 5.16**

Looking at the summary activity level, the proportion of men in Group 3 was lower in Inner London (32% age-standardised) than in the other area types (38%-40%). Among women the proportion in Group 3 did not vary significantly by area type. **Table 5.12**

5.4.2 Logistic regression of participation in physical activities

Separate logistic regressions were run for men and women, with the following independent variables: age group, social class of head of household, equivalised household income quintile, employment status and Health Authority area type. Six models were run (for each sex separately), with the dependent variables being participation in heavy housework, participation in heavy manual work/DIY, participation in walking, participation in sports and exercise, participation in physical activity at work, and participation in physical activity at activity Group 3. The odds ratios are presented in Tables 5.18 and 5.19, and are relative to average for each independent variable. An odds ratio of less than one means that the group was less likely to participate in the activity in question, and an odds ratio greater than one that the group was more likely. Independent variables with a 'p' value of 0.05 or less are significant predictors of the dependent variable at the 95% confidence level.

The variations noted between sub-groups in participation in the different activity types, and in physical activities overall, tended to be confirmed in the regression models.

For men, the odds of being in activity Group 3 were higher than average for those aged under 55 (particularly those aged 16-24), for those in the manual social classes, for those in the third and fourth income quintiles, and for those in employment. The lowest odds of being in activity Group 3 were for men aged 75 and over (0.20) or 65-74 (0.50), for men in Social Class I (0.59), and for the other economically inactive (0.47).

Taking into account all the other independent variables, participation in heavy housework was more likely among men aged 25-54 and among the unemployed and retired. Men in the youngest (16-24) and oldest (75 and over) age groups were less likely than average to participate in heavy manual work/DIY, as were the other economically active and those living in Inner London. The odds of participating in walking were higher for men aged under 55 (particularly those aged 16-24), those in the non-manual social classes, those in the two highest income quintiles, the unemployed and retired, and those in Mature and Prosperous area types. Participation in sports and exercise was more likely among men aged under 44 (particularly those aged 16-24), those in Social Classes I and II, and those in the top two income quintiles. The odds of participating in physical activity at work were higher than average for men aged 16-24 and 55-64, for men in the manual social classes, for those in the second and third income quintiles, and (of course) for those in employment.

For women, the odds of being in activity Group 3 were higher than average for those aged under 55 and for those in employment. Social class, household income and area type were not significant predictors of activity Group 3 for women.

Taking into account all the other independent variables in the models, participation in heavy housework was more likely than average among women aged 25-64, those in Social Class IIINM, in the bottom income quintile, among those in employment, and among those living in Urban and Rural area types. The odds of women participating in heavy manual work/DIY were higher among those aged 25-74, and in Prosperous and Rural areas. Participation in walking was more likely in those aged under 55, those in non-manual social classes, those in the top income quintile, the unemployed, and those living in Inner London and Prosperous areas. For sports and exercise, the odds of participation were higher in those aged under 55 (particularly those aged 16-34), the non-manual social classes, the top two income quintiles, the unemployed, and those living in Mature and Prosperous areas. The odds of women participating in physical activity at work were higher in Social Classes IV and V, the bottom three income quintiles, and those living in Urban and Mining and Industrial areas.

Table 5.18

Table 5.19

References and notes

1   *Saving Lives: Our Healthier Nation*, The Stationery Office, London, 1999.

2   See for example *The Health of the Nation. A strategy for health in England*, HMSO, London, 1992; *More people more active more often. Physical activity in England: A consultation paper*. Department of Health, London, June 1995.

3   See for example Shaper AG and Wanamathee G. *Physical activity and ischaemic heart disease in middle-aged British men*, British Heart Journal 1991; **66**:384-394;

    Powell KE, Thompson PD, Casperson CT et al. *Physical activity and the incidence of coronary heart disease,* Annual Review of Public Health 1987; **8**:235-287.

4   See for example Helmrich SP et al. *Physical activity and reduced occurrence of non-insulin-dependent diabetes mellitus*, New England Journal of Medicine 1991; **325**:147-152;

    Wolman R. *Osteoporosis and exercise*, British Medical Journal 1994; **309**:400-403.

5   Killoran A et al (eds). *Moving on: international perspectives on promoting physical activity*, Health Education Authority, London, 1995.

6   American College of Sports Medicine. *The recommended quantity and quality of exercise for developing and maintaining cardiorespiratory and muscular fitness in healthy adults*, Medicine and Science in Sports and Exercise 1990; **22**:265-274.

7   Blair SN and Connelly JC. *How much physical activity should we do? The case for moderate amounts and intensities of physical activity* in Killoran A et al (eds) ibid.

8   Pate R R et al. *Physical activity and public health: a recommendation from the Centres for Disease Control and Prevention and the American College of Sports Medicine*, Journal of the American Medical Association 1995; **273**:402-407.

9   *Strategy statement on physical activity*, Department of Health, London, 1996.

10 US Department of Health and Human Services. *Physical activity and health: a report of the Surgeon General*, Department of Health and Human Services, Centre for Disease Control and Prevention, National Centre for Chronic Disease Promotion and Health Promotion, Pittsburgh, 1996.

11 Gray R. *Physical Activity* in Colhoun H and Prescott-Clarke P (eds) *Health Survey for England 1994*, HMSO, London, 1994.

12 Prior G. *Physical Activity* in Prescott-Clarke P and Primatesta P (eds) *Health Survey for England '95-'97*, The Stationery Office, London, 1998.

13 *Allied Dunbar National Fitness Survey*, Health Education Authority and Sports Council, London, 1992.

14 **Sports and exercise – Energy cost**

Vigorous:

a) All occurrences of running/jogging, squash, boxing, kick boxing, skipping, trampolining.

b) Sports coded as vigorous intensity if they had made the informant out of breath or sweaty, but otherwise coded as moderate intensity, including: cycling, aerobics, keep fit, gymnastics, dance for fitness, weight training, football, rugby, swimming, tennis, badminton.

Moderate:

a) See 'vigorous' category b).

b) All occasions of a large number of activities including: basketball, canoeing, fencing, field athletics, hockey, ice skating, lacrosse, netball, roller skating, rowing, skiing, volleyball.

c) Sports coded as moderate intensity if they had made the informant out of breath or sweaty, but otherwise coded as light intensity, including: exercise (press-ups, sit-ups), dancing.

Light:

a) See 'moderate' category c).

b) All occasions of a large number of activities including: abseiling, baseball, bowls, cricket, croquet, darts, fishing, golf, riding, rounders, sailing, shooting, snooker, snorkelling, softball, table tennis, yoga.

15 **Home activities:**

Examples of 'heavy' gardening or DIY work classified as moderate intensity:

Digging, clearing rough ground, building in stone/bricklaying, mowing large areas with a hand mower, felling trees, chopping wood, mixing/laying concrete, moving heavy loads, refitting a kitchen or bathroom or any similar heavy manual work.

Examples of 'heavy' housework classified as moderate intensity:

Walking with heavy shopping for more than 5 minutes, moving heavy furniture, spring cleaning, scrubbing floors with a scrubbing brush, cleaning windows, or other similar heavy housework.

Examples of 'light' gardening or DIY work classified as light intensity:

Hoeing, weeding, pruning, mowing with a power mower, planting flowers/seeds, decorating, minor household repairs, car washing and polishing, car repairs and maintenance.

16 **Work activities:**

Vigorous:

Considers self very physically active in job and is in one of a small number of occupations defined as involving heavy work including:

fishermen/women, furnace operators, rollermen, smiths and forge workers, faceworking coal-miners, other miners, construction workers and forestry workers.

Moderate:

Considers self very physically active in job and is not in occupation groups listed above OR considers self fairly physically active in job and is in one of a small number of occupations involving heavy or moderate work including:

any listed above OR fire service officers, metal plate workers, shipwrights, riveters, steel erectors, benders, fitters, galvanisers, tin platers, dip platers, plasterers, roofers, glaziers, general building workers, road surfacers, stevedores, dockers, goods porters, refuse collectors.

Light:

Considers self fairly physically active in job and is not in one of the occupation groups listed above.

Tables

Table 5.1

Number of days' participation in different activities in the last four weeks, by age and sex

Aged 16 and over   *1998*

Number of days in the last four weeks (at least 15 minutes a day)	Age							Total
	16-24	25-34	35-44	45-54	55-64	65-74	75 +	
	%	%	%	%	%	%	%	%
Men								
Number of days Heavy Housework								
None	72	55	57	63	69	60	68	62
Any	28	45	43	37	31	40	32	38
1 to 3 days	17	22	21	19	14	17	12	18
4 to 11 days	9	19	19	14	14	17	15	16
12 to 19 days	1	2	2	2	2	3	3	2
20 days or more	1	1	2	1	1	4	2	2
Mean number of days[a]	1.2	2.1	2.1	1.7	1.6	2.5	1.8	1.9
Standard error of the mean	0.12	0.11	0.11	0.11	0.12	0.18	0.18	0.05
Number of days Heavy Manual/DIY								
None	84	66	63	65	69	66	83	69
Any	16	34	37	35	31	34	17	31
1 to 3 days	10	20	20	18	13	16	7	16
4 to 11 days	5	11	13	13	13	12	6	11
12 to 19 days	1	2	2	2	2	3	2	2
20 days or more	1	2	2	1	3	2	1	2
Mean number of days[a]	0.7	1.6	1.8	1.8	2.0	2.0	1.1	1.6
Standard error of the mean	0.08	0.11	0.11	0.11	0.15	0.15	0.15	0.05
Number of days Walking[b]								
None	47	57	64	68	78	84	91	68
Any	53	43	36	32	22	16	9	32
1 to 3 days	6	9	8	6	4	2	2	6
4 to 11 days	11	12	12	11	6	5	1	9
12 to 19 days	8	5	5	3	2	2	2	4
20 days or more	27	17	12	11	9	8	4	13
Mean number of days[a]	8.9	5.9	4.6	4.0	3.1	2.7	1.4	4.6
Standard error of the mean	0.37	0.26	0.23	0.23	0.24	0.26	0.24	0.10
Number of days Sports and Exercise								
None	23	38	50	64	77	83	93	58
Any	77	62	50	36	23	17	7	42
1 to 3 days	12	15	13	11	6	6	1	10
4 to 11 days	23	21	17	13	9	6	3	14
12 to 19 days	14	11	9	6	3	2	1	7
20 days or more	29	16	10	6	5	3	2	10
Mean number of days[a]	11.4	7.2	5.4	3.4	2.3	1.5	0.8	4.9
Standard error of the mean	0.36	0.26	0.23	0.19	0.20	0.17	0.16	0.10
Occupational activity								
None	72	71	72	75	78	97	99	78
Any	28	29	28	25	22	3	1	22
Mean number of days[a]	5.2	5.6	5.6	5.0	4.2	0.6	0.1	4.3
Standard error of the mean	0.29	0.24	0.25	0.24	0.26	0.11	0.05	0.10
Number of days all physical activities[c]								
None	8	8	12	19	30	33	54	20
Any	92	92	88	81	70	67	46	80
1 to 3 days	5	8	10	10	10	15	12	10
4 to 11 days	12	18	19	20	18	22	17	18
12 to 19 days	10	11	9	11	7	11	8	10
20 days or more	65	54	49	40	35	20	9	42
Mean number of days[a]	19.7	17.3	15.6	13.3	11.2	8.2	4.7	13.7
Standard error of the mean	0.35	0.29	0.31	0.31	0.36	0.34	0.34	0.13
Base								
Men	*875*	*1338*	*1305*	*1289*	*987*	*837*	*562*	*7193*

continued...

Table 5.1 *continued*

Number of days in the last four weeks (at least 15 minutes a day)	Age							Total
	16-24	25-34	35-44	45-54	55-64	65-74	75 +	
	%	%	%	%	%	%	%	%
Women								
Number of days Heavy Housework								
None	53	30	31	37	41	51	74	42
Any	47	70	69	63	59	49	26	58
1 to 3 days	23	26	26	25	21	21	12	23
4 to 11 days	19	33	31	27	29	21	11	26
12 to 19 days	2	5	5	6	5	4	2	4
20 days or more	3	6	6	6	5	3	1	5
Mean number of days[a]	2.5	4.6	4.6	4.2	3.8	2.9	1.4	3.6
Standard error of the mean	0.15	0.16	0.16	0.16	0.17	0.16	0.12	0.06
Number of days Heavy Manual/DIY								
None	94	86	85	85	87	88	96	88
Any	6	14	15	15	13	12	4	12
1 to 3 days	4	9	10	9	7	6	2	7
4 to 11 days	1	4	3	5	5	4	2	4
12 to 19 days	0	0	1	0	1	0	0	0
20 days or more	0	0	1	0	1	1	0	0
Mean number of days[a]	0.2	0.5	0.6	0.5	0.6	0.5	0.3	0.5
Standard error of the mean	0.03	0.05	0.07	0.05	0.07	0.07	0.07	0.02
Number of days Walking[b]								
None	65	70	69	74	81	86	94	76
Any	35	30	31	26	19	14	6	24
1 to 3 days	4	4	5	3	2	2	1	3
4 to 11 days	10	8	8	9	6	4	1	7
12 to 19 days	5	4	4	3	3	2	1	3
20 days or more	16	13	13	12	8	7	3	11
Mean number of days[a]	5.4	4.5	4.5	3.9	2.9	2.2	1.0	3.7
Standard error of the mean	0.29	0.22	0.22	0.22	0.21	0.21	0.15	0.09
Number of days Sports and Exercise								
None	43	50	57	64	74	84	96	64
Any	57	50	43	36	26	16	4	36
1 to 3 days	14	14	13	10	8	4	1	10
4 to 11 days	24	20	18	15	12	7	2	15
12 to 19 days	9	9	6	5	3	2	0	5
20 days or more	11	7	6	5	3	3	0	5
Mean number of days[a]	5.9	4.6	3.8	3.2	2.1	1.5	0.3	3.3
Standard error of the mean	0.26	0.18	0.17	0.17	0.15	0.15	0.07	0.07
Occupational activity								
None	85	87	83	82	88	99	100	88
Any	15	13	17	18	12	1	0	12
Mean number of days[a]	2.4	2.2	2.6	2.9	1.9	0.2	0.0	1.9
Standard error of the mean	0.19	0.14	0.15	0.17	0.15	0.06	0.02	0.06
Number of days all physical activities[c]								
None	15	11	12	16	24	41	69	24
Any	85	89	88	84	76	59	31	76
1 to 3 days	12	13	13	12	13	14	10	13
4 to 11 days	22	25	25	23	26	22	11	23
12 to 19 days	13	15	14	13	13	8	4	12
20 days or more	39	36	36	35	24	14	5	29
Mean number of days[a]	13.6	13.5	13.3	12.6	9.9	6.5	2.7	11.0
Standard error of the mean	0.35	0.26	0.27	0.28	0.30	0.29	0.21	0.11
Base								
Women	*1006*	*1630*	*1573*	*1484*	*1148*	*967*	*907*	*8715*

[a] Mean based on all informants.

[b] Walking at a 'Fairly brisk' or 'Fast' pace.

[c] Includes Heavy housework; Heavy manual/DIY; Walking; Sports and Exercise; and Occupational activity (counted as 20 days for full-time workers, 12 days for part-time workers).

Table 5.2

Average time spent participating in physical activities per week, by age and sex

Aged 16 and over   *1998*

Average time spent per week[a]	Age							Total
	16-24	25-34	35-44	45-54	55-64	65-74	75 +	
	%	%	%	%	%	%	%	%

Men

Heavy Housework								
No time	72	55	57	63	69	60	68	62
Less than 1 hour	18	24	22	18	14	17	17	19
1, less than 3 hours	7	15	13	11	11	14	9	12
3, less than 5 hours	2	3	5	4	3	3	4	3
5, less than 7 hours	1	1	1	2	1	2	1	1
7 hours or more	1	2	2	2	2	4	1	2
Mean number of hours[b]	0.4	0.8	0.8	0.8	0.7	1.1	0.5	0.8
Standard error of the mean	0.05	0.06	0.07	0.08	0.11	0.11	0.08	0.03
Heavy Manual/DIY								
No time	84	65	63	65	68	66	83	69
Less than 1 hour	5	8	8	6	6	8	5	7
1, less than 3 hours	5	13	12	13	10	12	7	11
3, less than 5 hours	3	5	6	6	5	4	1	5
5, less than 7 hours	1	2	3	2	3	2	1	2
7 hours or more	3	7	7	8	8	8	3	7
Mean number of hours[b]	0.6	1.6	1.7	1.9	1.9	1.8	0.7	1.5
Standard error of the mean	0.08	0.14	0.12	0.15	0.18	0.19	0.15	0.06
Walking[c]								
No time	47	57	64	68	78	84	91	68
Less than 1 hour	11	14	12	11	5	3	2	9
1, less than 3 hours	15	12	11	9	7	4	2	9
3, less than 5 hours	11	6	6	5	3	2	2	5
5, less than 7 hours	6	3	2	2	2	2	0	3
7 hours or more	10	8	6	5	5	6	2	6
Mean number of hours[b]	2.3	2.1	1.5	1.3	1.4	1.1	0.4	1.5
Standard error of the mean	0.16	0.19	0.15	0.12	0.18	0.16	0.10	0.06
Sports and Exercise								
No time	23	38	50	64	77	83	93	58
Less than 1 hour	14	20	17	14	9	8	3	13
1, less than 3 hours	22	20	20	14	7	5	2	14
3, less than 5 hours	13	10	7	4	3	2	0	6
5, less than 7 hours	9	5	3	2	2	0	0	3
7 hours or more	18	7	4	3	1	1	1	5
Mean number of hours[b]	3.7	1.9	1.3	0.8	0.5	0.3	0.1	1.3
Standard error of the mean	0.17	0.09	0.08	0.05	0.05	0.05	0.04	0.04
All physical activities[d]								
No time	8	8	12	19	30	32	54	20
Less than 1 hour	7	10	12	11	10	16	16	11
1, less than 3 hours	14	15	15	15	14	17	14	15
3, less than 5 hours	10	12	10	10	7	8	5	9
5, less than 7 hours	8	7	7	6	5	6	3	6
7 hours or more	54	47	44	39	35	21	7	38
Mean number of hours[b]	9.6	9.1	8.0	7.2	6.5	4.5	1.9	7.2
Standard error of the mean	0.31	0.28	0.25	0.26	0.30	0.29	0.22	0.11

Base								
Men	*875*	*1338*	*1305*	*1289*	*987*	*837*	*562*	*7193*

continued...

Table 5.2 *continued*

Average time spent per week[a]	Age							Total
	16-24	25-34	35-44	45-54	55-64	65-74	75 +	
	%	%	%	%	%	%	%	%

Women

Heavy Housework
No time	53	30	31	37	41	51	74	42
Less than 1 hour	22	25	21	20	21	20	13	21
1, less than 3 hours	15	24	25	22	20	18	8	20
3, less than 5 hours	4	8	10	9	7	5	3	7
5, less than 7 hours	2	4	4	4	4	2	1	3
7 hours or more	4	9	9	9	7	5	1	7
Mean number of hours[b]	1.2	2.0	2.3	2.3	1.8	1.2	0.5	1.7
Standard error of the mean	0.10	0.09	0.12	0.13	0.12	0.09	0.06	0.04

Heavy Manual/DIY
No time	94	86	85	85	87	88	96	88
Less than 1 hour	2	5	5	4	4	4	1	4
1, less than 3 hours	2	5	6	6	5	4	2	4
3, less than 5 hours	1	2	2	2	2	2	0	2
5, less than 7 hours	0	1	1	1	1	1	1	1
7 hours or more	0	2	2	1	1	1	1	1
Mean number of hours[b]	0.1	0.4	0.5	0.4	0.3	0.3	0.2	0.4
Standard error of the mean	0.04	0.06	0.06	0.06	0.05	0.06	0.05	0.02

Walking[c]
No time	65	70	69	74	81	85	94	76
Less than 1 hour	8	7	8	6	4	4	2	6
1, less than 3 hours	11	9	9	8	6	4	1	7
3, less than 5 hours	8	6	5	5	3	2	1	5
5, less than 7 hours	3	2	3	2	2	1	1	2
7 hours or more	5	5	6	5	4	4	1	4
Mean number of hours[b]	1.5	1.1	1.3	1.2	0.8	0.7	0.3	1.1
Standard error of the mean	0.20	0.08	0.09	0.10	0.09	0.11	0.07	0.04

Sports and Exercise
No time	42	50	57	64	74	84	96	64
Less than 1 hour	18	19	17	15	11	5	1	13
1, less than 3 hours	22	19	17	14	10	8	2	14
3, less than 5 hours	10	8	6	4	4	1	0	5
5, less than 7 hours	4	3	2	1	1	1	0	2
7 hours or more	5	2	2	1	1	1		2
Mean number of hours[b]	1.6	1.1	0.9	0.7	0.5	0.3	0.0	0.8
Standard error of the mean	0.10	0.05	0.06	0.05	0.04	0.03	0.01	0.02

All physical activities[d]
No time	15	11	12	16	24	41	69	24
Less than 1 hour	16	14	13	12	14	16	13	14
1, less than 3 hours	20	22	21	19	21	20	9	19
3, less than 5 hours	13	13	12	12	9	7	3	10
5, less than 7 hours	10	9	8	8	8	5	2	8
7 hours or more	27	31	33	32	23	12	4	25
Mean number of hours[b]	5.4	5.7	6.2	6.1	4.4	2.6	1.0	4.8
Standard error of the mean	0.23	0.17	0.20	0.21	0.19	0.17	0.11	0.08

Base
Women	*1006*	*1630*	*1573*	*1484*	*1148*	*967*	*907*	*8715*

[a] Minimum duration 15 minutes per day.

[b] Mean based on all informants.

[c] Walking at a 'Fairly brisk' or 'Fast' pace.

[d] Includes Heavy housework; Heavy manual/DIY; Walking; and Sports and Exercise; and Occupational activity

Table 5.3

Maximum intensity level attained, by age and sex

Aged 16 and over 1998

Maximum intensity level	Age							Total
	16-24	25-34	35-44	45-54	55-64	65-74	75 +	
	%	%	%	%	%	%	%	%
Men								
Inactive	2	2	2	5	10	13	25	7
Light	5	5	9	13	19	17	27	12
Moderate	26	41	51	58	59	64	46	49
Vigorous	67	52	37	25	13	6	2	32
Women								
Inactive	4	2	4	5	9	18	39	10
Light	10	7	8	9	13	20	26	12
Moderate	45	56	61	65	65	57	34	56
Vigorous	41	34	28	20	13	5	1	22
Bases								
Men	*875*	*1338*	*1305*	*1289*	*987*	*837*	*562*	*7193*
Women	*1006*	*1630*	*1573*	*1484*	*1148*	*967*	*907*	*8715*

Table 5.4

Physical activity at work, by age and sex

Aged 16 and over in paid work in the last four weeks 1998

Activities involved in job	Age					Total
	16-24	25-34	35-44	45-54	55 +	
	%	%	%	%	%	%
Men						
Mainly walking about	51	43	41	44	49	44
Climbing	31	28	29	31	29	30
Lifting and/or carrying heavy loads	66	52	47	45	42	49
At least two of these	50	40	37	39	37	40
None of these	21	33	36	34	31	32
Women						
Mainly walking about	45	36	41	40	50	41
Climbing	11	8	8	8	8	8
Lifting and/or carrying heavy loads	54	39	39	38	37	41
At least two of these	37	25	27	25	27	27
None of these	32	44	42	41	35	40
Bases						
Men	*875*	*1338*	*1305*	*1289*	*2386*	*7193*
Women	*1006*	*1630*	*1573*	*1484*	*3022*	*8715*

Table 5.5

Frequency-intensity activity level, by age and sex

Aged 16 and over								1998
Frequency-intensity level	Age							Total
	16-24	25-34	35-44	45-54	55-64	65-74	75 +	
	%	%	%	%	%	%	%	%
Men								
Level 0	9	10	14	21	34	36	57	23
Level 1	8	14	16	16	15	22	20	15
Level 2	12	15	15	15	12	14	8	14
Level 3	20	25	29	33	32	24	14	27
Level 4	20	18	13	7	4	2	1	10
Level 5	30	18	12	8	3	1	0	11
Level 3 and above	*70*	*61*	*55*	*48*	*40*	*28*	*15*	*48*
Women								
Level 0	18	14	14	19	28	45	71	26
Level 1	20	20	19	20	21	22	16	20
Level 2	16	19	20	17	18	13	5	16
Level 3	23	26	30	33	28	18	8	25
Level 4	14	13	12	7	4	2	0	8
Level 5	10	9	6	4	2	1	0	5
Level 3 and above	*46*	*47*	*47*	*45*	*34*	*20*	*8*	*38*
Bases								
Men	*875*	*1338*	*1305*	*1289*	*987*	*837*	*562*	*7193*
Women	*1006*	*1630*	*1573*	*1484*	*1148*	*967*	*907*	*8715*

Table 5.6

Trends in frequency-intensity activity level since 1994, by age and sex

Aged 16 and over								1994, 1998
Frequency-intensity level	Age							Total
	16-24	25-34	35-44	45-54	55-64	65-74	75 +	
	%	%	%	%	%	%	%	%
Men								
1994								
Level 0	7	8	11	15	24	29	53	17
Level 1	12	14	17	19	19	26	22	18
Level 2	14	17	17	16	17	17	13	16
Level 3	17	26	28	37	32	26	11	27
Level 4	22	19	15	7	5	1	1	11
Level 5	27	17	12	6	4	1	1	11
Level 3 and above	*67*	*62*	*55*	*50*	*40*	*28*	*12*	*49*
1998								
Level 0	9	10	14	21	34	36	57	23
Level 1	8	14	16	16	15	22	20	15
Level 2	12	15	15	15	12	14	8	14
Level 3	20	25	29	33	32	24	14	27
Level 4	20	18	13	7	4	2	1	10
Level 5	30	18	12	8	3	1	0	11
Level 3 and above	*70*	*61*	*55*	*48*	*40*	*28*	*15*	*48*
Women								
1994								
Level 0	11	8	9	12	18	33	62	19
Level 1	20	22	23	22	27	30	22	24
Level 2	21	22	23	21	19	17	8	20
Level 3	22	26	29	35	29	18	9	25
Level 4	17	16	12	8	5	1	0	9
Level 5	9	7	4	3	2	1	0	4
Level 3 and above	*47*	*49*	*45*	*45*	*36*	*20*	*9*	*38*
1998								
Level 0	18	14	14	19	28	45	71	26
Level 1	20	20	19	20	21	22	16	20
Level 2	16	19	20	17	18	13	5	16
Level 3	23	26	30	33	28	18	8	25
Level 4	14	13	12	7	4	2	0	8
Level 5	10	9	6	4	2	1	0	5
Level 3 and above	*46*	*47*	*47*	*45*	*34*	*20*	*8*	*38*
Bases								
Men 1994	*968*	*1434*	*1329*	*1127*	*1001*	*877*	*441*	*7178*
Men 1998	*875*	*1338*	*1305*	*1289*	*987*	*837*	*562*	*7193*
Women 1994	*1080*	*1723*	*1520*	*1300*	*1059*	*1120*	*825*	*8631*
Women 1998	*1006*	*1630*	*1573*	*1484*	*1148*	*967*	*907*	*8715*

Table 5.7

Summary of overall participation in physical activities, by age and sex

Aged 16 and over | | | | | | | | | *1998*

Average number of days of 30 minutes or more moderate-plus activity per week, and summary activity level[a]	Age							Total
	16-24	25-34	35-44	45-54	55-64	65-74	75+	
	%	%	%	%	%	%	%	%
Men								
None	10	11	15	22	34	38	59	24
Any	90	89	85	78	66	62	41	76
Less than one day a week	6	11	12	11	10	14	12	11
One or two days a week	15	19	20	21	17	21	14	19
Three or four days a week	11	11	9	10	7	10	7	9
Five or more days a week	58	48	43	36	32	17	7	37
Group 1 – Low	16	22	28	33	44	52	72	35
Group 2 – Medium	26	30	29	31	24	31	21	28
Group 3 – High	58	48	43	36	32	17	7	37
Women								
None	20	15	16	21	29	47	73	28
Any	80	85	84	79	71	53	27	72
Less than one day a week	13	13	14	13	13	14	9	13
One or two days a week	22	26	25	23	26	21	10	23
Three or four days a week	13	15	14	13	12	7	4	12
Five or more days a week	32	31	32	30	21	12	4	25
Group 1 – Low	33	28	29	34	42	61	82	41
Group 2 – Medium	35	41	39	37	37	28	14	34
Group 3 – High	32	31	32	30	21	12	4	25
Bases								
Men	*875*	*1338*	*1305*	*1289*	*987*	*837*	*562*	*7193*
Women	*1006*	*1630*	*1573*	*1484*	*1148*	*967*	*907*	*8715*

[a] Group 3 = 30 minutes or more on at least 5 days a week; Group 2 = 30 minutes or more on 1 to 4 days a week; Group 1 = lower level of activity.

Table 5.8

Trends in summary activity level since 1994, by age and sex

Aged 16 and over *1994, 1998*

Summary activity level[a]	Age							Total
	16-24	25-34	35-44	45-54	55-64	65-74	75 +	
	%	%	%	%	%	%	%	%
Men								
1994								
Group 1 – Low	17	19	24	28	37	46	67	30
Group 2 – Medium	33	36	33	32	33	38	26	34
Group 3 – High	50	45	43	40	30	16	7	37
1998								
Group 1 – Low	16	22	28	33	44	52	72	35
Group 2 – Medium	26	30	29	31	24	31	21	28
Group 3 – High	58	48	43	36	32	17	7	37
Women								
1994								
Group 1 – Low	27	24	25	27	37	51	75	35
Group 2 – Medium	44	49	49	46	43	39	21	43
Group 3 – High	29	28	27	27	21	10	5	22
1998								
Group 1 – Low	33	28	29	34	42	61	82	41
Group 2 – Medium	35	41	39	37	37	28	14	34
Group 3 – High	32	31	32	30	21	12	4	25
Bases								
Men 1994	*968*	*1434*	*1329*	*1127*	*1001*	*877*	*441*	*7177*
Men 1998	*875*	*1338*	*1305*	*1289*	*987*	*837*	*562*	*7193*
Women 1994	*1080*	*1723*	*1520*	*1300*	*1059*	*1120*	*825*	*8627*
Women 1998	*1006*	*1630*	*1573*	*1484*	*1148*	*967*	*907*	*8715*

[a] Group 3 = 30 minutes or more on at least 5 days a week; Group 2 = 30 minutes or more on 1 to 4 days a week; Group 1 = lower level of activity.

Table 5.9

Summary of participation in vigorous and moderate activity, by age and sex

Aged 16 and over 1998

Summary of participation in vigorous and moderate activity	Age							Total
	16-24	25-34	35-44	45-54	55-64	65-74	75 +	
	%	%	%	%	%	%	%	%
Men								
Activity level reached:								
20 minutes vigorous activity on 3 days a week, **and** 30 minutes moderate-plus activity on 5 days a week	25	14	9	6	3	1	-	9
20 minutes vigorous activity on 3 days a week only	5	4	3	2	0	0	0	2
30 minutes moderate-plus activity on 5 days a week only	32	34	34	31	29	16	7	28
Total reaching either guideline level	62	52	46	39	32	17	7	40
Not at guideline level but active on at least one day a week	29	39	40	41	35	47	36	38
Inactive[a]	9	9	14	21	33	36	57	22
Women								
Activity level reached:								
20 minutes vigorous activity on 3 days a week, **and** 30 minutes moderate-plus activity on 5 days a week	7	6	5	3	1	1	-	4
20 minutes vigorous activity on 3 days a week only	3	3	1	1	1	0	0	1
30 minutes moderate-plus activity on 5 days a week only	24	25	27	27	19	11	4	21
Total reaching either guideline level	35	34	34	31	22	12	4	26
Not at guideline level but active on at least one day a week	48	53	53	51	51	44	25	48
Inactive[a]	17	13	14	18	27	44	71	26
Bases								
Men	875	1338	1305	1289	987	837	562	7193
Women	1006	1630	1573	1484	1148	967	907	8715

[a] In this table 'inactive' includes those informants who did not report at least one occasion per week of moderate or vigorous activity of at least 20 minutes' duration.

Table 5.10

Summary activity level (observed and age-standardised), by social class of head of household and sex

Aged 16 and over 1998

Summary activity level[a]	Social class of head of household						Social class of head of household					
	I	II	IIINM	IIIM	IV	V	I	II	IIINM	IIIM	IV	V
	%	%	%	%	%	%	%	%	%	%	%	%
	Men						**Women**					
Observed												
Group 1 – Low	35	34	37	34	35	31	33	38	43	40	44	45
Group 2 – Medium	37	35	31	22	23	21	44	35	32	35	33	32
Group 3 – High	28	30	32	44	42	48	23	27	24	26	23	22
Standardised												
Group 1 – Low	33	33	36	32	34	29	37	40	41	42	43	40
Group 2 – Medium	36	35	31	22	23	20	42	34	33	33	33	35
Group 3 – High	31	32	33	46	44	50	21	26	26	25	24	25
Bases	503	2178	718	2265	1042	335	515	2499	1346	2209	1374	498

[a] Group 3 = 30 minutes or more on at least 5 days a week; Group 2 = 30 minutes or more on 1 to 4 days a week; Group 1 = lower level of activity.

Table 5.11

**Summary activity level (observed and age-standardised),
by equivalised household income and sex**

Aged 16 and over *1998*

Summary activity level[a]	Equivalised annual household income quintile				
	Up to £7,186	Over £7,186 to £10,834	Over £10,834 to £17,890	Over £17,890 to £27,705	Over £27,705
	%	%	%	%	%
Men					
Observed					
Group 1 – Low	44	46	32	27	28
Group 2 – Medium	26	22	26	29	38
Group 3 – High	30	32	42	44	35
Standardised					
Group 1 – Low	42	39	31	28	31
Group 2 – Medium	26	21	25	29	36
Group 3 – High	32	40	44	43	34
Women					
Observed					
Group 1 – Low	46	52	35	35	31
Group 2 – Medium	32	29	37	36	41
Group 3 – High	23	19	29	29	28
Standardised					
Group 1 – Low	45	43	37	41	39
Group 2 – Medium	32	32	36	33	37
Group 3 – High	23	24	27	26	24
Bases					
Men	*1002*	*1004*	*1441*	*1394*	*1362*
Women	*1413*	*1489*	*1653*	*1493*	*1385*

[a] Group 3 = 30 minutes or more on at least 5 days a week; Group 2 = 30 minutes or more on 1 to 4 days a week; Group 1 = lower level of activity.

Table 5.12

Summary activity level (observed and age-standardised), by Health Authority area type and sex

Aged 16 and over   *1998*

Summary activity level[a]	Health Authority area type					
	Inner London	Mining & Industrial	Urban	Mature	Prosperous	Rural
	%	%	%	%	%	%
Men						
Observed						
Group 1 – Low	41	38	37	32	33	33
Group 2 – Medium	25	26	26	30	29	28
Group 3 – High	34	36	37	38	38	38
Standardised						
Group 1 – Low	46	36	36	31	31	31
Group 2 – Medium	22	26	26	30	29	28
Group 3 – High	32	38	38	39	40	40
Women						
Observed						
Group 1 – Low	40	42	42	43	40	39
Group 2 – Medium	34	33	33	33	34	37
Group 3 – High	26	24	25	24	26	24
Standardised						
Group 1 – Low	44	42	42	42	41	39
Group 2 – Medium	32	33	33	33	34	36
Group 3 – High	23	25	25	25	25	24
Bases						
Men	*240*	*1106*	*1057*	*1100*	*1946*	*1744*
Women	*309*	*1295*	*1341*	*1309*	*2388*	*2073*

[a] Group 3 = 30 minutes or more on at least 5 days a week; Group 2 = 30 minutes or more on 1 to 4 days a week; Group 1 = lower level of activity.

Table 5.13

Summary activity level (observed and age-standardised), by region and sex

Aged 16 and over   *1998*

Summary activity level[a]	Region							
	Northern & Yorkshire	North West	Trent	West Midlands	Anglia & Oxford	North Thames	South Thames	South & West
	%	%	%	%	%	%	%	%
Men								
Observed								
Group 1 – Low	35	34	39	37	30	39	31	33
Group 2 – Medium	26	27	27	28	34	26	28	29
Group 3 – High	39	39	34	35	37	35	41	38
Standardised								
Group 1 – Low	33	33	37	36	29	37	30	30
Group 2 – Medium	27	27	27	28	33	26	27	30
Group 3 – High	40	40	36	37	37	37	42	41
Women								
Observed								
Group 1 – Low	41	40	43	41	39	42	41	40
Group 2 – Medium	35	33	35	36	36	33	32	35
Group 3 – High	24	27	22	22	25	25	27	25
Standardised								
Group 1 – Low	40	41	43	42	41	43	42	40
Group 2 – Medium	35	32	35	36	35	32	32	35
Group 3 – High	25	27	22	23	24	25	26	25
Bases								
Men	*1030*	*979*	*797*	*746*	*812*	*915*	*893*	*1021*
Women	*1249*	*1135*	*941*	*913*	*961*	*1118*	*1183*	*1215*

[a] Group 3 = 30 minutes or more on at least 5 days a week; Group 2 = 30 minutes or more on 1 to 4 days a week; Group 1 = lower level of activity.

Table 5.14

Components of activity (observed and age-standardised), by social class of head of household and sex

Aged 16 and over   1998

Mean number of days' participation in each type of activity in the last four weeks (at least 15 minutes a day)	Social class of head of household						Social class of head of household					
	I	II	IIINM	IIIM	IV	V	I	II	IIINM	IIIM	IV	V
	%	%	%	%	%	%	%	%	%	%	%	%
	Men						**Women**					
Heavy Housework												
Observed												
% who participated	37	39	42	36	36	35	55	57	60	60	57	54
Mean number of days[a]	1.7	1.9	2.1	1.8	2.0	1.9	3.1	3.4	3.7	4.0	3.7	3.9
Standard error of the mean	0.17	0.09	0.16	0.08	0.13	0.22	0.23	0.11	0.16	0.13	0.16	0.28
Standardised												
% who participated	38	39	42	36	37	36	51	54	61	58	59	58
Mean number of days[a]	1.7	1.8	2.1	1.8	2.0	1.9	2.9	3.2	3.8	3.8	3.8	4.3
Standard error of the mean	0.17	0.09	0.16	0.08	0.13	0.23	0.22	0.11	0.16	0.13	0.16	0.30
Heavy Manual/DIY												
Observed												
% who participated	30	32	27	32	29	27	14	14	13	11	10	9
Mean number of days[a]	1.3	1.6	1.5	1.8	1.6	1.7	0.5	0.5	0.6	0.4	0.5	0.4
Standard error of the mean	0.13	0.08	0.15	0.09	0.14	0.26	0.08	0.05	0.06	0.04	0.06	0.07
Standardised												
% who participated	29	31	28	32	30	27	13	13	13	11	11	9
Mean number of days[a]	1.2	1.5	1.5	.1.7	1.6	1.7	0.5	0.5	0.6	0.4	0.5	0.4
Standard error of the mean	0.13	0.08	0.15	0.09	0.14	0.25	0.09	0.04	0.06	0.04	0.06	0.08
Walking[b]												
Observed												
% who participated	42	38	36	25	28	31	33	29	25	22	20	16
Mean number of days[a]	5.4	5.1	5.1	3.7	4.1	4.9	4.6	4.1	3.9	3.5	3.2	2.6
Standard error of the mean	0.41	0.19	0.34	0.17	0.26	0.50	0.38	0.17	0.23	0.17	0.21	0.32
Standardised												
% who participated	44	39	37	27	29	32	30	28	26	22	20	18
Mean number of days[a]	5.6	5.4	5.1	4.0	4.3	5.1	4.3	4.0	4.1	3.4	3.2	2.9
Standard error of the mean	0.41	0.20	0.34	0.18	0.27	0.51	0.37	0.16	0.23	0.17	0.21	0.33
Sports and Exercise												
Observed												
% who participated	48	49	45	36	38	35	47	44	34	33	28	24
Mean number of days[a]	5.6	5.6	5.3	4.1	4.3	4.9	4.0	4.2	2.9	3.0	2.5	2.3
Standard error of the mean	0.39	0.19	0.32	0.16	0.25	0.49	0.28	0.14	0.17	0.14	0.16	0.26
Standardised												
% who participated	52	52	45	39	40	37	43	43	36	32	28	27
Mean number of days[a]	6.3	6.1	5.2	4.5	4.6	5.0	3.7	4.1	3.1	2.9	2.6	2.6
Standard error of the mean	0.40	0.19	0.32	0.17	0.26	0.49	0.28	0.14	0.17	0.13	0.16	0.28
Occupational activity												
% who participated	7	11	14	32	31	39	8	12	9	14	13	17
Mean number of days[a]	1.3	2.0	2.7	6.3	6.1	7.3	1.2	1.9	1.4	2.2	2.1	2.6
Standard error of the mean	0.22	0.13	0.25	0.19	0.28	0.51	0.19	0.11	0.13	0.12	0.15	0.27
All physical activities[c]												
Observed												
% who participated	83	82	80	78	78	77	84	80	76	77	72	68
Mean number of days[a]	12.9	13.0	13.1	14.2	14.1	15.4	11.7	11.9	10.7	11.0	10.3	9.9
Standard error of the mean	0.49	0.24	0.42	0.24	0.36	0.64	0.45	0.22	0.29	0.23	0.29	0.47
Standardised												
% who participated	84	83	80	79	80	79	80	77	78	75	73	73
Mean number of days[a]	13.5	13.6	13.2	14.8	14.6	15.9	10.8	11.5	11.2	10.6	10.5	10.9
Standard error of the mean	0.49	0.24	0.42	0.24	0.36	0.63	0.45	0.22	0.29	0.23	0.29	0.48
Bases	503	2178	718	2265	1042	335	515	2499	1346	2209	1374	498

[a] Mean based on all informants.   [b] Walking at a 'Fairly brisk' or 'Fast' pace.   [c] Includes Heavy housework; Heavy manual/DIY; Walking; Sports and Exercise; and Occupational activity (counted as 20 days for full-time workers, 12 days for part-time workers).

Table 5.15

Components of activity (observed and age-standardised), by equivalised household income and sex

Aged 16 and over   1998

Mean number of days' participation in each type of activity in the last four weeks (at least 15 minutes a day)	Equivalised annual household income quintile				
	Up to £7,186	Over £7,186 to £10,834	Over £10,834 to £17,890	Over £17,890 to £27,705	Over £27,705
	%	%	%	%	%
Men					
Heavy Housework					
Observed					
% who participated	35	36	38	40	41
Mean number of days[a]	2.2	2.1	1.9	1.7	1.7
Standard error of the mean	0.15	0.14	0.11	0.10	0.10
Standardised					
% who participated	37	35	38	40	39
Mean number of days[a]	2.4	2.1	1.8	1.7	1.6
Standard error of the mean	0.16	0.14	0.11	0.10	0.09
Heavy Manual/DIY					
Observed					
% who participated	23	27	34	35	34
Mean number of days[a]	1.3	1.7	1.8	1.7	1.5
Standard error of the mean	0.12	0.14	0.11	0.11	0.10
Standardised					
% who participated	25	28	33	34	31
Mean number of days[a]	1.3	1.7	1.8	1.7	1.4
Standard error of the mean	0.11	0.15	0.11	0.10	0.09
Walking[b]					
Observed					
% who participated	26	21	30	39	43
Mean number of days[a]	4.4	3.6	4.1	5.3	5.5
Standard error of the mean	0.29	0.26	0.22	0.25	0.24
Standardised					
% who participated	27	26	32	38	41
Mean number of days[a]	4.5	4.4	4.4	5.4	5.4
Standard error of the mean	0.29	0.29	0.22	0.25	0.25
Sports and Exercise					
Observed					
% who participated	30	32	38	48	58
Mean number of days[a]	4.0	3.6	4.2	5.5	6.5
Standard error of the mean	0.26	0.24	0.21	0.23	0.24
Standardised					
% who participated	31	40	41	47	55
Mean number of days[a]	4.0	4.6	4.6	5.5	6.3
Standard error of the mean	0.26	0.26	0.21	0.23	0.24
Occupational activity					
% who participated	14	19	30	27	15
Mean number of days[a]	2.4	3.8	6.0	5.3	3.0
Standard error of the mean	0.20	0.24	0.24	0.23	0.19
All physical activities[c]					
Observed					
% who participated	68	67	82	87	88
Mean number of days[a]	11.3	11.3	14.5	15.5	14.7
Standard error of the mean	0.36	0.37	0.30	0.30	0.29
Standardised					
% who participated	70	73	83	86	85
Mean number of days[a]	11.9	13.3	14.9	15.2	14.1
Standard error of the mean	0.36	0.37	0.30	0.30	0.30
Base					
Men	*1002*	*1004*	*1441*	*1394*	*1362*

[a] Mean based on all informants.

[b] Walking at a 'Fairly brisk' or 'Fast' pace.

[c] Includes Heavy housework; Heavy manual/DIY; Walking; Sports and Exercise; and Occupational activity (counted as 20 days for full-time workers, 12 days for part-time workers).

continued...

Table 5.15 *continued*

Mean number of days' participation in each type of activity in the last four weeks (at least 15 minutes a day)	Equivalised annual household income quintile				
	Up to £7,186	Over £7,186 to £10,834	Over £10,834 to £17,890	Over £17,890 to £27,705	Over £27,705
	%	%	%	%	%
Women					
Heavy Housework					
Observed					
% who participated	61	52	61	61	60
Mean number of days[a]	4.4	3.7	4.1	3.5	3.1
Standard error of the mean	0.18	0.16	0.15	0.14	0.13
Standardised					
% who participated	62	58	59	57	54
Mean number of days[a]	4.5	4.3	3.9	3.2	2.7
Standard error of the mean	0.18	0.17	0.15	0.14	0.12
Heavy Manual/DIY					
Observed					
% who participated	10	9	12	15	15
Mean number of days[a]	0.5	0.4	0.6	0.6	0.5
Standard error of the mean	0.06	0.04	0.06	0.06	0.05
Standardised					
% who participated	11	10	11	14	12
Mean number of days[a]	0.5	0.4	0.5	0.6	0.4
Standard error of the mean	0.06	0.05	0.06	0.06	0.05
Walking[b]					
Observed					
% who participated	19	18	25	28	35
Mean number of days[a]	3.4	2.9	3.7	4.2	4.9
Standard error of the mean	0.22	0.19	0.19	0.22	0.24
Standardised					
% who participated	19	22	24	26	30
Mean number of days[a]	3.4	3.6	3.6	3.9	4.4
Standard error of the mean	0.22	0.21	0.19	0.21	0.23
Sports and Exercise					
Observed					
% who participated	25	22	37	45	53
Mean number of days[a]	2.3	2.0	3.2	4.2	5.1
Standard error of the mean	0.16	0.14	0.16	0.18	0.20
Standardised					
% who participated	24	29	36	41	45
Mean number of days[a]	2.3	2.5	3.2	3.8	4.4
Standard error of the mean	0.15	0.15	0.16	0.18	0.20
Occupational activity					
% who participated	8	9	18	14	10
Mean number of days[a]	1.2	1.4	2.9	2.3	1.7
Standard error of the mean	0.11	0.12	0.16	0.15	0.14
All physical activities[c]					
Observed					
% who participated	72	64	80	84	87
Mean number of days[a]	10.0	8.7	12.1	12.4	12.9
Standard error of the mean	0.28	0.27	0.27	0.27	0.29
Standardised					
% who participated	72	73	78	79	78
Mean number of days[a]	10.1	10.8	11.7	11.4	11.3
Standard error of the mean	0.28	0.28	0.27	0.28	0.29
Base					
Women	*1413*	*1489*	*1653*	*1493*	*1385*

[a] Mean based on all informants.

[b] Walking at a 'Fairly brisk' or 'Fast' pace.

[c] Includes Heavy housework; Heavy manual/DIY; Walking; Sports and Exercise; and Occupational activity (counted as 20 days for full-time workers, 12 days for part-time workers).

Table 5.16

Components of activity (observed and age-standardised), by Health Authority area type and sex

Aged 16 and over   *1998*

Mean number of days' participation in each type of activity in the last four weeks (at least 15 minutes a day)	Health Authority area type					
	Inner London	Mining & Industrial	Urban	Mature	Prosperous	Rural
	%	%	%	%	%	%
Men						
Heavy Housework						
Observed						
% who participated	35	38	39	38	38	38
Mean number of days[a]	1.8	2.0	2.0	1.9	1.7	2.0
Standard error of the mean	0.27	0.13	0.13	0.12	0.09	0.11
Standardised						
% who participated	32	38	39	39	38	37
Mean number of days[a]	1.7	2.0	2.0	1.9	1.7	1.9
Standard error of the mean	0.27	0.13	0.13	0.12	0.08	0.10
Heavy Manual/DIY						
Observed						
% who participated	9	29	29	28	33	35
Mean number of days[a]	0.6	1.5	1.4	1.6	1.6	2.0
Standard error of the mean	0.18	0.12	0.11	0.12	0.09	0.11
Standardised						
% who participated	9	30	29	28	32	35
Mean number of days[a]	0.6	1.4	1.4	1.5	1.6	1.9
Standard error of the mean	0.19	0.12	0.11	0.12	0.09	0.11
Walking[b]						
Observed						
% who participated	36	26	28	35	36	32
Mean number of days[a]	6.2	3.9	4.2	4.9	4.9	4.4
Standard error of the mean	0.67	0.26	0.26	0.27	0.20	0.21
Standardised						
% who participated	32	28	29	36	38	34
Mean number of days[a]	5.7	4.3	4.3	5.1	5.2	4.6
Standard error of the mean	0.65	0.26	0.27	0.28	0.21	0.21
Sports and Exercise						
Observed						
% who participated	46	37	39	44	46	41
Mean number of days[a]	6.0	4.3	4.6	4.9	5.3	4.8
Standard error of the mean	0.59	0.25	0.25	0.25	0.19	0.20
Standardised						
% who participated	39	40	41	46	49	44
Mean number of days[a]	5.2	4.7	4.8	5.2	5.7	5.3
Standard error of the mean	0.57	0.25	0.25	0.26	0.20	0.21
Occupational activity						
% who participated	16	22	22	22	22	22
Mean number of days[a]	3.1	4.4	4.4	4.1	4.2	4.4
Standard error of the mean	0.45	0.25	0.25	0.24	0.18	0.20
All physical activities[c]						
Observed						
% who participated	73	74	77	80	83	81
Mean number of days[a]	13.2	12.6	13.4	13.9	14.2	13.9
Standard error of the mean	0.77	0.35	0.36	0.34	0.26	0.27
Standardised						
% who participated	68	76	78	82	85	82
Mean number of days[a]	12.0	13.2	13.7	14.4	14.7	14.4
Standard error of the mean	0.77	0.35	0.36	0.34	0.26	0.27
Base						
Men	*240*	*1106*	*1057*	*1100*	*1946*	*1744*

continued...

[a] Mean based on all informants.   [b] Walking at a 'Fairly brisk' or 'Fast' pace.   [c] Includes Heavy housework; Heavy manual/DIY; Walking; Sports and Exercise; and Occupational activity (counted as 20 days for full-time workers, 12 days for part-time workers).

Table 5.16 *continued*

Mean number of days' participation in each type of activity in the last four weeks (at least 15 minutes a day)	Health Authority area type					
	Inner London	Mining & Industrial	Urban	Mature	Prosperous	Rural
	%	%	%	%	%	%
Women						
Heavy Housework						
Observed						
% who participated	57	58	59	54	55	62
Mean number of days[a]	4.0	3.9	3.9	3.3	3.2	4.0
Standard error of the mean	0.37	0.17	0.17	0.15	0.11	0.13
Standardised						
% who participated	53	58	59	54	54	62
Mean number of days[a]	3.7	3.9	3.9	3.3	3.1	3.9
Standard error of the mean	0.35	0.17	0.17	0.15	0.11	0.13
Heavy Manual/DIY						
Observed						
% who participated	6	11	10	11	13	14
Mean number of days[a]	0.2	0.5	0.4	0.5	0.5	0.6
Standard error of the mean	0.07	0.06	0.05	0.06	0.04	0.05
Standardised						
% who participated	6	11	10	11	13	14
Mean number of days[a]	0.2	0.5	0.4	0.5	0.5	0.6
Standard error of the mean	0.06	0.06	0.05	0.06	0.04	0.05
Walking[b]						
Observed						
% who participated	28	20	20	25	29	24
Mean number of days[a]	4.9	2.9	3.2	3.7	4.3	3.6
Standard error of the mean	0.53	0.20	0.21	0.22	0.17	0.17
Standardised						
% who participated	26	20	20	25	28	24
Mean number of days[a]	4.6	3.0	3.2	3.8	4.3	3.5
Standard error of the mean	0.52	0.20	0.21	0.23	0.17	0.17
Sports and Exercise						
Observed						
% who participated	34	30	32	37	40	35
Mean number of days[a]	3.2	2.7	2.9	3.5	3.7	3.1
Standard error of the mean	0.37	0.17	0.17	0.19	0.14	0.14
Standardised						
% who participated	30	31	32	38	40	35
Mean number of days[a]	2.9	2.8	2.9	3.6	3.7	3.1
Standard error of the mean	0.35	0.17	0.17	0.19	0.14	0.14
Occupational activity						
% who participated	8	13	15	11	10	13
Mean number of days[a]	1.4	2.1	2.4	1.7	1.6	2.0
Standard error of the mean	0.28	0.16	0.16	0.14	0.10	0.12
All physical activities[c]						
Observed						
% who participated	76	73	75	74	78	79
Mean number of days[a]	11.5	10.4	10.7	11.0	11.2	11.1
Standard error of the mean	0.63	0.30	0.29	0.30	0.22	0.23
Standardised						
% who participated	70	73	75	74	77	78
Mean number of days[a]	10.6	10.5	10.7	11.0	11.0	11.1
Standard error of the mean	0.62	0.30	0.29	0.30	0.22	0.23
Base						
Women	*309*	*1295*	*1341*	*1309*	*2388*	*2073*

[a] Mean based on all informants.　[b] Walking at a 'Fairly brisk' or 'Fast' pace.　[c] Includes Heavy housework; Heavy manual/DIY; Walking; Sports and Exercise; and Occupational activity (counted as 20 days for full-time workers, 12 days for part-time workers).

Table 5.17

Components of activity (observed and age-standardised), by region and sex

Aged 16 and over 1998

Mean number of days' participation in each type of activity in the last four weeks (at least 15 minutes a day)	Region							
	Northern & Yorkshire	North West	Trent	West Midlands	Anglia & Oxford	North Thames	South Thames	South & West
	%	%	%	%	%	%	%	%
Men								
Heavy Housework								
Observed								
% who participated	40	40	35	38	39	36	37	37
Mean number of days[a]	2.1	2.2	1.7	2.1	1.7	1.8	1.7	1.7
Standard error of the mean	0.14	0.15	0.14	0.17	0.12	0.13	0.13	0.12
Standardised								
% who participated	40	40	36	38	39	36	37	38
Mean number of days[a]	2.1	2.2	1.7	2.1	1.7	1.8	1.7	1.7
Standard error of the mean	0.13	0.15	0.14	0.17	0.12	0.13	0.13	0.12
Heavy Manual/DIY								
Observed								
% who participated	29	31	31	36	34	26	29	32
Mean number of days[a]	1.4	1.7	1.7	1.7	1.7	1.5	1.7	1.6
Standard error of the mean	0.12	0.14	0.15	0.14	0.14	0.13	0.14	0.12
Standardised								
% who participated	30	30	31	36	34	25	28	32
Mean number of days[a]	1.4	1.7	1.7	1.6	1.7	1.4	1.6	1.6
Standard error of the mean	0.12	0.14	0.15	0.14	0.14	0.13	0.14	0.12
Walking[b]								
Observed								
% who participated	29	29	28	27	38	34	40	32
Mean number of days[a]	4.4	4.3	3.8	3.7	5.0	4.8	5.7	4.8
Standard error of the mean	0.28	0.28	0.29	0.30	0.31	0.30	0.32	0.28
Standardised								
% who participated	31	30	30	29	38	36	41	34
Mean number of days[a]	4.7	4.5	4.0	3.9	5.0	5.1	5.9	5.0
Standard error of the mean	0.28	0.28	0.29	0.30	0.31	0.30	0.32	0.29
Sports and Exercise								
Observed								
% who participated	36	42	39	37	48	42	45	46
Mean number of days[a]	4.6	4.8	4.4	4.1	5.6	4.8	5.4	5.2
Standard error of the mean	0.26	0.26	0.29	0.29	0.31	0.28	0.29	0.26
Standardised								
% who participated	39	44	42	40	49	45	47	49
Mean number of days[a]	5.0	5.0	4.8	4.5	5.7	5.2	5.8	5.7
Standard error of the mean	0.27	0.27	0.29	0.30	0.31	0.28	0.30	0.27
Occupational activity								
% who participated	23	23	21	21	19	19	22	24
Mean number of days[a]	4.6	4.6	4.1	4.2	3.8	3.6	4.3	4.7
Standard error of the mean	0.26	0.27	0.28	0.30	0.27	0.25	0.27	0.26
All physical activities[c]								
Observed								
% who participated	76	79	78	79	84	77	81	83
Mean number of days[a]	13.5	14.0	12.6	12.8	14.5	13.1	14.7	14.1
Standard error of the mean	0.36	0.37	0.40	0.41	0.39	0.38	0.38	0.35
Standardised								
% who participated	78	79	79	81	84	79	82	85
Mean number of days[a]	14.0	14.2	13.0	13.3	14.6	13.7	15.1	14.8
Standard error of the mean	0.36	0.37	0.40	0.41	0.39	0.38	0.38	0.35
Base								
Men	*1030*	*979*	*797*	*746*	*812*	*915*	*893*	*1021*

continued...

[a] Mean based on all informants. [b] Walking at a 'Fairly brisk' or 'Fast' pace. [c] Includes Heavy housework; Heavy manual/DIY; Walking; Sports and Exercise; and Occupational activity (counted as 20 days for full-time workers, 12 days for part-time workers).

Table 5.17 *continued*

Mean number of days' participation in each type of activity in the last four weeks (at least 15 minutes a day)	Region							
	Northern & Yorkshire	North West	Trent	West Midlands	Anglia & Oxford	North Thames	South Thames	South & West
	%	%	%	%	%	%	%	%
Women								
Heavy Housework								
Observed								
% who participated	60	56	62	60	59	55	56	55
Mean number of days[a]	4.2	3.8	3.7	4.1	3.2	3.3	3.5	3.3
Standard error of the mean	0.19	0.18	0.18	0.20	0.17	0.16	0.17	0.16
Standardised								
% who participated	60	55	62	60	58	54	55	55
Mean number of days[a]	4.2	3.7	3.6	4.1	3.1	3.2	3.4	3.2
Standard error of the mean	0.19	0.18	0.18	0.20	0.16	0.16	0.17	0.16
Heavy Manual/DIY								
Observed								
% who participated	11	12	11	13	14	11	11	13
Mean number of days[a]	0.4	0.5	0.4	0.5	0.6	0.4	0.5	0.5
Standard error of the mean	0.05	0.07	0.06	0.08	0.07	0.06	0.07	0.06
Standardised								
% who participated	11	12	11	13	14	11	11	13
Mean number of days[a]	0.4	0.5	0.4	0.5	0.6	0.4	0.5	0.5
Standard error of the mean	0.05	0.07	0.05	0.08	0.07	0.06	0.07	0.06
Walking[b]								
Observed								
% who participated	21	22	20	19	28	27	30	26
Mean number of days[a]	3.1	3.5	3.3	2.8	3.7	4.2	4.7	3.9
Standard error of the mean	0.21	0.24	0.25	0.23	0.25	0.26	0.26	0.24
Standardised								
% who participated	21	22	21	20	27	26	29	27
Mean number of days[a]	3.2	3.5	3.3	2.8	3.6	4.2	4.6	3.9
Standard error of the mean	0.22	0.24	0.25	0.23	0.25	0.26	0.26	0.24
Sports and Exercise								
Observed								
% who participated	31	34	32	31	39	36	39	40
Mean number of days[a]	2.8	3.4	2.7	2.4	3.8	3.4	3.8	3.5
Standard error of the mean	0.17	0.20	0.19	0.18	0.23	0.20	0.20	0.19
Standardised								
% who participated	32	34	33	32	37	36	39	40
Mean number of days[a]	2.9	3.3	2.8	2.5	3.6	3.4	3.7	3.6
Standard error of the mean	0.18	0.20	0.19	0.18	0.23	0.20	0.20	0.19
Occupational activity								
% who participated	14	14	10	14	12	10	11	12
Mean number of days[a]	2.2	2.3	1.6	2.2	2.0	1.5	1.7	1.8
Standard error of the mean	0.16	0.17	0.16	0.18	0.18	0.15	0.15	0.15
All physical activities[c]								
Observed								
% who participated	75	74	76	76	80	76	78	76
Mean number of days[a]	10.7	11.4	10.1	10.4	11.2	11.0	11.6	11.1
Standard error of the mean	0.30	0.33	0.34	0.34	0.34	0.32	0.32	0.31
Standardised								
% who participated	76	73	76	76	78	75	77	77
Mean number of days[a]	10.9	11.3	10.1	10.4	10.7	10.9	11.4	11.1
Standard error of the mean	0.30	0.33	0.34	0.34	0.34	0.32	0.32	0.31
Base								
Women	*1249*	*1135*	*941*	*913*	*961*	*1118*	*1183*	*1215*

[a] Mean based on all informants. [b] Walking at a 'Fairly brisk' or 'Fast' pace. [c] Includes Heavy housework; Heavy manual/DIY; Walking; Sports and Exercise; and Occupational activity (counted as 20 days for full-time workers, 12 days for part-time workers).

Table 5.18

Logistic regression models for physical activity measures among men

Men aged 16 and over   *1998*

Odds ratios[a]	Participation in:					Summary Group 3
	Heavy housework	Heavy manual/DIY	Walking	Sports and exercise	Physical activity at work	
Age group	**(p=0.0000)**	**(p=0.0000)**	**(p=0.0000)**	**(p=0.0000)**	**(p=0.0003)**	**(p=0.0000)**
16-24	0.77	0.49	3.60	8.02	1.89	3.64
25-34	1.67	1.31	2.08	2.88	1.15	1.75
35-44	1.56	1.38	1.50	1.80	1.19	1.46
45-54	1.20	1.32	1.29	0.97	1.10	1.10
55-64	0.85	1.21	0.79	0.60	1.78	1.00
65-74	0.87	1.28	0.43	0.35	0.91	0.50
75 and over	0.56	0.55	0.20	0.12	0.32	0.20
Social class of head of household	**(p=0.2076)**	**(p=0.4377)**	**(p=0.0000)**	**(p=0.0000)**	**(p=0.0000)**	**(p=0.0000)**
I	0.89	0.94	1.34	1.19	0.28	0.59
II	1.01	1.00	1.13	1.28	0.39	0.64
IIINM	1.17	0.92	1.10	1.03	0.59	0.74
IIIM	0.93	1.11	0.74	0.82	1.88	1.38
IV	1.02	1.07	0.83	0.92	2.09	1.33
V	1.01	0.97	0.97	0.84	3.95	1.96
Equivalised household income	**(p=0.2308)**	**(p=0.3504)**	**(p=0.0001)**	**(p=0.0000)**	**(p=0.0000)**	**(p=0.0001)**
Bottom quintile	0.91	0.92	0.88	0.66	0.90	0.83
Second quintile	0.93	0.94	0.78	0.96	1.20	1.00
Third quintile	0.99	1.09	0.97	0.91	1.30	1.17
Fourth quintile	1.07	1.07	1.18	1.11	1.09	1.19
Top quintile	1.13	0.99	1.27	1.57	0.65	0.87
Employment status	**(p=0.0000)**	**(p=0.0000)**	**(p=0.0000)**	**(p=0.0001)**	**(p=0.0000)**	**(p=0.0000)**
In employment	0.83	1.44	0.98	1.03	16.54	1.75
ILO unemployed	1.19	1.16	1.30	1.13	2.78	1.09
Retired	1.58	1.22	1.36	1.31	0.07	1.11
Other economically inactive	0.64	0.49	0.58	0.66	0.32	0.47
Health Authority area type	**(p=0.5419)**	**(p=0.0000)**	**(p=0.0011)**	**(p=0.2033)**	**(p=0.3107)**	**(p=0.3050)**
Inner London	0.87	0.35	1.07	0.95	0.72	0.90
Mining & Industrial	1.08	1.17	0.83	0.91	0.99	0.89
Urban	1.10	1.13	0.84	0.95	1.13	1.01
Mature	1.04	1.12	1.16	1.04	1.14	1.09
Prosperous	0.95	1.34	1.14	1.14	1.12	1.09
Rural	0.98	1.45	1.02	1.02	0.97	1.03

[a] Odds ratios are relative to average, not to a designated reference category.

Table 5.19

Logistic regression models for physical activity measures among women

Women aged 16 and over   *1998*

Odds ratios[a]	Participation in:					Summary Group 3
	Heavy housework	Heavy manual/DIY	Walking	Sports and exercise	Physical activity at work	
Age group	**(p=0.0000)**	**(p=0.0000)**	**(p=0.0000)**	**(p=0.0000)**	**(p=0.1161)**	**(p=0.0000)**
16-24	0.65	0.46	1.85	3.32	1.09	1.66
25-34	1.93	1.34	1.38	2.33	0.98	1.56
35-44	1.72	1.44	1.43	1.73	1.02	1.59
45-54	1.40	1.36	1.14	1.17	1.19	1.40
55-64	1.18	1.36	0.89	0.86	1.45	1.01
65-74	0.89	1.44	0.90	0.56	1.13	0.75
75 and over	0.32	0.42	0.30	0.13	0.47	0.23
Social class of head of household	**(p=0.0064)**	**(p=0.0775)**	**(p=0.0003)**	**(p=0.0000)**	**(p=0.0000)**	**(p=0.2351)**
I	0.81	1.08	1.21	1.15	0.74	0.84
II	0.93	1.11	1.15	1.29	1.01	1.10
IIINM	1.23	1.21	1.21	1.10	0.67	1.11
IIIM	1.02	0.91	0.95	0.92	1.04	1.01
IV	1.02	0.92	0.84	0.86	1.16	0.97
V	1.03	0.83	0.75	0.78	1.65	1.00
Equivalised household income	**(p=0.0095)**	**(p=0.3307)**	**(p=0.0063)**	**(p=0.0000)**	**(p=0.0000)**	**(p=0.0695)**
Bottom quintile	1.21	1.02	0.88	0.70	1.32	1.02
Second quintile	1.00	0.86	0.90	0.79	1.41	0.98
Third quintile	1.03	0.98	0.99	1.03	1.34	1.14
Fourth quintile	1.08	1.12	1.03	1.21	0.81	1.00
Top quintile	0.87	1.04	1.25	1.46	0.49	0.88
Employment status	**(p=0.0086)**	**(p=0.1724)**	**(p=0.0037)**	**(p=0.0003)**	**(p=0.0000)**	**(p=0.0000)**
In employment	1.14	1.00	1.08	1.01	14.93	1.40
ILO unemployed	1.02	1.35	1.32	1.36	7.59	1.09
Retired	0.94	0.83	0.80	0.90	0.06	0.74
Other economically inactive	0.91	0.89	0.88	0.81	0.15	0.90
Health Authority area type	**(p=0.0000)**	**(p=0.0017)**	**(p=0.0001)**	**(p=0.0077)**	**(p=0.0046)**	**(p=0.8695)**
Inner London	0.90	0.64	1.25	0.89	0.83	1.10
Mining & Industrial	0.96	0.96	0.82	0.89	1.17	0.98
Urban	1.12	0.95	0.80	0.93	1.26	1.00
Mature	0.90	1.03	1.07	1.12	0.96	1.01
Prosperous	0.91	1.27	1.16	1.18	0.81	0.99
Rural	1.25	1.31	0.98	1.03	1.05	0.93

[a] Odds ratios are relative to average, not to a designated reference category.

Self-reported health and psychosocial well-being

6

Richard Boreham and Clare Tait

SUMMARY

- 44% of both men and women reported a longstanding illness. This is an increase since 1994, when prevalence was 39% among men and 40% among women. Prevalence increased with age, as did the number of illnesses reported.

- The age-standardised prevalence of longstanding illness increased with decreasing household income and was higher in manual social classes.

- 25% of men and 27% of women reported a longstanding illness that limited their activities in some way.

- The prevalence of limiting longstanding illness increased more rapidly with age than did overall longstanding illness.

- Differences in the prevalence of limiting longstanding illness by social class and household income were similar to those for longstanding illness overall, but more strongly marked.

- 15% of men and 19% of women reported acute sickness in the two weeks before the interview. Prevalence was higher in 1998 than in 1994 (increasing from 12% to 15% among men and 15% to 19% among women).

- Among men, the prevalence of acute sickness was inversely related to household income, and showed a social class gradient with prevalence higher among manual social classes. Among women, there was no clear relationship with social class or household income.

- 75% of men and 73% of women rated their health as 'good' or 'very good', a decline from 78% of men and 75% in 1994. 19% of men and 20% of women rated their health 'fair'. 7% of each sex rated it as 'bad' or 'very bad'

- The proportion rating their health as 'good' or 'very good' declined with increasing age, and (less markedly) with decreasing household income and lower social class. It was below average in Inner London.

- The General Health Questionnaire (GHQ12) is a measure of psychiatric morbidity and a GHQ12 score of four or more is used to identify informants with a possible psychiatric disorder. Women (18%) were more likely than men (13%) to have a high GHQ12 score (of 4 or more). No trend since 1994 was seen.

- The prevalence of high GHQ12 did not appear to be related to social class. Among men, but not among women, it was inversely related to household income.

- The prevalence of a high GHQ12 score was higher in Inner London than other areas.

- Men (16%) were more likely than women (11%) to report a severe lack of social support. No clear trend since 1994 was observed.

- The proportion with a severe lack of social support was higher in the lower income quintiles, manual social classes, and in Inner London.

6.1 Introduction

This chapter covers self-reported illness (6.2) and acute sickness (6.3), self-assessed general health (6.4), and two measures of psychosocial health (GHQ12 and perceived social support) (6.5).

When considering the results presented in this chapter, it should be borne in mind that data based on self-assessments of health are measures of informants' subjective views that would not necessarily correspond to medical diagnoses, and also that some conditions, such as mental illness, have been shown to be under-reported in health surveys.[1] It should also be noted that those living in institutions, or unavailable for interview as a result of a serious medical problem, are not included in the sample.

Mental health has been set as a priority area for action by the government.[2] Information about the level of mental distress in the population is important for planning services and health promotion. Psychological factors are also associated with the development and outcome of some conditions, notably cardiovascular disease.[3]

Measures of psychosocial well-being have been included in every year of the Health Survey. In 1998 psychosocial well-being was assessed using two scales, administered in a self-completion questionnaire. These were the General Health Questionnaire (GHQ12) and a perceived social support scale.

6.2 Self-reported longstanding illness

6.2.1 Prevalence of self-reported longstanding illness

Informants were asked whether they had any longstanding illness, disability or infirmity that had troubled them over a period of time or was likely to affect them over a period of time. Those who said they had such an illness were asked about the nature of their condition. They were also asked whether the condition limited their activities in any way. This last question was introduced into the Health Survey series in 1996: the other questions were asked since the first survey in 1991. Trends are analysed back to 1994, except for limiting longstanding illness, where the series is not yet long enough.

By sex and age

44% of both men and women reported a longstanding illness. About a third of men, and more than a third of women, reporting a longstanding illness reported two or more such illnesses.

The prevalence of longstanding illness and number of reported longstanding illnesses increased with age. 21% of men aged 16-24 had a longstanding illness compared to 65% of men aged 75 and over. For women, comparable figures were 27% of those aged 16-24 and 72% of those aged 75 and over.   **Table 6.1**

By social class of head of household

The age-standardised prevalence of longstanding illness showed a social class gradient. Prevalence among men increased from 38% in Social Class I to 44% in Social Class V, with comparable figures for women being 41% to 46%.   **Table 6.3**

By equivalised household income

The age-standardised prevalence of longstanding illness increased as income decreased. 38% of men and 36% of women in the highest income quintile reported longstanding illness, compared with 52% of men and 48% of women in the lowest income quintile, as shown by the top line in Figure 6A.   **Table 6.4, Figure 6A**

By Health Authority area type

The age-standardised prevalence of longstanding illness was higher in the first three, more urban, area types (Inner London, Mining and Industrial, Urban). Among men, it ranged from 42% to 46% in this group, compared with 40% to 41% in other areas. For women prevalence in the urban group was in the range 46% to 48%, compared with 41% to 44% in the other three.   **Table 6.5**

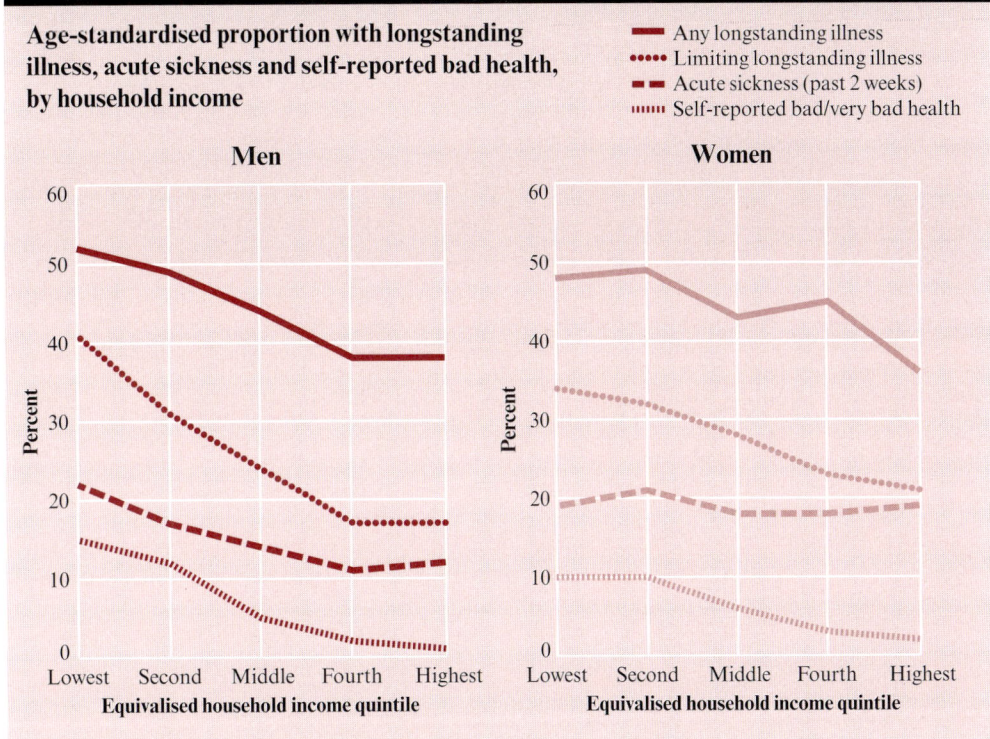

Figure 6A

Age-standardised proportion with longstanding illness, acute sickness and self-reported bad health, by household income

Legend:
— Any longstanding illness
••••• Limiting longstanding illness
– – Acute sickness (past 2 weeks)
||||||| Self-reported bad/very bad health

Men / Women charts, y-axis Percent (0–60), x-axis: Lowest, Second, Middle, Fourth, Highest — Equivalised household income quintile

6.2.2 Logistic regression of the prevalence of longstanding illness

Separate logistic regressions were run for men and women, with the following independent variables: age, social class of head of household, equivalised household income, employment status and Health Authority area type. The odds ratios are relative to average. An odds ratio of less than one means that the group was less likely than average to report a (limiting) longstanding illness, and an odds ratio greater than one indicates a greater than average likelihood of report a (limiting) longstanding illness.

After adjusting for the other variables in the model, age remained a strong predictor of longstanding illness. Men aged 75 and over were eight times as likely to report a longstanding illness as men aged 16-24 (odds ratios relative to average: 0.24 for men aged 16-24, 1.97 for men aged 75 and over), and women in the same age groups were five times as likely to report longstanding illness (odds ratios relative to average: 0.46 for women aged 16-24, 2.14 for women aged 75 and over).

Social class of head of household, household income and Health Authority area type effects were mostly not significant, and did not form clear patterns.

Employment status was analysed in the model, but not in cross-tabulations. Analysis was by four categories, in work, unemployed, retired and other economically inactive. The last of these groups includes those unable to work because of chronic illness, and not surprisingly had higher odds of longstanding illness in both sexes (particularly men). Among women, the retired had higher odds of longstanding illness than those economically active, but this was not the case for men. Unemployed men had higher odds of longstanding illness than men in work, but among women no difference between the unemployed and in work categories was seen.   **Table 6.7**

6.2.3 Limiting longstanding illness

Since more than half of those with a longstanding illness had a limiting longstanding illness, it is not surprising to find that limiting longstanding illness shows a similar pattern of relationships with sex, age and socio-economic variables. This section therefore reports on limiting longstanding illness relationships only where they are different from longstanding illness relationships, in direction or in strength. A logistic regression was run similar to that for longstanding illness, with the same independent variables.

25% of men and 27% of women reported a longstanding illness that limited their activities in some way (compared with 44% of each sex reporting any longstanding illness).

The increase in prevalence with age was steeper for limiting longstanding illness than for longstanding illness as a whole. Prevalences of longstanding illness quoted in Section 6.2.1 for the youngest and oldest groups were 21% to 65% for men and 27% to 72% for women. Comparable figures for limiting longstanding illness were 8% to 49% for men and 7% to 39% for women. The older a person was, the greater the likelihood of longstanding illness, and the greater the probability that this longstanding illness was limiting.   **Table 6.1**

Like longstanding illness, but to a more marked degree, the age-standardised prevalence of limiting longstanding illness varied by social class, increasing among men from 17% in Social Class I to 31% in Social Class V, corresponding prevalences for women being 24% and 30%.   **Table 6.3**

Similarly, variation by equivalised household income was more marked for limiting longstanding illness than for longstanding illness as a whole. The age-standardised proportion with limiting longstanding illness increased among men from 17% in the highest income quintile to 41% in the lowest income quintile, corresponding figures for women being 21% to 34%. The pattern is shown by the top two lines of Figure 6A.   **Table 6.4, Figure 6A**

In the logistic regression model, social class effects for limiting longstanding illness in both sexes were non-significant after adjusting for the other factors in the model. Significant income effects were seen, however, for both men and women after adjusting for the other factors in the model. Odds ratios (relative to average) for men ranged from 0.87 and 0.77 in the two highest income quintiles to 1.30 in the lowest quintile. For women, comparable figures were 0.76 and 0.90 to 1.15. The odds of limiting longstanding illness were particularly high for economically inactive men other than the retired: as noted in Section 6.2.2, this group contains those unable to work because of chronic illness. Among women, both the retired and the other economically inactive had above average odds of limiting longstanding illness.   **Table 6.7**

6.2.4 Types of longstanding illness

Illnesses were coded into broad categories which were then further aggregated into groups which correspond as far as possible to the chapter headings of the Ninth Revision of the International Classification of Diseases (ICD).[4]

It should be noted that, since the Health Survey classification of conditions is based on self-reported information, results will not correspond exactly with those that would be obtained by medical diagnosis. In addition the ICD is used mostly for coding conditions and diseases according to the cause, whereas the Health Survey classifies according to the reported symptoms.

The reported prevalence of longstanding conditions follows the pattern shown in earlier Health Survey reports, the most common being musculoskeletal problems, followed by heart and circulatory system conditions and respiratory conditions.   **Table 6.2**

6.2.5 Trends over time in self-reported longstanding illness

Analysis of longstanding illness trends is based on data from 1994 to 1998.

There was a significant upwards trend in the proportion of both men and women reporting a longstanding illness. In 1994 39% of men and 40% of women reported a longstanding illness, and these figures had increased to 44% of men and 44% of women in both 1997 and 1998, as shown by the top pair of lines in Figure 6B.   **Table 6.9, Figure 6B**

6.3 Self-reported acute sickness

6.3.1 Prevalence of acute sickness in the past two weeks

Acute sickness was defined as having to cut down, in the two weeks preceding the interview, on anything usually done about the house, at work, at school or in free time, because of illness or injury. Informants reporting acute sickness were asked for how many days their activities had been limited in this way (a measure of the severity of the acute sickness).

Figure 6B

Trends in self-reported health

— Longstanding illness
- - Acute sickness (past 2 weeks)
•••• Self-reported bad/very bad health

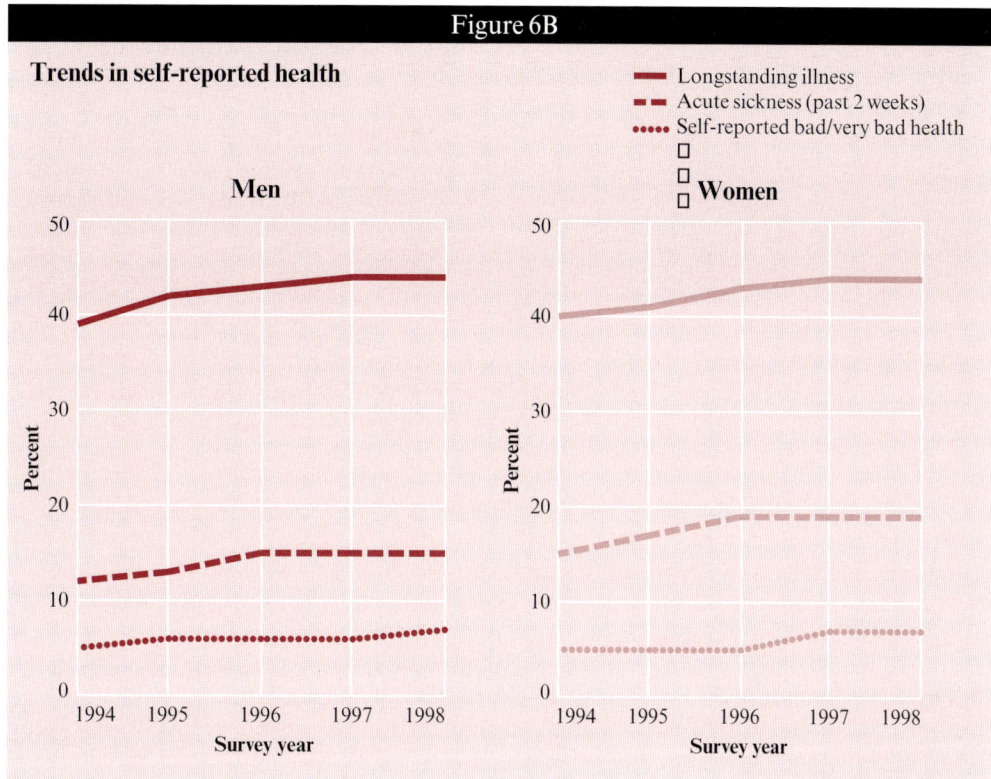

As for the other self-reported health measures in this chapter, a logistic regression model was run (separately for each sex) for the prevalence of acute sickness, the same independent variables being included. Results are incorporated with those on cross-tabulations.

By sex and age

15% of men and 19% of women reported that they had had an acute sickness in the past two weeks.

The prevalence of acute sickness in the past two weeks increased from 11% for the youngest men (aged 16-24) to 22% for the oldest (age 75 and over), and from 14% for the youngest women to 24% for the oldest.   **Table 6.10**

By social class of head of household and income

Among men, prevalence of acute sickness in the past two weeks increased as income decreased and was higher in manual social classes. This was not observed for women.

Tables 6.11, 6.12, Figure 6A

Logistic regression model of acute sickness prevalence

The observed relationship with age noted above remained significant in the model, odds ratios (relative to average) ranging from 0.50 among the youngest men to 1.60 among the oldest men, the range for women being from 0.73 (youngest) to 1.11 (oldest). Women aged 45-54 also had above-average odds (1.26), a feature not found among men.

Neither income nor social class were significant predictors of acute sickness after adjustment for other factors in the logistic regression model. Nor was Health Authority area type.

Odds of acute sickness were high among retired women (but not retired men). Unemployed men had higher odds than men in work, but this was not seen among women.   **Table 6.15**

6.3.2   Trends over time in self-reported acute sickness in the past two weeks

There was a significant upwards trend between 1994 and 1996 in the proportion of both men and women reporting acute sickness, as shown by the middle pair of lines in Figure 6B. In 1994 12% of men and 15% of women reported a longstanding illness, and these figures had increased to 15% of men and 19% of women by 1996. From 1996, the figures have remained unchanged.   **Table 6.16, Figure 6B**

6.4 Self-assessed general health

6.4.1 Prevalence of good and poor health

Informants were asked to rate their health in general on a five-point scale from 'very good' to 'very bad'. As for other self-report variables, a regression model has been run, using the same independent variables, but instead of choosing a point at which to divide self-reported health into good and bad and so create a dichotomous variable suitable for logistic regression, the technique of ordinal regression has been applied to the scale as a whole (see below). Since self-assessed health is a 5-category ordinal variable, modelling techniques that account for the ordinality are appropriate. There are various methods for ordinal regression modelling, but a continuation ratio model is presented here,[5,6] principally because it can be fitted, after some data manipulation, using the SPSS logistic regression procedure.

The interpretation of the odds ratio in a continuation ratio model is somewhat different to that of a logistic regression model. Whereas in a logistic regression model only one set of odds is estimated, namely odds of being in category 1 of a binary variable, in a continuation ratio model several odds are estimated simultaneously, each set of odds corresponding to a different split in the dependent ordinal variable. For example, for self-assessed health (which is defined as 1 if in 'very good' health, 2 if 'good' health, 3 if 'fair' health, 4 if 'bad' health and 5 if 'very bad' health), four sets of odds are estimated (corresponding to four splits in the data): the odds of being in 'very good' health; the odds of being in 'good' health if not in 'very good' health; the odds of being in 'fair' health if not in 'good' or 'very good' health; and the odds of being in 'bad' health if not in any of the three higher categories. Four binary comparisons are thus made 1 v 2345; 2 v 345; 3 v 45; 4 v 5. An odds ratio of greater than one for any group implies that, for each of the four comparisons, the group are more likely to be on the 'better' health side of the split. Conversely, an odds ratio of less than one implies that, for each of the four comparisons, the group are more likely to be on the 'worse' health side of the split. In what follows an odds ratio of greater than one is interpreted as implying 'better health' and an odds ratio of less than one as implying 'worse health'.

Two models were run (for each sex separately). In the first, the independent variables were the same as those used in the models for longstanding illness and acute sickness, namely age group, social class of head of household, equivalised household income quintile, employment status and Health Authority area type. The second model added longstanding illness and acute sickness, in order to explore their relation to self-assessed general health. Educational level was also added.

In both models, the odds ratio expresses the ratio of the odds to average, not to the odds in a reference category.

By sex and age

75% of men and 73% of women rated their health as 'good' or 'very good'. 19% of men and 20% of women rated their health 'fair'. 7% of each sex rated it as 'bad' or 'very bad'.

The proportion of men and women rating their health as 'good' or 'very good' decreased with increasing age. In the youngest and oldest groups (16-24 and 75 and over), the proportions of men rating their health as 'good' or 'very good' were 85% and 54%. Comparable figures for women were 82% and 50%.   **Table 6.17**

By social class of head of household and equivalised household income

The percentage of both men and women rating their health as 'good' or 'very good' increased with increasing household income and was higher in non-manual social classes.

The age-standardised proportion with 'good' or 'very good' health increased among men from 61% in Social Class V to 86% in Social Class I and among women from 64% to 81%.
                                                                    Table 6.18
The proportion with bad or very bad health, shown in Figure 6A in preference to the proportion with good health to permit more direct comparison with longstanding illness and acute sickness patterns, decreased among men from 15% in the lowest income quintile to 1% in the highest income quintile, corresponding figures for women being 10% and 2%.
                                                            Table 6.19, Figure 6A

By Health Authority area type

For both men and women, the highest age-standardised prevalence of 'good' or 'very good' health was in Prosperous areas (80% for men, 78% for women), whilst the lowest rating was in Inner London (64% for men, 63% for women).   Table 6.20

The first regression model

After adjustment for the other variables in the model, the relationship with age remained strong for both sexes, but stronger for men than women. Odds ratios (relative to average) for youngest and oldest groups were respectively 2.14 and 0.54 for men, and 1.41 and 0.68 for women.

After adjusting for the other factors in the model as well as for age, the social class and income effects both remained significant. Odds ratios of 'better' health, from lowest to highest income quintiles, ranged from 0.79 to 1.23 for men and from 0.82 to 1.34 for women. From Social Class V to Social Class I the odds ratio of 'better' health ranged from 0.75 to 1.29 for men and 0.79 to 1.22 for women. The income and social class gradients were thus very similar.

The regression model suggests, after adjustment by the other factors in the model, a division of the six Health Authority area types into two groups, with higher odds of 'better' health in the three less urban categories – Mature, Prosperous and Rural.

Self-assessed general health is not shown by employment status in the tables, but employment status is included in the regression model in Table 6.22. It will be seen that after adjusting for age group, social class of head of household, equivalised household income and Health Authority area type, there were statistically significant effects by employment status. Among men in work, the odds of 'better' health were well above average, and significantly higher than those for those out of work or the retired. The odds of 'better' health were low for the remainder of those not economically active (that is, other than the retired). It must be remembered that this group includes those unable to work because of chronic ill-health. Differences between employment status groups were less marked for women, but again those in work had significantly greater odds of 'better' health than economically active women. But the small difference observed between employed and unemployed women was not statistically significant.   Table 6.21

6.4.2 The second model: relation of self-assessed general health to self-reported illness

As noted in Section 6.4.1, the second model took the same five independent variables as the first model, but added three others, educational level, prevalence of limiting longstanding illness and prevalence of acute sickness. The inclusion of these factors yields a model in which odds ratios for the other factors may be different than for the first model, as a result of the additional adjustment factors.

The effects of age were attenuated for men in the second model (and non-significant for women), probably because of the presence of longstanding illness, which is associated with it. But variations by social class and equivalised household income were substantially the same in both models.

The second model shows higher odds of 'better' health among those with higher educational qualifications (odds ratio relative to average 1.27 among men with a degree, 0.78 among men with no qualifications – comparable figures for women 1.21 and 0.73).

It also shows marked differences in odds of 'better' health between longstanding illness categories (limiting, non-limiting, no illness). Relative to average, the odds ratio was 0.37 in men with limiting illness and 2.34 in men with no longstanding illness (among women, 0.33 and 2.67). Similarly, those had experienced acute sickness in the past two weeks had lower odds of 'better' health than of those without.   Table 6.23

6.4.3 Trends over time in self-assessed general health

There has been a steady decrease in the proportion of men reporting 'good' or 'very good' health from 78% in 1994 to 75% in 1998. Women also showed a decline from 75% in 1994 to 73% in 1998, although the trend was not as consistent or as marked as that for men. Like Figure 6A, the bottom two lines of Figure 6B present proportions with bad health rather than with good health for more direct comparison with acute sickness and longstanding illness patterns. They show an increase in self-reported bad or very bad health from 1994 to 1998.   Table 6.24, Figure 6B

6.5 The General Health Questionnaire (GHQ12)

GHQ12 was designed to detect possible psychiatric morbidity in the general population. The questionnaire is based on 12 questions about general level of happiness, depression, anxiety and sleep disturbance over the past four weeks. A score is constructed from the responses. As in previous Health Survey reports, a score of 4 or more was used as a threshold in the 1998 survey to identify informants with a possible psychiatric disorder,[7] and is referred to as a 'high GHQ12 score'.

Variations in the prevalence of a high GHQ12 by sex and age

Women were more likely than men to have a high GHQ12 score; 18% of women had a score of four or more, compared with 13% of men. This difference occurred throughout the age range, and has been displayed in previous health surveys.

There was an increase in the prevalence of high GHQ12 scores from 10% in men in the youngest group (16-24) to 14% among men aged 35-44, then a decline to 11% among men aged 65-74, and finally an increase to 16% among the oldest group (aged 75 and over). The results for women were essentially similar, but with the notable difference that those aged 16-24 presented an above-average figure, in contrast to the situation among men of that age.

Table 6.25

Variations in the prevalence of a high GHQ12 score by social class of head of household

There was no clear relationship between the prevalence of high GHQ12 and social class of the head of household, for either men or women. Some variations between social classes were observed, but did not form a clear pattern.

Table 6.26

Variations in the prevalence of a high GHQ12 score by equivalised household income

Among men, there was a marked inverse relationship between high GHQ12 and equivalised household income: the lower the income, the higher the proportion with a high GHQ12 score. The age-standardised proportion of men scoring 4 or more increased from 9% in the highest income quintile to 20% in the lowest income quintile.

A similar relationship was also found among women, but was weaker: the age-standardised proportion scoring 4 or more increased from 17% in the lowest income quintile to 21% in each of the two highest quintiles.

Table 6.27, Figure 6C

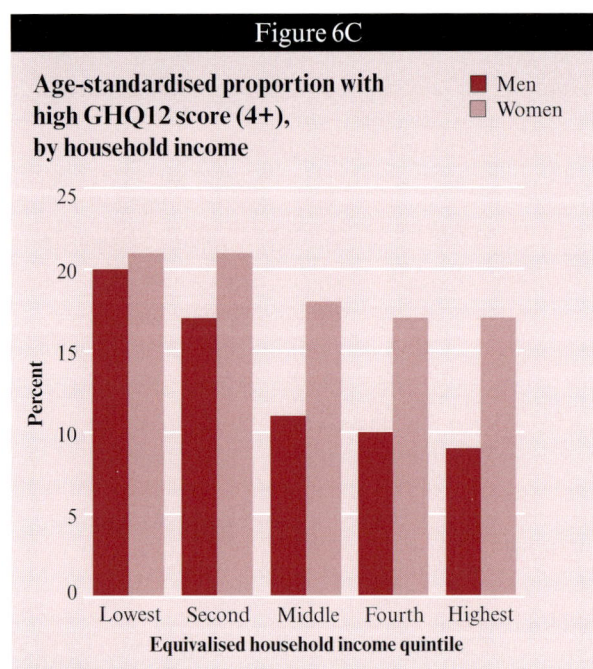

Figure 6C

Age-standardised proportion with high GHQ12 score (4+), by household income
■ Men
■ Women

Variations in the prevalence of a high GHQ12 score by Health Authority area type

In Inner London, age-standardised proportions with a high GHQ12 score (men 26%, women 26%) were significantly higher than in other area types.

Table 6.28

Trends over time in the prevalence of high GHQ12 scores

There was no evidence of a significant trend over time in high GHQ12 scores.   **Table 6.30**

Logistic regression model predicting high GHQ12

Following the above examination of bivariate relationships by means of cross-tabulations, this section explores the relationship between GHQ12 and socio-economic indicators when taken together, using logistic regression, with a GHQ12 score of 4 or more as the dependent variable. The independent variables were age, social class of head of household, equivalised household income, employment status and Health Authority area type. Logistic regressions were run separately for men and women. The results of the logistic regressions are shown in Table 6.31. The odds ratios are relative to a reference category, indicated on the table for each variable.

For both men and women, employment status was a strong predictor of a GHQ12 score of 4 or more, particularly among men, after adjustment by the other variables in the model. Economically inactive men (excluding the retired) were 3½ times as likely to score 4 or more as men in employment (odds ratio for economically inactive 3.59 relative to men in employment). Women currently unemployed and women economically inactive (again excluding the retired) were 1½ times more likely to have a high GHQ12 score than those in employment (relative to those in employment, odds ratio for economically inactive 1.57, for ILO unemployed 1.56).

Among men, Health Authority area type was also a predictor, those in Inner London being over twice as likely to score 4 or more as those in Rural areas (odds ratio for Inner London 2.46 relative to Rural areas).

Age was also significantly associated with high GHQ12 scores among men and women. The variations in odds by age reflected the pattern already commented on above.

The odds of a high GHQ12 score were higher for men in the two lowest equivalised household income quintiles. The same pattern was observed for women, but not at a statistically significant level.

There were no significant relationships between high GHQ12 scores and social class.

Table 6.31

6.6 Perceived social support

The perceived social support scale, originally used in the Health and Lifestyle survey,[8] asked informants about the amount of support and encouragement they received from family and friends. The scale is based on seven questions about physical and emotional aspects of social support. From these, a single scale was derived by assigning a score between one (lack of support) and three (no lack of support) for each of the seven questions. Informants with the maximum score of 21 were classified as having no lack of social support, those with a score of 18 to 20 were classified as having some lack of social support and those with a score under 18 as having a severe lack of social support.

Variations in social support by sex and age

Men were more likely to lack social support than women:

	Men	Women
Proportion with:		
No lack of social support	55%	64%
Some lack of social support	29%	24%
Severe lack of social support	16%	11%

There was no clear pattern of social support lack by age.   **Table 6.32**

Variations in social support by social class of head of household

The perceived social support scale scores were found to be strongly associated with the social class of the head of household. Men and women in Social Class V were much more likely to be classified as having a severe lack of social support than men or women in Social Class I. The (age-standardised) proportion classified as having a severe lack of social support rose from 10% of men and 6% of women in Social Class I to 27% of men and 16% of women in Social Class V.   **Table 6.33, Figure 6D**

Figure 6D

Age-standardised proportion with severe lack of social support, by social class

Legend: ■ Men ■ Women

Y-axis: Percent (0–30)

X-axis: Social class of head of household (I, II, IIINM, IIIM, IV, V)

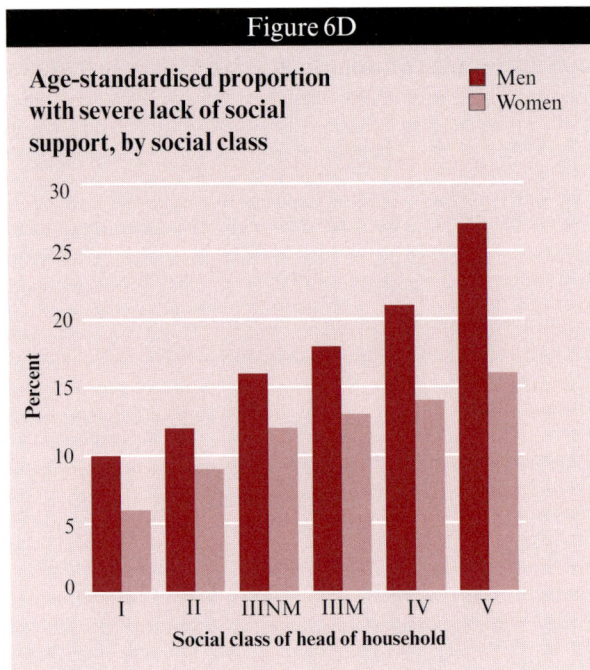

Variations in social support by household income

There was a strong inverse relationship between perceived social support and equivalised household income for both men and women. The (age-standardised) proportion of men classified as having a severe lack of social support rose from 11% in the highest income quintile to 25% in the lowest quintile. The proportion of women classified as having a severe lack of social support increased from 7% in each of the top two income quintiles to 19% in the lowest income quintile.

Table 6.34, Figure 6E

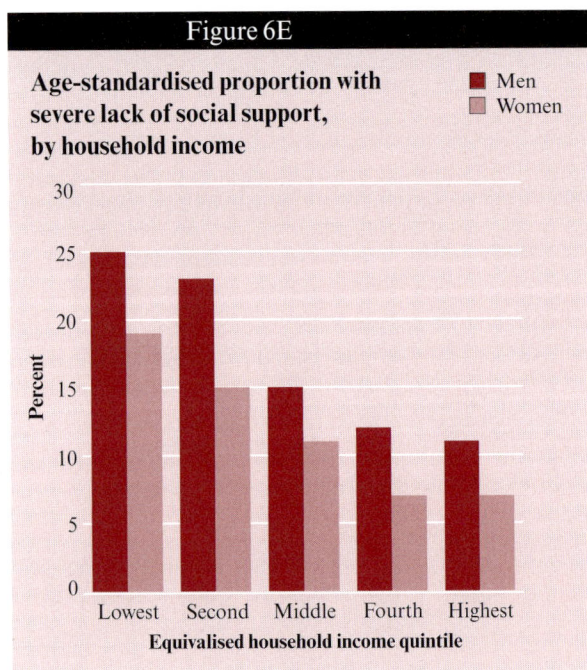

Figure 6E

Age-standardised proportion with severe lack of social support, by household income

Legend: ■ Men ■ Women

Y-axis: Percent (0–30)

X-axis: Equivalised household income quintile (Lowest, Second, Middle, Fourth, Highest)

Variations in perceived social support by Health Authority area type

The (age-standardised) proportion classified as having a severe lack of social support was significantly higher for men (24%) and women (18%) in Inner London than in other area types.

Table 6.35

Trends over time in social support

No clear trend over time was seen, among either men or women, in Table 6.37, which shows perceived lack of social support as reported in the Health Surveys for 1994, 1995 and 1998.

Table 6.37

Logistic regression of the prevalence of severe lack of social support

The relationships between perceived social support and socio-economic factors were also explored using logistic regression. The dependent variable was severe lack of social support, and the independent variables were age, social class, equivalised household income, Health Authority area type and employment status. The models were analysed separately for men and women.

Equivalised household income was a strong predictor of severe lack of social support among both men and women. Those in the lowest household income quintile were nearly twice as likely to have a severe lack of social support as those in the highest household income quintile among men (odds ratio for lowest household income quintile 1.96 relative to highest income quintile). Among women, they were $2^1/_2$ times more likely to have a severe lack of social support (odds ratio for lowest household income quintile 2.67 relative to highest income quintile).

Social class was a predictor of severe lack of social support, odds increasing from Social Class I to Social Class V (odds ratio for Social Class 1 was 0.42 relative to Social Class V). This pattern was more marked among men than among women.

Among Health Authority area type categories, the odds of severe lack of social support were highest in Inner London.

Odds did not differ significantly between employment status categories. **Table 6.38**

6.7 Comparisons of prevalence of high GHQ12 and severe lack of social support

The 1994 Health Survey report showed that these two measures were associated in those aged 65 and over. This analysis has been extended to the whole sample in 1998 and a strong association was again seen, in spite of much wider age range covered. The proportions were as follows:

	Level of perceived social support		
	No lack	Some lack	Severe lack
	%	%	%
Percent of each sex (within each of the social support categories) with a GHQ12 score of 4 or more			
Men	10	13	21
Women	14	20	37

Patterns of differences between population groups were in many respects similar for both high GHQ12 and severe lack of social support, but there were differences.

These are best examined in the logistic regressions that adjust for other variables in the model, these independent variables being age, social class, equivalised household income, employment status and Health Authority area type. Separate models were run for each sex. Patterns are summarised below.

- Higher odds of high GHQ12 among women than among men, but the reverse with severe lack of social support

- Higher odds of high GHQ12 among the unemployed than among those in work (also observed, but not reaching statistical significance, for severe lack of social support)

- Odds increasing with decreasing income: more marked for severe lack of social support than for GHQ12, and not reaching significance for women in the latter case

- Higher odds in Inner London than in other Health Authority area types

- Severe lack of social support strongly associated with social class, odds increasing from

Social Class I to Social Class V among men and to Social Class IIIM among women (all three manual classes for women having similar odds), whereas high GHQ12 was not significantly related to social class

● A clear if not strongly marked age pattern for high GHQ12 among men, with odds rising into middle age then falling before a final increase in the oldest group. Similar for women except for higher odds among the youngest women. No clear pattern in either sex for severe lack of social support.

There were also interesting similarities and differences in their relation to self-reported general health measures, as shown in Table 6.14 of the 1994 report. A repetition of this analysis produced the following:

Self-reported health	% of each self-reported health group who had high GHQ12		% of each self-reported health group who perceived severe lack of social support	
	Men	Women	Men	Women
Very good/good	8	12	14	9
Fair	21	28	23	17
Poor/very poor	48	52	22	23
Limiting illness	25	31	20	16
Non-limiting illness	9	16	14	11
No longstanding illness	9	13	15	10
Acute sickness in past 2 weeks	29	35	20	13
No acute sickness	10	14	16	11

The prevalence of high GHQ12 was much higher among those with poor or very poor self-reported health than among those reporting good health. The prevalence of severe lack of social support shows a similar type of relationship, but it was considerably less marked. The relation between high GHQ12 and longstanding illness was fairly strong, but the relationship between severe lack of social support and longstanding illness was relatively weak. The same is true in relation to acute sickness. It is not possible from the figures to infer the direction and nature of causality. It may be, for example, that a recent acute sickness will affect responses to GHQ12 but not (to the same extent) responses about lack of social support. Or the underlying condition that gives rise to responses that score high on GHQ12 may be one that makes the informant more liable to acute sickness.

References and notes

1 Reasons why available statistics may underestimate the extent of mental illness in the population are given in *The Health of the Nation: Key Area Handbook on Mental Health*, Department of Health, London, 1993.

2 Secretary of State for Health. *Saving Lives: Our Healthier Nation*. The Stationery Office, London, 1999.

3 Shapiro PA. *Psychiatric aspects of cardiovascular disease*. Psychiatr Clin North Am. 1996; **19/3**:613-626.

4 *The International Classification of Diseases and Related Health Problems (Ninth Revision)*, WHO, Geneva, 1977.

5 Fienberg SE, Mason WM. *Identification and estimation of age-period-cohort models in the analysis of discrete archival data*. Sociological Methodology: 1979:1-67.

6 Berridge DM. *A review of methods for modelling ordered categorical survey data* in Westlake A, Banks R, Payne C, Orchard T (eds), Survey and Statistical Computing, North-Holland, Amsterdam, 1992.

7 Each item in the GHQ12 has four possible answers. In scoring, each item is treated as a bimodal response scale so that only pathological deviations from normal signal possession of the iitem. Thus each informant scores 1 or 0 on each questionnaire item, and the total possible score for the GHQ12 is 12. See Goldberg D, Williams PA. *User's Guide to the General Health Questionnaire*. NFER-NELSON, 1988, pp 11-12 for further discussion of the scoring method.

8 Cox BD et al. *The Health and Lifestyle Survey*. The Health Promotion Research Trust, London, 1987.

Tables

Table 6.1

Longstanding illness and limiting longstanding illness, by age and sex

Aged 16 and over   *1998*

Longstanding illness and limiting longstanding illness	Age							Total
	16-24	25-34	35-44	45-54	55-64	65-74	75 +	
	%	%	%	%	%	%	%	%
Men								
Longstanding illness	21	30	38	45	60	65	65	44
Limiting longstanding illness	8	15	19	24	38	41	49	25
Number of longstanding illnesses:								
1	16	25	30	31	35	37	33	29
2 or more	4	5	8	14	25	28	33	15
Mean number of illnesses[a]	1.3	1.2	1.3	1.4	1.6	1.6	1.8	1.5
Standard error of the mean	0.04	0.02	0.03	0.03	0.03	0.04	0.05	0.01
Women								
Longstanding illness	27	28	36	42	55	65	72	44
Limiting longstanding illness	13	13	21	25	34	42	54	27
Number of longstanding illnesses:								
1	20	21	26	27	31	33	33	27
2 or more	7	7	10	15	24	32	39	17
Mean number of illnesses[a]	1.3	1.3	1.4	1.5	1.6	1.7	1.8	1.6
Standard error of the mean	0.04	0.03	0.03	0.03	0.03	0.04	0.04	0.01
Bases								
Men	*873*	*1337*	*1305*	*1287*	*986*	*836*	*562*	*7186*
Women	*1006*	*1630*	*1572*	*1482*	*1148*	*967*	*907*	*8712*

[a] Mean number of illnesses is based on those with a longstanding illness.

Table 6.2

Rate per thousand reporting longstanding illness conditions, by age and sex

Aged 16 and over   1998

Condition group (ICD chapters)[a]	Age							Total
	16-24	25-34	35-44	45-54	55-64	65-74	75 +	
	Rate per 1000							
Men								
I Infectious disease	1	1	2	4	1	2	4	2
II Neoplasms & benign growths	2	2	7	7	17	29	23	11
III Endocrine & metabolic	2	14	26	47	71	69	66	39
IV Blood & related organs	2	2	2	3	8	5	9	4
V Mental disorders	19	23	32	23	28	13	14	23
VI Nervous system	22	27	29	44	37	32	43	33
VI Eye complaints	13	5	9	16	28	48	105	25
VI Ear complaints	7	11	17	36	55	47	79	32
VII Heart & circulatory system	6	17	33	90	214	267	286	109
VIII Respiratory system	104	84	93	72	104	122	136	97
IX Digestive system	3	28	42	56	73	72	79	48
X Genito-urinary system	5	8	7	14	32	53	41	19
XII Skin complaints	17	21	23	18	12	18	14	18
XIII Musculoskeletal system	53	122	153	201	276	281	263	184
Other complaints	1	-	-	2	2	1	2	1
Women								
I Infectious disease	2	2	2	3	1	3		2
II Neoplasms & benign growths	1	6	11	24	25	36	21	17
III Endocrine & metabolic	15	17	30	46	95	115	107	55
IV Blood & related organs	5	6	5	8	6	10	15	7
V Mental disorders	19	26	40	44	35	20	19	31
VI Nervous system	35	39	35	52	48	36	41	41
VI Eye complaints	7	6	13	9	23	49	91	24
VI Ear complaints	5	11	16	14	17	27	64	20
VII Heart & circulatory system	13	16	36	67	166	245	280	101
VIII Respiratory system	128	87	82	74	87	110	109	94
IX Digestive system	14	34	38	52	63	107	115	56
X Genito-urinary system	17	22	30	27	20	24	31	25
XII Skin complaints	26	22	15	15	7	18	8	16
XIII Musculoskeletal system	61	76	135	189	289	341	417	197
Other complaints	-	1	1	1	1	2	1	1
Bases:								
Men	*873*	*1337*	*1305*	*1287*	*986*	*836*	*562*	*7186*
Women	*1006*	*1630*	*1572*	*1482*	*1148*	*967*	*907*	*8712*

[a] ICD Chapters refer to the ninth revision (1977).

Table 6.3

Longstanding illness and limiting longstanding illness (observed and age-standardised), by social class of head of household and sex

Aged 16 and over   *1998*

Longstanding illness and limiting longstanding illness	Social class of head of household											
	I	II	IIINM	IIIM	IV	V	I	II	IIINM	IIIM	IV	V
	%	%	%	%	%	%	%	%	%	%	%	%
	Men						**Women**					
Observed												
Longstanding illness	40	42	42	46	46	46	38	40	45	43	49	49
Limiting longstanding illness	18	21	23	28	31	32	20	22	29	27	32	33
Standardised												
Longstanding illness	38	40	41	44	45	44	41	41	44	44	48	46
Limiting longstanding illness	17	20	23	26	29	31	24	23	27	29	31	30
Bases	*503*	*2177*	*718*	*2263*	*1042*	*335*	*515*	*2499*	*1346*	*2209*	*1374*	*498*

Table 6.4

Longstanding illness and limiting longstanding illness (observed and age-standardised), by equivalised household income and sex

Aged 16 and over   *1998*

Longstanding illness and limiting longstanding illness	Equivalised annual household income quintile				
	Up to £7,186	Over £7,186 to £10,834	Over £10,834 to £17,890	Over £17,890 to £27,705	Over £27,705
	%	%	%	%	%
Men					
Observed					
Longstanding illness	52	54	46	37	37
Limiting longstanding illness	41	36	25	16	16
Standardised					
Longstanding illness	52	49	44	38	38
Limiting longstanding illness	41	31	24	17	17
Women					
Observed					
Longstanding illness	48	56	42	40	31
Limiting longstanding illness	33	37	26	19	15
Standardised					
Longstanding illness	48	49	43	45	36
Limiting longstanding illness	34	32	28	23	21
Bases					
Men	*1001*	*1004*	*1440*	*1394*	*1362*
Women	*1413*	*1489*	*1653*	*1493*	*1385*

Table 6.5

Longstanding illness and limiting longstanding illness (observed and age-standardised), by Health Authority area type and sex

Aged 16 and over 1998

Longstanding illness and limiting longstanding illness	Health Authority area type					
	Inner London	Mining & Industrial	Urban	Mature	Prosperous	Rural
	%	%	%	%	%	%
Men						
Observed						
Longstanding illness	39	48	46	43	42	43
Limiting longstanding illness	25	31	27	25	22	24
Standardised						
Longstanding illness	42	46	45	41	40	41
Limiting longstanding illness	29	29	26	23	21	23
Women						
Observed						
Longstanding illness	42	48	46	44	41	43
Limiting longstanding illness	26	31	30	28	24	25
Standardised						
Longstanding illness	46	48	46	44	41	43
Limiting longstanding illness	30	31	30	28	25	25
Bases						
Men	*240*	*1106*	*1052*	*1100*	*1944*	*1744*
Women	*309*	*1295*	*1338*	*1309*	*2388*	*2073*

Table 6.6

Longstanding illness and limiting longstanding illness (observed and age-standardised), by region and sex

Aged 16 and over 1998

Longstanding illness and limiting longstanding illness	Region							
	Northern & Yorkshire	North West	Trent	West Midlands	Anglia & Oxford	North Thames	South Thames	South & West
	%	%	%	%	%	%	%	%
Men								
Observed								
Longstanding illness	46	47	49	43	38	42	40	44
Limiting longstanding illness	28	29	29	25	19	24	22	25
Standardised								
Longstanding illness	44	46	48	41	38	40	39	42
Limiting longstanding illness	27	28	28	24	19	23	21	23
Women								
Observed								
Longstanding illness	46	50	47	41	43	42	40	43
Limiting longstanding illness	30	30	31	27	23	25	24	25
Standardised								
Longstanding illness	45	50	47	40	44	42	40	42
Limiting longstanding illness	29	30	31	27	24	25	24	25
Bases								
Men	*1030*	*979*	*797*	*745*	*812*	*914*	*889*	*1020*
Women	*1249*	*1135*	*941*	*913*	*961*	*1117*	*1181*	*1215*

Table 6.7

Estimated odds ratios for prevalence of longstanding illness

Aged 16 and over 1998

Independent variables	Men			Women		
	N	Odds ratio[a]	95% CI	N	Odds ratio[a]	95% CI
Age		p=0.0000			p=0.0000	
16-24	691	0.24	0.20 - 0.30	801	0.46	0.39 - 0.54
25-34	1148	0.63	0.54 - 0.73	1444	0.52	0.46 - 0.59
35-44	1177	0.84	0.73 - 0.97	1387	0.78	0.69 - 0.88
45-54	1105	1.12	0.98 - 1.29	1259	1.04	0.92 - 1.18
55-64	831	1.71	1.48 - 1.96	925	1.42	1.25 - 1.61
65-74	697	2.04	1.65 - 2.53	761	1.71	1.44 - 2.03
75 and over	445	1.97	1.53 - 2.54	646	2.14	1.78 - 2.59
Social class of head of household		p=0.5252			p=0.2946	
I	433	0.97	0.81 - 1.17	440	1.05	0.88 - 1.26
II	1872	1.02	0.91 - 1.14	2128	0.97	0.88 - 1.08
IIINM	618	0.93	0.80 - 1.09	1153	1.05	0.94 - 1.19
IIIM	1967	1.07	0.96 - 1.19	1894	0.94	0.85 - 1.04
IV	895	1.12	0.97 - 1.28	1171	1.12	1.00 - 1.27
V	309	0.91	0.73 - 1.13	436	0.98	0.82 - 1.17
Equivalised household income		p=0.2124			p=0.0007	
Bottom quintile	959	0.95	0.82 - 1.09	1328	1.04	0.93 - 1.16
Second quintile	988	1.06	0.93 - 1.20	1421	1.16	1.04 - 1.30
Middle quintile	1424	1.10	0.99 - 1.22	1631	0.98	0.89 - 1.07
Fourth quintile	1375	0.92	0.83 - 1.03	1467	1.07	0.97 - 1.19
Top quintile	1348	0.98	0.87 - 1.11	1375	0.79	0.71 - 0.89
Employment status		p=0.0000			p=0.0000	
In employment	3962	0.52	0.46 - 0.59	3698	0.75	0.67 - 0.83
ILO unemployed	342	0.78	0.64 - 0.96	287	0.76	0.61 - 0.94
Retired	1218	0.82	0.66 - 1.01	1406	1.30	1.11 - 1.53
Other economically inactive	572	3.00	2.51 - 3.59	1831	1.35	1.22 - 1.51
Health Authority area type		p=0.5419			p=0.0085	
Inner London	178	0.95	0.72 - 1.26	255	0.90	0.71 - 1.13
Mining & Industrial	966	1.09	0.96 - 1.25	1100	1.19	1.05 - 1.34
Urban Centres	904	1.07	0.94 - 1.23	1111	1.10	0.97 - 1.24
Mature	889	0.95	0.83 - 1.10	1025	0.95	0.84 - 1.08
Prosperous	1657	0.94	0.84 - 1.06	1998	0.89	0.81 - 0.99
Rural	1500	0.99	0.89 - 1.12	1733	1.01	0.91 - 1.12

[a] Odds ratios are relative to average, not to a designated reference category.

Table 6.8

Estimated odds ratios for prevalence of limiting longstanding illness

Aged 16 and over   *1998*

Independent variables	Men			Women		
	N	Odds ratio[a]	95% CI	N	Odds ratio[a]	95% CI
Age		p=0.0000			p=0.0000	
16-24	691	0.15	0.11 - 0.19	801	0.42	0.34 - 0.51
25-34	1148	0.70	0.58 - 0.84	1444	0.51	0.44 - 0.60
35-44	1177	0.88	0.74 - 1.05	1387	0.92	0.80 - 1.05
45-54	1105	1.10	0.93 - 1.30	1259	1.21	1.05 - 1.39
55-64	831	1.54	1.32 - 1.80	925	1.43	1.25 - 1.64
65-74	697	2.26	1.80 - 2.84	761	1.37	1.15 - 1.62
75 and over	445	2.88	2.22 - 3.74	646	2.16	1.81 - 2.59
Social class of head of household		p=0.1943			p=0.1538	
I	433	0.87	0.69 - 1.09	440	1.02	0.82 - 1.26
II	1872	1.06	0.93 - 1.21	2128	0.87	0.77 - 0.98
IIINM	618	1.08	0.90 - 1.31	1153	0.99	0.87 - 1.14
IIIM	1967	1.07	0.95 - 1.21	1894	1.00	0.89 - 1.12
IV	895	1.19	1.02 - 1.39	1171	1.13	0.99 - 1.29
V	309	1.04	0.82 - 1.33	436	1.01	0.83 - 1.22
Equivalised household income		p=0.0004			p=0.0013	
Bottom quintile	959	1.30	1.12 - 1.51	1328	1.15	1.02 - 1.30
Second quintile	988	1.09	0.95 - 1.25	1421	1.13	1.01 - 1.27
Middle quintile	1424	1.04	0.92 - 1.18	1631	1.11	1.00 - 1.24
Fourth quintile	1375	0.77	0.67 - 0.89	1467	0.90	0.80 - 1.02
Top quintile	1348	0.87	0.75 - 1.02	1375	0.76	0.66 - 0.89
Employment status		p=0.0000			p=0.0000	
In employment	3962	0.44	0.38 - 0.51	3698	0.60	0.53 - 0.68
ILO unemployed	342	0.78	0.61 - 0.99	287	0.81	0.62 - 1.05
Retired	1218	0.61	0.49 - 0.77	1406	1.30	1.10 - 1.53
Other economically inactive	572	4.67	3.89 - 5.61	1831	1.59	1.41 - 1.79
Health Authority area type		p=0.7072			p=0.0058	
Inner London	178	1.06	0.77 - 1.46	255	0.92	0.71 - 1.20
Mining & Industrial	966	1.07	0.92 - 1.25	1100	1.19	1.04 - 1.36
Urban Centres	904	1.03	0.88 - 1.21	1111	1.11	0.97 - 1.27
Mature	889	0.97	0.82 - 1.14	1025	1.03	0.89 - 1.18
Prosperous	1657	0.92	0.80 - 1.05	1998	0.87	0.78 - 0.98
Rural	1500	0.96	0.83 - 1.09	1733	0.91	0.81 - 1.03

[a] Odds ratios are relative to average, not to a designated reference category.

Table 6.9

Trends in longstanding illness, by sex

Longstanding illness	Survey year					Survey year				
	1994	1995	1996	1997	1998	1994	1995	1996	1997	1998
	%	%	%	%	%	%	%	%	%	%
	Men					**Women**				
Longstanding illness	39	42	43	44	44	40	41	43	44	44
Limiting longstanding illness	a	a	25	25	25	a	a	27	28	27
Number of longstanding illnesses:										
1	28	27	29	29	29	27	26	27	27	27
2 or more	11	15	14	15	15	13	15	16	17	17
Mean number of illnesses[b]	1.4	1.5	1.5	1.5	1.5	1.4	1.5	1.5	1.5	1.6
Standard error of the mean	0.01	0.01	0.01	0.02	0.01	0.01	0.01	0.01	0.02	0.01
Bases	*7173*	*7335*	*7485*	*3894*	*7186*	*8623*	*8719*	*8956*	*4681*	*8712*

[a] Not asked.

[b] Mean number of illnesses is based on those with a longstanding illness.

Table 6.10

Acute sickness, by age and sex

Acute sickness	Age							Total
	16-24	25-34	35-44	45-54	55-64	65-74	75 +	
	%	%	%	%	%	%	%	%
Men								
Had acute sickness	11	12	13	14	19	18	22	15
1-3 days	4	6	5	3	4	3	2	4
4-6 days	1	2	2	2	2	2	2	2
7-13 days	3	2	2	3	2	3	3	3
a full 2 weeks	2	3	4	6	10	10	14	6
No acute sickness	89	88	87	86	81	82	78	85
Mean number of days[a]	0.6	0.7	0.9	1.2	1.8	1.8	2.4	1.2
Standard error of the mean	0.08	0.07	0.08	0.10	0.14	0.15	0.21	0.04
Mean number of days[b]	6.1	5.9	7.0	8.7	9.7	10.0	11.1	8.4
Standard error of the mean	0.48	0.37	0.39	0.37	0.38	0.39	0.39	0.16
Women								
Had acute sickness	14	16	16	20	20	22	24	19
1-3 days	6	6	5	6	5	3	3	5
4-6 days	3	3	2	3	3	2	2	3
7-13 days	2	3	3	3	4	4	4	3
a full 2 weeks	2	3	5	8	8	13	16	7
No acute sickness	86	84	84	80	80	78	76	81
Mean number of days[a]	0.8	1.0	1.2	1.6	1.7	2.3	2.7	1.5
Standard error of the mean	0.08	0.07	0.09	0.10	0.12	0.15	0.17	0.04
Mean number of days[b]	5.8	6.2	7.5	8.0	8.5	10.4	11.2	8.3
Standard error of the mean	0.39	0.29	0.32	0.29	0.33	0.31	0.29	0.13
Bases								
Men	*874*	*1337*	*1305*	*1288*	*987*	*837*	*561*	*7189*
Women	*1006*	*1630*	*1573*	*1481*	*1148*	*967*	*907*	*8712*

[a] Mean number of days based on all informants.

[b] Mean number of days based on those with acute sickness.

Table 6.11

Acute sickness (observed and age-standardised), by social class of head of household and sex

Aged 16 and over 1998

Acute sickness	Social class of head of household							Social class of head of household					
	I	II	IIINM	IIIM	IV	V		I	II	IIINM	IIIM	IV	V
	%	%	%	%	%	%		%	%	%	%	%	%
	Men							**Women**					
Acute sickness													
Observed	11	13	14	17	16	16		16	17	19	19	19	21
Standardised	11	13	14	16	15	16		18	17	19	19	19	21
Bases	*503*	*2178*	*718*	*2265*	*1042*	*335*		*515*	*2499*	*1346*	*2209*	*1374*	*498*

Table 6.12

Acute sickness (observed and age-standardised), by equivalised household income and sex

Aged 16 and over 1998

Acute sickness	Equivalised annual household income quintile				
	Up to £7,186	Over £7,186 to £10,834	Over £10,834 to £17,890	Over £17,890 to £27,705	Over £27,705
	%	%	%	%	%
Men					
Acute sickness					
Observed	21	18	14	11	11
Standardised	22	17	14	11	12
Women					
Acute sickness					
Observed	19	22	18	17	18
Standardised	19	21	18	18	19
Bases					
Men	*1002*	*1004*	*1441*	*1394*	*1362*
Women	*1413*	*1489*	*1653*	*1493*	*1385*

Table 6.13

Acute sickness (observed and age-standardised), by Health Authority area type and sex

Aged 16 and over   *1998*

Acute sickness	Health Authority area type					
	Inner London	Mining & Industrial	Urban	Mature	Prosperous	Rural
	%	%	%	%	%	%
Men						
Acute sickness						
Observed	16	18	16	14	14	14
Standardised	16	17	15	14	14	13
Women						
Acute sickness						
Observed	21	19	20	18	19	17
Standardised	22	19	20	18	19	17
Bases						
Men	*240*	*1106*	*1054*	*1100*	*1946*	*1744*
Women	*309*	*1295*	*1339*	*1309*	*2388*	*2073*

Table 6.14

Acute sickness (observed and age-standardised), by region and sex

Aged 16 and over   *1998*

Acute sickness	Region							
	Northern & Yorkshire	North West	Trent	West Midlands	Anglia & Oxford	North Thames	South Thames	South & West
	%	%	%	%	%	%	%	%
Men								
Acute sickness								
Observed	18	16	15	14	12	16	13	14
Standardised	17	15	15	14	12	16	13	14
Women								
Acute sickness								
Observed	20	21	18	18	19	18	18	17
Standardised	19	21	18	18	19	18	18	17
Bases								
Men	*1030*	*979*	*797*	*746*	*812*	*915*	*890*	*1021*
Women	*1249*	*1135*	*941*	*913*	*961*	*1117*	*1182*	*1215*

Table 6.15

Estimated odds ratios for prevalence of acute sickness

Aged 16 and over *1998*

Independent variables	Men			Women		
	N	Odds ratio[a]	95% CI	N	Odds ratio[a]	95% CI
Age		p=0.0001			p=0.0022	
16-24	692	0.50	0.39 - 0.65	801	0.73	0.60 - 0.90
25-34	1148	0.93	0.75 - 1.13	1444	0.94	0.81 - 1.09
35-44	1177	0.99	0.81 - 1.21	1387	1.06	0.91 - 1.23
45-54	1105	0.99	0.81 - 1.20	1259	1.26	1.09 - 1.46
55-64	831	0.99	0.82 - 1.19	925	1.03	0.89 - 1.20
65-74	698	1.40	1.05 - 1.86	761	1.06	0.87 - 1.29
75 and over	445	1.60	1.15 - 2.22	645	1.11	0.90 - 1.36
Social class of head of household		p=0.5351			p=0.6482	
I	433	0.90	0.69 - 1.18	440	0.93	0.74 - 1.16
II	1873	1.03	0.88 - 1.20	2128	0.91	0.81 - 1.04
IIINM	618	1.04	0.84 - 1.29	1153	1.04	0.91 - 1.20
IIIM	1968	1.14	0.99 - 1.31	1894	0.98	0.86 - 1.10
IV	895	1.07	0.89 - 1.28	1171	1.03	0.89 - 1.19
V	309	0.85	0.64 - 1.14	436	1.13	0.92 - 1.39
Equivalised household income		p=0.7439			p=0.1860	
Bottom quintile	960	1.07	0.91 - 1.27	1328	0.87	0.76 - 1.00
Second quintile	988	1.00	0.85 - 1.17	1421	1.08	0.95 - 1.23
Middle quintile	1425	1.02	0.88 - 1.17	1631	0.96	0.86 - 1.09
Fourth quintile	1375	0.90	0.77 - 1.06	1467	1.00	0.88 - 1.14
Top quintile	1348	1.02	0.86 - 1.21	1375	1.09	0.94 - 1.26
Employment status		p=0.0000			p=0.0000	
In employment	3962	0.54	0.46 - 0.63	3698	0.82	0.71 - 0.94
ILO unemployed	343	0.94	0.73 - 1.22	287	0.70	0.52 - 0.94
Retired	1219	0.70	0.52 - 0.93	1406	1.23	1.02 - 1.49
Other economically inactive	572	2.83	2.36 - 3.40	1831	1.41	1.24 - 1.61
Health Authority area type		p=0.7320			p=0.3111	
Inner London	178	1.11	0.79 - 1.57	255	1.12	0.86 - 1.46
Mining & Industrial	966	1.08	0.91 - 1.28	1100	1.02	0.89 - 1.18
Urban Centres	905	1.00	0.84 - 1.19	1111	1.09	0.95 - 1.26
Mature	889	0.95	0.79 - 1.14	1025	0.92	0.79 - 1.07
Prosperous	1658	0.97	0.83 - 1.13	1998	0.97	0.86 - 1.10
Rural	1500	0.90	0.77 - 1.06	1733	0.89	0.78 - 1.01

[a] Odds ratios are relative to average, not to a designated reference category.

Table 6.16

Trends in acute sickness, by sex

Aged 16 and over 1994-1998

Acute sickness	Survey year						Survey year				
	1994	1995	1996	1997	1998		1994	1995	1996	1997	1998
	%	%	%	%	%		%	%	%	%	%
	Men						**Women**				
Had acute sickness	12	13	15	15	15		15	17	19	19	19
1-3 days	4	4	5	5	4		5	5	6	6	5
4-6 days	3	2	2	3	2		4	3	3	3	3
7-13 days	1	2	2	2	3		1	3	3	3	3
a full 2 weeks	4	5	6	5	6		5	6	7	7	7
No acute sickness	88	87	85	85	85		85	83	81	81	81
Mean number of days[a]	0.9	1.0	1.2	1.2	1.2		1.2	1.3	1.5	1.5	1.5
Standard error of the mean	0.04	0.04	0.04	0.05	0.04		0.04	0.04	0.04	0.06	0.04
Mean number of days[b]	7.7	7.8	8.1	7.5	8.4		7.7	7.6	7.8	7.8	8.3
Standard error of the mean	0.18	0.16	0.16	0.21	0.16		0.14	0.13	0.13	0.17	0.13
Bases	*7153*	*7335*	*7482*	*3895*	*7189*		*8588*	*8717*	*8957*	*4683*	*8712*

[a] Mean number of days based on all informants.

[b] Mean number of days based on those with acute sickness.

Table 6.17

Self-assessed general health, by age and sex

Aged 16 and over 1998

Self-assessed general health	Age							Total
	16-24	25-34	35-44	45-54	55-64	65-74	75+	
	%	%	%	%	%	%	%	%
Men								
Very good	42	40	40	35	28	26	22	35
Good	43	44	42	41	37	35	32	40
Good/very good	*85*	*84*	*82*	*76*	*65*	*61*	*54*	*75*
Fair	13	14	15	18	22	27	31	19
Bad	2	2	3	5	9	8	11	5
Very bad	-	0	0	2	4	4	4	2
Bad/very bad	*2*	*2*	*3*	*6*	*13*	*12*	*15*	*7*
Women								
Very good	34	38	36	32	28	22	17	31
Good	48	48	44	43	39	37	32	42
Good/very good	*82*	*86*	*80*	*76*	*67*	*59*	*50*	*73*
Fair	16	12	15	17	23	30	37	20
Bad	2	2	3	5	8	9	10	5
Very bad	1	0	1	2	3	2	4	2
Bad/very bad	*3*	*3*	*4*	*7*	*10*	*11*	*14*	*7*
Bases								
Men	*875*	*1338*	*1305*	*1289*	*987*	*836*	*562*	*7192*
Women	*1006*	*1630*	*1573*	*1484*	*1148*	*967*	*907*	*8715*

Table 6.18

Self-assessed general health (observed and age-standardised), by social class of head of household and sex

Aged 16 and over   *1998*

Self-assessed general health	Social class of head of household							Social class of head of household					
	I	II	IIINM	IIIM	IV	V		I	II	IIINM	IIIM	IV	V
	%	%	%	%	%	%		%	%	%	%	%	%
	Men							**Women**					
Observed													
Very good or good	86	82	78	71	65	59		84	82	72	71	65	60
Fair	12	14	17	21	25	28		14	14	21	21	25	28
Very bad or bad	3	3	5	9	9	13		2	4	7	8	11	12
Standardised													
Very good or good	86	83	78	73	67	61		81	81	73	70	65	64
Fair	11	14	16	20	24	27		16	15	20	22	24	26
Very bad or bad	2	3	5	8	8	12		3	4	7	8	10	11
Bases	*503*	*2178*	*718*	*2264*	*1042*	*335*		*515*	*2499*	*1346*	*2209*	*1374*	*498*

Table 6.19

Self-assessed general health (observed and age-standardised), by equivalised household income and sex

Aged 16 and over   *1998*

Self-assessed general health	Equivalised annual household income quintile				
	Up to £7,186	Over £7,186 to £10,834	Over £10,834 to £17,890	Over £17,890 to £27,705	Over £27,705
	%	%	%	%	%
Men					
Observed					
Very good or good	56	61	76	86	87
Fair	29	26	18	12	12
Very bad or bad	15	13	6	2	1
Standardised					
Very good or good	56	65	77	86	87
Fair	29	23	18	12	12
Very bad or bad	15	12	5	2	1
Women					
Observed					
Very good or good	62	61	75	83	88
Fair	28	27	18	14	11
Very bad or bad	10	12	6	3	2
Standardised					
Very good or good	62	67	74	81	85
Fair	28	23	19	16	12
Very bad or bad	10	10	6	3	2
Bases					
Men	*1001*	*1004*	*1441*	*1394*	*1362*
Women	*1413*	*1489*	*1653*	*1493*	*1385*

Table 6.20

Self-assessed general health (observed and age-standardised), by Health Authority area type and sex

Aged 16 and over   *1998*

Self-assessed general health	Health Authority area type					
	Inner London	Mining & Industrial	Urban	Mature	Prosperous	Rural
	%	%	%	%	%	%
Men						
Observed						
Very good or good	66	68	73	75	79	76
Fair	21	21	19	20	17	18
Very bad or bad	13	10	8	5	4	6
Standardised						
Very good or good	64	70	74	76	80	78
Fair	21	20	19	19	16	17
Very bad or bad	15	10	8	5	4	5
Women						
Observed						
Very good or good	66	68	69	74	79	74
Fair	25	22	23	20	17	20
Very bad or bad	9	10	9	6	5	6
Standardised						
Very good or good	63	69	69	74	78	74
Fair	27	22	23	20	17	20
Very bad or bad	10	9	9	6	5	6
Bases						
Men	*240*	*1106*	*1056*	*1100*	*1946*	*1744*
Women	*309*	*1295*	*1341*	*1309*	*2388*	*2073*

Table 6.21

Self-assessed general health (observed and age-standardised), by region and sex

Aged 16 and over   *1998*

Self-assessed general health	Region							
	Northern & Yorkshire	North West	Trent	West Midlands	Anglia & Oxford	North Thames	South Thames	South & West
	%	%	%	%	%	%	%	%
Men								
Observed								
Very good or good	69	73	72	76	82	73	77	76
Fair	21	20	20	18	14	19	18	19
Very bad or bad	10	7	7	6	3	8	5	5
Standardised								
Very good or good	71	74	74	77	82	75	78	77
Fair	20	19	20	17	14	18	18	19
Very bad or bad	9	7	7	6	3	7	5	4
Women								
Observed								
Very good or good	69	71	69	72	77	75	77	76
Fair	21	21	24	20	18	18	18	19
Very bad or bad	10	9	8	8	5	7	4	4
Standardised								
Very good or good	70	70	69	73	76	75	77	77
Fair	21	21	24	19	19	19	19	19
Very bad or bad	10	9	8	8	6	7	4	4
Bases								
Men	*1030*	*979*	*797*	*746*	*812*	*914*	*893*	*1021*
Women	*1249*	*1135*	*941*	*913*	*961*	*1118*	*1183*	*1215*

Table 6.22

Estimated odds ratios for ordinal regression of self-assessed general health (first model)

Aged 16 and over   *1998*

Independent variables	Men			Women		
	N^b	Odds ratio^a	95% CI	N^b	Odds ratio^a	95% CI
Age		p=0.0000			p=0.0000	
16-24	1187	2.14	1.87 - 2.45	1478	1.41	1.26 - 1.59
25-34	2034	1.33	1.19 - 1.48	2563	1.48	1.35 - 1.62
35-44	2148	1.21	1.08 - 1.35	2605	1.14	1.04 - 1.25
45-54	2166	0.94	0.85 - 1.05	2511	0.86	0.79 - 0.95
55-64	1816	0.90	0.81 - 1.00	1993	0.85	0.78 - 0.93
65-74	1573	0.64	0.54 - 0.75	1757	0.83	0.74 - 0.94
75 and over	1065	0.54	0.45 - 0.65	1599	0.68	0.60 - 0.78
Social class of head of household		p=0.0000			p=0.0000	
I	752	1.29	1.12 - 1.49	786	1.22	1.06 - 1.40
II	3362	1.22	1.12 - 1.32	3877	1.23	1.14 - 1.32
IIINM	1179	1.10	0.98 - 1.24	2309	1.08	0.99 - 1.18
IIIM	4064	0.92	0.85 - 0.99	3935	0.94	0.87 - 1.01
IV	1929	0.83	0.76 - 0.92	2596	0.84	0.77 - 0.91
V	703	0.75	0.65 - 0.87	1003	0.79	0.69 - 0.89
Equivalised household income		p=0.0000			p=0.0000	
Bottom quintile	2267	0.79	0.72 - 0.87	2996	0.82	0.76 - 0.89
Second quintile	2234	0.82	0.75 - 0.90	3240	0.81	0.75 - 0.87
Middle quintile	2804	0.97	0.90 - 1.05	3261	0.97	0.91 - 1.04
Fourth quintile	2391	1.29	1.18 - 1.40	2676	1.15	1.06 - 1.24
Top quintile	2293	1.23	1.13 - 1.36	2333	1.34	1.23 - 1.47
Employment status		p=0.0000			p=0.0000	
In employment	6949	1.70	1.55 - 1.86	6612	1.33	1.23 - 1.44
ILO unemployed	660	1.24	1.07 - 1.43	530	1.21	1.04 - 1.41
Retired	2782	1.31	1.12 - 1.54	3286	0.86	0.77 - 0.97
Other economically inactive	1598	0.36	0.32 - 0.41	4078	0.72	0.67 - 0.78
Health Authority area type		p=0.0029			p=0.0000	
Inner London	390	0.71	0.59 - 0.87	531	0.88	0.75 - 1.04
Mining & Industrial	2046	0.99	0.90 - 1.09	2363	0.92	0.84 - 1.00
Urban Centres	1830	1.02	0.92 - 1.12	2345	0.91	0.83 - 0.99
Mature	1718	1.09	0.99 - 1.21	2036	1.73	1.58 - 1.90
Prosperous	3125	1.11	1.03 - 1.21	3744	1.22	1.13 - 1.32
Rural	2880	1.13	1.04 - 1.23	3487	1.05	0.97 - 1.13

^{a} Odds ratios are relative to average, not to a designated reference category.

^{b} The bases on this table represent the numbers of comparisons made in the ordinal regression procedure (see text Section 6.4.1), and not the number of informants, since some informants will be involved in more than one comparison. For the same reason, the ratios of the bases for different sub-groups do not necessarily reflect the ratios of the numbers of informants in those groups.

Table 6.23

Estimated odds ratios for ordinal regression of self-assessed general health (second model)

Aged 16 and over   *1998*

Independent variables	Men			Women		
	N^b	Odds ratio^a	95% CI	N^b	Odds ratio^a	95% CI
Age		p=0.0009			p=0.1444	
16-24	1179	1.34	1.16 - 1.55	1477	0.95	0.84 - 1.08
25-34	2034	1.09	0.97 - 1.23	2559	1.11	1.00 - 1.23
35-44	2141	1.12	1.00 - 1.26	2600	1.03	0.93 - 1.13
45-54	2166	0.94	0.84 - 1.05	2511	0.92	0.83 - 1.01
55-64	1815	1.02	0.92 - 1.14	1993	1.02	0.92 - 1.13
65-74	1569	0.84	0.71 - 1.00	1757	1.04	0.91 - 1.19
75 and over	1063	0.75	0.61 - 0.92	1597	0.96	0.83 - 1.11
Social class of head of household		p=0.0000			p=0.0000	
I	752	1.13	0.97 - 1.33	786	1.19	1.02 - 1.38
II	3356	1.19	1.08 - 1.30	3877	1.17	1.08 - 1.27
IIINM	1176	1.10	0.97 - 1.24	2309	1.08	0.98 - 1.18
IIIM	4058	0.97	0.89 - 1.06	3930	0.94	0.87 - 1.02
IV	1922	0.91	0.82 - 1.01	2595	0.87	0.80 - 0.96
V	703	0.77	0.65 - 0.90	997	0.81	0.71 - 0.93
Equivalised household income		p=0.0000			p=0.0000	
Bottom quintile	2267	0.83	0.75 - 0.92	2990	0.82	0.75 - 0.90
Second quintile	2225	0.84	0.76 - 0.93	3238	0.84	0.78 - 0.92
Middle quintile	2793	1.00	0.92 - 1.08	3257	0.99	0.92 - 1.07
Fourth quintile	2389	1.23	1.12 - 1.34	2676	1.15	1.05 - 1.25
Top quintile	2293	1.17	1.06 - 1.30	2333	1.27	1.15 - 1.40
Employment status		p=0.0000			p=0.0000	
In employment	6935	1.31	1.19 - 1.44	6608	1.13	1.04 - 1.23
ILO unemployed	658	1.13	0.97 - 1.33	530	1.05	0.89 - 1.24
Retired	2778	1.21	1.02 - 1.44	3284	0.98	0.87 - 1.11
Other economically inactive	1596	0.56	0.49 - 0.63	4072	0.86	0.79 - 0.93
Health Authority area type		p=0.0028			p=0.0003	
Inner London	390	0.67	0.55 - 0.82	531	0.84	0.70 - 1.00
Mining & Industrial	2041	1.03	0.93 - 1.14	2360	0.97	0.88 - 1.07
Urban Centres	1826	1.05	0.95 - 1.17	2345	0.95	0.86 - 1.04
Mature	1716	1.08	0.97 - 1.21	2030	1.05	0.96 - 1.16
Prosperous	3120	1.11	1.02 - 1.22	3744	1.20	1.11 - 1.31
Rural	2874	1.14	1.05 - 1.25	3484	1.02	0.94 - 1.11
Highest educational qualification		p=0.0000			p=0.0000	
Degree/NVQ5	1589	1.27	1.14 - 1.42	1347	1.21	1.08 - 1.35
A Level/NVQ 3/4	2693	1.02	0.95 - 1.11	2450	1.06	0.98 - 1.16
O Level/NVQ1/2	3762	0.98	0.92 - 1.06	4952	1.06	0.99 - 1.13
No qualifications	3923	0.78	0.71 - 0.85	5745	0.73	0.68 - 0.80
Limiting longstanding illness		p=0.0000			p=0.0000	
Limiting longstanding illness	4311	0.37	0.35 - 0.40	5229	0.33	0.31 - 0.36
Non-limiting longstanding illness	2216	1.14	1.06 - 1.23	2517	1.13	1.06 - 1.22
No longstanding illness	5440	2.34	2.19 - 2.51	6748	2.67	2.51 - 2.85
Acute sickness		p=0.0000			p=0.0000	
Yes	2372	0.70	0.66 - 0.74	3428	0.69	0.66 - 0.73
No	9595	1.43	1.35 - 1.52	11066	1.44	1.37 - 1.52

^{a} Odds ratios are relative to average, not to a designated reference category.

^{b} The bases on this table represent the numbers of comparisons made in the ordinal regression procedure (see text Section 6.4.1), and not the number of informants, since some informants will be involved in more than one comparison. For the same reason, the ratios of the bases for different sub-groups do not necessarily reflect the ratios of the numbers of informants in those groups.

Table 6.24

Trends in self-assessed general health, by sex

Aged 16 and over   *1994-1998*

Self-assessed general health	Survey year									
	1994	1995	1996	1997	1998	1994	1995	1996	1997	1998
	%	%	%	%	%	%	%	%	%	%
	Men					**Women**				
Very good	36	38	37	35	35	32	33	33	31	31
Good	42	39	40	40	40	43	43	42	42	42
Good/very good	*78*	*77*	*77*	*76*	*75*	*75*	*76*	*75*	*73*	*73*
Fair	17	18	17	19	19	20	20	20	20	20
Bad	4	4	5	4	5	4	4	4	5	5
Very bad	1	1	1	2	2	1	1	1	1	2
Bad/very bad	*5*	*6*	*6*	*6*	*7*	*5*	*5*	*5*	*7*	*7*
Bases	*7175*	*7332*	*7485*	*3895*	*7192*	*8622*	*8719*	*8956*	*4682*	*8715*

Table 6.25

GHQ12 score, by age and sex

Aged 16 and over   *1998*

GHQ12 score	Age							Total
	16-24	25-34	35-44	45-54	55-64	65-74	75 +	
	%	%	%	%	%	%	%	%
Men								
0	60	60	62	66	67	71	57	63
1-3	30	28	25	21	20	19	26	24
4 or more	10	12	14	13	13	11	16	13
Women								
0	45	53	57	56	60	60	52	55
1-3	34	29	24	24	26	26	30	27
4 or more	22	18	20	19	14	15	18	18
Bases								
Men	*823*	*1279*	*1257*	*1231*	*926*	*785*	*501*	*6802*
Women	*970*	*1563*	*1512*	*1425*	*1083*	*904*	*797*	*8254*

Table 6.26

GHQ12 score (observed and age-standardised), by social class of head of household and sex

Aged 16 and over 1998

GHQ12 score	Social class of head of household											
	I	II	IIINM	IIIM	IV	V	I	II	IIINM	IIIM	IV	V
	%	%	%	%	%	%	%	%	%	%	%	%
	Men						**Women**					
Observed												
0	63	65	60	64	62	63	60	57	53	55	53	50
1-3	24	24	26	23	24	21	23	27	27	27	28	29
4 or more	13	11	14	12	14	16	17	16	20	18	19	21
Standardised												
0	62	64	60	64	63	63	58	56	52	54	53	51
1-3	26	25	26	24	24	21	24	28	27	27	28	28
4 or more	13	11	14	12	13	16	18	16	21	19	19	21
Bases	*478*	*2099*	*684*	*2128*	*966*	*309*	*494*	*2399*	*1287*	*2083*	*1278*	*465*

Table 6.27

GHQ12 score (observed and age-standardised), by equivalised household income and sex

Aged 16 and over 1998

GHQ12 score	Equivalised annual household income quintile				
	Up to £7,186	Over £7,186 to £10,834	Over £10,834 to £17,890	Over £17,890 to £27,705	Over £27,705
	%	%	%	%	%
Men					
Observed					
0	53	61	64	68	66
1-3	28	22	25	22	25
4 or more	19	17	11	10	10
Standardised					
0	52	61	63	68	66
1-3	28	22	25	22	24
4 or more	20	17	11	10	9
Women					
Observed					
0	51	51	55	58	56
1-3	28	28	26	25	27
4 or more	21	20	18	17	16
Standardised					
0	51	51	55	57	57
1-3	28	28	27	27	26
4 or more	21	21	18	17	17
Bases					
Men	*902*	*964*	*1380*	*1340*	*1335*
Women	*1279*	*1460*	*1577*	*1430*	*1357*

Table 6.28

GHQ12 score (observed and age-standardised), by Health Authority area type and sex

Aged 16 and over *1998*

GHQ12 score	Health Authority area type					
	Inner London	Mining & Industrial	Urban	Mature	Prosperous	Rural
	%	%	%	%	%	%
Men						
Observed						
0	47	62	62	62	65	67
1-3	27	24	26	25	24	22
4 or more	26	14	12	13	12	11
Standardised						
0	47	62	61	62	64	66
1-3	26	24	26	26	24	23
4 or more	26	14	12	12	12	11
Women						
Observed						
0	48	52	52	56	56	57
1-3	27	28	27	27	28	27
4 or more	24	20	21	17	17	16
Standardised						
0	47	52	52	56	55	56
1-3	27	28	26	27	28	27
4 or more	26	20	21	17	17	16
Bases						
Men	*221*	*1041*	*1004*	*1042*	*1863*	*1631*
Women	*283*	*1223*	*1271*	*1240*	*2291*	*1946*

Table 6.29

GHQ12 score (observed and age-standardised), by region and sex

Aged 16 and over   *1998*

GHQ12 score	Region							
	Northern & Yorkshire	North West	Trent	West Midlands	Anglia & Oxford	North Thames	South Thames	South & West
	%	%	%	%	%	%	%	%
Men								
Observed								
0	62	59	67	68	65	59	64	65
1-3	25	25	21	22	24	27	24	23
4 or more	13	16	12	10	11	14	12	12
Standardised								
0	62	59	66	67	65	59	64	64
1-3	25	26	22	22	25	27	24	23
4 or more	13	15	12	10	11	14	12	13
Women								
Observed								
0	55	51	54	54	54	57	57	55
1-3	25	28	28	27	29	27	26	27
4 or more	20	20	18	18	18	16	17	18
Standardised								
0	54	51	54	54	53	57	57	55
1-3	25	29	29	28	29	28	26	27
4 or more	20	20	18	18	17	16	17	18
Bases								
Men	*990*	*905*	*744*	*687*	*790*	*862*	*845*	*979*
Women	*1189*	*1060*	*882*	*859*	*925*	*1059*	*1130*	*1150*

Table 6.30

Proportion with GHQ12 score of 4 or more in 1994, 1995, 1997 and 1998, by age and sex

Aged 16 and over   *1994,1995,1997,1998[a]*

GHQ12 score of 4 or more	Age							Total
	16-24	25-34	35-44	45-54	55-64	65-74	75 +	
	%	%	%	%	%	%	%	%
Men								
1994	12	12	15	13	12	10	14	12
1995	12	12	16	17	14	13	14	14
1997	11	13	14	12	12	10	15	12
1998	10	12	14	13	13	11	16	13
Women								
1994	21	19	21	21	15	14	21	19
1995	21	21	21	21	19	15	20	20
1997	23	19	19	22	16	15	17	19
1998	22	18	20	19	14	15	18	18
Bases								
Men								
1994	*950*	*1402*	*1304*	*1104*	*974*	*842*	*405*	*6981*
1995	*960*	*1372*	*1343*	*1161*	*963*	*879*	*458*	*7109*
1997	*472*	*713*	*713*	*673*	*516*	*429*	*230*	*3746*
1998	*823*	*1279*	*1257*	*1231*	*926*	*785*	*501*	*6802*
Women								
1994	*1058*	*1684*	*1486*	*1256*	*1017*	*1070*	*780*	*8354*
1995	*1058*	*1697*	*1477*	*1351*	*1093*	*1014*	*754*	*8444*
1997	*543*	*889*	*805*	*779*	*563*	*515*	*409*	*4503*
1998	*970*	*1563*	*1512*	*1425*	*1083*	*904*	*797*	*8254*

[a] The General Health Questionnaire (GHQ12) was not included in the 1996 survey.

Table 6.31

Estimated odds ratios for prevalence of GHQ12 score of 4 or more

Aged 16 and over *1998*

Independent variables	Men			Women		
	N[b]	Odds ratio[a]	95% CI	N[b]	Odds ratio[a]	95% CI
Age		p=0.0001			p=0.0003	
16-24[a]	654	1		775	1	
25-34	1105	1.72	1.24 - 2.40	1395	0.85	0.68 - 1.07
35-44	1138	2.08	1.50 - 2.87	1337	1.05	0.83 - 1.31
45-54	1057	1.89	1.36 - 2.62	1215	1.04	0.83 - 1.32
55-64	790	1.37	0.97 - 1.95	881	0.65	0.50 - 0.86
65-74	664	1.27	0.75 - 2.15	723	0.57	0.40 - 0.80
75 and over	404	1.83	1.05 - 3.21	577	0.72	0.51 - 1.02
Social class of head of household		p=0.2533			p=0.3278	
I	414	1.24	0.79 - 1.95	425	0.88	0.61 - 1.26
II	1810	0.98	0.67 - 1.41	2057	0.80	0.60 - 1.05
IIIN	592	1.01	0.67 - 1.52	1111	0.98	0.74 - 1.30
IIIM	1862	0.83	0.58 - 1.19	1796	0.88	0.67 - 1.16
IV	845	0.97	0.66 - 1.41	1100	0.84	0.63 - 1.11
V[a]	289	1		414	1	
Equivalised household income		p=0.0026			p=0.5264	
Bottom quintile	887	1.53	1.12 - 2.09	1239	1.11	0.87 - 1.41
Second quintile	919	1.70	1.26 - 2.28	1338	1.22	0.96 - 1.53
Middle quintile	1355	1.13	0.86 - 1.49	1564	1.09	0.88 - 1.34
Fourth quintile	1342	1.12	0.86 - 1.45	1427	1.04	0.84 - 1.27
Top quintile[a]	1309	1		1335	1	
Employment status		p=0.0000			p=0.0000	
In employment[a]	3821	1		3595	1	
ILO unemployed	322	1.67	1.18 - 2.38	282	1.56	1.15 - 2.11
Retired	1145	1.31	0.85 - 2.02	1311	1.30	0.98 - 1.71
Other economically inactive	524	3.59	2.79 - 4.63	1715	1.57	1.34 - 1.84
Health Authority area type		p=0.0008			p=0.0016	
Inner London	171	2.46	1.66 - 3.65	239	1.61	1.16 - 2.23
Mining & Industrial	916	1.22	0.95 - 1.58	1046	1.24	1.01 - 1.51
Urban Centres	871	1.07	0.82 - 1.40	1068	1.43	1.17 - 1.74
Mature	850	1.10	0.84 - 1.44	978	1.13	0.92 - 1.40
Prosperous	1592	1.16	0.92 - 1.46	1931	1.07	0.89 - 1.27
Rural[a]	1412	1		1641	1	

[a] Reference category.

Table 6.32

Perceived social support, by age and sex

Aged 16 and over *1998*

Perceived social support	Age							Total
	16-24	25-34	35-44	45-54	55-64	65-74	75 +	
	%	%	%	%	%	%	%	%
Men								
No lack	49	58	55	57	52	57	53	55
Some lack	33	28	29	28	31	27	28	29
Severe lack	19	14	16	15	17	16	19	16
Women								
No lack	63	64	63	63	67	66	69	64
Some lack	25	24	25	26	23	23	21	24
Severe lack	12	13	12	11	10	11	10	11
Bases								
Men	*827*	*1288*	*1252*	*1236*	*927*	*787*	*505*	*6822*
Women	*973*	*1568*	*1516*	*1421*	*1087*	*910*	*802*	*8277*

Table 6.33

Perceived social support (observed and age-standardised), by social class of head of household and sex

Aged 16 and over *1998*

Perceived social support	Social class of head of household							Social class of head of household					
	I	II	IIINM	IIIM	IV	V		I	II	IIINM	IIIM	IV	V
	%	%	%	%	%	%		%	%	%	%	%	%
	Men							**Women**					
Observed													
No lack	64	60	56	52	47	44		72	69	65	61	60	61
Some lack	26	28	28	31	32	30		21	22	24	26	26	25
Severe lack	10	12	16	18	21	26		6	9	12	13	14	15
Standardised													
No lack	64	60	56	52	47	44		72	69	65	62	59	59
Some lack	26	28	28	31	32	30		23	22	24	25	26	25
Severe lack	10	12	16	18	21	27		6	9	12	13	14	16
Bases	*478*	*2102*	*690*	*2137*	*971*	*305*		*495*	*2394*	*1292*	*2099*	*1289*	*459*

Table 6.34

Perceived social support (observed and age-standardised), by equivalised household income quintile and sex

Aged 16 and over   *1998*

Perceived social support	Equivalised annual household income quintile				
	Up to £7,186	Over £7,186 to £10,834	Over £10,834 to £17,890	Over £17,890 to £27,705	Over £27,705
	%	%	%	%	%
Men					
Observed					
No lack	46	47	53	60	65
Some lack	31	30	31	28	25
Severe lack	23	23	15	12	10
Standardised					
No lack	45	46	53	59	64
Some lack	31	31	32	28	25
Severe lack	25	23	15	12	11
Women					
Observed					
No lack	54	63	62	70	73
Some lack	27	23	27	23	21
Severe lack	19	14	11	7	7
Standardised					
No lack	54	60	62	69	71
Some lack	27	24	27	23	23
Severe lack	19	15	11	7	7
Bases					
Men	*905*	*971*	*1387*	*1336*	*1334*
Women	*1283*	*1476*	*1578*	*1426*	*1360*

Table 6.35

Perceived social support (observed and age-standardised), by Health Authority area type and sex

Aged 16 and over   *1998*

Perceived social support	Health Authority area type					
	Inner London	Mining & Industrial	Urban	Mature	Prosperous	Rural
	%	%	%	%	%	%
Men						
Observed						
No lack	49	52	54	53	56	58
Some lack	28	31	29	30	28	29
Severe lack	24	17	17	17	16	14
Standardised						
No lack	48	52	53	54	56	57
Some lack	28	31	29	30	28	29
Severe lack	24	17	17	17	16	14
Women						
Observed						
No lack	57	63	64	62	66	66
Some lack	24	26	25	25	23	23
Severe lack	18	12	11	13	10	11
Standardised						
No lack	58	63	64	62	66	66
Some lack	24	25	25	25	23	23
Severe lack	18	12	11	13	10	11
Bases						
Men	*220*	*1038*	*1013*	*1047*	*1867*	*1637*
Women	*287*	*1224*	*1274*	*1247*	*2298*	*1947*

Table 6.36

Perceived social support (observed and age-standardised), by region and sex

Aged 16 and over   *1998*

Perceived social support	Region							
	Northern & Yorkshire	North West	Trent	West Midlands	Anglia & Oxford	North Thames	South Thames	South & West
	%	%	%	%	%	%	%	%
Men								
Observed								
No lack	54	54	56	55	58	51	57	54
Some lack	31	30	28	29	28	30	25	30
Severe lack	16	16	16	16	14	19	17	15
Standardised								
No lack	54	53	57	55	58	51	57	54
Some lack	31	30	28	29	28	30	26	31
Severe lack	16	17	15	16	14	18	17	15
Women								
Observed								
No lack	63	64	63	66	66	62	67	66
Some lack	27	25	24	22	24	25	22	23
Severe lack	10	12	13	12	10	13	11	10
Standardised								
No lack	62	64	63	66	66	62	67	66
Some lack	27	25	24	22	24	25	22	24
Severe lack	11	12	13	12	10	13	11	10
Bases								
Men	*994*	*909*	*744*	*697*	*784*	*862*	*845*	*987*
Women	*1189*	*1063*	*881*	*859*	*928*	*1068*	*1122*	*1167*

Table 6.37

Perceived social support in 1994, 1995 and 1998, by age and sex

Aged 16 and over								1994,1995,1998[a]
Perceived social support	**Age**							**Total**
	16-24	25-34	35-44	45-54	55-64	65-74	75 +	
	%	%	%	%	%	%	%	%
Men								
No lack								
1994	45	54	54	55	54	56	57	53
1995	48	55	52	55	49	47	49	51
1998	49	58	55	57	52	57	53	55
Some lack								
1994	36	31	28	30	31	27	24	30
1995	35	31	33	29	33	33	31	32
1998	33	28	29	28	31	27	28	29
Severe lack								
1994	19	15	18	15	16	17	19	17
1995	18	15	15	15	17	20	20	17
1998	19	14	16	15	17	16	19	16
Women								
No lack								
1994	54	58	62	62	68	62	65	61
1995	57	60	59	62	60	57	57	59
1998	63	64	63	63	67	66	69	64
Some lack								
1994	32	29	26	25	22	28	21	26
1995	29	29	29	27	27	27	27	28
1998	25	24	25	26	23	23	21	24
Severe lack								
1994	14	12	12	13	10	10	14	12
1995	14	11	13	11	13	16	16	13
1998	12	13	12	11	10	11	10	11
Bases								
Men								
1994	*955*	*1413*	*1298*	*1096*	*974*	*847*	*409*	*6992*
1995	*913*	*1376*	*1352*	*1167*	*969*	*881*	*498*	*7156*
1998	*827*	*1288*	*1252*	*1236*	*927*	*787*	*505*	*6822*
Women								
1994	*1060*	*1703*	*1496*	*1262*	*1030*	*1075*	*788*	*8417*
1995	*1065*	*1710*	*1479*	*1360*	*1093*	*1032*	*773*	*8512*
1998	*973*	*1568*	*1516*	*1421*	*1087*	*910*	*802*	*8277*

[a] The perceived social support scale was not included in the 1996 and 1997 surveys.

Table 6.38

Estimated odds ratios for prevalence of severe lack of social support

Aged 16 and over   *1998*

Independent variables	Men			Women		
	N^b	Odds ratio^a	95% CI	N^b	Odds ratio^a	95% CI
Age		p=0.6106			p=0.0203	
16-24^a	658	1		777	1	
25-34	1113	0.90	0.68 - 1.18	1399	1.35	1.01 - 1.81
35-44	1133	1.10	0.84 - 1.44	1343	1.26	0.94 - 1.69
45-54	1063	0.95	0.72 - 1.25	1214	1.39	1.03 - 1.88
55-64	790	1.09	0.81 - 1.45	881	1.05	0.74 - 1.47
65-74	662	1.06	0.68 - 1.66	726	0.93	0.62 - 1.41
75 and over	406	1.20	0.74 - 1.96	582	0.69	0.44 - 1.09
Social class of head of household		p=0.0001			p=0.0127	
I	414	0.42	0.27 - 0.64	427	0.56	0.33 - 0.92
II	1814	0.48	0.35 - 0.66	2052	0.73	0.52 - 1.03
IIIN	596	0.57	0.40 - 0.81	1115	0.89	0.64 - 1.25
IIIM	1869	0.62	0.46 - 0.83	1810	1.04	0.76 - 1.42
IV	847	0.70	0.51 - 0.96	1109	0.97	0.70 - 1.35
V^a	285	1		409	1	
Equivalised household income		p=0.0000			p=0.0000	
Bottom quintile	890	1.96	1.47 - 2.61	1242	2.67	1.97 - 3.61
Second quintile	926	2.08	1.58 - 2.73	1355	1.88	1.39 - 2.55
Middle quintile	1363	1.48	1.15 - 1.89	1563	1.58	1.19 - 2.10
Fourth quintile	1338	1.17	0.91 - 1.50	1423	1.10	0.82 - 1.48
Top quintile^a	1308	1		1339	1	
Employment status		p=0.0680			p=0.2147	
In employment^a	3831	1		3592	1	
ILO unemployed	323	1.23	0.90 - 1.68	281	1.34	0.92 - 1.95
Retired	1144	0.87	0.59 - 1.27	1319	1.23	0.88 - 1.71
Other economically inactive	527	1.34	1.04 - 1.72	1730	1.18	0.97 - 1.43
Health Authority area type		p=0.0078			p=0.0101	
Inner London	168	1.57	1.04 - 2.39	243	1.92	1.33 - 2.77
Mining & Industrial	914	1.18	0.93 - 1.49	1048	1.06	0.82 - 1.36
Urban Centres	876	1.28	1.01 - 1.62	1071	1.06	0.83 - 1.36
Mature	857	1.49	1.17 - 1.89	984	1.30	1.01 - 1.67
Prosperous	1594	1.41	1.14 - 1.74	1940	1.13	0.90 - 1.41
Rural^a	1416	1		1636	1	

^{a} Reference category.

Use of health services and prescribed medicines

7

Madhavi Bajekal

SUMMARY

- 13% of men and 18% of women had contacted their (NHS) GP in the two weeks before interview, yielding an estimated average of 4 (men) and 6 (women) consultations per person per year. In the previous year, a third of each sex had visited an outpatient or casualty department, 6% of each sex had had a day patient stay, and 8% of men and 11% of women had been admitted as an inpatient.

- The use of health services increased with age for both men and women. Compared to men, women in the reproductively active ages of 16-44 had consistently higher rates of GP consultation and inpatient attendance, probably due to pregnancy and childbirth. From the age of 45 onwards and for services not related to maternity, such as day patient and outpatient attendance (which exclude ante-natal visits), the pattern of service use for men and women was similar.

- Utilisation of all healthcare services increased markedly with increasing levels of self-reported morbidity as measured by self-assessed general health status and longstanding illness. For example, age-standardised GP consultation rates for men rose from 9% for men with good (self-assessed) health to 38% for men with bad health. The equivalent figures for women were 14% and 41%. Similarly, for outpatient and day patient visits, attendance rates in both sexes were two to three times as high for those in bad health as for those in good health. The gradient for inpatient attendance was particularly steep, rising from 5% for men (8% for women) in good health to 25% for men (28% for women) in bad health.

- About two in five men (39%) and half of all women (49%) were taking prescribed medicines. From age 45, use of prescribed medicines rose steeply with age. From age 75, 81% of men and 86% of women were on prescribed medication, with more than two in five of those on medication taking four or more drugs.

- The age-standardised proportion using prescribed medicine was more than twice as high among those in bad or very bad health (men 77%, women 87%) as among those assessing their health as good or very good (men 29%, women 41%). For those on medication, the mean number of drugs taken also rose significantly with increasing severity of self-reported morbidity for both men and women.

- Overall, there has been a slight upward trend since 1994 in the proportions of adults who took any medication. There was no significant change in the distribution of medicines taken by broad British National Formulary (BNF) categories over the period 1995 to 1998.

- 9% of women were on hormone replacement therapy (HRT) when interviewed and 6% had been users in the past. The proportion of women ever having used HRT increased sharply with age to 39% at age 45-54, and 41% at age 55-64, falling to 12% at 65-74 and 3% at 75 and over.

- Most users (62%) started on HRT between the ages of 45 and 54 and, on average, spent 5 years on the therapy.

- A significantly higher proportion of women in Social Class I households reported having used HRT (31%) than of women in Social Class V households (20%). Similarly, women in households in the highest income quintile were more likely to have used HRT (33%) than women in the lowest income quintile (20%).

7.1 Introduction

Consultation rates and admissions to hospital provide measures of primary and secondary health service usage that have an important role in health care planning. The General Household Survey (GHS) has provided such measures in a long-running annual data series on general health services utilisation.[1] The health service utilisation module in the 1998 Health Survey for England included the same questions as those in the GHS series. Additionally, informants who reported having a CVD condition were also asked if utilisation was in respect of their CVD condition. The Health Surveys for 1995, 1996 and 1997 dealt with utilisation only in respect of the specific conditions that provided the focus of those surveys. The 1994 Health Survey, like the 1998 survey, focused on cardiovascular conditions, and also included a utilisation module.

However, the questionnaires used in 1994 and 1998 differ in important respects which limit possibilities for assessing trends in health service utilisation over time. In 1994, for example, informants were asked only to state the total number of consultations they had with a doctor (other than during a visit to hospital) on their own behalf in the two weeks prior to interview. All consultations in 1994 were assumed to have been with a National Health Service (NHS) general practitioner (GP), and details of the site of consultation were not recorded. In 1998, NHS consultations were separated out, and site details were recorded. Outpatient visits and day patient stays were separated out in 1998, but not in 1994. While the definition of an inpatient stay was the same in both surveys, the 1998 survey also included details of the duration of each stay (to a maximum of 6) in the past year.

This chapter examines the use of GP services (7.2) and hospital services (7.3), followed by the use of prescribed medicines (7.4), contraceptive pills (7.5) and hormone replacement therapy (7.6).

7.2 GP consultations

7.2.1 The measures used

Informants were asked whether they had talked to a doctor in person or by telephone, other than during a visit to a hospital, in the two weeks prior to interview. For each consultation, informants were asked on whose behalf the consultation was made; whether it was on the NHS or paid for privately; whether the doctor consulted was a GP or a specialist; the site of consultation and whether the doctor had issued a prescription. This section focuses on consultations on the informant's own behalf with a GP under the NHS in the two weeks prior to interview. These constitute 88% of all consultations recorded, the remainder being on behalf of others (2%), or on behalf of the informant but either paid for privately (3%) or with a doctor other than a GP (6%).

The proportion having had an NHS GP consultation in the previous two weeks is referred to below as the GP 'consultation rate'. The number of consultations (the 'contact rate') is somewhat in excess of the consultation rate, since some informants had more than one consultation in the two-week reference period. Multiplying this two-week contact rate by 26 gives an 'annual contact rate' - the estimated number of consultations during a whole year. This provides an estimate of a central aspect of GP workload. The calculation is similar to that used in the GHS, which is known to overestimate contact rates when compared to actual annual contact rates recorded in the national morbidity survey in general practice (MSGP4).[2] The contact rate is the product of two quantities, the consultation rate and the number of contacts per person consulting. If the mean of the latter does not vary between sample sub-groups, sub-groups' contact rates will be in direct proportion to their consultation rates. This is broadly the case, so that the relative GP workloads to which various sample sub-groups give rise are fairly well summarised by the consultation rate alone, and the commentary below focuses mainly on this. The tables annexed to this chapter, however, give both the consultation rate and the annual contact rate (estimated mean number of consultations per year).

7.2.2 GP consultations by age and sex

In 1998, the proportion consulting an NHS GP in the past two weeks was 13% for men and 18% for women. Among women, the consultation rate did not vary greatly between age groups. Consultation rates for men remained at around 9% up to age 45, when they began to increase, reaching 21% for men aged 75 and over.

Women aged under 65 had a much higher consultation rate than men did, the difference being greatest for those aged under 35 (9% for men, 19% for women). Many of these consultations were likely to have been related to pregnancy and birth control rather than illness. From age 65 onwards, GP consultation rates for men and women converged. **Table 7.1**

7.2.3 Site of consultation by age and sex

5% of men and 6% of women who had had contact with a GP in the past two weeks had done so at home, with 7% and 8% respectively making contact by phone. The great majority of contacts took place at a surgery or health centre.

Those aged 75 and over were the most likely to be visited at home, the proportion being higher in the case of women (26%) than of men (16%). **Table 7.2**

7.2.4 GP consultation rates and reported levels of morbidity

Among men, there were marked differences in the age-standardised GP consultation rate between categories of self-assessed general health: 9% among those with good health, 19% among those with fair health and 38% among those with bad health. There was a similar but less marked pattern in relation to longstanding illness (8% among men with no illness, 13% among men with non-limiting illness and 22% among men with limiting illness). Because consultation rates were higher for women, the age-standardised proportions consulting were significantly higher for women than men across all categories, ranging from 14% among those with good (self-assessed) health to 41% among those with bad health, and from 13% for women with no illness to 30% for those with limiting longstanding illness. **Table 7.3, Figures 7A, 7B**

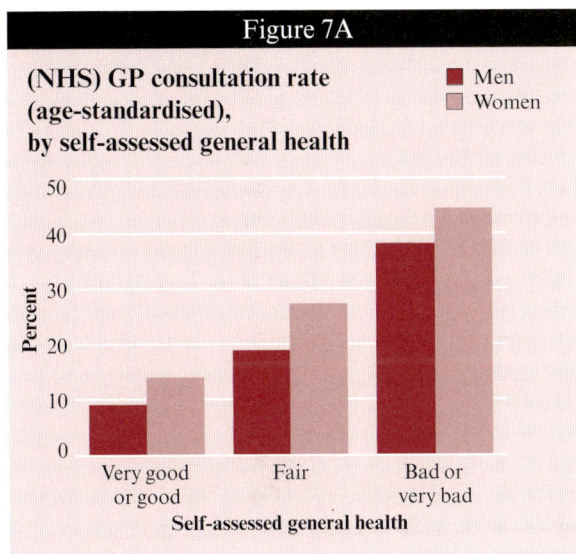

Figure 7A

(NHS) GP consultation rate (age-standardised), by self-assessed general health

■ Men
■ Women

Percent
Self-assessed general health: Very good or good / Fair / Bad or very bad

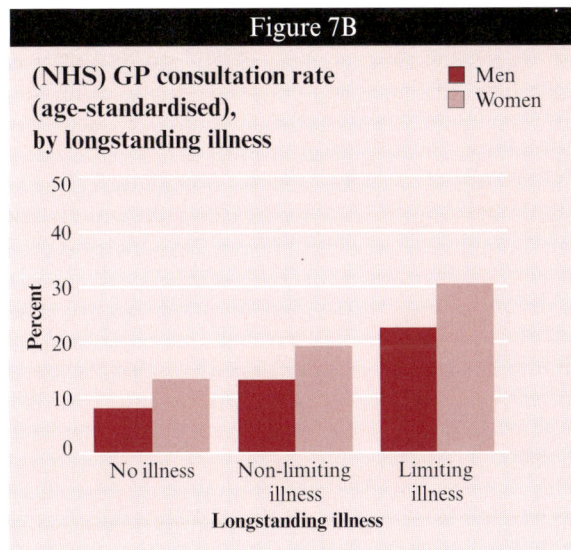

Figure 7B

(NHS) GP consultation rate (age-standardised), by longstanding illness

■ Men
■ Women

Percent
Longstanding illness: No illness / Non-limiting illness / Limiting illness

As the proportions above show, the relationship of the GP consultation rate with self-assessed health was stronger than its relationship with longstanding illness, for both men and women. The steeper increase in the former measure of morbidity may partly be explained by factors which influence informants' perception of their current general health at the time of interview – such as a recent bout of acute illness – which in turn was more likely to have resulted in a GP consultation in the two week reference period.

Not only were people with higher levels of reported morbidity more likely to consult their GP, the average number of consultations per person consulting was also generally higher. Annual contact rates thus increased with self-reported morbidity more rapidly than consultation rates did, as the following table shows (age-standardised figures):

	Men		Women	
	% who consulted in the past two weeks	Mean contact rate per person per year	% who consulted in the past two weeks	Mean contact rate per person per year
Self-assessed general health:				
Good/very good	9	3	14	4
Fair	19	6	27	9
Bad/very bad	38	12	41	15
Longstanding illness:				
No illness	8	2	13	4
Non-limiting	13	4	19	6
Limiting	22	7	30	10

The additional GP workload entailed by increased morbidity was broadly similar for both men and women. For instance, men and women with non-limiting longstanding illness had on average 2 extra consultations per year and those with a limiting illness 5 to 6 extra consultations per year compared to those with no limiting illness. **Table 7.3**

7.2.5 GP consultation rates by social class, household income and Health Authority area type

Age-standardised GP consultation rates varied by social class of head of household. The manual/non-manual divide formed a natural break in the pattern of consultation, with the constituent social class groups within each of these two categories having very similar consultation rates. The observed increase in consultation rates from Social Class IIINM to Social Class IIIM was significant for women (16% to 20%), but not for men (12% to14%). **Table 7.4**

Men's age-standardised consultation rates went up with decreasing (equivalised) household income, from 9% in the top income quintile to 18% percent in the bottom quintile. The increase among women was slightly shallower, from 15% to 21%. For both sexes, these differences were similar in magnitude to the differences in annual contact rates per person. **Table 7.5**

Health authorities categorised as 'Mature' had the lowest age-standardised consultation rates for both men (10%) and women (17%). Inner London consultation rates were high for women, but not significantly so. There was no consistent pattern for the other area types. **Table 7.6**

7.3 Hospital utilisation

7.3.1 Measures of hospital utilisation

Informants were asked whether they had attended an outpatient or casualty department, or been admitted to hospital as a day patient or as an inpatient (overnight or longer), during the last year. Those who said they had attended as outpatients were asked about the number of visits in each of the three months prior to interview. Those who had attended as a day patient were asked to recall the number of days they had been in hospital over the last year. Similarly, informants who had been admitted as inpatients during the past year were asked about the number of nights spent in hospital on each occasion in the six most recent stays. Fewer than one percent of inpatients had more than six inpatient stays during the past year, and for these informants only the stays beyond the sixth were not recorded, so the stays that were recorded comprised the great majority (97.4%) of all stays. Sections 7.3.2 to 7.3.4 examine variations by socio-demographic and health status factors in the proportion attending hospital as outpatients, day patients and inpatients. Section 7.3.5 provides further detail about inpatient stays.

7.3.2 Outpatient attendance

As in 1994, a third of all informants in 1998 (33% of men and 32% of women) had attended hospital as outpatients in the 12 months before interview. A slightly higher proportion of men than women had made an outpatient visit in all age groups except 45-54 and 55-64. **Table 7.8**

More than twice as high a proportion of men and women with bad self-reported health than of those with good health attended an outpatient or casualty department in the past year. Standardised for age, the proportion of men attending outpatient clinics rose from 27% among those with very good or good self-assessed health to 59% among those with bad or very bad health. It also rose from 23% among those with no longstanding illness to 49% among those with limiting longstanding illness. The pattern was similar for women:

Figure 7C

Outpatient attendance in the past year (age-standardised), by self-assessed general health

■ Men
■ Women

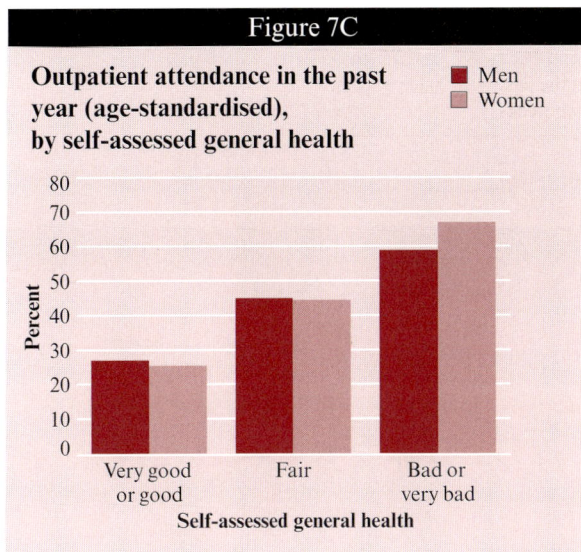

Self-assessed general health (Very good or good, Fair, Bad or very bad)

Figure 7D

Outpatient attendance in the past year (age-standardised), by longstanding illness

■ Men
■ Women

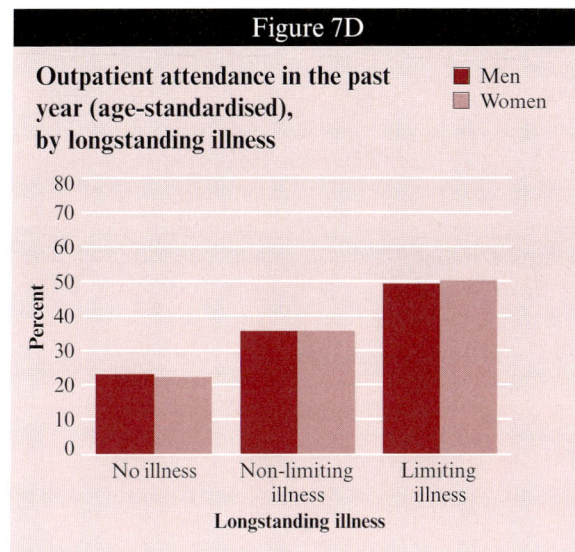

Longstanding illness (No illness, Non-limiting illness, Limiting illness)

the corresponding figures were 26% to 67% for self-assessed health and 22% to 50% for longstanding illness.

Table 7.9, Figures 7C, 7D

There was no significant difference in outpatient visit rates by social class for either men or women. Among men, there was a slight upward trend in (age-standardised) outpatient attendance with decreasing (equivalised) household income, ranging from 30% in the highest income quintile to 37% in the lowest quintile. No clear pattern was observed among women.

Tables 7.10, 7.11

None of the different types of hospital attendance proportions show any clear pattern of variation by Health Authority area type.

Table 7.12

7.3.3 Day patient attendance

During the 12 months before the interview, 6% of both men and women had been admitted to hospital for treatment as day patients.

Table 7.8

On average, day patients each spent two days in hospital over the year (table not shown).

There was a strong association between the day patient attendance rates and self-assessed general health. Age-standardised proportions attending as day patients varied from 4% among men with good or very good health to 13% among men with bad or very bad health, comparable figures being 5% to 14% for women. Day patient attendance was also strongly associated with longstanding illness, though the association was not as strong as in the case of self-assessed general health. Of men and women with no longstanding illness, 4% had been day patients in the past year: among those with limiting longstanding illness the figure was 9% among men and 10% among women.

Table 7.9

There was no significant variation in day patient attendance by social class, household income quintile or Health Authority area type for either men or women.   **Tables 7.10, 7.11, 7.12**

7.3.4 Inpatient attendance

8% of men and 11% of women had been inpatients in the preceding 12 months. Women aged 16-44 were more likely than men of the same age to have been inpatients, with those in the primary child-bearing age group of 25-34 having almost three times as high a rate of admission as men in that age group (14% for women and 5% for men). This is probably because stays relating to maternity are included in inpatient stays. From age 55 onwards, the gender differences were reversed and admissions for men were generally higher than for women.

Table 7.8

As with the other measures of health service utilisation, the proportion of people attending as inpatients was strongly associated with increasing levels of self-reported morbidity for both men and women. 5% (age-standardised) of men reporting good or very good health had been inpatients compared with 25% of those reporting bad or very bad health. Comparable figures for women were 8% and 28%.

4% of men with no limiting illness had an inpatient stay, compared with 16% of those with limiting longstanding illness, proportions for women being 8% and 16% respectively.

The tendency for a higher proportion (age-standardised) of women than of men to have had inpatient stays was more marked among those with low levels of self-reported morbidity than among those with high levels, where the sex difference largely disappeared.

Table 7.9, Figures 7E, 7F

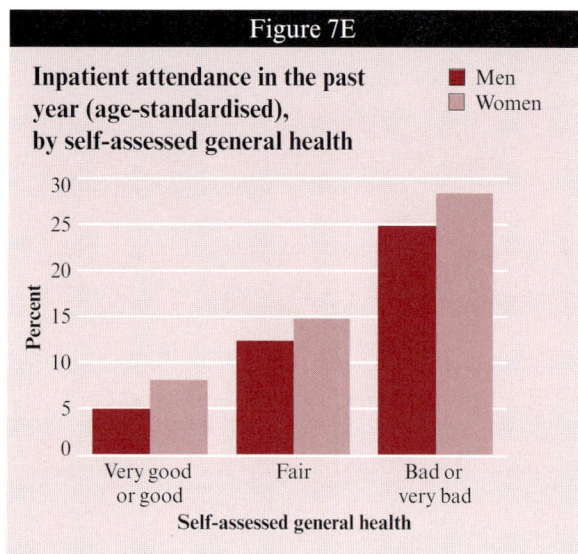

Figure 7E

Inpatient attendance in the past year (age-standardised), by self-assessed general health
■ Men ▢ Women

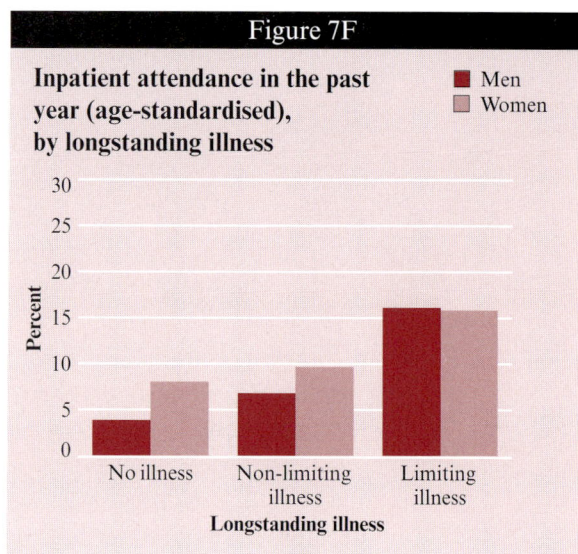

Figure 7F

Inpatient attendance in the past year (age-standardised), by longstanding illness
■ Men ▢ Women

7.3.5 Inpatient stays

Three measures summarising the intensity of hospital use per inpatient were derived, based on the number of informants admitted as inpatients (p), the total number of inpatient stays (s), and the total number of nights spent in hospital in the last year (n). The three derived measures were mean number of stays per inpatient (frequency of stay), mean nights per stay (length of stay per admission) and mean nights per inpatient per year (annual duration of stay).

	Men	Women
Per 100 men/women		
Number of inpatients (p)	8.1	10.7
Number of inpatient stays (s)	11.2	14.2
Number of nights as inpatient(n)	79.6	90.5
Derivations		
Mean stays per inpatient (s/p) (frequency of stay)	1.38	1.33
Mean nights per stay (n/s) (length of stay per admission)	7.12	6.37
Mean nights per inpatient per year (n/p) (annual duration of stay)	9.81	8.47

Age and sex variation in inpatient usage has been examined for all three of the dimensions of inpatient attendance derived above. For the purpose of presenting age-standardised comparisons of socio-economic and health status groups, the last summary measure – mean nights per inpatient per year – has been selected as being probably the best indicator of the severity of illness.

Until the age of 44, almost all men who were admitted as inpatients had only one stay over the year. From age 55 onwards, however, almost a quarter of men admitted to hospital had more than one inpatient stay. The increase in the proportion of men attending hospital as inpatients from age 55 onwards (noted in Section 7.3.4), coupled with increasing frequency of attendance, resulted in the mean number of stays per 100 men rising from around 7 in the 16-54 age group to 15 in the 55-64 age group and 34 per 100 among those aged 75 and over.

Among women aged 16-44, both inpatient attendance and frequency of stay were higher than for men in the age group 16-44. However, from 45 onwards, the proportion admitted and mean number of stays were broadly similar in both sexes.

Table 7.14

Not only the number of inpatient stays but also their average duration increased with age. On average, the median length of stay in hospital per admission was 4 nights for both men and women. However, more than 2 out of 5 stays for persons aged 75 and over lasted over a week.

Among those aged 16-34, although the *median* length of stay for women (3 nights) was higher than for men (2 nights), the *mean* length of stay was almost a night longer for men than for women (5.8 vs. 4.7). This was because in this age group, the distribution of nights spent per hospital stay is more skewed to the right for men, with a higher percentage of stays lasting 8 nights or more.   **Table 7.15**

On average, men inpatients spent 10 nights per year in hospital and women 9 nights. But because prevalence was higher among women, on a per capita basis women (90 nights per 100 women) spent more nights in hospital than men (80 nights per 100 men). And since women form a larger proportion of the population than men, they accounted for appreciably over half of all hospital nights (table not shown).

This per capita figure (mean nights per 100 persons per year) is a product of the proportion attending hospital as inpatients and the frequency and duration of admission. Since all of these increased with age, the mean per capita figure increased even faster with age than any of the separate components. For men, it increased more than six-fold, from 42 per 100 in the youngest age group to 273 per 100 in the oldest, while proportion admitted to hospital increased only four-fold (5% to 20%). For women the increase in the per capita figure was less steep than for men, rising from 50 in the youngest group to 226 in the oldest.   **Table 7.16**

Mean nights per inpatient varied between morbidity groups. On average, inpatients with good self-assessed health and with no chronic illness spent 6 nights in hospital per year. Those with poor self-assessed health or with a limiting illness, on the other hand, spent on average 12 to 14 nights per year as inpatients. This difference further accentuates the already significant variation in inpatient prevalence illustrated in Figures 7E and 7F.

Table 7.17, Figures 7E, 7F

There was little difference in mean nights per inpatient per year by social class, equivalised household income and Health Authority area type (tables not shown).

7.4 Prescribed medication

7.4.1 Introduction

Following the practice of previous Health Surveys, information on prescribed medicines was collected as part of the nurse visit, and the name of each type of prescribed medication was recorded. Medicines were allocated a 6-digit code corresponding to the British National Formulary (BNF)[3] listing, by the nurse. Any medicines that nurses were unable to code were checked by office coding staff. As the proportion of individuals taking a specific type of medication was fairly small, for analysis purposes medicines have been collapsed into 13 pharmacological groups, corresponding to BNF chapters. Contraceptives were not included as prescribed medicines.

7.4.2 Proportions taking prescribed medicines

Overall, about two in five men (39%) and half of all women (49%) were taking prescribed medicines. From age 45, use of prescribed medicines rose steeply with age. By age 75, more than 4 in 5 of all informants (81% men, 86% women) were on prescribed medication.

Under age 65, considerably more women than men were using prescribed medicines. Around age 55, the increase in the proportion of men taking prescribed medicines was particularly marked and from age 65 the proportion on medication was similar for men and women.

Of those taking prescribed medicines, more than 60% of all informants were taking more than one medicine. The average number of medicines per taker was 2.6 for both men and women. This average rose with age: steadily for men (from 1.5 in the 16-24 age group to 3.3 for those aged 75 and over); while for women the average stayed constant at about 2.0 until age 55, rising steadily thereafter to 3.5 among those aged 75 and over. By age 75, about a third of all informants (and 2 in 5 of those on medication) were taking 4 or more prescribed medicines.   **Table 7.18, Figure 7G**

The proportion (age-standardised) taking prescribed medicine more than doubled between those assessing their health as good compared with those in bad or very bad health for men (29% vs. 77%) and women (41% vs. 87%). An increase of a similar magnitude is seen for those with limiting longstanding illness, with the proportions for men rising from 1 in 5 for

Figure 7G

Proportion taking prescribed medication, by age

Legend: 4 drugs, 3 drugs, 2 drugs, 1 drug

Men

Women

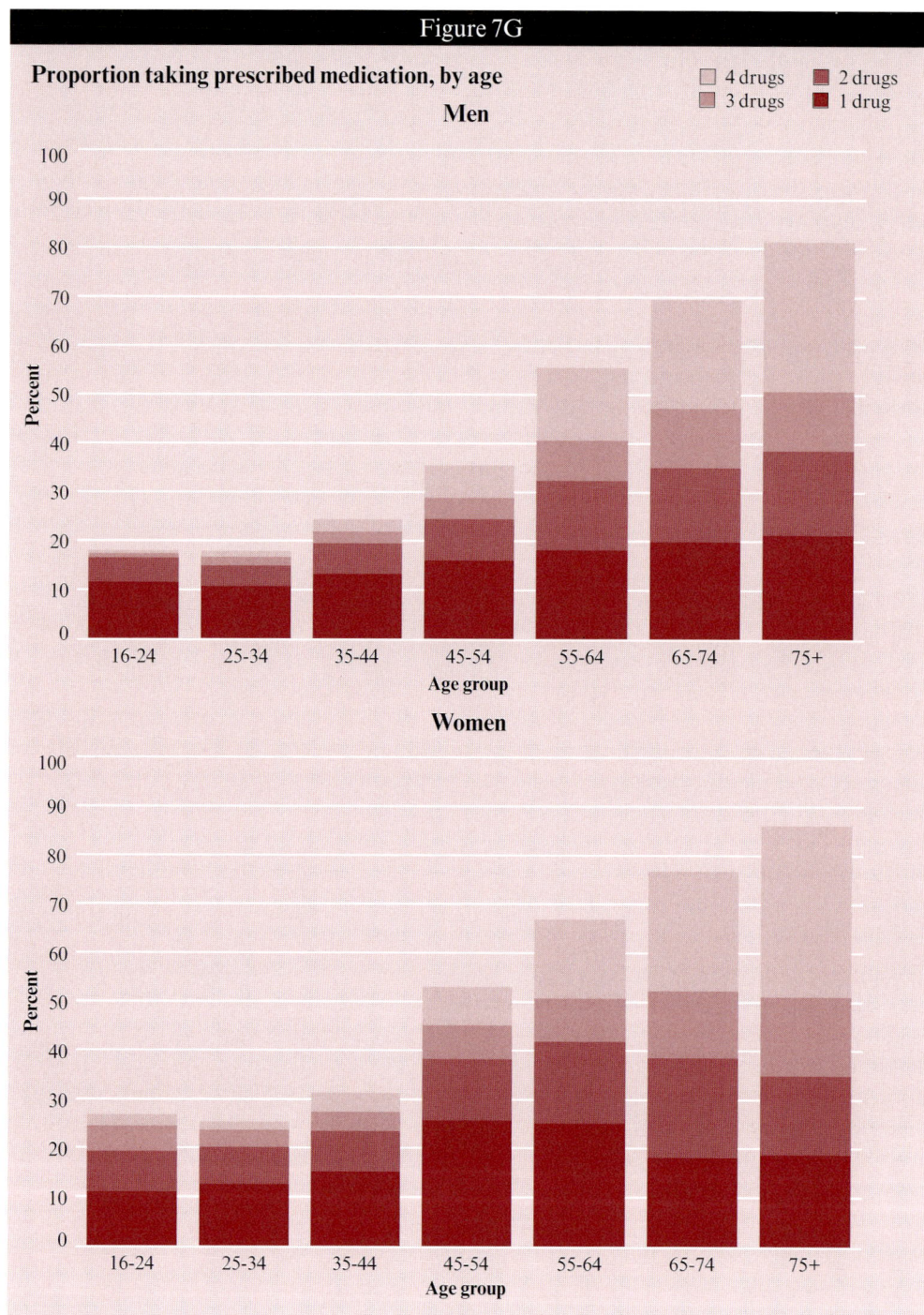

those with no illness to 3 in 5 for those with a limiting illness. The corresponding increase for women in the proportions taking medicines was from 1 in 3 for those with no illness to over 2 in 3 of those with a limiting longstanding illness. The mean number of drugs taken by those on medication also rose significantly with severity of self-rated morbidity for both men and women.   **Table 7.19**

The age-standardised proportion taking medicine increased with declining (equivalised) household income: from 32% of men and 43% of women in the highest income quintile to 43% of men and 52% of women in the lowest income quintile. The average number of drugs taken by those on medication rose from about 2.0 in the highest income quintile in both sexes to 3.0 in the lowest quintile for men, 3.7 for women.   **Table 7.20**

There was no marked difference in the age-standardised proportion taking medicine by social class or Health Authority area types (tables not shown).

7.4.3 Category of prescribed medicine taken

Table 7.21 shows type of medicine taken (based on all informants) by 13 broad pharmacological groups. The most frequently taken types of medicine for both men and women were those for cardiovascular disease and for the central nervous system.

As shown above, women were more likely than men to be taking prescribed medication. Nevertheless, for most drug groups there was little difference in the proportions of men and women using them. A higher proportion of women than men were using medicines prescribed for the endocrine system. This could be due to women receiving hormone replacement therapy (HRT); the age group with the highest proportion of women taking this group of medicines (28%) was aged 45-64. Women, particularly older women, were also more likely than men to be taking medicines for the central nervous system.

For both men and women the proportions taking cardiovascular, gastrointestinal and central nervous system drugs showed the most marked increases with age. For example, about 2% of men and women in the 16-44 age group had been prescribed cardiovascular drugs, compared with over half of those aged 75 and over. The proportion using respiratory drugs displays a U-shaped curve with age for both sexes, being highest among the youngest (16-24) and oldest age groups. **Table 7.21**

7.4.4 Trends in type of medication 1994-1998

Overall there has been a slight upward trend since 1994 in the proportions of men and women who took any prescribed medication: 33% of men and 44% of women did so in 1994 compared with 39% and 49%, respectively, in 1998. There was a change in coding practice in the Health Survey series in 1995[4] which accounts for the increase in the proportions taking cardiovascular and musculoskeletal drugs between 1994 and 1995. From 1995 onwards the proportion of adults taking medicines for the central nervous system increased slightly, by 3% for men and 2% for women. For all other categories of medicines, there was no significant change in the proportion on each type of medication over the period 1995 to 1998. **Table 7.22**

7.5 Contraceptive pill use

Women aged 16 and over were asked, on the self-completion questionnaire, whether they were taking the contraceptive pill or having a contraceptive injection or implant. Those who were taking oral contraceptives or having a contraceptive injection or implant were asked to give the brand name of the contraceptive, and to indicate whether it was an injection, mini pill, combined pill or implant (Norplant). Pill brands were allocated a 6-digit BNF code. The data discussed in the following two paragraphs are based on women aged 16-54, for consistency with earlier Health Surveys, and are derived from pill brand names.

More than a quarter (27%) of women aged 16-54 were using contraceptive pills, injections or implants. Over half of women aged 16-24 (52%) were using contraceptive pills, injections or implants. Contraceptive pill use was lowest among those aged 45-54 (3%).

The most common type of contraceptive drug used was the combined pill, which was used by 22% of all women aged 16-54. Only 5% were using the mini pill or contraceptive injections and implants. (It is not possible to separate out use of the mini pill from contraceptive injections and implants when using data derived from pill brand names, as both are progestogen-only contraceptives and so were allocated the same 6-digit BNF code.) **Table 7.23**

7.6 Hormone replacement therapy use

7.6.1 Introduction

Women aged 16 and over were asked, on a self-completion questionnaire, whether they were currently, or had been, on hormone replacement therapy (HRT). All HRT users were asked at what age they had started on HRT and past users were asked what age they stopped using HRT. All women were also asked whether they were menstruating or whether their periods had stopped. Women whose periods had stopped were then asked; *'Did your periods stop as a result of an operation?'* It has been assumed in the analysis that given the sequence of questions, most informants would have understood 'an operation' to mean a hysterectomy and women who answered in the affirmative have therefore been categorised as having had a surgical menopause. Of those who were current or past users ('ever users') of HRT, 36% had had a hysterectomy, 39% were post-menopausal, and a substantial proportion (25%) reported to be still menstruating (pre-menopausal).

With the exception of Table 7.24, which shows the distribution of HRT usage for women aged 16 and over, all the other tables in this section only include women aged 35 to 74. Young (16-34) and older (75 and over) women have been excluded because the number who had ever used HRT in these age groups was small (3%).

7.6.2 HRT use by age

Overall, 9% of women aged 16 and over were on HRT when interviewed and 6% had been users in the past. However, these figures were much higher for older women. The proportion currently using HRT increased sharply to 27% at age 45-54, and 22% at age 55-64, falling to 5% at 65-74 and 1% at 75 and over. The proportion who had used HRT at all (currently or in the past) in these four age groups was respectively 38%, 41%, 13% and 3%. In the absence of any trend in HRT uptake over time, these figures would be expected to increase cumulatively, and the fact that they do not indicates the presence of a cohort effect with progressively higher rates of usage in younger cohorts.   **Table 7.24**

The age pattern is shown graphically in Figure 7H. The overall height of the shaded area in the figure indicates, by year of age, the proportion who have ever used HRT. Within the shaded area, the lower part indicates current users, while the upper part indicates those who have used in the past but not currently. In examining these patterns it is necessary to bear in

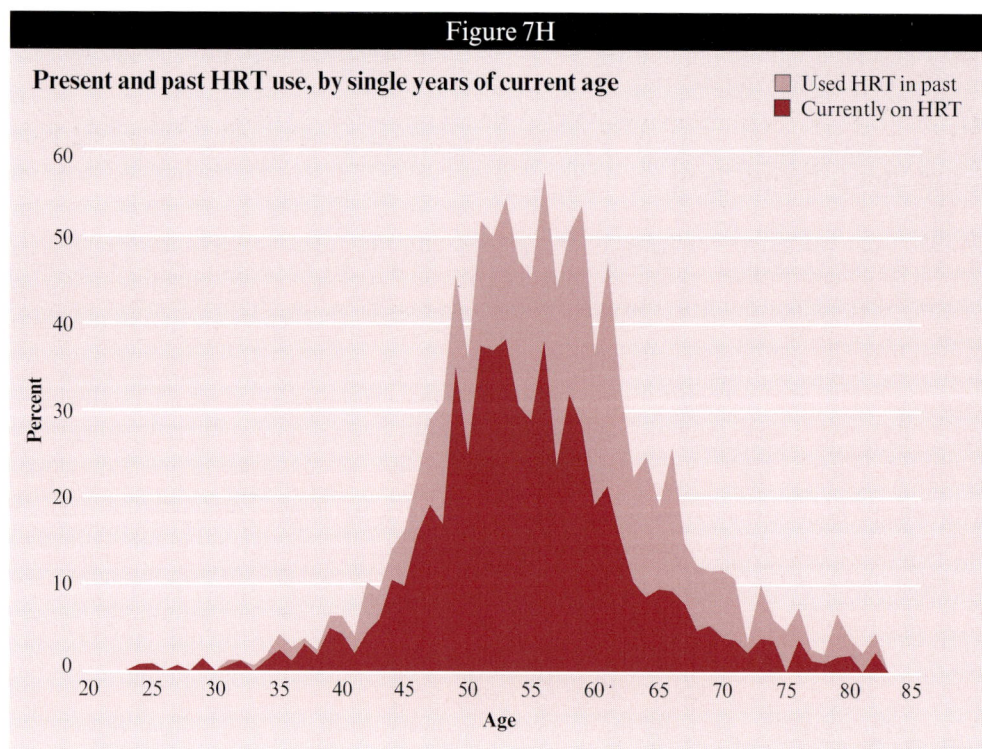

Figure 7H

Present and past HRT use, by single years of current age

mind that HRT use has changed over time, so that the results for different age groups are not comparable: for example, results for those aged over 55 cannot be used to predict future use by those currently younger.   **Figure 7H**

7.6.3 Age started HRT and mean duration of use

Most users (62%) in the sample started on HRT between the age of 45 to 54 years, although a quarter (26%) started at a younger age. The median age at which women started was almost identical for current and past users (48 and 49 years respectively). On average women spent 5 years on the therapy with women starting younger spending significantly more years on HRT.

**Those who have ever used HRT:
age started HRT and mean duration of use**

Age started HRT	% of ever users	Mean years on HRT (SE)
16-34	4	9.4 (1.2)
35-44	22	6.5 (0.5)
45-54	62	4.5 (0.2)
55-64	12	3.6 (0.3)
65 and over	1	1.6 (0.5)
Total	100	4.9 (0.2)

Looking at duration of use by current age for women in the sample who were currently on HRT or had been in the past, 16% had used HRT for under a year and 58% for under five years. Long term usage, defined as being on HRT for 10 years or more, rose steadily with advancing age. As a result, mean duration increased from 3 years in the 35-44 age group to 8 years in the 65-74 age range.   **Table 7.25**

7.6.4   HRT use by health status, social class, income and Health Authority area type

The age-standardised proportion of women who had ever used HRT was significantly higher for women with self-assessed bad health (29%) and limiting long term illness (29%) than for those in good health (23%) or with no illness (22%).   **Table 7.26**

There was an inverse relationship in HRT use by social class and equivalised household income. A significantly higher (age-standardised) proportion of women living in households in Social Class I reported having used HRT (31%) than of women in households in Social Class V (20%). Similarly, women resident in households in the highest household income quintile were more likely to have used HRT (33%) than of women in the lowest income quintile (20%).   **Tables 7.27, 7.28, Figures 7I, 7J**

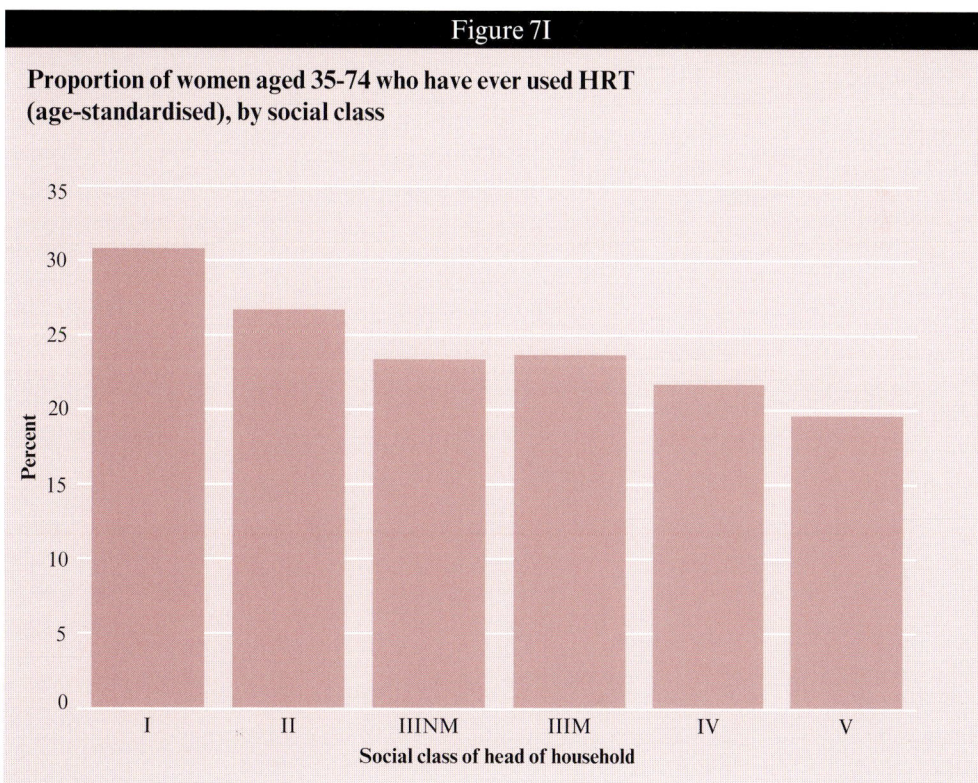

Figure 7I

Proportion of women aged 35-74 who have ever used HRT (age-standardised), by social class

Women living in the Health Authority area type classified as 'Prosperous' were more likely than others to be using, or to have used, HRT.   **Table 7.29**

Figure 7J

Proportion of women aged 35-74 who have ever used HRT (age-standardised), by household income

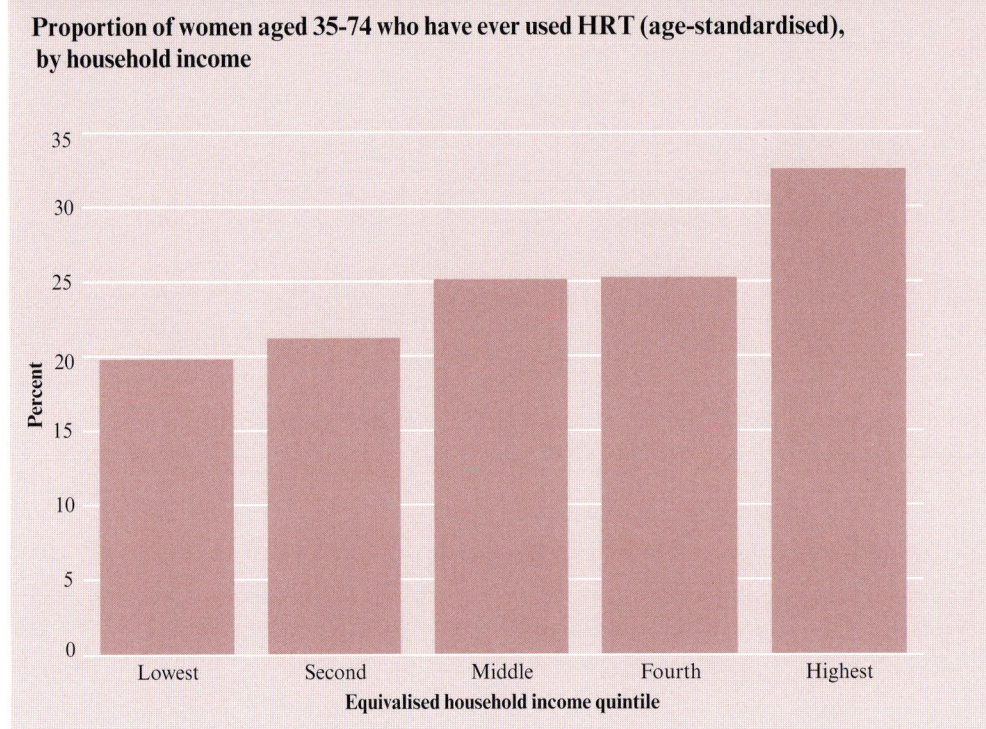

Percent (y-axis, 0 to 35)

Equivalised household income quintile (x-axis): Lowest, Second, Middle, Fourth, Highest

References and notes

1 *Living in Britain: results from the 1996 General Household Survey*. The Stationery Office, London, 1997.

2 McCormick A, Fleming D, Charlton J. *Morbidity Statistics from General Practice. Fourth National Study 1991-1992*. HMSO, London, 1995.

3 *British National Formulary*. British Medical Association and Royal Pharmaceutical Society of Great Britain, London, September 1997.

4 Prior G and Di Salvo P. *General health, psychosocial well-being and prescribed medicines*, in Prescott-Clarke P and Primatesta P (eds.) *Health Survey for England 1995. Volume 1: Findings*. The Stationery Office, London, 1997.

Tables

Table 7.1

(NHS) GP consultations in the two weeks before interview and mean number of consultations per year, by age and sex

Aged 16 and over   *1998*

Consulting GP on own behalf	Age							Total
	16-24	25-34	35-44	45-54	55-64	65-74	75 +	
	%	%	%	%	%	%	%	%
Men								
Consulted a GP in past two weeks	9	9	10	12	17	20	21	13
1 consultation	8	8	8	11	14	17	17	11
2 consultations	1	0	2	1	3	3	4	2
3 or more consultations	0	0	0	0	0	1	0	0
Did not consult a GP in past two weeks	91	91	90	88	83	80	79	87
Estimated mean number of consultations per year[a]	3	3	3	4	5	6	7	4
Standard error of the mean	0.33	0.24	0.28	0.28	0.42	0.47	0.61	0.13
Women								
Consulted a GP in past two weeks	18	19	15	18	20	20	21	18
1 consultation	16	17	12	14	17	17	17	15
2 consultations	2	2	2	3	2	3	3	2
3 or more consultations	0	1	0	1	1	1	1	1
Did not consult a GP in past two weeks	82	81	85	82	80	80	79	82
Estimated mean number of consultations per year[a]	5	6	5	6	6	7	7	6
Standard error of the mean	0.41	0.33	0.31	0.34	0.41	0.49	0.53	0.15
Bases								
Men	*874*	*1336*	*1305*	*1287*	*987*	*837*	*562*	*7188*
Women	*1006*	*1630*	*1572*	*1483*	*1148*	*967*	*907*	*8713*

[a] Annualised by multiplying mean rate for all informants in the past two weeks by 26. Based on total sample, not on those consulting.

Table 7.2

Site of (NHS) GP consultation in past two weeks, by age and sex

Aged 16 and over who consulted an (NHS) GP in the past two weeks   *1998*

Site of GP consultation[a]	Age							Total
	16-24	25-34	35-44	45-54	55-64	65-74	75 +	
Men								
At home	1	2	3	1	5	5	16	5
By telephone	9	6	10	7	7	7	4	7
Surgery, health centre or elsewhere	91	94	90	92	91	91	81	90
Women								
At home	2	2	3	4	5	8	26	6
By telephone	8	9	9	6	7	7	9	8
Surgery, health centre or elsewhere	91	91	92	94	90	87	70	89
Bases								
Men	*82*	*121*	*125*	*156*	*170*	*171*	*117*	*942*
Women	*182*	*312*	*231*	*263*	*229*	*198*	*191*	*1606*

[a] Percentages add up to more than 100 because some people consulted at more than one site during the reference period.

Table 7.3

Percentage of people consulting a (NHS) GP and mean number of consultations per year (observed and age-standardised), by reported health status and sex

Aged 16 and over   *1998*

Consulting GP on own behalf	Self-assessed general health			Longstanding illness		
	Very good or good	Fair	Bad or very bad	No illness	Non-limiting illness	Limiting illness
Men						
% consulting in past two weeks						
Observed	9	21	39	8	13	25
Standardised	9	19	38	8	13	22
Estimated mean number of consultations per year[a]						
Observed	3	7	13	2	4	8
Standard error	0.12	0.40	0.84	0.13	0.29	0.37
Standardised	3	6	12	2	4	7
Standard error	0.12	0.39	0.82	0.13	0.29	0.36
Women						
% consulting in past two weeks						
Observed	14	27	41	13	19	29
Standardised	14	27	41	13	19	30
Estimated mean number of consultations per year[a]						
Observed	4	9	15	4	6	10
Standard error	0.14	0.38	0.90	0.16	0.32	0.37
Standardised	4	9	15	4	6	10
Standard error	0.14	0.38	0.88	0.16	0.32	0.36
Bases						
Men	*5366*	*1349*	*472*	*4036*	*1332*	*1817*
Women	*6385*	*1732*	*596*	*4895*	*1480*	*2337*

[a] Annualised by multiplying mean rate for all informants in the past two weeks by 26. Based on total sample, not on those consulting.

Table 7.4

Percentage of people consulting a (NHS) GP and mean number of consultations per year (observed and age-standardised), by social class of head of household and sex

Aged 16 and over   *1998*

Consulting GP on own behalf	Social class of head of household						Social class of head of household					
	I	II	IIINM	IIIM	IV	V	I	II	IIINM	IIIM	IV	V
	%	%	%	%	%	%	%	%	%	%	%	%
	Men						**Women**					
% consulting in past two weeks												
Observed	11	11	12	15	16	16	15	16	16	20	21	23
Standardised	11	11	12	14	15	16	15	16	16	20	21	22
Estimated mean number of consultations per year[a]												
Observed	3	3	4	5	5	5	4	5	5	6	7	7
Standard error	0.47	0.21	0.41	0.26	0.36	0.69	0.47	0.26	0.35	0.30	0.38	0.66
Standardised	3	3	4	4	5	5	4	5	5	6	7	7
Standard error	0.47	0.21	0.40	0.26	0.35	0.70	0.46	0.26	0.35	0.31	0.38	0.64
Bases	*503*	*2178*	*718*	*2265*	*1041*	*335*	*515*	*2499*	*1346*	*2209*	*1374*	*498*

[a] Annualised by multiplying mean rate for all informants in the past two weeks by 26. Based on total sample, not on those consulting.

Table 7.5

Percentage of people consulting a (NHS) GP and mean number of consultations per year (observed and age-standardised), by equivalised household income and sex

Aged 16 and over   *1998*

Consulting GP on own behalf	Equivalised annual household income quintile				
	Up to £7,186	Over £7,186 to £10,834	Over £10,834 to £17,890	Over £17,890 to £27,705	Over £27,705
	%	%	%	%	%
Men					
% consulting in past two weeks					
Observed	18	19	13	10	9
Standardised	18	17	12	10	9
Estimated mean number of consultations per year[a]					
Observed	6	6	4	3	3
Standard error	0.41	0.42	0.28	0.24	0.26
Standardised	6	5	4	3	3
Standard error	0.41	0.39	0.28	0.25	0.28
Women					
% consulting in past two weeks					
Observed	21	21	19	17	15
Standardised	21	20	19	17	15
Estimated mean number of consultations per year[a]					
Observed	7	7	6	5	4
Standard error	0.39	0.38	0.36	0.32	0.31
Standardised	7	6	6	5	5
Standard error	0.39	0.37	0.38	0.32	0.35
Bases					
Men	*1002*	*1004*	*1440*	*1394*	*1362*
Women	*1413*	*1489*	*1653*	*1493*	*1385*

[a] Annualised by multiplying mean rate for all informants in the past two weeks by 26. Based on total sample, not on those consulting.

Table 7.6

Percentage of people consulting a (NHS) GP and mean number of consultations per year (observed and age-standardised), by Health Authority area type and sex

Aged 16 and over						1998
Consulting GP on own behalf	**Health Authority area type**					
	Inner London	Mining & Industrial	Urban	Mature	Prosperous	Rural
	%	%	%	%	%	%
Men						
% consulting in past two weeks						
Observed	13	15	16	10	12	12
Standardised	14	15	16	10	12	12
Estimated mean number of consultations per year[a]						
Observed	4	5	5	3	4	4
Standard error	0.76	0.36	0.38	0.34	0.24	0.25
Standardised	5	5	5	3	4	4
Standard error	0.80	0.36	0.38	0.33	0.23	0.24
Women						
% consulting in past two weeks						
Observed	22	18	20	17	18	18
Standardised	23	18	20	17	19	18
Estimated mean number of consultations per year[a]						
Observed	7	6	6	5	6	6
Standard error	0.90	0.38	0.39	0.36	0.27	0.30
Standardised	8	6	6	5	6	6
Standard error	0.93	0.38	0.39	0.36	0.27	0.30
Bases						
Men	240	1106	1053	1100	1946	1743
Women	309	1295	1339	1309	2388	2073

[a] Annualised by multiplying mean rate for all informants in the past two weeks by 26. Based on total sample, not on those consulting.

Table 7.7

Percentage of people consulting a (NHS) GP and mean number of consultations per year (observed and age-standardised), by region and sex

Aged 16 and over   *1998*

Consulting GP on own behalf	Region							
	Northern & Yorkshire	North West	Trent	West Midlands	Anglia & Oxford	North Thames	South Thames	South & West
	%	%	%	%	%	%	%	%
Men								
% consulting in past two weeks								
Observed	14	14	15	16	12	12	10	12
Standardised	14	14	14	15	12	12	10	12
Estimated mean number of consultations per year[a]								
Observed	5	4	5	5	4	4	3	4
Standard error	0.40	0.32	0.42	0.43	0.38	0.36	0.39	0.32
Standardised	4	4	4	5	4	4	3	3
Standard error	0.39	0.32	0.41	0.42	0.37	0.35	0.39	0.31
Women								
% consulting in past two weeks								
Observed	19	20	19	17	17	18	19	18
Standardised	19	20	19	17	17	18	19	18
Estimated mean number of consultations per year[a]								
Observed	6	6	6	6	5	6	6	5
Standard error	0.41	0.40	0.43	0.47	0.43	0.42	0.39	0.36
Standardised	6	6	6	6	5	6	6	5
Standard error	0.40	0.41	0.43	0.48	0.44	0.42	0.40	0.36
Bases								
Men	*1030*	*979*	*796*	*746*	*812*	*915*	*889*	*1021*
Women	*1249*	*1135*	*941*	*913*	*961*	*1118*	*1181*	*1215*

[a] Annualised by multiplying mean rate for all informants in the past two weeks by 26. Based on total sample, not on those consulting.

Table 7.8

Hospital attendance in the past year as an outpatient, day patient or inpatient, by age and sex

Aged 16 and over   *1998*

Outpatient/Day patient/ Inpatient	Age							Total
	16-24	25-34	35-44	45-54	55-64	65-74	75 +	
	%	%	%	%	%	%	%	%
Men								
Outpatient	31	30	28	28	36	41	47	33
Day patient	4	4	5	6	8	7	7	6
Inpatient	5	5	5	6	11	13	20	8
Women								
Outpatient	26	25	25	33	38	38	41	32
Day patient	4	7	6	7	6	7	7	6
Inpatient	9	14	8	7	9	13	16	11
Bases								
Men	*874*	*1337*	*1305*	*1287*	*987*	*837*	*562*	*7189*
Women	*1006*	*1630*	*1572*	*1482*	*1148*	*966*	*906*	*8710*

Table 7.9

Proportion attending hospital as outpatients, day patients or inpatients in the past year (observed and age-standardised), by reported health status and sex

Aged 16 and over   *1998*

Outpatient/Day patient/ Inpatient	Self-assessed general health			Longstanding illness		
	Very good or good	Fair	Bad or very bad	No illness	Non-limiting illness	Limiting illness
	%	%	%	%	%	%
Men observed						
Outpatient	27	47	65	23	36	53
Day patient	4	8	15	4	6	10
Inpatient	5	14	28	4	7	19
Men standardised						
Outpatient	27	45	59	23	36	49
Day patient	4	7	13	4	6	9
Inpatient	5	12	25	4	7	16
Women observed						
Outpatient	25	45	66	21	36	50
Day patient	5	9	13	4	7	10
Inpatient	8	15	29	8	9	17
Women standardised						
Outpatient	26	44	67	22	36	50
Day patient	5	9	14	4	7	10
Inpatient	8	15	28	8	10	16
Bases [a]						
Men	*5366*	*1350*	*472*	*4037*	*1332*	*1817*
Women	*6384*	*1730*	*596*	*4893*	*1479*	*2337*

[a] Bases vary slightly: those shown are for outpatient attendance.

Table 7.10

Proportion attending hospital as outpatients, day patients or inpatients in the past year (observed and age-standardised), by social class of head of household and sex

Aged 16 and over — *1998*

Outpatient/Day patient/ Inpatient	Social class of head of household							Social class of head of household					
	I	II	IIINM	IIIM	IV	V		I	II	IIINM	IIIM	IV	V
	%	%	%	%	%	%		%	%	%	%	%	%
	Men observed							**Women** observed					
Outpatient	32	30	35	34	34	35		30	30	32	31	33	35
Day patient	5	5	6	6	6	5		6	7	7	6	6	7
Inpatient	7	7	10	9	8	10		9	9	11	11	13	13
	Men standardised							**Women** standardised					
Outpatient	32	30	35	34	33	35		32	30	32	32	32	33
Day patient	5	5	6	6	6	5		5	7	7	6	6	8
Inpatient	6	6	9	8	8	9		11	9	10	11	13	12
Bases [a]	503	2178	718	2265	1042	335		515	2498	1345	2208	1374	498

[a] Bases vary slightly: those shown are for outpatient attendance.

Table 7.11

Proportion attending hospital as outpatients, day patients or inpatients in the past year (observed and age-standardised), by equivalised household income and sex

Aged 16 and over — *1998*

Outpatient/Day patient/ Inpatient	Equivalised annual household income quintile				
	Up to £7,186	Over £7,186 to £10,834	Over £10,834 to £17,890	Over £17,890 to £27,705	Over £27,705
	%	%	%	%	%
Men observed					
Outpatient	38	36	33	32	28
Day patient	8	6	5	5	5
Inpatient	11	11	8	6	6
Men standardised					
Outpatient	37	35	33	33	30
Day patient	7	6	5	5	5
Inpatient	10	8	8	6	7
Women observed					
Outpatient	31	36	31	29	29
Day patient	7	6	6	6	7
Inpatient	12	13	11	9	8
Women standardised					
Outpatient	31	34	32	31	33
Day patient	7	6	6	5	7
Inpatient	12	13	11	10	10
Bases [a]					
Men	1002	1004	1441	1394	1362
Women	1413	1489	1652	1493	1384

[a] Bases vary slightly: those shown are for outpatient attendance.

Table 7.12

Proportion attending hospital as outpatients, day patients or inpatients in the past year (observed and age-standardised), by Health Authority area type and sex

Aged 16 and over   *1998*

Outpatient/Day patient/ Inpatient	Health Authority area type					
	Inner London	Mining & Industrial	Urban	Mature	Prosperous	Rural
	%	%	%	%	%	%
Men observed						
Outpatient	34	36	33	36	31	32
Day patient	8	7	5	7	6	5
Inpatient	8	9	9	8	7	8
Men standardised						
Outpatient	36	36	32	35	31	31
Day patient	8	7	5	6	5	5
Inpatient	9	8	9	8	7	7
Women observed						
Outpatient	28	32	36	32	32	29
Day patient	7	7	6	8	6	6
Inpatient	11	10	11	9	10	12
Women standardised						
Outpatient	29	31	36	32	32	29
Day patient	7	7	6	8	6	6
Inpatient	12	10	11	9	10	12
Bases [a]						
Men	*240*	*1106*	*1053*	*1100*	*1946*	*1744*
Women	*308*	*1294*	*1339*	*1309*	*2388*	*2072*

[a] Bases vary slightly: those shown are for outpatient attendance.

Table 7.13

Proportion attending hospital as outpatients, day patients or inpatients in the past year (observed and age-standardised), by region and sex

Aged 16 and over								*1998*
Outpatient/Day patient/ Inpatient	**Region**							
	Northern & Yorkshire	North West	Trent	West Midlands	Anglia & Oxford	North Thames	South Thames	South & West
	%	%	%	%	%	%	%	%
Men observed								
Outpatient	33	34	36	30	30	35	34	31
Day patient	6	7	4	6	4	5	8	7
Inpatient	9	9	10	7	7	7	8	8
Men standardised								
Outpatient	33	34	35	29	30	34	34	31
Day patient	6	6	4	6	4	4	8	6
Inpatient	8	9	9	7	7	7	7	7
Women observed								
Outpatient	32	35	32	30	32	30	33	28
Day patient	6	8	5	6	6	6	7	7
Inpatient	11	12	12	11	11	10	9	10
Women standardised								
Outpatient	32	36	31	30	32	30	33	28
Day patient	6	8	5	7	6	6	7	6
Inpatient	11	12	12	11	12	10	10	10
Bases [a]								
Men	*1030*	*979*	*797*	*746*	*812*	*915*	*889*	*1021*
Women	*1249*	*1134*	*941*	*913*	*961*	*1117*	*1181*	*1214*

[a] Bases vary slightly: those shown are for outpatient attendance.

Table 7.14

Number of stays in hospital in the past year, by age and sex

Aged 16 and over

Inpatient stays	Age							1998 Total
	16-24	25-34	35-44	45-54	55-64	65-74	75 +	
	%	%	%	%	%	%	%	%
Men								
0	95	95	95	94	89	87	80	92
1	5	4	4	5	9	10	15	7
2	0	0	0	1	2	2	3	1
3 or more	0	0	0	0	1	1	2	1
Mean number of stays per 100 persons	6	6	7	8	15	18	34	11
Standard error	1.06	0.78	1.18	0.94	1.59	1.88	5.39	0.63
Women								
0	91	86	92	93	91	87	84	89
1	8	11	7	6	7	10	13	9
2	0	1	1	1	1	2	3	1
3 or more	1	1	0	0	1	1	1	1
Mean number of stays per 100 persons	12	19	10	8	13	19	21	14
Standard error	1.47	1.53	1.06	0.91	1.53	2.12	1.75	0.55
Bases								
Men	*873*	*1337*	*1304*	*1286*	*987*	*836*	*561*	*7184*
Women	*1006*	*1630*	*1571*	*1482*	*1148*	*965*	*906*	*8708*

Table 7.15

Number of nights in hospital per inpatient stay, by age and sex

Inpatient stays by those aged 16 and over

Inpatient duration	Age							1998 Total
	16-24	25-34	35-44	45-54	55-64	65-74	75 +	
	%	%	%	%	%	%	%	%
Men								
% of inpatient stays that were								
1-3 nights	72	62	40	55	47	36	20	43
4-7 nights	15	24	41	22	33	32	38	31
8 or more nights	13	14	18	23	20	32	43	26
Median length of stay	2	2	4	3	4	5	7	4
Mean length of stay	6.8	5.1	8.0	6.8	6.0	8.2	9.6	7.5
Standard error	2.33	0.94	1.62	1.04	0.74	1.05	0.73	0.41
Women								
% of inpatient stays that were								
1-3 nights	64	59	48	50	39	44	27	47
4-7 nights	29	32	32	35	33	29	28	31
8 or more nights	7	9	21	15	28	27	45	21
Median length of stay	3	3	4	4	5	4	7	4
Mean length of stay	4.1	4.9	7.4	5.1	7.3	6.1	11.1	6.6
Standard error	0.57	0.49	1.12	0.75	0.70	0.52	0.91	0.29
Bases (number of stays)								
Men	*53*	*78*	*87*	*99*	*144*	*146*	*160*	*767*
Women	*122*	*299*	*164*	*124*	*144*	*175*	*185*	*1213*

Table 7.16

Mean nights per inpatient per year and mean nights per 100 persons per year, by age and sex

Aged 16 and over   *1998*

Inpatient duration	Age							Total
	16-24	25-34	35-44	45-54	55-64	65-74	75 +	
Men								
Mean nights per inpatient per year[a]	8.3	6.1	11.2	8.4	8.0	10.7	13.8	9.8
Standard error	3.42	1.20	2.61	1.46	1.09	1.48	1.68	0.66
Mean nights per 100 persons per year[b]	42	30	53	52	87	143	273	80
Standard error	18.1	6.9	14.0	10.7	14.2	23.4	40.5	6.2
Women								
Mean nights per inpatient per year[a]	5.4	6.5	8.5	6.3	9.8	8.5	14.0	8.5
Standard error	1.13	1.44	1.57	1.17	1.18	0.85	1.30	0.53
Mean nights per 100 persons per year[b]	50	90	71	42	91	112	226	90
Standard error	11.5	20.8	14.3	8.9	13.8	14.5	27.1	6.3
Bases								
Men								
Inpatients	*44*	*66*	*62*	*80*	*107*	*112*	*111*	*582*
All	*873*	*1337*	*1304*	*1286*	*987*	*836*	*561*	*7184*
Women								
Inpatients	*93*	*227*	*131*	*100*	*107*	*127*	*146*	*931*
All	*1006*	*1630*	*1571*	*1482*	*1148*	*965*	*906*	*8708*

[a] Base inpatients.

[b] Base all informants.

Table 7.17

Mean number of nights spent in hospital as an inpatient per year (observed and age-standardised), by reported health status and sex

Inpatients aged 16 and over   *1998*

Nights per inpatient per year	Self-assessed general health			Longstanding illness		
	Very good or good	Fair	Bad or very bad	No illness	Non-limiting illness	Limiting illness
Men						
Observed mean	6.6	11.5	13.9	5.9	5.8	12.7
Standard error	0.73	1.35	1.49	0.87	0.78	1.02
Standardised mean	6.3	11.1	11.9	5.7	5.3	13.8
Standard error	0.78	1.37	1.40	0.86	0.71	1.24
Women						
Observed mean	5.8	9.8	14.3	5.2	6.9	12.3
Standard error	0.39	1.44	1.49	0.41	1.08	1.10
Standardised mean	6.1	9.7	13.0	5.9	7.0	12.0
Standard error	0.40	1.62	1.61	0.43	1.12	1.39
Bases						
Men	*260*	*192*	*130*	*149*	*97*	*336*
Women	*509*	*251*	*171*	*403*	*136*	*392*

Table 7.18

Number of prescribed medicines taken, by age and sex

Aged 16 and over — *1998*

Number of medicines taken	Age							Total
	16-24	25-34	35-44	45-54	55-64	65-74	75 +	
	%	%	%	%	%	%	%	%
Men								
None	82	82	76	64	44	31	19	61
1	11	11	13	16	18	20	21	15
2	5	4	6	9	14	15	17	9
3	1	2	2	4	8	12	12	5
4 or more	1	1	2	7	15	22	31	9
Mean number of prescribed drugs								
Per person (base all)	0.3	0.3	0.5	0.8	1.6	2.1	2.7	1.0
Standard error	0.03	0.03	0.03	0.04	0.07	0.08	0.11	0.02
Per taker (base taking medication)	1.5	1.7	1.9	2.3	2.9	3.0	3.3	2.6
Standard error	0.09	0.09	0.09	0.09	0.10	0.10	0.12	0.04
Women								
None	73	75	69	47	33	23	14	51
1	11	13	15	26	25	18	19	18
2	8	8	8	13	17	20	16	12
3	5	4	4	7	9	14	16	7
4 or more	2	2	4	8	16	24	35	11
Mean number of prescribed drugs								
Per person (base all)	0.5	0.5	0.6	1.1	1.7	2.4	3.0	1.3
Standard error	0.04	0.03	0.03	0.04	0.07	0.08	0.09	0.02
Per taker (base taking medication)	2.0	1.8	2.0	2.1	2.6	3.2	3.5	2.6
Standard error	0.08	0.06	0.07	0.06	0.08	0.09	0.10	0.03
Bases								
Men								
All	698	1132	1129	1138	857	730	480	6164
Currently taking prescribed medication	125	202	275	404	476	507	390	2379
Women								
All	836	1392	1356	1297	999	818	722	7420
Currently taking prescribed medication	224	353	424	688	668	628	622	3607

Table 7.19

Proportion taking prescribed medication and mean number of drugs taken (observed and age-standardised), by reported health status and sex

Aged 16 and over   *1998*

Taking prescribed medication	Self-assessed general health			Longstanding illness		
	Very good or good	Fair	Bad or very bad	No illness	Non-limiting illness	Limiting illness
	%	%	%	%	%	%
Men						
% taking medication[a]						
Observed	28	61	90	17	57	71
Standardised	29	53	77	19	54	60
Mean number of drugs per taker[b]						
Observed	2.0	2.8	4.3	1.6	2.2	3.3
Standard error	0.04	0.07	0.15	0.05	0.05	0.07
Standardised	2.0	2.6	3.6	1.7	2.1	2.9
Standard error	0.04	0.08	0.16	0.04	0.05	0.07
Women						
% taking medication[a]						
Observed	38	73	92	28	68	79
Standardised	41	66	87	33	66	71
Mean number of drugs per taker[b]						
Observed	1.9	3.1	4.3	1.7	2.3	3.4
Standard error	0.03	0.07	0.12	0.03	0.05	0.06
Standardised	2.0	2.9	3.8	1.9	2.3	3.2
Standard error	0.03	0.07	0.12	0.04	0.05	0.06
Bases						
Men						
All	*4608*	*1147*	*408*	*3380*	*1187*	*1591*
Currently taking prescribed medication	*1309*	*704*	*366*	*569*	*682*	*1127*
Women						
All	*5450*	*1483*	*487*	*4131*	*1292*	*1995*
Currently taking prescribed medication	*2081*	*1080*	*446*	*1147*	*885*	*1573*

[a] Based on all informants.

[b] Based on those currently taking prescribed medication.

Table 7.20

Proportion taking prescribed medication and mean number of drugs taken (observed and age-standardised), by equivalised household income and sex

Aged 16 and over   *1998*

Taking prescribed medication	Equivalised annual household income quintile				
	Up to £7,186	Over £7,186 to £10,834	Over £10,834 to £17,890	Over £17,890 to £27,705	Over £27,705
	%	%	%	%	%
Men					
% taking medication[a]					
Observed	48	52	42	31	28
Standardised	43	41	39	33	33
Mean number of drugs per taker[b]					
Observed	3.1	2.9	2.6	2.2	1.9
Standard error	0.13	0.10	0.09	0.09	0.07
Standardised	3.0	2.7	2.6	2.3	2.1
Standard error	0.13	0.11	0.09	0.09	0.07
Women					
% taking medication[a]					
Observed	51	62	48	41	36
Standardised	52	52	50	47	43
Mean number of drugs per taker[b]					
Observed	2.7	3.1	2.4	2.2	2.0
Standard error	0.09	0.08	0.07	0.07	0.07
Standardised	2.7	2.9	2.5	2.5	2.4
Standard error	0.09	0.08	0.07	0.08	0.08
Bases					
Men					
All	*833*	*858*	*1269*	*1238*	*1207*
Currently taking prescribed medication	*400*	*444*	*528*	*382*	*334*
Women					
All	*1170*	*1263*	*1469*	*1328*	*1213*
Currently taking prescribed medication	*597*	*786*	*711*	*549*	*435*

[a] Based on all informants.

[b] Based on those currently taking prescribed medication.

Table 7.21

Category of prescribed medicine taken, by age and sex

Aged 16 and over   *1998*

Medicine category[a]	Age							Total
	16-24	25-34	35-44	45-54	55-64	65-74	75 +	
	%	%	%	%	%	%	%	%
Men								
Cardiovascular	-	1	3	13	30	45	56	17
Gastrointestinal	0	2	4	6	10	14	20	7
Respiratory	10	7	6	6	10	11	14	8
Central nervous system	3	5	8	11	17	20	30	12
Infections	3	2	2	3	2	2	2	2
Endocrine	0	1	1	3	6	9	9	4
Gynaecological/Urinary	-	-	0	1	1	3	3	1
Cytotoxic	-	0	0	0	1	1	1	1
Nutrition and blood	0	0	0	1	2	3	4	1
Musculoskeletal	0	2	4	7	11	14	16	7
Eye, ear, nose and throat	1	1	2	2	3	6	7	3
Skin	3	2	3	3	2	3	4	3
Other	-	-	0	0	-	-	-	0
No medicine taken	82	82	76	65	45	31	19	61
Women								
Cardiovascular	0	1	4	11	26	47	60	17
Gastrointestinal	2	2	3	6	10	18	25	8
Respiratory	12	6	9	8	11	11	11	9
Central nervous system	5	7	10	18	22	30	40	17
Infections	4	4	2	3	3	3	3	3
Endocrine	1	3	7	28	28	18	16	14
Gynaecological/Urinary	0	0	0	1	1	1	2	1
Cytotoxic	-	0	0	2	2	2	2	1
Nutrition and blood	2	3	2	2	3	6	9	3
Musculoskeletal	2	2	5	7	13	14	17	8
Eye, ear, nose and throat	2	1	2	2	3	4	7	3
Skin	6	3	2	1	2	4	4	3
Other	-	-	-	-	-	-	-	-
No medicine taken	73	75	69	47	33	23	14	51
Bases								
Men	*698*	*1132*	*1129*	*1138*	*857*	*730*	*480*	*6164*
Women	*836*	*1392*	*1356*	*1297*	*999*	*818*	*722*	*7420*

[a] Percentages may add to more than 100 as informants may have been taking more than one type of medicine.

Table 7.22

Category of prescribed medecine taken, by survey year and sex

Aged 16 and over   *1994-1998*

Medicine category[a]	Survey year						Survey year				
	1994	1995	1996	1997	1998		1994	1995	1996	1997	1998
	%	%	%	%	%		%	%	%	%	%
	Men						**Women**				
Cardiovascular	13	16	15	15	17		15	16	16	17	17
Gastrointestinal	6	6	6	6	7		6	7	7	7	8
Respiratory	7	8	10	9	8		7	10	11	10	9
Central nervous system	12	9	10	10	12		18	15	15	16	17
Infections	3	3	3	3	2		4	4	4	3	3
Endocrine	3	4	4	3	4		12	13	13	13	14
Gynaecological/Urinary	0	0	0	1	1		0	0	0	1	1
Infections	0	0	0	0	1		1	1	1	1	1
Nutrition and blood	1	1	1	1	1		3	3	3	3	3
Musculoskeletal	2	6	5	6	7		1	6	7	7	8
Eye, ear, nose and throat	2	3	3	3	3		2	3	3	3	3
Skin	3	3	3	3	3		3	3	4	4	3
Other	5	0	0	0	0		0		0	-	
None of these	64	62	63	63	61		56	53	52	52	51
Bases	*6285*	*6350*	*6600*	*3484*	*6164*		*7430*	*7497*	*7829*	*4116*	*7420*

[a] Percentages may add to more than 100 as informants may have been taking more than one type of medicine.

Table 7.23

Contraceptive pill use, derived from brand name, by age

Women aged 16-54   *1998*

Contraceptive use, derived from brand name	Age				Total
	16-24	25-34	35-44	45-54	
	%	%	%	%	%
Uses contraceptives	52	41	17	3	27
Mini-pill, injection or implant	6	6	6	3	5
Combined pill	46	35	11	1	22
Don't know contraceptive type	1	1	0	0	0
Contraceptives not used	47	58	83	96	72
Bases					
Women	*1006*	*1630*	*1573*	*1484*	*5693*

Table 7.24

Proportion of women on hormone replacement therapy (HRT), by age

Women aged 16 and over   *1998*

HRT use	Age							Total
	16-24	25-34	35-44	45-54	55-64	65-74	75 +	
	%	%	%	%	%	%	%	%
Currently on HRT	0	1	4	27	22	5	1	9
Had surgery[a]	-	0	2	10	8	2	1	4
Did not have surgery[b]	0	0	2	16	14	3	0	6
Used HRT in the past	-	0	2	12	19	7	2	6
Had surgery[a]	-	-	1	3	5	3	1	2
Did not have surgery[b]	-	0	2	9	13	4	1	4
Ever used HRT	0	1	6	38	41	13	3	15
Bases								
Women	*718*	*1563*	*1517*	*1418*	*1084*	*906*	*789*	*7995*

[a] Periods stopped due to operation (surgical menopause).

[b] Includes women who were menstruating as well as those whose periods had stopped.

Table 7.25

Duration of HRT use, by age

Women aged 35-74 ever used HRT   *1998*

Years on HRT	Age				Total
	35-44	45-54	55-64	65-74	
	%	%	%	%	%
<1 year	23	18	13	14	16
1 to <2 years	30	16	9	8	14
2 to <5 years	24	33	24	21	28
5 to <10 years	17	26	36	23	29
10 years or more	6	8	18	34	14
Mean duration (years)	3.0	3.9	5.8	8.0	4.9
Standard error	0.53	0.21	0.28	0.75	0.17
Bases					
Women	*90*	*547*	*439*	*113*	*1189*

Table 7.26

HRT usage (observed and age-standardised), by reported health status

Women aged 35-74   *1998*

Ever used HRT	Self-assessed general health			Longstanding illness		
	Very good or good	Fair	Bad or very bad	No illness	Non-limiting illness	Limiting illness
	%	%	%	%	%	%
Ever used HRT						
Observed	23	29	29	22	25	29
Standardised	23	29	29	22	24	29
Bases						
Women	*3567*	*1003*	*374*	*2599*	*923*	*1419*

Table 7.27

**HRT usage (observed and age-standardised),
by social class of head of household**

Women aged 35-74   *1998*

Ever used HRT	Social class of head of household					
	I	II	IIINM	IIIM	IV	V
	%	%	%	%	%	%
Ever used HRT						
Observed	31	27	22	24	22	21
Standardised	31	27	24	24	22	20
Bases						
Women	*315*	*1559*	*708*	*1304*	*699*	*272*

Table 7.28

HRT usage (observed and age-standardised), by equivalised household income

Women aged 35-74   *1998*

Ever used HRT	Equivalised annual household income quintile				
	Up to £7,186	Over £7,186 to £10,834	Over £10,834 to £17,890	Over £17,890 to £27,705	Over £27,705
	%	%	%	%	%
Ever used HRT					
Observed	18	20	25	26	30
Standardised	20	21	25	25	33
Bases					
Women	*706*	*781*	*1007*	*912*	*831*

Table 7.29

HRT usage (observed and age-standardised), by Health Authority area type

Women aged 35-74   *1998*

Ever used HRT	Health Authority area type					
	Inner London	Mining & Industrial	Urban	Mature	Prosperous	Rural
	%	%	%	%	%	%
Ever used HRT						
Observed	23	23	24	24	27	24
Standardised	25	23	23	23	26	24
Bases						
Women	*145*	*747*	*711*	*727*	*1410*	*1204*

Table 7.30

HRT usage (observed and age-standardised), by region

Women aged 35-74   *1998*

Ever used HRT	Region							
	Northern & Yorkshire	North West	Trent	West Midlands	Anglia & Oxford	North Thames	South Thames	South & West
	%	%	%	%	%	%	%	%
Ever used HRT								
Observed	23	24	22	24	25	24	28	26
Standardised	23	23	22	25	25	24	28	26
Bases								
Women	*721*	*617*	*531*	*527*	*555*	*638*	*659*	*696*

Health Survey for England:
Cardiovascular Disease '98

Volume 2: Methodology & Documentation

A survey carried out on behalf of The Department of Health

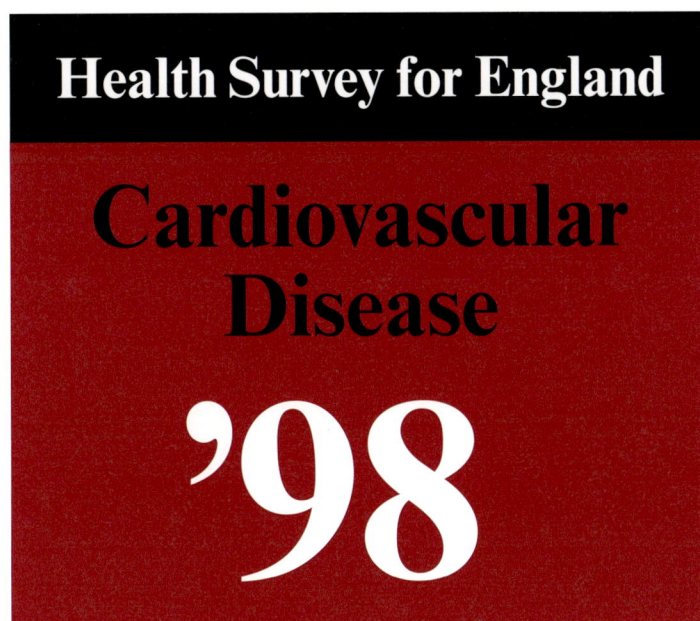

Health Survey for England

Cardiovascular Disease

'98

Volume 2: Methodology & Documentation

Edited by
Bob Erens
Paola Primatesta

Principal Authors
Madhavi Bajekal, Richard Boreham
Bob Erens, Emanuela Falaschetti
Vasant Hirani, Paola Primatesta
Gillian Prior, Clare Tait

Joint Health Surveys Unit
National Centre for Social Research
Department of Epidemiology and Public Health
at the Royal Free and University College Medical School

LONDON: THE STATIONERY OFFICE

Published with permission of the Department of Health
on behalf of the Controller of Her Majesty's Stationery Office

ISBN 0 11 322 307 2

Designed by Davenport Associates
Printed in the United Kingdom for The Stationery Office
J99580 C8 12/99 9385 11749

Contents

Volume II: Methodology and documentation

Survey methodology and response

8

*Richard Boreham, Marion Brookes, Bob Erens,
Johanna Laiho, Paola Primatesta and Gillian Prior*

SUMMARY

- 9,208 households took part in the 1998 survey (74% of eligible households).

- 15,908 adults were interviewed (69% of adults in eligible households and 92% of adults in co-operating households).

- 3,746 children were interviewed (75% of sampled children in eligible households and 96% in co-operating households). Response was slightly higher for children aged 2-12 (the age at which parents acted as proxy informants) than for children aged 13-15 (the age at which the child rather than the parent was interviewed).

- 13,586 adults saw a nurse (59% of adults in eligible households and 79% of adults in co-operating households).

- 3,213 children saw a nurse (64% of sampled children in eligible households and 83% of sampled children in co-operating households).

- 10,773 adults gave a blood sample (47% of all adults in eligible households and 62% of adults in co-operating households).

- 268 children aged 11-15 gave a blood sample (32% of sampled children aged 11-15 in eligible households and 41% of children in co-operating households aged 11-15).

- Response to the interview was higher among women than among men. However, more interviewed men than women were willing to see a nurse and were eligible and willing to give a blood sample.

- There was no significant difference in response between boys and girls to being interviewed or to seeing a nurse.

- Response to providing a blood sample was significantly greater among boys than girls aged 11 to 15 (in co-operating households samples were obtained from 48% of boys and 32% of girls).

- Response varied by region, with response being lowest in the North West and in London (North Thames and South Thames).

- The laboratory used for blood analysis was different to that used in the four preceding years.

8.1 Overview of survey design

The 1998 Health Survey for England was designed to provide data at both national and regional level about the population aged 2 and over living in private households in England. The sample for the 1998 survey, as in previous years, was drawn from the Postcode Address File (PAF). Sampled addresses were selected from 720 postal sectors, with 60 sectors covered each month. Each sector was covered by an interviewer/nurse team.

At each address all persons aged 2 and over were eligible for inclusion in the survey. Where there were three or more children aged 2-15, two were selected at random. Information was obtained directly from those aged 13 or over. Information about children aged 2-12 was obtained from a parent, with the child present. An interview with each eligible person (Stage 1) was followed by a visit by a nurse (Stage 2), who made a number of measurements and requested permission to obtain a sample of blood from those aged 11 and over. Saliva samples were also collected from those aged 4 and over. Blood and saliva samples were sent to a laboratory for analysis.

Interviewing was conducted throughout the year to take account of seasonal differences.

Computer-assisted interviewing was used by both interviewers and nurses.

8.2 Sample design

8.2.1 Summary of sample design in the Health Survey series

The surveys in the Health Survey series have all adopted a similar multi-stage stratified probability sampling design.

The population surveyed has been the population living in private households. Those living in institutions have not been covered. They are likely to be older and, on average, in poorer health than those in private households, and this should be borne in mind when considering the Health Survey's account of the population's health.

The sampling frame has been the small user Postcode Address File (PAF). The very small proportion of households living at addresses not on PAF (less than 1%) have not been covered.

In all years, with the exception of 1997, postcode sectors have been the primary sampling units (PSUs). In 1993 the number of PSUs was 504; in 1994 to 1996 and in 1998 there were 720. In 1997 half-sectors were adopted as PSUs and the sample was drawn from 648 half sectors.[1]

In 1995 children were introduced into the Health Survey for the first time. This change was accommodated within the same sample design by reducing the lower age limit of eligibility within each household from 16 to 2. Children have been included in all subsequent years.

8.2.2 Sample selection in 1998: primary sampling units

720 postcode sectors (similar in size to electoral wards) were selected as the primary sampling units. Before selection, the list of postal sectors was stratified in order to maximise the precision of the sample. Postal sectors with fewer than 1,000 PAF 'delivery points' were first combined with neighbouring sectors so as to avoid any tight clustering of sampled addresses.

Two stratification levels were used. Postal sectors were first sorted by Health Authority and then, within Health Authority, listed in order of the percentage of households with the household head in a non-manual occupation (SEG 1-6, 13). Thus, in addition to ensuring that each Health Authority was correctly represented in the sample, a correct regional balance was achieved. The data used to classify postal sectors by the proportion of household heads in non-manual occupations was taken from the 1991 Census of Population.

720 sectors were then selected systematically with each postcode sector being given a probability of selection proportional to its total number of 'delivery points' (addresses).

The sample was then systematically sub-divided, each PSU being assigned to a month of the year. This was done so that fieldwork conducted in each quarter of the year was carried out with a fully representative sub-set of the total sample.

8.2.3 **Sampling delivery points (addresses)**

The small user Postcode Address File (PAF) was used as the sampling frame for addresses.

19 delivery points (addresses) were systematically selected from each selected PSU, yielding a total selected sample of 13,680 addresses. Selecting sectors with probability proportionate to number of delivery points (addresses), and then selecting a fixed number of addresses from each, gives every address an equal chance of inclusion.

When visited by interviewers, 10% of the selected addresses were found to contain no private households. Examples include businesses and institutions, vacant properties, demolished addresses and those still in the process of being built. These addresses were thus ineligible and were excluded from the survey sample.

A small proportion of addresses on PAF contain more than one household. Interviewers were instructed to include in the sample all households at addresses with one, two or three households. In the rare event of an address containing more than three households, the interviewer was given a special procedure to follow, using random selection digits provided. This procedure resulted in a random selection of three households from among all households at the address. All three selected were included in the survey sample, the other households being omitted. Theoretically, the sample should be weighted to take account of the omitted households. In practice, because there are so few cases, the complications introduced by this weighting would not be justified.

8.2.4 **Sampling individuals within addresses**

In order to limit the burden on households where there were three or more children aged 2 to 15, two of these children were randomly selected for the survey. No interviews were attempted with the other children. As 21% of contacted households containing children aged 2-15 had 3 or more children in this age group, 15% of all children were omitted from the sample. The application of weights is therefore required to compensate for the omissions (see Section 8.8.2).

8.3 Topic coverage

8.3.1 **Documentation**

Copies of all survey data collection documents are included in Appendix A. Measurement and saliva and blood sample collection protocols are given in Appendix B. The content of the Stage 1 interview and the Stage 2 nurse visit is summarised below.

8.3.2 **Stage 1: the interview**

Data was collected at two levels - household and individual. Figure 8A summarises the content of the household and individual interviews.

The main focus in 1998 for adults was cardiovascular disease (CVD) and related risk factors. The questions on CVD were based on those adopted in 1993 and 1994. Questions on the use of health services were revised in 1998 to bring them into line with those adopted for the General Household Survey series. The questions adopted for physical activity among adults were those used in 1993 and 1994 with some slight modifications to allow for changes in physical activity guidelines to be measured. Physical activity questions for children were based on those used in the 1997 Health Survey. A revised module of questions on eating habits was introduced in order to measure fat and fibre intake. Additional questions were introduced into the alcohol consumption module in order to examine drinking in the last week.

Informants aged 8 and over were asked to complete a self-completion booklet during the interview. There were four booklets - one for adults, one for young adults aged 16 to 17, one for teenagers aged 13-15 and one for children aged 8-12. The information obtained in this way is shown below.

Adults booklet	CAGE questions on drinking experience, perceived current weight status, GHQ12, social support, contraceptive pill and HRT use
Young adults	Smoking, drinking (including CAGE), perceived current weight status, GHQ12, social support, contraceptive pill use and HRT use
13-15 year olds	Smoking, drinking, perceived current weight status, GHQ12
8-12 year olds	Smoking, drinking, perceived current weight status, cycle helmet use.

8.3.3 Stage 2: the nurse visit

Nurses collected information about use of prescribed medicines, vitamin or mineral supplements and nicotine replacement products. They took blood pressure, waist, hip, upper arm circumference and demi-span measurements. Each measurement was limited to a particular age range, as shown in Figure 8A. A saliva sample for cotinine assay was requested from those aged 4 and over.

8.3.4 Collecting blood samples

Nurses also requested a small sample of blood by venepuncture from those aged 11 and over and obtained appropriate consents. All sampled informants aged 18 and over were eligible to provide a blood sample. However, informants aged 11 to 17 (minors) were eligible only if they had been sampled in PSUs allocated to the second half of the fieldwork year (July to December) or in 10 of the 60 June PSUs. Informants aged 11 to 17 sampled in PSUs allocated to the earlier part of the year were not asked to provide a blood sample, as a new protocol for obtaining blood from informants under 18 was being developed and approval was being sought from the Royal College of Paediatrics and Child Health. The new protocol included offering informants under 18 the option of an anaesthetic cream. This protocol was piloted in 10 PSUs in June and then introduced for all those aged 11 to 17 in PSUs covered in July to December.

Samples were analysed for total cholesterol, HDL-cholesterol, haemoglobin, ferritin, fibrinogen, and C-reactive protein. Nurses also sought agreement to the storage of a small sample of blood for possible future analysis. **Figure 8A**

8.3.5 Defining age for data collection and other purposes

A considerable part of the data collected in the 1998 Health Survey is age specific, with different questions directed to different age groups. The informant's date of birth was ascertained. For data collection purposes, an informant's age was defined as their age on their last birthday before the interview. The nurse, who visited them later, treated them as being of the same age as at the interview.

Age is a continuous variable, and an exact age variable on the data file expresses it as such (so that, for example, someone whose 14th birthday was on January 1 1998 and was interviewed on October 1 1998 would be classified as being aged 14.75 ($14^3/4$)).

The presentation of tabular data involves classifying the sample into year bands. There are two main ways of doing this:

- *age last birthday* (the child in the above example would be classified as being aged 14), corresponding to everyday usage.

- *'rounded age'*, in which the child's exact age is rounded to the nearest integer (the child in the above example being classified as aged 15). In rounded age, all children aged $14^1/2$ to $15^1/2$ are counted as being aged 15.

Rounded age was used for certain analyses of children in the 1995 and 1996 Health Survey reports, but in the present report all references to age are to age at last birthday.

8.4 Ethical clearance

Ethical approval for the 1998 survey was obtained from the North Thames Multi-centre Research Ethics Committee (MREC) and from all Local Research Ethics Committees (LRECs) in England. Approval for the revised blood protocol for minors was obtained from LRECs covering the PSUs in which the protocol was adopted (see Section 8.3.4).

1998 Health Survey for England – Contents

Household level data

Household size, composition and relationships
Accommodation tenure and number of bedrooms
Household cooking and heating appliances
Smoking in household

Car and telephone ownership
Income of household/income sources
Economic status/occupation of head of household
Type of dwelling and area

Individual level data	Age								
	2-3	4	5-6	7	8-10	11-12	13-15	16-64	65+
Interviewer visit									
General health, longstanding illness, limiting longstanding illness, acute sickness	●	●	●	●	●	●	●	●	●
Use of health services	●	●	●	●	●	●	●	●	●
MRC respiratory questionnaire								●	●
Chest pain								●	●
CVD, including use of services								●	●
Physical activity	●	●	●	●	●	●	●	●	●
Eating habits								●	●
Smoking					●[a]	●[a]	●[a]	●[b]	●
Drinking (including CAGE if 16+)					●[a]	●[a]	●[a]	●[b]	●
Reported birthweight	●	●	●	●	●	●	●		
Economic status/occupation								●	●
Educational attainment								●	●
Ethnic origin	●	●	●	●	●	●	●	●	●
Parental history								●	●
Height/weight measurements	●	●	●	●	●	●	●	●	●
Perception of current weight					●[a]	●[a]	●[a]	●[a]	●[a]
GHQ12							●[a]	●[a]	●[a]
Social support								●[a]	●[a]
Use of contraceptive pill								●[a]	●[a]
Hormone replacement therapy								●[c]	●[c]
Nurse visit									
Prescribed drugs and vitamin supplements	●	●	●	●	●	●	●	●	●
Nicotine replacements								●	●
Waist and hip circumference								●	●
Upper arm circumference	●	●	●	●	●	●	●		
Demi-span									●
Blood pressure			●	●	●	●	●	●	●
Blood sample- total cholesterol, HDL-cholesterol, haemoglobin, ferritin						●	●	●[d]	●
Blood sample – fibrinogen, C-reactive protein								●[d]	●
Saliva sample - cotinine		●	●	●	●	●	●	●	●

[a] These modules were administered by self-completion.

[b] This module was administered by self-completion for those aged 16-17 and some aged 18-19.

[c] This module was administered by self-completion and directed to women aged 18 and over only.

[d] From those aged 18+ in all sample points and those aged 16/17 in 310 sample points.

8.5 Fieldwork procedures

8.5.1 Advance letters

Each sampled address was sent an advance letter which introduced the survey and stated that an interviewer would be calling to seek permission to interview.

8.5.2 Making contact

At initial contact, the interviewer established how many households lived at the address. If there were three or fewer, all were included in the sample. If there were more than three, three were selected for inclusion in the survey, using a random number selection procedure.

The interviewer then made contact with each household and attempted to interview all adults and up to two eligible children (see below).

8.5.3 Collecting data

At each co-operating eligible household the interviewer first completed a Household Questionnaire, information being obtained from the head of household or their partner wherever possible. This questionnaire obtained information about all members of the household, regardless of age. If there were one or two children aged 2-15, they were automatically included in the sample for further interview. If there were three or more children aged 2 to 15, the computer program used random numbers to select two for interview. Individual Questionnaires were created by the computer program for these two children only.

An Individual Questionnaire interview was carried out with all adults and with sampled children. In order to reduce the amount of time spent in a household, interviews could be carried out concurrently, the program allowing for up to 4 informants to be interviewed in a session.

Height and weight measurements were obtained towards the end of the interview.

At the end of the interview informants were asked for their agreement to the second stage of the survey, the follow-up visit by a nurse. In the case of children aged 2-12, it was the parent's permission that was sought (see Section 8.5.6 for fuller details). Wherever possible an appointment was made for the nurse to visit within a few days of the interview. At this visit the nurse carried out the measurements specified in Section 8.3.3 and obtained the saliva and blood samples.

Before a blood sample was taken, written consent was obtained from the informant. If the informant was aged 11-17, the additional written consent of a parent or guardian (with legal parental responsibility) was required. Nurses also asked informants for consent to store part of the blood sample for additional analyses at some future date. If the informant agreed, a written consent was obtained. All informants aged 11-17 who consented to give a blood sample were given the option of having an anaesthetic cream applied beforehand. Those requesting the use of anaesthetic cream had to wait at least 60 minutes after application for venepuncture to take place.

In addition to an advance letter, informants were given two leaflets describing the purpose of the survey and of the associated measurements. Interviewers handed out one describing the purpose of the interview, and nurses handed out one explaining the purpose of their visit. Copies of these two documents are appended. Informants were also given a leaflet summarising some findings from previous surveys.

8.5.4 Feedback to informants

Each informant was given a Measurement Record Card in which the interviewer and the nurse entered the informant's height, weight, waist, hip, upper arm circumference, demi-span and blood pressure measurements. Informants were also sent (if they wished) the results of their blood sample analyses. Informants who saw a nurse were asked if they would like their blood pressure readings and blood sample analyses sent to their GP. If the answer was in the affirmative, written consent was obtained. Nurses were issued with a set of guidelines to follow when commenting on informants' blood pressure readings (see Appendix B for details). In summary, if an adult's blood pressure reading was severely raised, nurses were instructed to contact the Survey Doctor at the earliest opportunity. They were instructed not to comment on a child's reading but to leave the Survey Doctor to assess whether any action was required. Where permission had been given for results to be sent to an informant's GP, the Survey Doctor contacted the GP if any blood pressure or blood sample results were abnormal.

8.5.5 Quality control measures

Training interviewers and nurses

Interviewers were fully briefed on the administration of the survey, and were given training in measuring height and weight (including a practice session).

All nurses were professionally qualified and proficient in taking blood before joining the

Health Survey team. They attended a two-day training session at which they received equipment training and were briefed on the specific requirements of the survey with respect to taking blood pressure, making anthropometric measurements and taking saliva and blood samples.

Full sets of written instructions, covering both survey procedures and measurement protocols, were provided for both interviewers and nurses (Appendix B contains a copy of the measurement protocols).

Interviewers and nurses who had worked on the previous year's survey attended full day refresher training sessions, where the emphasis was on improving measurement skills and gaining informant co-operation.

All interviewers and nurses new to the Health Survey were accompanied by an interviewer or a nurse supervisor during the early stages of their work to ensure that interviews and protocols were being correctly administered. Routine supervision of the work of both interviewers and nurses was carried out thereafter.

Checking interview and measurement quality

A large number of quality control measures were built into the survey at both data collection and subsequent stages to check on the quality of interviewer and nurse performance.

Recalls to check on the work of both interviewers and nurses were carried out at 10% of productive households.

The computer program used by interviewers had in-built soft and hard checks, which included messages querying uncommon or unlikely answers. For example, if someone aged 16 or over had a height entered in excess of 1.93 metres, a message asked the interviewer to confirm that this was a correct entry. For children, the checks were age specific.

At the end of each survey month, the measurements made by each interviewer and nurse were inspected. For example, if a nurse had obtained a number of abnormally low readings this could be an indication of inadequate instructions to informants on how to perform a particular test. Supervisors discussed such results with the relevant nurse or interviewer.

8.5.6 **Interviewing and measuring children**

Children aged 13-15 were interviewed directly by interviewers, permission having first been obtained from the child's parent or guardian. Interviewers were instructed to ensure that the child's parent or guardian was present in the home throughout the interview. Information about younger children was collected from a parent. Younger children were present while their parent answered questions about their health. This was partly because the interviewer had to measure their height and weight and, in the case of those aged 8 and over, to ask the child to complete a short self-completion booklet during the interview. It also ensured that the child could contribute information.

Permission for a nurse to carry out any measurements on a child aged 2-15 had to be obtained from the child's parent or someone else with legal parental responsibility for that child. This person had to be present during the nurse visit. In 14 households there was a child for whom no-one claimed such responsibility, and no nurse visit was therefore arranged.

Written consent to send information to a child's GP was obtained from the parent.

8.6 Survey response

8.6.1 Response analysis

The sample design, described in Section 8.2, requires all adults and up to two children aged 2-15 to be interviewed. Non-informants to the survey fall into two groups, those living in households where no-one co-operated with the survey and those living in households where at least one person was interviewed.

This section looks first at the response of sampled households, then at that of eligible individuals within these households and then at variation in response by region, area and household type.

As informants were asked to co-operate in a sequence of operations, beginning with a face-to-face interview, progressing to a nurse visit and ending with a request for saliva and blood samples, individual non-response accumulated through the survey stages. Individual response for adults and children is looked at in two ways: overall response by all eligible individuals and response by individuals within co-operating households.

Not every measurement obtained by an interviewer or a nurse was subsequently considered valid for analysis purposes. For example, informants who reported eating, drinking or smoking in the 30 minutes prior to the blood pressure measurement were excluded from analysis, as were those for whom less than three blood pressure readings were obtained (the average of the last two readings forming the basis of analyses). Full details of the numbers of measurements used for analysis, the number of exclusions and the reasons for them are given at the start of each relevant chapter.

8.6.2 Household response

Table 8.1 shows the household response by calendar quarter.

The row labelled 'Total eligible households' shows the number of private residential households found at these addresses (after selection of three households, if more than three were found).

Households described as 'co-operating' are those where at least one eligible person was interviewed at Stage 1. Households described as 'all interviewed' are those where all eligible persons were interviewed. Those described as 'fully co-operating' are where all of those eligible for interview were interviewed, had their height and weight measured and agreed to see the nurse. Households where an informant was ineligible for a height or weight measurement because of a functional impairment or pregnancy are counted as partially co-operating for this response analysis.

74% of eligible households (9,208) took part in the 1998 survey. At 65% of households all eligible adults and children were interviewed.   **Table 8.1**

8.6.3 Individual response - adults

Overall response

There were 15,908 individual interviews with adults, 13,586 saw a nurse and 10,773 gave a blood sample.

The numerator of the response rate - the number of productive outcomes - is of course known (though, as already noted, there are a variety of different outcomes). The denominator - the total number of adults in the sampled households - is not known and must be estimated. There are three groups of households to consider: co-operating households (17,240 adults in 9,208 households, average 1.87), non co-operating households where information on number of adults is known (3,787 adults in 2,141 households, average 1.77), and non co-operating households about which nothing is known (1,097 households). The most reasonable assumption is to impute to the last group the same average number of adults (1.85) as for all households where the number is known (the sum of the first two groups). This assumption gives an estimated total of 23,085 adults (the 'set' sample). The assumption is likely to be conservative, and the estimated number thus too large. Non co-operating households where the number is not known are more likely to resemble non co-operating households where it is known than co-operating households.

Using this estimate as a denominator, the response rates for adults at various stages (Table 8.4) were:

    69% were interviewed
    66% had their height measured
    64% had their weight measured
    59% saw a nurse
    58% had their waist-hip measured
    58% had their blood pressure measured
    57% gave a saliva sample
    49% agreed to give a blood sample
    47% gave a blood sample

12% of those seeing a nurse did not give a blood sample either because it was not possible to obtain a sample from them, for example because of collapsed veins (4%), or because they were ineligible to give blood (8%). Ineligible informants include those aged 16 or 17 who were sampled in survey months in which blood was not taken from minors as well as those ineligible because of pregnancy, drug treatment or a specified health condition.

A further assumption is needed to provide separate response rates for men and women. In non co-operating households where the number of adults was known, the separate numbers of men and women were usually not obtained. However, it can simply be assumed that the proportion of men and women in the estimated total is the same as for the adults in the 9,237 households where the sex split is known (the 9,208 co-operating, plus another 29 who provided a household questionnaire but no individual interviews). The proportions are 47.2% men and 52.8% women. Applying these proportions to the estimated total of adults gives 'set samples' of 10,885 men and 12,200 women. These numbers are shown as bases in Table 8.4.

Response to the interview stage was higher among women (71%) than among men (66%).

Although a smaller proportion of men than women responded to the interview, higher proportions of men than women agreed to see a nurse and agreed to have their blood pressure measured.

Table 8.4

Adult response in co-operating households

As adults' ages and other personal characteristics are not known in non co-operating households, indications of response differences by these characteristics are confined to those households that did co-operate. Tables 8.6 and 8.7 show the proportion of men and women in co-operating households who responded to the key survey stages. These are summarised below:

	Men	Women	All adults
	%	%	%
Interviewed	88	96	92
Height measured	85	92	89
Weight measured	84	88	86
Saw a nurse	76	81	79
Waist and hip measured	75	79	77
Blood pressure measured	75	79	77
Saliva sample obtained	75	78	77
Agreed to give blood	64	67	65
Blood sample obtained	62	63	62

2% of men and 1% of women in co-operating households were ineligible to give a blood sample because they were aged 16 or 17 and sampled in the survey months in which blood was not taken from minors. A further 3% of men and 5% of women were ineligible because of a clotting or other disorder or because of pregnancy. A blood sample was obtained from 66% of eligible men and 67% of eligible women in co-operating households.

In co-operating households, interview response was highest among those aged 65 and over (96% of men and 98% of women) and lowest among those aged under 25 (83% of men and 89% of women), who were also less inclined to co-operate with subsequent survey stages.

Tables 8.6, 8.7

8.6.4 Individual response - children

Overall response

Interviews were carried out with 3,746 children (in the case of those aged 2-12 the information was obtained from a parent). 3,213 children were seen by a nurse and 268 children aged 11 to 15 gave a blood sample.

To compute the response rate the number of eligible children in sampled households (the 'set sample') is needed as the denominator. 25.80% of contacted households contained children aged 2-15. If it is assumed that the proportions of all sampled households containing 0, 1, 2.. children aged 2-15 were the same as among households contacted, then 3,211 households contained at least one child aged 2-15, and the number of children to be interviewed (a maximum of two per household) was 4,999. This is the 'set sample'. (The total number of children in these households would be slightly greater as some households would have contained more than two children.)

Almost all non-responding children were in households where no-one (child or adult) co-operated with the survey.

Among the 'set' sample of 4,999 children response rates at various stages were:

75%	were interviewed
71%	had their height measured
71%	had their weight measured
64%	saw a nurse
64%	had their upper arm circumference measured

Table 8.5

Blood pressure measurements were limited to those aged 5-15, saliva samples to those aged 4-15 and blood samples to those aged 11-15 in PSUs where blood was taken from minors. As the age distribution of children in non-responding households is not known, a further estimate has to be made to obtain the relevant denominator in each case. On the assumption that the age distribution of children in the 'set sample' is the same as that of children living in interviewed households, responses to these measurements were:

62%	of those aged 5-15 had their blood pressure measured
61%	of those aged 4-15 provided a saliva sample
32%	of eligibles aged 11 to 15 provided a blood sample

A further estimate has to be made to provide separate response rates by sex of child. The 'set sample' of boys and girls in Table 8.5 has been derived by assuming that the 4,999 children were split between boys and girls in the same proportions as in households which provided a household questionnaire (51.03% boys and 48.97% girls). Although there were no significant differences in interview and measurement response by sex of child, there were considerable differences between boys and girls aged 11 to 15 in their response to the request for a blood sample. This is discussed further in the following section.

Child response in co-operating households

Child response rates, like adult response rates, have been calculated on a co-operating household base. The proportion interviewed was high overall. There were slight differences in response to the interview stage between children aged 13-15, where the interview was conducted with the child, and those aged 2-12, where a parent acted as proxy informant at the interview stage. Interview data was collected from 93% of children aged 13-15, and from parents in respect of 98 % of those aged 2-12.

	Boys	Girls	All children
	%	%	%
Interviewed	96	97	96
Height measured	93	91	92
Weight measured	92	91	91
Saw a nurse	83	83	83
Mid-upper arm measured	82	82	82
Blood pressure measured (aged 5 and over)	81	81	81
Gave a saliva sample (aged 4 and over)	81	81	81
Agreed to a blood sample (aged 11-15)	56	42	49
Blood sample obtained (aged 11-15)	51	34	43

The great majority of children in all age groups co-operated with the measurements and provided a saliva sample.

The change in protocol introduced in 1998 for obtaining a blood sample from minors (see Section 8.3.4) appears to have considerably affected the willingness of children aged 11 to 15 to agree to venepuncture. The proportion of children aged 11 to 15 agreeing to provide a blood sample was substantially lower than in previous survey years (41% in 1998 as compared with 53% in 1996 and 50% in 1995). The marked difference between boys and girls aged 11 to 15 in their willingness to provide a blood sample was also not found in previous survey years. This gender difference is almost entirely due to the far higher proportion of girls than boys saying they did not wish to give a sample - of those seeing a nurse 31% of boys and 43% of girls refused to co-operate in this respect. **Tables 8.8, 8.9**

8.6.5 Variations in survey response

Regional variations in response

As in previous years, response varied by region (NHS Regional Offices). Household response was lowest in the North West, North Thames and South Thames regions. It was highest in Northern & Yorkshire region.   Table 8.2

Response by type of dwelling

Table 8.3 analyses the household response by the type of building housing the address (as classified by interviewers).

Response was highest among households living in detached houses (77%) and lowest among households living in flats (particularly those located on or above the 4th floor or in converted properties - 64%).   Table 8.3

8.7 Sample profile of those interviewed in 1998

8.7.1 Non-response

Non-response bias is of particular concern in a survey where informants can opt out of the survey at different stages. This section compares the basic socio-demographic profile of responding households and responding adults and children at two survey stages (interview and nurse visit). Table 8.19 provides age and sex comparisons with mid-1998 population estimates (it should be noted that these population estimates cover both institutional and private residential populations, whereas the Health Survey only covers the private residential population).

The 1996 Health Survey report contains a fuller analysis of non-responders to the Health Survey (Chapter 11, Section 11.10.1).

8.7.2 Age and sex of adults

The proportion men form of all adults, according to the 1998 mid-year population estimates, is 48.7%. The proportion of men in the interviewed sample of adults in the 1998 Health Survey was 45.2%. Of those seeing a nurse, 45.4% were men.

Table 8.19 compares the age distribution of the responding adult sample with mid-1998 population estimates. Men aged 34 and under are under-represented at both interview and nurse visit. Men aged 65 and over are slightly over-represented. Women under 24 are under-represented at both stages, as are women aged 75 and over.   Table 8.19

8.7.3 Ethnic origin of responding adults

Table 8.20 shows the ethnic origin of responding adults at the two survey stages. Of those who responded at Stage 1, black ethnic groups were less likely than others to participate in Stage 2 of the survey or to provide a blood sample.   Table 8.20

8.8 Weighting the data

8.8.1 Adult sample

At the start of the Health Survey series it was decided not to weight the adult sample. The profile of the responding sample was judged to be sufficiently close to the estimated population distribution to make weighting unnecessary. This policy of not reweighting to compensate for response rate differences has remained unchanged.

8.8.2 The child sample

Results for children are not presented in this report, but to assist users of the child tables on the Department of Health website (see Chapter 1, Section 1.6.6), the child sample weighting procedures are described in this section.

When children aged 2-15 were introduced into the survey series in 1995 it became necessary to apply a 'child weight' to the child sample to compensate for limiting the number of children interviewed in a household to two (the sampling fraction therefore being lower in households containing three or more children).

In principle, the 'child weight' could have three components: (a) for the unequal selection probabilities, (b) for chance deviations in the selection of two children where there were more than two, and (c) for differences in response rates. The policy of not weighting for differential response levels that had been adopted for adults (see above) was extended to children also, so (c) was not applied. This left only (a) and (b) as the two components of the 'child weight'.

Component (a) is required only where there were more than two eligible children, and is attached to each child selected for interview (whether or not actually interviewed). The weight is the total number of children aged 2-15 in the household divided by the number of selected children in the household. Weighting by component (a) can be expected to result in the weighted sample having a sex/age distribution close to that of the aggregate of all children in the co-operating households, any deviations being due to the effects of chance in the selection process. The match was found to be close, but it was decided to eliminate such random differences as there were by adding a second weighting component, (b), which was applied separately for each cell of the sex/age distribution. It was computed as m/n, where m is the aggregate number of children aged 2-15 in the cell (summing those recorded in all co-operating households) and n is the number in the corresponding sex/age cell of the selected sample after weighting by component (a). The average value of the 'child weight', incorporating both components, is about 1.13.

8.9 Estimating errors in complex sample designs: design factors

The Health Survey uses a multi-stage design involving the stratified selection of a sample of postal sectors. The addresses selected for the survey are confined to these sectors and are thus geographically clustered. In addition, since more than one interview may be made at one address, there is clustering of interviews within addresses as well as within postal sectors.

Clustering is almost always employed in national survey designs in the UK. For reasons explained below, clustered sample designs are subject to sampling errors that are larger (for a given sample size) than those of a simple random sample. But this is more than offset by the fact that their lower cost per interview permits a larger sample for the same financial outlay. Clustered designs are therefore usually more cost-effective.

The reason that estimates from a clustered sample are likely to have larger sampling errors than those from a simple random sample of the same size is that there tend to be greater similarities, in some respects at least, between members of the same cluster than between independently selected sample members. This tendency is measured by the intra-cluster correlation coefficient for the variable concerned. Selecting an additional member from the same cluster adds less new information than would a completely independent selection, and the clustered sample thus achieves less precision (for a given number of interviews) than a simple random sample.

Practical sample designs differ from simple random samples in other ways than the use of clustering. For example, stratification is typically used (which tends to reduce sampling errors).

The net effect of clustering, stratification and other factors is that the standard errors of these 'complex' sample designs tend to be greater than those of a simple random sample (which is rarely encountered in practice). The ratio of the standard error of the complex sample to that of a simple random sample of the same size is known as the design factor. This design factor, usually abbreviated to 'deft', is therefore the factor by which the standard error of an estimate from a simple random sample has to be multiplied to give the true standard error of the complex design.

Defts vary from one estimate to another within the same survey. They are affected by the average number of interviews per sampling point within the sub-group being analysed: the smaller this is, the lower the deft will tend to be (provided the interviews are evenly spread across sampling points). But an uneven spread of interviews between sampling points will tend to increase defts, as can be the case with, for example, a social class group.

The standard errors of complex samples have been calculated using a Taylor Series expansion method implemented in the package STATA. They have been calculated for adults (aged 16 and over) only. The deft values presented in Tables 8.10 to 8.18 (which are themselves estimates subject to random sampling error) are for survey estimates based on all males or females. Defts for small sub-samples are likely to be smaller than those shown in the tables, with the notable exception of sub-groups (such as a region) that are concentrated within a sub-set of sampling points.

The tables deal in turn with a number of different variables used in the analysis for this report. For each, the first column shows the proportion (or mean) as estimated by the sample. The second column shows the size of the sample (or sub-sample) on which it is based. The third column shows the weighted sample size. The fourth column shows its estimated true standard error. The fifth column shows the 95% confidence interval. The final column shows the estimated deft.

97% of defts in Tables 8.10 to 8.18 are less than 1.2 (78% are less than 1.1). Defts of this order are usually considered to be small. **Tables 8.10-8.18**

8.10 Quality control of blood and saliva analytes

8.10.1 Introduction

This section describes the assay of analytes, quality control and quality assessment that were carried out during the survey period. Details of procedures used in the collection, processing and transportation of the specimens are described in Appendix B.

8.10.2 Change of analysing laboratories

Blood samples collected during the 1998 Health Survey were analysed by The Royal Victoria Infirmary (RVI) laboratories in Newcastle upon Tyne. RVI was also responsible for analysing samples taken in the 1991 to 1993 Health Surveys. However, analysis of blood samples collected in the 1994 to 1997 Health Surveys had been undertaken by the laboratories of the West Middlesex University Hospital (WMUH). Possible implications of the use of different laboratories in 1994 and 1998 are discussed below. The Nicotine Laboratory at New Cross Hospital have analysed levels of cotinine in blood, and more recently saliva, samples since 1993.

Following written consent from eligible informants, three blood samples (one 6ml plain, a 4ml EDTA and a 4.5ml citrate tube for adults; a 6ml plain and two 2ml EDTA tubes for children) and one saliva sample were collected and despatched to the Department of Clinical Biochemistry at RVI that acted as the co-ordinating department for transport of samples to the individual departments undertaking the analysis.

8.10.3 Samples collected

Samples collected in the 6ml plain tube for serum

This provided the sample for total cholesterol, HDL-cholesterol and ferritin analysis for those aged 11 and above and C-reactive protein (CRP) analysis for informants aged 16 and above. If written consent was given by the informant, a minimum of 0.5ml of the remaining serum was stored in a freezer at minus 70°C ± 5°C for possible future analysis.

Samples collected in the 4ml EDTA (ethylene diamine tetra-acetic acid) tube

This provided the sample for haemoglobin analysis for informants aged 11 and above. If written consent was given by the informant, approximately 1ml of whole blood was stored in a freezer at minus 20°C ± 5°C for possible future analysis.

Samples collected in the 4.5ml citrate tube

This provided the sample for fibrinogen analysis for informants aged 16 and above.

Saliva tube

This provided the sample for cotinine analysis for informants aged 4 and above.

8.10.4 Methodology

Methods used for each analyte at the RVI were similar to that used at the WMUH, although there were some differences which are described below. To compare the two laboratories and assess the extent of agreement between them a cross-over study was considered. Nevertheless since most of the techniques of analysis were different in the two laboratories the comparison study was deemed not applicable and was not carried out.

All analyses were carried out according to Standard Operating Procedures by State Registered Medical Laboratory Scientific Officers (MLSOs) under the supervision of the Senior MLSO. All results were routinely checked by the duty Biochemist and seriously abnormal results were immediately faxed to the Survey Doctor at UCL. The informant and their General Practitioner were then notified and advised as appropriate.

Total cholesterol

Total cholesterol analysis was carried out using the DAX Cholesterol Oxidase assay method calibrated to the Centre for Disease Control standard (CDC) by the Biochemistry Department at RVI.

The same method (cholesterol oxidase) was used by both laboratories in 1994 (WMUH) and 1998 (RVI), although the equipment used was different. Both laboratories participate in external quality control schemes and perform within the acceptable range of assay performance (See Tables 8.20 and 8.27 for the RVI internal quality control and external quality assessment results). Some caution should nevertheless be applied when comparing the results.

HDL-cholesterol

HDL-cholesterol analysis was carried out using the DAX Cholesterol Oxidase assay method calibrated to CDC after PTA precipitation by the Biochemistry Department at RVI. Samples were not analysed in 1994 for HDL-cholesterol.

C-reactive protein (CRP)

CRP analysis was carried out using the N Latex CRP mono Immunoassay on the Behring Nephelometer II Analyzer by the Biochemistry Department at RVI. Samples were not analysed in 1994 for C-reactive protein.

Ferritin

Ferritin analysis was carried out by the Haematology Department at RVI using the Abbott Microparticle Enzyme Immunoassay (MEIA)/IMX ferritin assay method, the same method used in 1996 and 1997 by WMUH. In 1994 and 1995 WMUH used the Boehringer Enzymun method for ferritin analysis. Results from a comparison study carried out at the WMUH in 1996 were presented in the 1996 Health Survey.[2] Given the wide inter-laboratory variability of immunoassays, the ferritin data in the 1998 report are not directly comparable with those in 1994.

Haemoglobin

The majority of the haemoglobin analysis was carried out by the Department of Haematology at RVI using one of two Coulter Electronics Ltd Model STKS analysers designated as STKSA. Occasional analysis was carried out using the second analyser designated as STKSB (see Table 8.25). Both analysers had two test and two blank spectrophotometric readings taken at 525 ± 30nm in an Isoton III diluent.

The methodology for this analysis has not changed since 1994.

Fibrinogen

Fibrinogen analysis was carried out using the Organon Teknika MDA 180 analyser, using a modification of the Clauss thrombin clotting method by the Department of Haematology at RVI.

In 1994 WMUH used the nephelometric method (clot turbidity) for fibrinogen analysis whilst at Newcastle a modification of the most commonly used Clauss method is used. This change in methodology does affect comparability with the 1994 fibrinogen results.

Cotinine

Cotinine analysis was carried out using a Hewlett Packard hp5890 gas chromatograph machine, with a rapid-liquid chromatography technique by the Nicotine Laboratory at New Cross Hospital. This method has been used since 1993, although in 1993 to 1997 cotinine levels for adults were analysed in serum.

Saliva samples received at RVI are checked for correct identification, assigned a laboratory accession number and stored at 4°C. Samples are checked for details and despatched weekly in polythene bags (20 samples per bag) by Red Star courier for overnight delivery to New Cross.

8.10.5 Internal quality control (IQC)

In order to ensure the accuracy and reliability of analyses, internal quality control (IQC) was carried out by laboratory staff in the Biochemistry and Haematology Departments at the RVI and at New Cross Hospital.

The first purpose of IQC is to estimate errors in an analytical run and to prevent release of data if the errors are unacceptably high. The second purpose is to monitor the performance of the assay over a period of time and detect trends.

For each analyte or group of analytes, the laboratory obtains a supply of quality control materials, usually at more than one concentration of analyte. A target (mean) value and target standard deviation are assigned for each analyte. Target assignment includes evaluation of values obtained by the laboratory from replicate measurements (over several runs) in conjunction with target values provided by manufacturers of IQC materials, if available. The standard deviation and the coefficient of variation (C.V.) are measures of imprecision and are presented here.

Total cholesterol

Low, Medium and High control materials are assayed with every 50 samples. Table 8.21 shows the monthly internal quality control results for total cholesterol. **Table 8.21**

HDL-cholesterol

A control is precipitated with each batch prior to assay on the DAX where Low, Medium and High control materials are assayed with every 50 samples. Table 8.22 shows the monthly internal quality control results for HDL-cholesterol. **Table 8.22**

C-reactive protein (CRP)

Based on materials in use in the department, the laboratory anticipated achieving levels of reproducibility comparable to company literature, i.e. coefficient of variation less than 3%. Table 8.23 shows the monthly internal quality control results for C-reactive protein. **Table 8.23**

Ferritin

IMX Ferritin calibrator and Low, Medium and High controls are included in each assay run of 21 samples and are calibrated against reagent and reaction cell batches. Table 8.24 shows the monthly internal quality control results for ferritin. **Table 8.24**

Haemoglobin

The analyser is calibrated using material provided by the manufacturer Coulter. Indices are checked at least daily using Coulter controls at three levels. In-house preparations, normal level, abnormal level I (ABNI) and abnormal level II (ABNII), are used to monitor within batch and between batch variation during the day. Reproducibility is assessed by 15 random samples being tested on 6 different occasions over a 6-hour period. Table 8.25 shows the monthly internal quality control results for haemoglobin. **Table 8.25**

Fibrinogen

Control plasmas are assayed at regular intervals and instrument function tests are monitored continuously. The control interval is specified as every 4 hours or 100 specimens. Significant deviations from specified limits are flagged and must be acknowledged by the operator. Table 8.26 shows the monthly internal quality control results for fibrinogen. **Table 8.26**

Cotinine

The Medical Toxicology Unit at New Cross does participate in inter-laboratory split analyses to ensure comparable results. A summary of these monthly results is outlined in Table 8.27.

Table 8.27

8.10.6 External quality assessment (EQA)

The RVI Biochemistry and Haematology Departments and the New Cross Hospital laboratory both participate in external quality assessment (EQA) schemes.

EQA permits comparison of results between laboratories measuring the same analyte. An EQA scheme for an analyte or group of analytes distributes aliquots of the same samples to participating laboratories, who are blind to the concentration of the analytes. The usual practice is to participate in a scheme for a full year during which samples are distributed at regular frequency (monthly or bimonthly for example); the number of samples in each distribution and the frequency differ between schemes. The samples contain varying concentrations of analytes. The same samples may or may not be distributed more than once.

Samples are assayed shortly after they arrive at the laboratory. Depending on the frequency of distribution there may be weeks or months in which no EQA samples are analysed. Results are returned to the scheme organisers, who issue a laboratory specific report giving at least the following data:

- Mean values, usually for all methods and for method groups;

- A measure of the between-laboratory precision;

- The bias of the results obtained by that laboratory.

EQA is a retrospective process of assessment of performance, particularly of inaccuracy or bias with respect to mean values; unlike IQC, it does not provide control of release of results at the time of analysis.

The United Kingdom National External Quality Assessment Schemes (UKNEQAS) is a network of EQA schemes run by UK clinical laboratories. The Welsh External Quality Assessment Schemes (WEQAS), the Coulter Interlaboratory QA programme, National External Quality Assessment Scheme for Haematology, the Cambridge External Quality Assessment Schemes (EQAS) and the Central Quality Assessment Schemes (QAS) are all schemes in which the laboratories participate on a routine basis.

As the methods and equipment used have been found to produce internal quality control and external quality assessment results within specified limits (see below), it can be concluded that the laboratories at RVI and New Cross performed acceptably for these analytes.

Total cholesterol

The Clinical Biochemistry laboratory participates in UKNEQAS and WEQAS schemes. Table 8.28 shows the monthly external quality assessment results for total cholesterol. The target and achieved values are shown.

Table 8.28

HDL-cholesterol

The Clinical Biochemistry laboratory participates in the WEQAS scheme. Table 8.29 shows the monthly external quality assessment results for HDL-cholesterol. The target and achieved values are shown.

Table 8.29

C-reactive protein (CRP)

The Clinical Biochemistry laboratory participates in UKNEQAS schemes. Table 8.30 shows the monthly external quality assessment results for C-reactive protein. The target and achieved values are shown.

Table 8.30

Ferritin

The Haematology laboratory participates in the UKNEQAS scheme receiving monthly surveys of 2 samples each. Table 8.31 shows the external quality assessment results for ferritin for each month. The target and achieved values are shown.

Table 8.31

Haemoglobin

The Haematology laboratory participates in Coulter Interlaboratory QA Program where results from 'normal' level material are submitted monthly to Coulter who produce reports to the 890 participants. UKNEQAS supply 2 samples monthly to a group of 235 participants and Cambridge EQAS schemes supplying a weekly sample to the 72 participants in the group. Table 8.32 shows the UKNEQAS monthly external quality assessment results for haemoglobin.

Table 8.32

Fibrinogen

The Haematology laboratory participates in UKNEQAS, 4 surveys per year and Central QAS schemes fortnightly. Table 8.33 shows the external quality assessment results for fibrinogen for each quarter.

Table 8.33

Cotinine

There was no external quality control scheme available in 1998 to analyse cotinine but, as stated in Section 8.10.5, the Medical Toxicology Unit participates in inter-laboratory split analyses to ensure comparable results.

8.10.7 Reference ranges

Table 8.34 shows the reference ranges for the analytes measured in the 1998 Health Survey.

Table 8.34

8.10.8 Maintenance

Each analyser has a schedule of Planned Preventative Maintenance carried out jointly by the manufacturers and the laboratory. Records are kept of when maintenance is due and carried out.

References and notes

1 See *Chapter 13: Survey Methodology and Response* in Prescott-Clarke P, Primatesta P (eds). *The health of young people 1995-97*. The Health Survey for England 1997. The Stationery Office, London, 1998.

2 See Section 10.2.3 of *Chapter 10: Quality Control of Blood Analytes* in Prescott-Clarke P, Primatesta P (eds). *The Health Survey for England 1996*. The Stationery Office, London, 1997.

Tables

Table 8.1

Household response, by quarter

Selected addresses/eligible households   *1998*

Address and household outcome	Jan-Mar		Apr-Jun		Jul-Sep		Oct-Dec		Annual	
Address and household outcome	N		N		N		N		N	
Selected addresses	3420		3420		3420		3420		13680	
Ineligible addresses[a]	381		319		341		389		1430	
Addresses at which interview sought	3039		3101		3079		3031		12250	
Extra households sampled at multi-household addresses	51		42		48		55		196	
Total eligible households	3090		3143		3127		3086		12446	
Household response		%		%		%		%		%
Co-operating households[b]:	2234	72	2314	74	2368	76	2292	74	9208	74
all interviewed	1969	64	2023	64	2082	67	2004	65	8078	65
fully co-operating[c]	1889	61	1932	61	1971	63	1906	62	7698	62
Non-responding households	856	28	829	26	759	24	794	26	3238	26
Base: all eligible households	*3090*		*3143*		*3127*		*3086*		*12446*	

[a] Address where no private households were found.

[b] Households where at least one person interviewed.

[c] All eligible household members were interviewed, had height and weight measured and agreed to a nurse visit.

Table 8.2

Household response, by region

Selected addresses/eligible households   *1998*

Region																	Total
	Northern & Yorkshire		North West		Trent		West Midlands		Anglia & Oxford		North Thames		South Thames		South & West		
	N	%	N	%	N	%	N	%	N	%	N	%	N	%	N	%	N	%
Address and household outcome																	
Selected addresses	1786		1863		1424		1453		1489		1863		1919		1883		13680	
Ineligible addresses[a]	184		212		145		137		137		223		176		216		1430	
Addresses at which interview sought	1602		1651		1279		1316		1352		1640		1743		1667		12250	
Extra households sampled at multi-household addresses	8		13		7		3		7		100		39		19		196	
Total eligible households	1610		1664		1286		1319		1359		1740		1782		1686		12446	
Household response																	
Co-operating households[b]:	1298	81	1188	71	1007	78	957	73	1012	74	1232	71	1214	68	1300	77	9208	74
all interviewed	1182	73	1064	64	899	70	837	63	899	66	1034	59	1017	57	1146	68	8078	65
fully co-operating[c]	1139	71	1006	60	843	66	781	59	868	64	992	57	974	55	1095	65	7698	62
Non-responding households	312	19	476	29	279	22	362	27	347	26	508	29	568	32	386	23	3238	26
Base: all eligible households	*1610*		*1664*		*1286*		*1319*		*1359*		*1740*		*1782*		*1686*		*12446*	

[a] Address where no private households were found.

[b] Households where at least one person interviewed.

[c] All eligible household members were interviewed, had height and weight measured and agreed to a nurse visit.

Table 8.3

Household response, by dwelling type

Eligible households   *1998*

Household response	Dwelling type							Total[a]
	Detached house	Semi-detached	Terraced house house	Purpose built flat[b] basement-3rd floor	Purpose built flat[b] 4th floor or above	Converted flat/rooms in a house	Other type	
	%	%	%	%	%	%	%	%
Co-operating households:	77	76	76	73	64	64	80	74
all interviewed	66	67	66	67	57	58	74	65
fully co-operating	62	64	63	65	55	56	71	62
Non-responding households	23	24	24	27	36	36	20	26
Base: all eligible households	*2615*	*4038*	*3475*	*1314*	*183*	*481*	*122*	*12446*

[a] Includes 218 households where type of dwelling not recorded.

[b] Includes maisonette.

Table 8.4

Summary of adults' individual response to the survey, by sex

Estimated adult sample ('set' sample of adults aged 16 and over)   *1998*

Individual response	Men		Women		All adults	
	N	%	N	%	N	%
Interviewed	7193	66	8715	71	15908	69
Non-responders:						
In co-operating households	935	9	397	3	1332	6
In non-responding households	2750	25	3082	25	5832	25
Saw nurse	6165	57	7421	61	13586	59
Responded to:						
Self-completion	6904	63	8415	69	15319	66
Height	6930	64	8386	69	15316	66
Weight	6824	63	8035	66	14859	64
Waist/Hip	6122	56	7190	59	13312	58
Blood pressure	6120	56	7190	59	13310	58
Saliva	6118	56	7122	58	13240	57
Blood sample:						
Obtained	5078	47	5695	47	10773	47
Attempted, not obtained	158	1	370	3	528	2
Ineligible[a]	403	4	600	5	1003	4
Base: set sample[b]	*10885*		*12200*		*23085*	

[a] Includes those aged 16 and 17 in sample points in which blood was not taken from minors, as well as those ineligible because of pregnancy or medical condition.

[b] For the method of estimating the adult 'set' sample, see Section 8.6.3. Estimated bases have been rounded.

Table 8.5

Summary of children's individual response to the survey, by sex

Estimated child sample aged 2-15 ('set' sample of children)   *1998*

Individual response	Boys		Girls		All children	
	N	%	N	%	N	%
Interviewed	1905	75	1841	75	3746	75
Non-responders:						
In co-operating households	86	3	61	2	147	3
In non-responding households	551	22	549	22	1100	22
Saw nurse	1642	64	1571	64	3213	64
Responded to:						
Height	1837	72	1734	71	3571	71
Weight	1811	71	1721	70	3532	71
Mid-upper arm circumference	1625	64	1553	63	3178	64
Base: set sample[a]	*2551*		*2448*		*4999*	

[a] For the method of estimating the child 'set' sample, see Section 8.6.4.

Table 8.6

Men in co-operating households: response to the stages of the survey, by age

Men aged 16 or over in co-operating households   *1998*

Individual response	Age							Total
	16-24	25-34	35-44	45-54	55-64	65-74	75 +	
	%	%	%	%	%	%	%	%
Interviewed[1]								
Interviewed	83	86	87	88	90	96	96	88
Not-contacted/refused	17	14	13	12	10	4	4	12
Height[1]								
Measured	80	83	85	85	87	92	88	85
Measurement not attempted	1	1	1	1	1	2	6	1
Not-contacted/refused[a]	19	16	14	14	12	6	6	13
Weight[1]								
Measured	79	82	83	84	85	90	88	84
Measurement not attempted	2	2	2	3	3	4	7	3
Not-contacted/refused[a]	19	16	14	14	12	6	5	13
Nurse visit[1]								
Co-operated with nurse visit	66	73	75	78	79	84	82	76
Not interviewed	17	14	13	12	10	4	4	12
Refused/no contact at nurse visit	17	13	12	10	12	12	14	13
Waist/Hip[1]								
Measured	66	72	75	77	78	83	80	75
No nurse visit[b]	34	27	25	22	21	16	18	24
Refused/not obtained	0	1	0	0	1	0	2	1
Blood pressure[1]								
Measured	66	72	75	77	78	83	80	75
No nurse visit[b]	34	27	25	22	21	16	18	24
Refused/not obtained	0	0	0	0	1	1	2	1
Saliva sample[1]								
Measured	66	72	75	77	78	83	81	75
No nurse visit[b]	34	28	25	23	22	17	19	25
Refused/not obtained	0	0	0	0	0	0	0	0
Blood sample[1]								
Blood sample taken	41	59	65	67	68	72	67	62
Unsuccessful attempt at sample	1	1	1	2	2	3	3	2
Ineligible – medical grounds	3	3	2	3	3	4	6	3
Ineligible – minors not asked for sample	12	-	-	-	-	-	-	2
Refused	12	9	6	5	5	4	5	7
No nurse visit[b]	32	27	25	22	21	16	18	24
Demi-span[2]								
Measured						83	80	82
No nurse visit[b]						16	18	17
Refused/not attempted						1	2	1
Bases								
[1] *Men aged 16 and over in co-operating households*	*1053*	*1560*	*1502*	*1464*	*1092*	*873*	*584*	*8128*
[2] *Men aged 65 and over in co-operating households*						*873*	*584*	*1457*

[a] Includes non-responders to interview as well as those refusing measurement.

[b] Includes non-responders to interview.

Table 8.7

Women in co-operating households: response to the stages of the survey, by age

Women aged 16 or over in co-operating households   *1998*

Individual response	Age							Total
	16-24	25-34	35-44	45-54	55-64	65-74	75 +	
	%	%	%	%	%	%	%	%
Interviewed[1]								
Interviewed	89	95	97	97	96	97	98	96
Not-contacted/refused	11	5	3	3	4	3	2	4
Height[1]								
Measured	87	93	95	94	92	92	87	92
Measurement not attempted	0	1	0	1	2	3	9	2
Not-contacted/refused[a]	13	6	4	5	6	5	4	6
Weight[1]								
Measured	81	86	90	92	90	91	87	88
Measurement not attempted	6	8	4	2	4	4	8	5
Not-contacted/refused[a]	13	7	6	6	6	6	4	7
Nurse visit[1]								
Co-operated with nurse visit	74	81	83	85	84	82	78	81
Not interviewed	11	5	3	3	4	3	2	4
Refused/no contact at nurse visit	15	14	13	12	12	15	20	14
Waist/Hip[1]								
Measured	69	75	82	84	83	81	76	79
No nurse visit[b]	30	24	18	15	16	18	22	20
Refused/not obtained	0	0	0	0	1	1	2	1
Blood pressure[1]								
Measured	69	75	81	84	83	81	76	79
No nurse visit[b]	26	19	17	15	16	18	22	19
Refused/not obtained	0	0	1	1	1	1	2	1
Ineligible: pregnant	4	6	1	-	-	-	-	2
Saliva sample[1]								
Measured	69	75	81	84	82	80	75	78
No nurse visit[b]	31	25	19	16	18	20	24	22
Refused/not obtained	0	0	0	0	0	0	1	0
Blood sample[1]								
Blood sample taken	41	57	67	73	69	66	61	63
Unsuccessful attempt at sample	4	4	5	4	5	2	4	4
Ineligible – pregnant/medical grounds	8	9	4	3	4	4	5	
Ineligible – minors not asked for sample	9	-	-	-	-	-	-	1
Refused	13	10	7	6	6	10	8	8
No nurse visit[b]	25	19	17	15	16	18	22	18
Demi-span[2]								
Measured						82	77	79
No nurse visit[b]						18	22	20
Refused/not attempted						1	1	1
Bases								
[1] *Women aged 16 and over in co-operating households*	*1132*	*1714*	*1626*	*1530*	*1193*	*995*	*922*	*9112*
[2] *Women aged 65 and over in co-operating households*						*995*	*922*	*1917*

[a] Includes non-responders to interview as well as those refusing measurement.

[b] Includes non-responders to interview.

Table 8.8

Boys in co-operating households: response to the stages of the survey, by age

Eligible boys aged 2-15 in co-operating households					1998
Individual response	**Age**				**Total**
	2-4	5-6	7-10	11-15	
	%	%	%	%	%
Interviewed[1]					
Interviewed	98	99	98	92	96
Not-contacted/refused	2	1	2	8	4
Height[1]					
Measured	92	96	95	90	93
Measurement not attempted	4	2	2	0	2
Not-contacted/refused[a]	3	2	3	10	5
Weight[1]					
Measured	90	95	93	89	92
Measurement not attempted	6	3	3	1	3
Not-contacted/refused[a]	3	2	3	10	5
Nurse visit[1]					
Co-operated with nurse visit	84	86	85	79	83
Not interviewed	2	1	2	8	4
Refused/no contact at nurse visit	14	14	13	12	13
Mid-upper arm circumference[1]					
Measured	82	85	84	79	82
No nurse visit[b]	16	14	15	21	17
Refused/not obtained	2	1	1	0	1
Saliva sample[2]					
Saliva sample taken		80	84	79	81
No nurse visit[b]		15	15	21	17
Refused/not obtained		5	1	1	2
Blood pressure[3]					
Measured		79	84	79	81
No nurse visit[b]		14	15	21	17
Refused/not obtained		7	1	1	2
Blood sample[4]					
Blood sample taken				48	48
Unsuccessful attempt at sample				5	5
Ineligible – medical grounds				4	4
Refused				25	25
No nurse visit[b]				19	19
Bases					
[1] All eligible boys in co-co-operating households	448	284	596	651	1979
[2] Eligible boys aged 4-15 in co-operating households		423	596	651	1670
[3] Eligible boys aged 5-15 in co-operating households		284	596	651	1531
[4] Eligible boys aged 11-15 in co-operating households where blood samples were taken				330	330

[a] Includes non-responders to interview as well as those refusing measurement.

[b] Includes non-responders to interview.

Table 8.9

Girls in co-operating households: response to the stages of the survey, by age

Eligible girls aged 2-15 in co-operating households · *1998*

Individual response	Age				Total
	2-4	5-6	7-10	11-15	
	%	%	%	%	%
Interviewed[1]					
Interviewed	99	96	97	96	97
Not-contacted/refused	1	4	3	4	3
Height[1]					
Measured	91	90	92	92	91
Measurement not attempted	5	5	3	1	3
Not-contacted/refused[a]	5	5	5	7	6
Weight[1]					
Measured	93	88	91	90	91
Measurement not attempted	3	7	4	2	4
Not-contacted/refused[a]	4	5	4	8	6
Nurse visit[1]					
Co-operated with nurse visit	86	81	85	80	83
Not interviewed	1	4	3	4	3
Refused/no contact at nurse visit	13	15	13	16	14
Mid-upper arm circumference[1]					
Measured	82	81	85	80	82
No nurse visit[b]	14	19	15	20	17
Refused/not obtained	4	0	0	0	1
Saliva sample[2]					
Saliva sample taken		79	84	79	81
No nurse visit[b]		17	15	20	18
Refused/not obtained		4	1	1	2
Blood pressure[3]					
Measured		79	84	79	81
No nurse visit[b]		19	15	20	18
Refused/not obtained		2	1	1	1
Blood sample[4]					
Blood sample taken				32	32
Unsuccessful attempt at sample				8	8
Ineligible – medical grounds				5	5
Refused				34	34
No nurse visit[b]				20	20
Bases					
[1] *All eligible girls in co-operating households*	408	304	536	650	1898
[2] *Eligible girls aged 4-15 in co-operating households*		438	536	650	1624
[3] *Eligible girls aged 5-15 in co-operating households*		304	536	650	1490
[4] *Eligible girls aged 11-15 in co-operating households where blood samples were taken*				325	325

[a] Includes non-responders to interview as well as those refusing measurement.

[b] Includes non-responders to interview.

Table 8.10

True standard errors and 95% confidence intervals for CVD variables

Base	Characteristic	% (p)	Sample size	True standard error	95% confidence interval	1998 Deft
	CVD conditions					
Men	Ever had angina	5.6	404	0.28	5.1 - 6.2	1.01
	Ever had heart attack	4.5	323	0.26	4.0 - 5.0	1.05
	Ever had heart murmur	3.5	249	0.23	3.0 - 3.9	1.05
	Ever had abnormal heart rhythm	7.8	559	0.32	7.2 - 8.4	1.01
	Ever had other heart trouble	1.8	130	0.16	1.5 - 2.1	0.99
	Ever had stroke	2.4	173	0.19	2.0 - 2.8	1.02
	Ever had diabetes	3.4	241	0.23	2.9 - 3.8	1.07
Women	Ever had angina	4.2	361	0.22	3.7 - 4.6	1.03
	Ever had heart attack	2.1	179	0.15	1.8 - 2.4	1.01
	Ever had heart murmur	4.0	351	0.22	3.6 - 4.5	1.02
	Ever had irregular heart rhythm	7.9	685	0.32	7.2 - 8.5	1.13
	Ever had other heart trouble	1.7	145	0.14	1.4 - 1.9	1.05
	Ever had stroke	2.2	194	0.16	1.9 - 2.5	1.01
	Ever had diabetes	3.1	267	0.19	2.7 - 3.4	1.01
Men	Had cardiovascular condition	27.9	2008	0.54	26.9 - 29.0	1.01
	Had IHD (angina or heart attack)	7.1	508	0.32	6.4 - 7.7	1.07
	Had CVD (angina, heart attack or stroke)	8.5	612	0.35	7.8 - 9.2	1.05
Women	Had cardiovascular condition	27.8	2415	0.49	26.8 - 28.7	1.02
	Had IHD (angina or heart attack)	4.6	402	0.23	4.2 - 5.1	1.01
	Had CVD (angina, heart attack or stroke)	6.2	540	0.25	5.7 - 6.7	0.98
	Severity of CVD conditions					
Men	Only heart murmur, irregular heart rhythm or other heart trouble	3.5	250	0.23	3.0 - 3.9	1.05
	Only high blood pressure or diabetes	16.0	1149	0.43	15.1 - 16.8	0.99
	Angina but not heart attack or stroke	2.6	184	0.18	2.2 - 2.9	0.95
	Heart attack or stroke	6.0	428	0.29	5.4 - 6.5	1.04
	None of these	72.0	5178	0.53	71.0 - 73.1	1.01
Women	Only heart murmur, irregular heart rhythm or other heart trouble	4.2	369	0.21	3.8 - 4.7	0.99
	Only high blood pressure or diabetes	17.4	1512	0.41	16.6 - 18.2	1.00
	Angina but not heart attack or stroke	2.5	215	0.18	2.1 - 2.8	1.08
	Heart attack or stroke	3.7	325	0.19	3.4 - 4.1	0.95
	None of these	72.2	6286	0.49	71.2 - 73.2	1.02

Table 8.11

True standard errors and 95% confidence intervals for alcohol consumption variables

1998

Base	Characteristic	Mean/%	Sample size	True standard error	95% confidence interval	Deft
	Number of alcohol units consumed per week					
Men	Mean number of alcohol units usually consumed per week	18.0	7129	0.30	17.4-18.6	1.09
Women	Mean number of alcohol units usually consumed per week	7.2	8666	0.13	6.9-7.4	1.07
	Levels exceeded					
Men	Drink more than 21 units a week (%)	30.9	7129	0.60	29.7 - 32.1	1.09
Women	Drink more than 14 units a week (%)	17.6	8666	0.44	16.7 - 18.4	1.08

Table 8.12

True standard errors and 95% confidence intervals for cigarette smoking variables

1998

Base	Characteristic	Mean/%	Sample size	True standard error	95% confidence interval	Deft
	Number of cigarettes smoked					
Men	Mean number of cigarettes smoked per smoker per day (current smokers)	15.6	2018	0.23	15.2-16.1	1.04
Women	Mean number of cigarettes smoked per smoker per day (current smokers)	13.6	2337	0.18	13.3-14.0	1.04
Men	Per capita mean number of cigarettes per day	4.4	7156	0.11	4.2-4.6	1.08
Women	Per capita mean number of cigarettes per day	3.7	8683	0.09	3.5-3.8	1.14
	Cigarette smoking status					
Men	Used to smoke cigarettes regularly (%)	31.4	7163	0.53	30.3-32.4	0.97
	Current cigarette smoker (%)	28.3	7163	0.60	27.1-29.4	1.13 *
	Never smoked cigarettes/used to smoke cigarettes occasionally (%)	40.4	7163	0.63	39.1-41.6	1.08
Women	Used to smoke cigarettes regularly (%)	21.2	8694	0.46	20.3-22.2	1.05
	Current cigarette smoker (%)	27.0	8694	0.54	25.9-28.0	1.13
	Never smoked cigarettes/used to smoke cigarettes occasionally (%)	51.8	8694	0.59	50.6-52.9	1.11

Table 8.13

True standard errors and 95% confidence intervals for anthropometric measurement variables

1998

Base	Characteristic	Mean/%	Sample size	True standard error	95% confidence interval	Deft
	Height					
Men	Mean height (cm)	174.4	6801	0.10	174.2-174.6	1.13
Women	Mean height (cm)	161.0	8204	0.09	160.9-161.2	1.16
	Weight					
Men	Mean weight (kg)	80.8	6709	0.19	80.4-81.1	1.09
Women	Mean weight (kg)	68.3	7887	0.16	68.0-68.6	1.03
	Body mass index					
Men	Mean body mass index (kg/m^2)	26.5	6600	0.05	26.4-26.6	1.08
Women	Mean body mass index (kg/m^2)	26.4	7730	0.06	26.2-26.5	1.04
Men	20 kg/m^2 or less (%)	3.6	6600	0.24	3.2-4.1	1.02
	Over 20-25 kg/m^2 (%)	33.5	6600	0.59	32.4-34.7	1.02
	Over 25-30 kg/m^2 (%)	45.5	6600	0.63	44.3-46.8	1.03
	Over 30 kg/m^2 (%)	17.3	6600	0.49	16.4-18.3	1.05
Women	20 kg/m^2 or less (%)	6.6	7730	0.30	6.0-7.2	1.06
	Over 20-25 kg/m^2 (%)	40.0	7730	0.61	38.8-41.2	1.10
	Over 25-30 kg/m^2 (%)	32.1	7730	0.54	31.1-33.2	1.02
	Over 30 kg/m^2 (%)	21.2	7730	0.46	20.3-22.1	1.00
	Waist and hip					
Men	Mean waist (cm)	94.4	6099	0.18	94.0 - 94.7	1.20
	Mean hip (cm)	103.7	6107	0.13	103.4 - 103.9	1.25
	Mean waist/hip ratio	0.9	6095	0.00	0.9 - 0.9	1.20
Women	Mean waist (cm)	83.2	7160	0.18	82.9 - 83.5	1.19
	Mean hip (cm)	104.2	7151	0.14	103.9 - 104.5	1.14
	Mean waist/hip ratio	0.8	7140	0.00	0.8 - 0.8	1.27
	Demi-span					
Men[a]	Mean demi-span (cm)	80.6	1159	0.12	80.4 - 80.9	1.03
Women[a]	Mean demi-span (cm)	73.2	1455	0.10	73.0 - 73.4	1.01

[a] Aged 65 and over only.

Table 8.14

True standard errors and 95% confidence intervals for blood pressure measurement variables

Base	Characteristic	Mean/%	Sample size	True standard error	95% confidence interval	1998 Deft
Men	Mean systolic blood pressure	136.8	7193	0.26	136.3-137.3	1.06
	Mean diastolic blood pressure	76.2	7193	0.19	75.8-76.6	1.11
	% with high blood pressure (1998 definition)	40.8	7193	0.68	39.5 - 42.1	1.18
	% with high blood pressure (pre-1998 definition)	18.4	7913	0.51	17.4-19.4	1.12
Women	Mean systolic blood pressure	132.5	8715	0.28	132.0-133.1	1.07
	Mean diastolic blood pressure	72.3	8715	0.17	71.9-72.6	1.14
	% with high blood pressure (1998 definition)	32.9	8715	0.58	31.8 - 34.1	1.16
	% with high blood pressure (pre-1998 definition)	18.4	8715	0.49	17.5-19.4	1.18

Table 8.15

True standard errors and 95% confidence intervals for blood analyte variables

Base	Characteristic	Mean/%	Sample size	True standard error	95% confidence interval	1998 Deft
	Cotinine					
Men	0<15 (ng/ml) (%)	67.5	5054	0.74	66.1-69.0	1.12
	15+ (ng/ml) (%)	32.5	5054	0.74	31.0-33.9	1.12
Women	0<15 (ng/ml) (%)	72.9	5478	0.64	71.6-74.1	1.07
	15+ (ng/ml) (%)	27.1	5478	0.64	25.9-28.4	1.07
	Total cholesterol					
Men	Mean total cholesterol (mmol/l)	5.5	4874	0.02	5.4 - 5.5	0.96
Women	Mean total cholesterol (mmol/l)	5.6	5458	0.02	5.5 - 5.6	1.08
	HDL-cholesterol					
Men	Mean HDL-cholesterol (mmol/l)	1.3	4862	0.01	1.3 - 1.3	0.96
Women	Mean HDL-cholesterol (mmol/l)	1.6	5442	0.01	1.6 - 1.6	1.08
	Ferritin					
Men	Mean ferritin (ng/ml)	110.8	4892	1.47	107.9 - 113.7	1.01
Women	Mean ferritin (ng/ml)	53.6	5378	0.73	52.2 - 55.0	0.95
	Haemoglobin					
Men	Mean haemoglobin (g/dl)	14.7	4948	0.02	14.7 - 14.8	0.88
Women	Mean haemoglobin (g/dl)	13.2	5472	0.01	13.2 - 13.2	0.97
	Fibrinogen					
Men	Mean fibrinogen (g/l)	2.6	4480	0.01	2.6 - 2.6	0.92
Women	Mean fibrinogen (g/l)	2.8	4926	0.01	2.8 - 2.8	0.98
	C-reactive protein					
Men	Mean C-reactive protein (mg/l)	3.0	4938	0.08	2.9 - 3.2	0.93
Women	Mean C-reactive protein (mg/l)	3.6	5502	0.09	3.4 - 3.8	1.06

Table 8.16

True standard errors and 95% confidence intervals for summary physical activity level variable

Base	Characteristic	% (p)	Sample size	True standard error	95% confidence interval	*1998* Deft
	Summary physical activity level					
Men	Group 1 – Low	34.6	7178	0.57	33.5-35.7	1.01
	Group 2 – Medium	28.0	7178	0.54	27.0-29.1	1.02
	Group 3 – High	37.4	7178	0.58	36.2-38.5	1.02
Women	Group 1 – Low	40.9	8699	0.52	39.8-41.9	1.00
	Group 2 – Medium	34.4	8699	0.53	33.3-35.4	1.04
	Group 3 – High	24.8	8699	0.50	23.8-25.8	1.08

Table 8.17

True standard errors and 95% confidence intervals for general health variables

Base	Characteristic	% (p)	Sample size	True standard error	95% confidence interval	*1998* Deft
	Longstanding illness/acute sickness					
Men	Longstanding illness/disability	43.8	7186	0.69	42.5-45.2	1.17
	Limiting longstanding illness	25.3	7186	0.58	24.2-26.4	1.13
	Self-reported acute sickness	14.8	7186	0.43	14.0-15.7	1.04
Women	Longstanding illness/disability	43.8	8712	0.61	42.6-45.0	1.15
	Limiting longstanding illness	26.8	8712	0.54	25.8-27.9	1.13
	Self-reported acute sickness	18.6	8712	0.44	17.7-19.4	1.06
	Self-reported general health					
Men	Very good/Good	74.7	7192	0.59	73.5-75.8	1.15
	Fair	18.8	7192	0.50	17.8-19.8	1.09
	Bad/Very bad	6.6	7192	0.32	5.9-7.2	1.09
Women	Very good/Good	73.3	8715	0.51	72.3-74.3	1.07
	Fair	19.9	8715	0.45	19.0-20.8	1.04
	Bad/Very bad	6.8	8715	0.28	6.3-7.4	
	Perceived social support					
Men	No lack	54.8	6822	0.63	53.5 - 56.0	1.05
	Some lack	29.1	6822	0.54	28.0 - 30.1	0.98
	Severe lack	16.1	6822	0.47	15.2 - 17.1	1.04
Women	No lack	64.5	8277	0.56	63.4 - 65.6	1.07
	Some lack	24.0	8277	0.49	23.1 - 25.0	1.05
	Severe lack	11.5	8277	0.38	10.7 - 12.2	1.09
	GHQ12 score					
Men	0	63.4	6802	0.65	62.1 - 64.6	1.11
	1-3	24.0	6802	0.50	23.0 - 25.0	0.97
	4 or more	12.6	6802	0.43	11.8 - 13.5	1.07
Women	0	54.7	8254	0.60	53.6 - 55.9	1.09
	1-3	27.2	8254	0.49	26.2 - 28.1	1.00
	4 or more	18.1	8254	0.44	17.2 - 19.0	1.03

Table 8.18

True standard errors and 95% confidence intervals for use of health services and medication variables

Base	Characteristic	% (p)	Sample size	True standard error	95% confidence interval	*1998* Deft
Men	Any inpatient stay in last 12 months	8.1	7185	0.33	7.5 - 8.8	1.03
Women	Any inpatient stay in last 12 months	10.7	8709	0.35	10.0 - 11.4	1.05
Men	NHS GP consultations in last 2 weeks	0.2	7188	0.01	0.1 - 0.2	1.04
Women	NHS GP consultations in last 2 weeks	0.2	8713	0.01	0.2 - 0.2	1.03
Men	Prescribed medicines	1.0	6164	0.02	1.0 - 1.0	1.06
Women	Prescribed medicines	1.3	7420	0.02	1.2 - 1.3	1.04
Women	Ever been on HRT	15.6	8015	0.43	14.7 - 16.4	1.06

Table 8.19

Age distribution of Health Survey responding adult sample compared to mid-1998 population estimates for England

Responding adults aged 16 and over   *1998*

Age	At interview %	At nurse visit %	Providing blood sample %	Mid-1998 population estimates[a] %
Men				
16-24	12	11	8	14
25-34	19	18	18	21
35-44	18	18	19	19
45-54	18	18	19	17
55-64	14	14	15	13
65-74	12	12	12	10
75 and over	8	8	8	7
Women				
16-24	12	11	8	13
25-34	19	19	17	19
35-44	18	18	19	17
45-54	17	17	20	16
55-64	13	13	14	12
65-74	11	11	12	11
75 and over	10	10	10	12
Bases				
Men	*7193*	*6165*	*5122*	*19206*
Women	*8715*	*7421*	*5729*	*20206*

[a] *Population Estimates, England and Wales, mid-1998* (Series PE no 1). Office for National Statistics, 1998. Base figures shown in thousands.

Table 8.20

Ethnic origin of adults responding to interview, nurse visit and blood sample

Responding adults aged 16 and over   *1998*

Ethnic group	Health Survey interviewed adults	Health Survey adults who saw the nurse	Health Survey adults who provided a blood sample
	%	%	%
White	94.1	94.6	95.1
Indian	1.5	1.4	1.4
Pakistani	0.9	0.8	0.7
Bangladeshi	0.3	0.3	0.3
Black (Caribbean/ African/Other)	1.9	1.7	1.4
Other	1.3	1.2	1.1
Bases	*15881*	*13573*	*10761*

Table 8.21

Internal quality control results for total cholesterol

1998

Date	Level (mmol/l) Target/ Achieved	Acceptable Range	S.D. (mmol/l) Achieved	C.V (%) Achieved
January 1998	3.2/3.17	3.1-3.3	0.05	1.4
	4.9/4.89	4.8-5.0	0.07	1.5
	6.8/6.82	6.7-7.0	0.07	1.0
February	3.2/3.17	3.1-3.3	0.04	1.3
	4.9/4.89	4.8-5.0	0.05	0.9
	6.8/6.81	6.7-7.0	0.07	1.0
March	3.2/3.17	3.1-3.3	0.05	1.5
	4.9/4.88	4.8-5.0	0.07	1.4
	6.8/6.78	6.7-7.0	0.10	1.5
April	3.2/3.18	3.1-3.3	0.04	1.2
	4.9/4.89	4.8-5.0	0.05	0.9
	6.8/6.80	6.7-7.0	0.06	1.0
May	3.2/3.18	3.1-3.3	0.05	1.5
	4.9/4.90	4.8-5.0	0.07	1.4
	6.8/6.80	6.7-7.0	0.26	1.3
June	3.2/3.16	3.1-3.3	0.05	1.5
	4.9/4.87	4.8-5.0	0.07	1.4
	6.8/6.76	6.7-7.0	0.09	1.4
July	3.2/3.19	3.1-3.3	0.04	1.3
	4.9/4.90	4.8-5.0	0.07	1.5
	6.8/6.83	6.7-7.0	0.09	1.3
August	2.9/2.92	2.8-3.0	0.06	2.1
	4.6/4.64	4.5-4.7	0.07	1.4
	6.4/6.34	6.2-6.5	0.07	1.1
September	2.9/2.92	2.8-3.0	0.03	0.9
	4.6/4.64	4.5-4.7	0.04	0.9
	6.4/6.33	6.2-6.5	0.05	0.9
October	2.9/2.92	2.8-3.0	0.04	1.5
	4.6/4.66	4.5-4.7	0.06	1.3
	6.4/6.37	6.2-6.5	0.08	1.3
November	2.9/2.91	2.8-3.0	0.04	1.1
	4.6/4.64	4.5-4.7	0.10	2.1
	6.4/6.34	6.2-6.5	0.08	1.2
December	2.9/2.92	2.8-3.0	0.05	1.7
	4.6/4.65	4.5-4.7	0.06	1.0
	6.4/6.35	6.2-6.5	0.08	1.0
January 1999	2.9/2.91	2.8-3.0	0.05	1.6
	4.6/4.65	4.5-4.7	0.06	1.4
	6.4/6.37	6.2-6.5	0.08	1.3
February	2.9/2.91	2.8-3.0	0.05	1.6
	4.6/4.62	4.5-4.7	0.19	4.2
	6.4/6.33	6.2-6.5	0.09	1.4

Table 8.22

Internal quality control results for HDL-cholesterol

Date	Level (mmol/l) Target/ Achieved	Acceptable Range	S.D. (mmol/l) Achieved	C.V (%) Achieved 1998
January 1998	2.1/2.24	1.8-2.4	0.16	7.0
February	2.1/2.18	1.8-2.4	0.17	7.9
March	2.1/2.15	1.8-2.4	0.18	8.4
April	2.1/2.03	1.8-2.4	0.18	9.1
May	1.8/1.80	1.6-2.0	0.08	4.4
June	1.8/1.82	1.6-2.0	0.10	5.4
July	1.8/1.82	1.6-2.0	0.13	7.2
August	1.8/1.81	1.6-2.0	0.11	6.2
September	1.8/1.85	1.6-2.0	0.08	4.5
October	1.8/1.77	1.6-2.0	0.09	5.0
November	1.8/1.80	1.6-2.0	0.06	3.5
December	1.8/1.75	1.6-2.0	0.11	6.5
January 1999	1.8/1.82	1.6-2.0	0.09	4.7
February	1.8/1.85	1.6-2.0	0.12	6.7

Table 8.23

Internal quality control results for C-reactive protein (CRP)

Date	Level (mg/l) Target/ Achieved	Acceptable Range	S.D. (mg/l) Achieved	C.V (%) Achieved 1998
February 1998				
Low	1.7/1.80	1.6-1.9	0.08	4.5
1	16.8/16.99	15.6-18.1	0.68	4.0
2	40.4/41.38	37.9-41.6	1.25	3.0
3	91.0/95.85	83.3-98.7	4.44	4.6
March				
Low	1.7/1.68	1.6-1.9	0.04	2.4
1	16.8/16.92	15.6-18.1	0.64	3.8
2	40.4/40.58	37.9-41.6	1.15	2.8
3	91.0/92.71	83.3-98.7	4.61	5.0
April				
Low	1.7/1.70	1.6-1.9	0.06	3.7
1	16.8/16.81	15.6-18.1	0.64	3.8
2	40.4/40.23	37.9-41.6	1.32	3.3
3	91.0/90.39	83.3-98.7	3.38	3.7
May				
Low	1.7/1.76	1.6-1.9	0.07	4.2
1	15.8/15.72	14.4-17.1	0.65	4.1
2	27.1/27.17	25.0-29.2	1.05	3.9
3	37.6/37.67	35.4-39.8	1.16	3.1
June				
Low	1.7/1.79	1.6-1.9	0.09	5.2
1	15.8/15.93	14.4-17.1	0.61	3.8
2	27.1/27.64	25.0-29.2	1.00	3.6
3	37.6/38.27	35.4-39.8	1.07	2.8
July				
Low	1.7/1.76	1.6-1.9	0.09	5.1
1	15.8/15.68	14.4-17.1	0.45	2.9
2	27.1/27.35	25.0-29.2	0.62	2.3
3	37.6/38.30	35.4-39.8	1.02	2.7
August				
Low	1.7/1.79	1.6-1.9	0.09	5.1
1	15.8/15.87	14.4-17.1	0.43	2.7
2	27.1/27.91	25.0-29.2	0.65	2.3
3	37.6/39.19	35.4-39.8	1.11	2.8
September				
Low	1.7/1.70	1.6-1.9	0.08	4.7
1	15.8/15.62	14.4-17.1	0.59	3.8
2	27.1/27.79	25.0-29.2	0.87	2.6
3	37.6/39.24	35.4-39.8	1.06	2.7
October				
Low	1.7/1.69	1.6-1.9	0.07	3.9
1	15.8/15.32	14.4-17.1	0.44	2.8
2	27.1/27.58	25.0-29.2	0.69	2.5
3	37.6/38.76	35.4-39.8	1.15	3.0
November				
Low	1.7/1.69	1.6-1.9	0.08	4.8
1	15.8/15.34	14.4-17.1	0.57	3.7
2	27.1/27.57	25.0-29.2	0.83	3.0
3	37.6/38.69	35.4-39.8	1.10	2.8

continued...

Table 8.23 *continued*

	1998			
Date	Level (mg/l) Target/ Achieved	Acceptable Range	S.D. (mg/l) Achieved	C.V (%) Achieved
December				
Low	1.70/1.69	1.60-1.90	0.08	4.8
1	15.80/15.50	14.40-17.10	0.64	4.2
2	27.10/27.41	25.00-29.20	1.06	3.9
3	37.60/38.41	35.40-39.80	1.31	3.4
January 1999				
Low	1.50/1.48	1.30-1.60	0.08	5.6
1	15.80/14.95	14.40-17.10	0.71	4.8
2	27.10/26.61	25.00-29.20	1.02	3.8
3	37.60/37.47	35.40-39.80	1.32	3.5
February				
Low	1.50/1.50	1.30-1.60	0.07	4.4
1	15.80/15.85	14.40-17.10	0.52	3.3
2	27.10/27.59	25.00-29.20	0.83	3.0
3	37.60/38.11	35.40-39.80	1.21	3.2

Table 8.24

Internal quality control results for ferritin

	1998			
Date	Level (ng/ml) Target/ Achieved	Acceptable Range	S.D. (ng/ml) Achieved	C.V (%) Achieved
February 1998				
Low	20.00/20.83	17.4-22.6	1.10	5.30
Normal	150.00/154.07	130-170	5.66	3.68
High	400.00/420.21	348-452	27.67	6.59
March				
Low	20.00/20.56	17.4-22.6	0.75	3.67
Normal	150.00/154.00	130-170	5.32	3.46
High	400.00/418.59	348-452	23.92	5.72
April				
Low	20.00/20.44	17.4-22.6	1.40	6.87
Normal	150.00/149.81	130-170	4.67	3.11
High	400.00/419.70	348-452	19.87	4.74
May				
Low	20.00/20.25	17.4-22.6	1.20	5.94
Normal	150.00/153.10	130-170	6.30	4.12
High	400.00/411.73	348-452	21.77	5.29
June				
Low	20.00/20.19	17.4-22.6	0.96	4.74
Normal	150.00/153.51	130-170	6.30	4.11
High	400.00/412.06	348-452	15.33	3.72
July				
Low	20.00/20.05	17.4-22.6	0.92	4.58
Normal	150.00/150.52	130-170	7.12	4.73
High	400.00/428.79	348-452	29.69	6.92
August				
Low	20.00/20.39	17.4-22.6	1.24	6.09
Normal	150.00/151.15	130-170	5.41	3.58
High	400.00/417.10	348-452	21.43	5.14
September				
Low	20.00/20.63	17.4-22.6	1.04	5.06
Normal	150.00/154.29	130-170	6.91	4.48
High	400.00/422.51	348-452	20.17	4.77
October				
Low	20.00/20.43	17.4-22.6	2.15	10.52
Normal	150.00/159.49	130-170	6.09	3.82
High	400.00/412.13	348-452	19.99	4.85
December				
Low	20.00/19.85	17.4-22.6	1.60	8.07
Normal	150.00/150.62	130.0-170.0	7.80	5.18
High	400.00/385.44	348.0-452.0	25.74	6.68
January 1999				
Low	20.00/19.76	17.4-22.6	1.02	5.16
Normal	150.00/153.03	130.0-170.0	6.07	3.97
High	400.00/396.07	348.0-452.0	23.55	5.95
February				
Low	20.00/20.59	17.4-22.6	1.54	7.46
Normal	150.00/152.73	130.0-170.0	6.74	4.41
High	400.00/398.31	348.0-452.0	26.70	6.70

Table 8.25

Internal quality control results for haemoglobin

1998

Date	Level (g/dl) Target/ Achieved	Acceptable Range	S.D. (g/dl) Achieved	C.V (%) Achieved
January 1998	5.3[a]/5.32	5.0-5.6	0.04	0.84
	12.8[b]/12.96	12.4-13.2	0.10	0.74
	16.4[c]/16.62	15.8-17.0	0.23	1.39
	16.4[d]/16.60	15.8-17.0	0.24	1.48
February	5.3[a]/5.36	5.0-5.6	0.09	1.74
	12.8[b]/13.07	12.4-13.2	0.09	0.69
	16.4[c]/16.72	15.8-17.0	0.17	1.01
	16.4[d]/16.58	15.8-17.0	0.13	0.79
	5.2[a]/5.36	4.9-5.5	0.10	1.82
	12.5[b]/12.93	12.1-12.9	0.08	0.63
	16.5[c]/16.93	15.9-17.1	0.23	1.33
	16.5[d]/16.51	15.9-17.1	0.17	1.01
March	5.2[a]/5.31	4.9-5.5	0.10	1.87
	12.5[b]/12.71	12.1-12.9	0.19	1.46
	16.5[c]/16.58	15.9-17.1	0.36	2.14
	16.5[d]/16.41	15.9-17.1	0.22	1.33
	16.7[d]/16.71	16.3-17.1	0.21	1.26
April	5.2[a]/5.30	4.9-5.5	0.00	0.00
	12.5[b]/12.80	12.1-12.9	0.00	0.00
	16.5[c]/16.65	15.9-17.1	0.07	0.42
	16.7[d]/16.60	16.3-17.1	0.20	1.20
	5.2[a]/5.25	4.9-5.5	0.13	2.46
	12.9[b]/13.10	12.5-13.3	0.13	1.01
	16.4[c]/16.57	15.8-17.0	0.17	1.00
	16.3[d]/16.00	15.7-16.9	0.23	1.44
May	5.2[a]/5.4	4.9-5.5	na	na
	12.9[b]/13.10	12.5-13.3	0.00	0.00
	16.4[c]/16.44	15.8-17.0	0.09	0.56
	16.3[d]/16.00	15.7-16.9	0.29	1.79
	5.1[a]/5.18	4.8-5.4	0.09	1.79
	12.8[b]/12.99	12.4-13.2	0.10	0.80
	16.3[c]/16.42	15.7-16.9	0.20	1.21
	5.2[a]/5.13	4.9-5.5	0.06	1.12
	12.9[b]/12.73	12.5-13.3	0.21	1.63
June	5.2[a]/4.99	4.9-5.5	0.18	3.67
	12.9[b]/12.82	12.5-13.3	0.22	1.69
	16.3[c]/16.30	15.7-16.9	0.24	1.50
	16.3[d]/16.25	15.7-16.9	0.22	1.33
	5.1[a]/4.98	4.8-5.4	0.19	3.81
	12.4[b]/12.64	12.0-12.8	0.14	1.08
	16.2[c]/16.26	15.6-16.8	0.24	1.46
	16.2[d]/16.13	15.6-16.8	0.33	2.05
July	5.1[a]/4.95	4.8-5.4	0.14	2.74
	12.4[b]/12.51	12.0-12.8	0.17	1.33
	16.2[c]/16.53	15.6-16.8	0.21	1.24
	16.2[d]/15.98	15.6-16.8	0.30	1.88
	16.1[c]/16.13	15.5-16.7	0.17	1.05
	16.1[d]/16.08	15.5-16.7	0.15	0.92

[a] Coulter Analyser STKSA, using abnormal control II.

[b] Coulter Analyser STKSA, using abnormal control I.

[c] Coulter Analyser STKSA, using normal control.

[d] Coulter Analyser STKSB, using normal control.

continued…

Table 8.25 continued

1998

Date	Level (g/dl) Target/ Achieved	Acceptable Range	S.D. (g/dl) Achieved	C.V (%) Achieved
August	5.1[a]/5.00	4.8-5.4	0.09	1.79
	12.4[b]/12.55	12.0-12.8	0.13	1.03
	16.1[c]/16.16	15.5-16.7	0.17	1.04
	16.1[d]/15.92	15.5-16.7	0.24	1.50
	5.2[a]/5.22	4.9-5.5	0.08	1.51
	12.8[b]/12.96	12.4-13.2	0.13	1.00
	16.2[c]/16.36	15.6-16.8	0.18	1.10
	16.2[d]/16.11	15.6-16.8	0.17	1.04
September	5.2[a]/5.23	4.9-5.5	0.10	1.83
	12.8[b]/12.50	12.4-13.2	0.57	4.53
	16.2[c]/16.27	15.6-16.8	0.29	1.18
	16.2[d]/16.36	15.6-16.8	0.18	1.11
	5.1[a]/5.14	4.8-5.4	0.07	1.30
	12.6[b]/12.59	12.2-13.0	0.12	0.98
	16.3[c]/16.30	15.7-16.9	0.20	1.20
	16.3[d]/16.15	15.7-16.9	0.33	2.07
October	5.1[a]/5.07	4.8-5.4	0.16	3.25
	12.6[b]/12.59	12.2-13.0	0.18	1.40
	16.3[c]/16.25	15.7-16.9	0.25	1.54
	16.3[d]/16.09	15.7-16.9	0.14	0.90
November	5.0[a]/4.90	4.7-5.3	0.14	2.80
	12.7[b]/12.59	12.3-13.1	0.22	1.73
	16.3[c]/15.94	15.7-16.9	0.34	2.14
	16.3[d]/16.08	15.7-16.9	0.23	1.41
December	5.0[a]/4.96	4.7-5.3	0.09	1.85
	12.7[b]/12.78	12.3-13.1	0.28	2.16
	16.3[c]/16.09	15.7-16.9	0.39	2.43
	16.3[d]/16.19	15.7-16.9	0.25	1.57
	5.1[a]/5.04	4.8-5.4	0.11	2.22
	12.8[b]/12.80	12.4-13.2	0.16	1.24
	16.4[c]/16.41	15.8-17.0	0.15	0.92
	16.5[d]/16.26	15.9-17.1	0.08	0.48
January 1999	5.1[a]/5.17	4.8-5.4	0.12	2.26
	12.8[b]/12.81	12.4-13.2	0.10	0.77
	16.4[c]/16.43	15.8-17.0	0.38	2.31
	16.5[d]/16.28	15.9-17.1	0.14	0.87
	12.7[b]/12.73	12.3-13.1	0.06	0.51
	16.3[c]/16.37	15.7-16.9	0.19	1.19
	16.2[d]/16.26	15.6-16.8	0.16	1.00
February	5.0[a]/5.15	4.7-5.3	0.13	2.49
	12.8[b]/12.74	12.4-13.2	0.09	0.68
	16.4[c]/16.31	15.8-17.0	0.15	0.90
	16.4[d]/16.21	15.8-17.0	0.15	0.94
	5.0[a]/5.19	4.7-5.3	0.08	1.51
	12.8[b]/12.84	12.4-13.2	0.18	1.41
	16.4[c]/16.20	15.8-17.0	0.32	1.98
	16.4[d]/16.25	15.8-17.0	0.13	0.81

[a] Coulter Analyser STKSA, using abnormal control II.

[b] Coulter Analyser STKSA, using abnormal control I.

[c] Coulter Analyser STKSA, using normal control.

[d] Coulter Analyser STKSB, using normal control.

Table 8.26

Internal quality control results for fibrinogen

Date	Level (g/l) Target/ Achieved	Acceptable Range	S.D. (g/l) Achieved	C.V (%) Achieved 1998
March 1998				
Low	1.30/1.31	1.10-1.50	0.13	9.82
Normal	2.70/2.93	2.26-2.92	0.26	8.89
April				
Low	1.30/1.26	1.10-1.50	0.10	8.19
Normal	2.70/2.71	2.26-2.92	0.19	6.86
May				
Low	1.30/1.20	1.10-1.50	0.10	8.60
Normal	2.70/2.48	2.26-2.92	0.16	6.60
June				
Low	1.30/1.28	1.10-1.50	0.11	8.33
Normal	2.70/2.67	2.26-2.92	0.17	6.52
July				
Low	1.30/1.21	1.10-1.50	0.10	8.08
Normal	2.70/2.61	2.26-2.92	0.16	6.23
August				
Low	1.30/1.25	1.10-1.50	0.10	8.19
Normal	2.70/2.72	2.26-2.92	0.16	6.06
September				
Low	1.30/1.26	1.10-1.50	0.14	11.01
Normal	2.70/2.69	2.26-2.92	0.21	7.94
October				
Low	1.30/1.28	1.10-1.50	0.12	9.49
Normal	2.70/2.48	2.26-2.92	0.15	6.19
November				
Low	1.30/1.27	1.10-1.50	0.13	10.14
Normal	2.60/2.58	2.34-2.86	0.17	6.61
December				
Low	1.30/1.20	1.10-1.50	0.12	10.22
Normal	2.60/2.49	2.34-2.86	0.20	7.88
January 1999				
Low	1.30/1.33	1.10-1.50	0.11	8.16
Normal	2.60/2.66	2.34-2.86	0.21	8.06
February				
Low	1.30/1.28	1.10-1.50	0.12	9.40
Normal	2.60/2.63	2.34-2.86	0.20	7.52

Table 8.27

Internal quality results for cotinine

Date	Target/Achieved (ng/ml)	S.D. Achieved (ng/ml)	C.V Achieved (%) 1998
January 1998	0.50/0.47	0.09	19.02
	1.00/1.09	0.12	10.67
	5.00/5.09	0.25	4.84
	100.00/100.28	0.97	0.97
February	0.50/0.46	0.08	17.87
	1.00/0.99	0.13	13.05
	5.00/5.07	0.28	5.49
	100.00/99.96	1.74	1.74
	600.00/598.02	7.46	1.25
March	1.00/0.97	0.11	10.90
	5.00/5.03	0.22	4.31
	100.00/99.99	2.44	2.44
	600.00/597.68	7.12	1.19
April	1.00/0.96	0.12	12.56
	5.00/4.97	0.22	4.39
	100.00/99.51	2.40	2.42
	600.00/595.98	9.32	1.56
May	1.00/0.99	0.14	14.55
	5.00/4.92	0.21	4.22
	100.00/98.37	2.98	3.03
	600.00/593.18	8.84	1.49
June	1.00/1.02	0.12	11.77
	5.00/5.03	0.23	4.67
	100.00/99.71	3.20	3.21
	600.00/596.56	9.08	1.52
July	1.00/0.97	0.12	12.61
	5.00/5.00	0.24	4.89
	100.00/99.62	2.96	2.97
	400.00/402.17	11.04	2.74
	600.00/596.69	9.55	1.60
August	1.00/1.01	0.12	11.54
	5.00/5.00	0.24	4.80
	20.00/19.78	0.96	4.85
	100.00/99.95	2.32	2.32
	400.00/403.60	11.81	2.93
	600.00/594.74	17.27	2.90
September	1.00/0.96	0.10	10.85
	5.00/5.00	0.20	4.02
	20.00/19.80	0.79	3.98
	100.00/99.30	2.62	2.63
	400.00/401.67	8.77	2.18
	600.00/596.71	8.93	1.50
October	1.00/0.93	0.10	11.13
	5.00/4.91	0.21	4.30
	20.00/19.86	1.04	5.23
	100.00/98.96	2.92	2.95
	400.00/398.04	9.55	2.40
	600.00/594.17	7.22	1.22

continued...

Table 8.27 *continued*

Date	Target/Achieved (ng/ml)	S.D. Achieved (ng/ml)	C.V Achieved (%)
November	1.00/0.95	0.10	10.44
	5.00/4.96	0.25	5.01
	20.00/20.12	1.20	5.99
	100.00/100.22	2.86	2.86
	400.00/402.47	7.91	1.97
	600.00/600.38	8.11	1.35
December	1.00/0.99	0.11	11.21
	5.00/4.99	0.22	4.48
	20.00/20.15	0.65	3.21
	100.00/99.49	2.02	2.03
	400.00/402.51	7.90	1.96
	600.00/594.90	8.61	1.45
January 1999	1.00/0.97	0.11	11.12
	5.00/5.07	0.22	4.28
	20.00/20.44	0.60	2.94
	100.00/100.50	2.93	2.92
	400.00/403.15	9.43	2.34
	600.00/599.98	8.62	1.44
February 1999	1.00/0.99	0.07	7.55
	5.00/5.01	0.21	4.18
	20.00/20.01	0.70	3.49
	100.00/100.32	4.11	4.10
	400.00/402.26	10.05	2.50
	600.00/599.53	12.10	2.02

Table 8.28

External quality assessment results for total cholesterol

Date	Target value[a] (mmol/l)	Assayed value (mmol/l)
January 1998	3.12	3.1
February	2.24	2.1
	1.79	2.0
March	3.65	3.6
	3.18	3.1
	2.06	2.1
April	2.95	2.9
May	2.96	2.9
	3.10	3.1
June	2.75	2.8
	3.87	3.9
July	3.97	3.8
	1.76	2.1
August	3.65	3.6
	3.81	3.8
September	4.97	4.8
	3.61	3.5
October	2.75	2.7
	3.94	3.9
November	2.07	2.1
	3.66	3.6
	2.98	3.0
December	2.16	2.2
January 1999	3.97	3.9
	3.79	3.7
February	2.05	2.1
	2.97	3.0
March	3.99	4.0
	3.25	3.3

[a] Method trimmed mean.

Table 8.29

**External quality assessment results
for HDL-cholesterol**

Date	Target value[a] (mmol/l)	*1998* Assayed value (mmol/l)
January 1998	1.19	1.3
	0.94	1.1
	1.17	1.3
	1.16	1.3
February	1.16	1.2
	1.18	1.3
	1.81	1.9
	1.18	1.3
	1.16	1.3
March	1.19	1.3
	1.55	1.6
	1.37	1.5
	1.20	1.3
April	1.31	1.3
	1.28	1.3
	1.42	1.4
	1.42	1.4
	1.38	1.4
May	1.40	1.4
	1.22	1.3
	1.41	1.4
	1.29	1.3
	1.44	1.4
June	1.39	1.5
	1.19	1.3
	1.31	1.4
	1.57	1.6
July	1.40	1.6
	1.23	1.3
	1.22	1.4
	1.41	1.5
August	1.55	1.6
	1.28	1.3
	1.42	1.4
	1.41	1.4
	1.30	1.4
September	1.42	1.5
	1.27	1.4
	1.21	1.3
	1.39	1.5
October	1.38	1.4
	1.28	1.2
	1.36	1.4
	1.54	1.5
	1.19	1.2
November	1.19	1.10
	1.18	1.20
	1.53	1.50
	1.03	1.30

[a] Overall mean.

continued ...

Table 8.29 *continued*

Date	Target value[a] (mmol/l)	*1998* Assayed value (mmol/l)
December	1.19	1.20
	1.48	1.50
	1.58	1.60
	1.32	1.30
	1.17	1.20
January 1999	1.50	1.60
	1.30	1.40
	1.33	1.40
	1.07	1.10
	1.48	1.50
February 1999	1.49	1.60
	1.58	1.70
	1.50	1.70
	1.48	1.60
	1.32	1.40
March	1.33	1.40
	1.20	1.20
	1.07	1.00
	1.17	1.20
	1.31	1.30

[a] Overall mean.

Table 8.30

External quality assessment results for C-reactive protein

Date	Target value[a] (mg/l)	1998 Assayed value (mg/l)
January 1998	37.5	45.0
February	62.3	79.4
March	72.7	88.5
April	82.6	87.7
May	97.4	108.0
June	117.4	118.0
August	147.2	152.0
September	11.5	13.5
October	21.7	24.2
November	33.6	36.6
December	59.3	59.3
January 1999	79.6	82.0
February	80.2	85.4
March	22.6	26.4

[a] All laboratory trimmed mean.

Table 8.31

External quality assessment results for ferritin

Date	Target value[a] (ng/ml)	1998 Assayed value (ng/ml)
February 1998	52.0	49.0
	33.0	33.0
March	175.0	145.0
	28.4	26.1
April	103.4	93.0
	2220.0	2073.0
May	16.9	17.6
	33.0	34.0
June	102.8	91.8
	103.0	88.1
July	28.6	26.0
	14.5	13.9
August	921.2	986.0
	8.3	8.3
September	40.9	41.0
	7.6	8.7
October	89.0	83.0
	139.0	129.0
November	27.2	23.3
	37.8	32.7
January 1999	2607.0	2505.0
	19.1	16.0
February	73.1	69.0
	30.1	27.0
March	36.1	30.0
	10.4	9.0

[a] All laboratory trimmed mean.

Table 8.32

External quality assessment results for haemoglobin

Date	Target value[a] (g/dl)	1998 Assayed value (g/dl)
January 1998	124.5	127.0
	118.3	120.0
March	94.6	96.0
	149.8	152.0
April	124.8	125.0
May	111.8	112.0
June	116.3	116.0
July	105.8	108.0
August	83.4	85.0
September	108.0	110.0
October	121.0	121.0
November	74.0	76.0
December	113.0	115.0
January 1999	114.0	114.0
February	82.0	82.0

[a] All laboratory trimmed mean.

Table 8.33

External quality assessment results for fibrinogen

Date	Target value[a] (g/l)	1998 Assayed value (g/l)
January 1998	2.70	2.70
May	2.55	2.60
November	2.15	2.0
January 1999	2.50	2.70

[a] All laboratory trimmed mean.

Table 8.34

Reference intervals for analytes

Analyte	Reference interval	1998 Units
Total cholesterol		
Males	3.5-6.4	mmol/l
Females	3.5-6.4	mmol/l
HDL-cholesterol		
Males	1.0-1.5	mmol/l
Females	1.2-1.8	mmol/l
C-reactive protein		
Males	0-12	mg/l
Females	0-12	mg/l
Ferritin		
Males	25-400	ng/ml
Females (Pre-menopausal <50)	6-85	ng/ml
Females (Post-menopausal ≥50)	20-200	ng/ml
Haemoglobin		
Males	13.2-16.9	g/dl
Females	11.5-16.5	g/dl
Fibrinogen		
Males	1.46-3.80	g/l
Females	1.46-3.80	g/l

Appendix A: Fieldwork documents

Stage 1 leaflet: Interviewer

Stage 2 leaflet: Nurse

Household questionnaire

Individual questionnaire

Show cards

Self-completion booklets
  8-12 year olds
  13-15 year olds
  Young adults
  Adults

Nurse schedule

Consent sheets

THE HEALTH SURVEY FOR ENGLAND

On behalf of the Department of Health

SCPR
SOCIAL & COMMUNITY PLANNING RESEARCH

UCL
MEDICAL
SCHOOL

THE HEALTH SURVEY FOR ENGLAND: 1998

*T*his survey is being carried out for the Department of Health, by SCPR (Social & Community Planning Research), an independent research institute, and the Department of Epidemiology and Public Health at UCL (University College London).

This leaflet tells you more about the survey and why it is being done.

• *What is it about?*

*T*he Department of Health wants information about the health of adults and children in England. This is so that new and better ways can be developed to help people maintain good health and provide the necessary services for people who need treatment at times of ill-health.

The Health Survey for England is an annual survey designed to provide this information. Each year a fresh set of people is interviewed.

This year the questions are concentrating on heart disease and related behaviour such as smoking, drinking and physical activity. The Department of Health is particularly interested in having this information because at the present time England has one of the highest rates of heart disease in the world. The survey also collects, if you agree, some physical measurements, such as height, weight, blood pressure, a saliva sample and (if you are aged 11 or over) a blood sample. Some personal details such as age, sex and employment are needed to interpret this information.

• *Why have we come to your household?*

*T*o visit every household in England would take too long and cost too much money. Instead we select a sample of addresses in such a way that all addresses in the country have an equal chance of being selected. Yours is one of those chosen for the 1998 survey. You will represent thousands of other people in the country. The addresses were taken from the Postcode Address File, a list compiled by the Post Office of addresses to which mail is delivered.

Once an address is selected, we cannot change one address with another, nor one individual with anyone else. If we did so, we could not be sure that all types of people were represented in the survey. The community consists of a great many different types of people and we need to represent them all in our survey. The results will present a more accurate picture if everyone we approach agrees to take part, and we hope you will.

• Is the survey confidential?

Yes. We take very great care to protect the confidentiality of the information we are given. The survey results will not be in a form which can reveal your identity. This will only be known to the SCPR/UCL research team.

If you agree, however, your name, address and date of birth, but no other information, will be passed to the National Health Service Central Register. This would help us if we wanted to follow you up in future.

• Is the survey compulsory?

No. In all our surveys we rely on voluntary co-operation. The success of the survey depends on the goodwill and co-operation of those asked to take part. The more people who do take part, the more representative and accurate the results will be. However, you are free to withdraw from any part of the survey at any time.

• What will happen after the interview?

After the interview, if you agree, the interviewer will arrange for a qualified nurse to visit - at a time convenient for you - so that some measurements can be taken. The nurse will measure your waist and hip circumferences (if you are aged 16 or over), your upper arm circumference (if you are aged under 16), the length of your arm (if you are aged 65 or over), and your blood pressure. For those aged 4 and over, the nurse will ask your agreement to take a sample of saliva (spit).

If you are aged 11 or over the nurse will also ask your agreement to take a small blood sample from your arm. The nurse will have to get your written permission before a blood sample can be taken. You are of course free to choose not to give a blood sample, even if you are willing to help the nurse with everything else.

The analysis of all the measurements and blood samples will tell us a lot about the health of the population. During the visit, the nurse will be able to explain the importance of these measurements and answer any questions.

• Do I get anything from the survey?

If you wish, you may have a record of your measurements and the results of the blood tests. Also, if you wish, your blood pressure and blood sample results will be sent to your GP who will be able to interpret them for you and give you advice if necessary. Your GP may also want to include the results in any future report about you.

Other benefits from the survey will be indirect and in due course will come from any improvements in health and in health services which result from the survey.

• If I have any other questions?

We hope this leaflet answers the questions you may have, and that it shows the importance of the survey. If you have any other questions, please do not hesitate to ring one of the contacts listed below.

Your co-operation is very much appreciated.

Andrea Nove   Dr Paola Primatesta
SCPR   Department of Epidemiology
35 Northampton Square   and Public Health
London   University College London
EC1V 0AX   1-19 Torrington Place
                                     London WC1E 6BT

Tel: 0171 250 1866   Tel: 0171 391 1733

Thank you very much for your help with this important survey.

MEASUREMENTS

- **Blood pressure (Age 5 years and over)**

High blood pressure can be a health problem. However, blood pressure is difficult to measure accurately. A person's blood pressure is influenced by age and can vary from day to day with emotion, meals, tobacco, alcohol, medication, temperature and pain. Although the nurse will tell you your blood pressure along with an indication of its meaning, a diagnosis cannot be made on a measurement taken on a single occasion. Blood pressure is measured using an inflatable cuff that goes around the upper arm.

- **Waist-to-hip ratio (Age 16 years and over)**

Lately there has been much discussion about the relationship between weight and health. We have already recorded your weight and height but another important factor is thought to be the distribution of weight over the body. The ratio of your waist to hip measurements is most useful for assessing this.

- **Mid-upper arm circumference (Age 2 -15 years)**

The circumference of the arm is measured using a tape measure. This will provide important information on changes over time in the size of children in the population.

- **Demi-span (Age 65 years and over)**

The demi-span is the length of the arm stretching from the bottom of the middle finger and ring finger to the sternal notch (the gap between the collar bones). It is strongly related to a person's height and is particularly useful if height cannot be measured easily. It simply involves measuring the length of the arm with a tape measure.

- **Saliva sample (Age 4 years and over)**

We would like to take a sample of saliva (spit). This simply involves dribbling saliva down a straw into a tube, or sucking on a piece of cotton wool. The sample will be analysed for cotinine. Cotinine is related to the intake of cigarette smoke and is of particular interest to see whether non-smokers may have raised levels as a result of 'passive' smoking.

- **Blood sample (Age 11 years and over)**

We would be very grateful if you would agree to provide us with a sample of blood. This is an important part of the survey, as the analysis of the blood

---

THE HEALTH SURVEY FOR ENGLAND

On behalf of the Department of Health

UCL
MEDICAL
SCHOOL

SCPR
SOCIAL & COMMUNITY
PLANNING RESEARCH

THE HEALTH SURVEY FOR ENGLAND: 1998

This survey is being carried out for the Department of Health, by SCPR (Social & Community Planning Research) and the Department of Epidemiology and Public Health at UCL (University College London). You have already taken part in the first stage of the survey which consisted of an interview and some measurements (height and weight).

This leaflet tells you more about the second stage of the survey.

THE SECOND STAGE

A registered nurse will ask you some further questions and will ask permission to take some measurements. The measurements are described overleaf. You need not have any measurements taken if you do not wish but, of course, we very much hope you will agree to them as they are a very important part of this survey. If the survey results are to be useful to the Department of Health, it is important that we obtain information from all types of people in all states of health.

samples will tell us a lot about the health of the population. You are of course free to choose not to give a blood sample, and the nurse will ask for your written permission before a blood sample is taken.

This part of the survey involves taking a small amount of blood (no more than 15ml) from your arm by a qualified nurse. The blood sample will be sent to a medical laboratory for testing total cholesterol, HDL cholesterol, haemoglobin and ferritin. For respondents aged 16 and over it will also be tested for fibrinogen and C-reactive protein.

Cholesterol is a type of fat present in the blood, related to diet. Too much cholesterol in the blood increases the risk of heart disease. Fibrinogen is a protein necessary for blood clotting and high levels are also associated with a higher risk of heart disease.

Haemoglobin is the red pigment in the blood which carries oxygen. A low level of haemoglobin is called anaemia. One reason for a low level of haemoglobin may be a shortage of iron. Ferritin is a measure of the body's iron stores.

The level of C-reactive protein in the blood gives information on inflammatory activity in the body, and it is also associated with risk of heart disease.

We would like to store a small amount of blood. Medical tests of blood samples are becoming more advanced and specialised. This means that we may be able to learn more about the health of the population by re-testing blood in the future. We will ask separately for permission to store blood.

The sample will **not** be tested for viruses such as the HIV (Aids) virus.

LETTING YOUR GP KNOW THE RESULTS

With your agreement we would like to send your blood pressure and blood sample results to your GP because we believe that this may help you to take steps to keep in good health. Your GP can interpret the results in the light of your medical history. We believe that this may help to improve your health.

If the GP considers your results to be satisfactory, then nothing further will be done.

If your results showed, for example, that your blood pressure was above what is usual for someone of your sex and age, your GP may wish to measure it again. Often it is possible to reduce blood pressure by treatment or by changing your diet. It is for you and your GP to decide what is the best action to take, if any.

Might there be implications for insurance cover?

If you agree to your results being sent to your GP, then she/he may use them in medical reports about you. This may occur if you apply for a new life assurance policy, or for a new job. Insurance companies may ask those who apply for new policies if they have had any medical tests. If so, the insurance company may ask if they can obtain a medical report from the GP. Because of the Access to Medical Reports Act 1988 an insurance company **cannot** ask your GP for a medical report on you without your permission. Having given your permission, you then have the right to see the report before your GP sends it to the insurance company and you can ask for the report to be amended if you consider it to be incorrect or misleading.

The purpose of a medical report is for the company to judge whether to charge normal premiums, whether to charge higher premiums or whether, in exceptional circumstances, to turn down life insurance on account of the person's health.

Insurance companies look for a history of illness or factors affecting health and some things concern them more than others. One measurement from the survey is very unlikely by itself to affect the company's decision. Please remember that we are **not** testing for the AIDS virus (HIV) or for any other virus.

We believe that the chances of anyone being refused life insurance or being charged higher premiums on life insurance as a result of the survey are very small. Existing life insurance policies would **not** be affected in any way. We hope that you will be willing to have your results sent to your GP. If you have any questions please discuss them with the nurse.

SCPR is insured for negligent injury to people who take part in the study.

ANSWERING OTHER QUESTIONS

We hope this leaflet answers many of the questions you may have. If you have others, please contact one of the people listed below:-

Andrea Nove
Social & Community Planning Research
35 Northampton Square
London EC1V 0AX

Dr Paola Primatesta
Department of Epidemiology
and Public Health
University College London
1-19 Torrington Place
London WC1E 6BT

Tel: 0171 250 1866   Tel: 0171 391 1733

Thank you very much for your help with this important survey.

National Centre for Social Research
Formerly SCPR
Charity No 298538

Head Office
35 Northampton Square
London EC1V 0AX
Telephone 0171 250 1866
Fax 0171 250 1524

Operations Department
100 Kings Road, Brentwood
Essex CM14 4LX
Telephone 01277 200 600
Fax 01277 214 117

P1727

The Health Survey for England 1998

Program Documentation

Household Questionnaire

Point
SAMPLE POINT NUMBER.
Range: 1..997

Address
ADDRESS NUMBER.
Range: 1..97

Hhold
HOUSEHOLD NUMBER.
Range: 1..3

AdrField
PLEASE ENTER ENTER THE FIRST TEN CHARACTERS OF THE FIRST LINE OF THE ADDRESS TAKEN FROM
A.R.F. ADDRESS LABEL. MAKE SURE TO TYPE IT EXACTLY AS IT IS PRINTED.
Text: Maximum 10 characters

First
INTERVIEWER FOR INFORMATION.... You are in the Questionnaire for
Point no: (Point number)
Address no: (Address number)
Household no: (Household number)

IntDate
PLEASE ENTER THE DATE OF THIS INTERVIEW.
ENTER DAY OF MONTH IN NUMBERS, NAME OF MONTH IN WORDS (FIRST THREE LETTERS), YEAR IN
NUMBERS, EG. 2 Jan 72::
Date

WhoHere
INTERVIEWER: COLLECT NAMES OF PEOPLE IN THIS HOUSEHOLD

IF First person in household OR More=Yes THEN
Name
What is the name of person number (1-14)?
ENTER PERSON'S FORENAME

More
Is there anyone else in this household?
1 Yes
2 No
ENDIF

(Name and More repeated for up to 14 household members)

HHSize
Household size.
Range: 0..14

SizeConf
So, can I check, altogether there are ((x) number) people in your household?
1 Yes
2 No, more than (x)
3 No, less than (x)

HOUSEHOLD COMPOSITION GRID FOR ALL HOUSEHOLD MEMBERS (MAXIMUM 14)

Person
Person number in Household Grid.
Range: 0..14

Name
First name from WhoHere

Sex
INTERVIEWER: CODE (name of respondent's) SEX.
1 Male
2 Female

DoB
What is (name of respondent's) date of birth?
Enter Day of month in numbers, Name of month in words (first three letters), Year in numbers Eg. 2 Jan 72
Variable names for date of birth are DOBday, DOBmonth, DOByear.

AgeOf
Can I check, what was (name of respondent's) age last birthday?
Range: 0..120

IF Age of Respondent is 16 or over THEN
Marital
Are you (is he/she)...
ASK OR RECORD. CODE FIRST THAT APPLIES.
1 ...single, that is never married,
2 married and living with husband/wife,
3 married and separated from husband/wife,
4 divorced,
5 or, widowed?
ENDIF

IF Age of respondent is 16 or 17 years THEN
LegPar
Can I check, do either of (name of respondent's) parents, or someone who has legal parental
responsibility for him/her, live in this household?
1 Yes
2 No
ENDIF

IF (Age of Respondent is 0 to 15 years) OR (LegPar = Yes) THEN
Par1
Which of the people in this household are (name of respondent's) parents or have legal parental
responsibility for him/her on a permanent basis?
CODE FIRST PERSON AT THIS QUESTION. IF Not a household member/dead, CODE 97
Range: 1..14, 97

The Health Survey for England – 1998 – Household Questionnaire

IF Par1 IN [1..14] THEN
Par2
Which other person in this household is *(name of respondent's)* parent or have legal parental responsibility for him/her on a permanent basis?
CODE SECOND PERSON AT THIS QUESTION. IF No-one else in the household, CODE 97
Range: 1..14, 97
ENDIF
ENDIF

RELATIONSHIPS BETWEEN HOUSEHOLD MEMBERS, COLLECTED FOR ALL HOUSEHOLD MEMBERS TO EACH OTHER

R
SHOW CARD A.
What is *(Name's)* RELATIONSHIP TO *(Name)*. Just tell me the number on this card.
1 Husband/Wife
2 partner/cohabitee
3 natural son/daughter
4 adopted son/daughter
5 foster child
6 stepson/daughter/child of partner
7 Son/daughter-in-law
8 natural parent
9 adoptive parent
10 foster parent
11 stepparent/parents partner
12 parent-in-law
13 natural brother/sister
14 half-brother/sister
15 step-brother/sister
16 adopted brother/sister
17 foster brother/sister
18 brother/sister-in-law
19 grandchild
20 grandparent
21 other relative
22 other non-relative
96 *(self – imputed for first person in household only)*

END OF HOUSEHOLD COMPOSITION GRID

ASK ALL

HHldr
In whose name is the accommodation owned or rented?
PROBE: Anyone else? CODE ALL THAT APPLY.
(Code frame of all household members)
1-14 Person numbers of household members
97 Not a household member

HoHNum
INTERVIEWER: CODE PERSON NUMBER OF HEAD OF HOUSEHOLD, USING STANDARD RULES.
(Code frame of adult household members)

HHResp
INTERVIEWER CODE: WHO WAS THE PERSON RESPONSIBLE FOR ANSWERING THE GRIDS IN THIS QUESTIONNAIRE?
(Code frame of adult household members)

The Health Survey for England – 1998 – Household Questionnaire

HQResp
Status of person answering grids.
1 Head of Household
2 Spouse / partner of HoH
3 Other adult

Tenure1
SHOW CARD B
Now, I'd like to get some general information about your household. In which of these ways does your household occupy this accommodation? Please give an answer from this card.
1 Own it outright
2 Buying it with the help of a mortgage or loan
3 Pay part rent and part mortgage (shared ownership)
4 Rent it
5 Live here rent free (including rent free in relative's/friend's property; excluding squatting)
6 Squatting

IF Tenure1=Rent it OR Live here rent free THEN
JobAccom
Does the accommodation go with the job of anyone in the household?
1 Yes
2 No

Landlord
Who is your landlord?
READ OUT AND CODE FIRST THAT APPLIES
1 ...the local authority/council/ New Town Development,
2 a housing association or co-operative or charitable trust,
3 employer (organisation) of a household member,
4 another organisation,
5 relative/friend (before you lived here) of a household member,
6 employer (individual) of a household member,
7 another individual private landlord?

Furn1
Is the accommodation provided...READ OUT.
1 ...furnished,
2 partly furnished (e.g. curtains and carpets only),
3 or, unfurnished?
ENDIF

ASK ALL

Bedrooms
How many bedrooms does your household have, including bedsitting rooms and spare bedrooms?
EXCLUDE BEDROOMS CONVERTED TO OTHER USES (eg. bathroom). INCLUDE BEDROOMS TEMPORARILY USED FOR OTHER THINGS (eg. study, playroom).
Range: 0..20

PasSm
Does anyone smoke **inside** this (house/flat) on most days?
INTERVIEWER: INCLUDE NON-HOUSEHOLD MEMBERS WHO SMOKE IN THE HOUSE OR FLAT. EXCLUDE HOUSEHOLD MEMBERS WHO ONLY SMOKE OUTSIDE THE HOUSE OR FLAT.
1 Yes
2 No

IF PasSm = Yes THEN
  NumSm
  How many people smoke inside this (house/flat) on most days?
    Range: 1..20
ENDIF

ASK ALL

Car
Is there a car or van **normally** available for use by you or any members of your household?
INCLUDE: ANY PROVIDED BY EMPLOYERS IF NORMALLY AVAILABLE FOR PRIVATE USE BY RESPONDENT OR MEMBERS OF HOUSEHOLD.
  1 Yes
  2 No

IF Car = Yes THEN
  NumCars
  How many are available?
    1 One
    2 Two
    3 Three or more
ENDIF

IF HQResp=Head of Household OR Spouse/Partner of Head of Household THEN
  SrcInc
  There has been a lot of talk about health and income. I would like to get some idea of your household's income.
  SHOW CARD C.
  This card shows various possible sources of income. Can you please tell me which kinds of income you *(and your husband/wife/partner)* receive?
  PROBE: FOR ALL SOURCES. CODE ALL THAT APPLY.
    1 Earnings from employment or self-employment
    2 State retirement pension
    3 Pension from former employer
    4 Child benefit
    5 Job-Seekers allowance
    6 Income Support
    7 Family Credit
    8 Housing Benefit
    9 Other state benefits
    10 Interest from savings and investments (eg stocks & shares)
    11 Other kinds of regular allowance from outside your household (eg maintenance, student's grants, rent
    12 No source of income

JntInc
SHOW CARD D.
This card shows incomes in weekly, monthly and annual amounts. Which of the groups on this card represents *(your/you and your husband/wife/partner's)* income from all these sources, before any deductions for income tax, National Insurance, etc? Just tell me the number beside the row that applies to *(you/your joint incomes)*.
ENTER BAND NUMBER. DON'T KNOW = 96, REFUSED = 97.
  Range: 1..97

IF 2 adults in household who are not Spouse/partner, or if 3 or more adults in household
(IF (NAdults>=2 AND PartHoH = 0) OR (NAdults>=3) THEN
  OthInc
  Can I check, does anyone else in the household have an income from any source?
    1 Yes
    2 No

IF (OthInc = Yes) THEN
  IF (JntInc IN [1..97]) THEN
    HHInc
    SHOW CARD D
    Thinking of the income of your household as a whole, which of the groups on this card represents the total income of the whole household before deductions for income tax, National Insurance, etc.
    ENTER BAND NUMBER. DON'T KNOW = 96, REFUSED = 97.
      Range: 1..97
  ENDIF
ENDIF
ENDIF

EMPLOYMENT DETAILS OF HEAD OF HOUSEHOLD COLLECTED

NHActiv
SHOW CARD E
Which of these descriptions applies to what *you/name* (Head of Household) were doing last week, that is in the seven days ending *(date last Sunday)*?
CODE FIRST TO APPLY.
  1 Going to school or college full-time (including on vacation)
  2 In paid employment or self-employment (or away temporarily)
  3 On a Government scheme for employment training
  4 Doing unpaid work for a business that you own, or that a relative owns
  5 Waiting to take up paid work already obtained
  6 Looking for paid work or a Government training scheme
  7 Intending to look for work but prevented by temporary sickness or injury (CHECK 28 DAYS OR LESS)
  8 Permanently unable to work because of long-term sickness or disability (USE ONLY FOR MEN AGED 16-64 OR WOMEN AGED 16-59)
  9 Retired from paid work
  10 Looking after the home or family
  11 Doing something else (SPECIFY)

IF NHActiv=Doing something else THEN
  NHActivO
  OTHER: PLEASE SPECIFY.
  Text: Maximum 60 characters
ENDIF

IF NHActiv=Going to school or college full-time THEN
  HStWork
  Did *you/name* (Head of Household) do any paid work in the seven days ending *(date last Sunday)*, either as an employee or self-employed?
    1 Yes
    2 No
ENDIF

IF (NHActiv=Intending to look for work but prevented by temporary sickness or injury, Retired from paid work, Looking after the home or family or Doing something else OR HStWork=No) AND (Head of Household aged under 65 (men)/60 (women)) THEN
  H4WkLook
  Thinking now of the 4 weeks ending *(date last Sunday)*, were *you/name* (Head of Household) looking for any paid work or Government training scheme at any time in those four weeks?
    1 Yes
    2 No
ENDIF

IF NHActiv=Looking for paid work or a government training scheme OR H4WkLook=Yes THEN

H2WkStrt

If a job or a place on a Government training scheme had been available in the *(7 days/four weeks)* ending *(date last Sunday)*, would *you/name* (Head of Household) have been able to start within two weeks?

  1 Yes
  2 No

ENDIF

IF (NHActiv IN [Looking for work or a government training scheme...Doing something else] OR HStWork = No) THEN

HEverJob

Have *you/name* (Head of Household) ever been in paid employment or self-employed?

  1 Yes
  2 No

ENDIF

IF NHActiv=Waiting to take up paid employment already obtained THEN

HOthPaid

Apart from the job *you/name* (Head of Household) are waiting to take up, have *you/name* (Head of Household) ever been in paid employment or self-employed?

  1 Yes
  2 No

ENDIF

IF (HEverJob = Yes) OR (NHActiv IN [In paid employment or self-employment...Waiting to take up a job already obtained]) OR (HStWork=Yes) THEN

HJobTitl

I'd like to ask you some details about the job *you/name* (Head of Household) were doing last week *(your most recent job/the main job you had/the job you are waiting to take up)*. What is (was/will be) the name or title of the job?

    Text: Maximum 60 characters

HFtPtime

Were/Are/Will you/name (Head of Household) *be* working full-time or part-time?
(FULL-TIME = MORE THAN 30 HOURS/PART-TIME = 30 HOURS OR LESS)

  1 Full-time
  2 Part-time

HWtWork

What kind of work *do/did/will you/name* (Head of Household) do most of the time?

    Text: Maximum 50 characters

HMatUsed

IF RELEVANT: What materials or machinery *do/did/will you/name* (Head of Household) use?
IF NONE USED, WRITE IN 'NONE'.

    Text: Maximum 50 characters

HSkilNee

What skills or qualifications are *(were)* needed for the job?

    Text: Maximum 120 characters

HEmploye

Were/Are/Will you/name (Head of Household) *be...*READ OUT...

  1 an employee,
  2 or, self-employed?

IF (HEmploye = SelfEmp) THEN

HDirctr

Can I just check, in this job *are/were/will you/name* (Head of Household) *be* a Director of a limited company?

  1 Yes
  2 No

ENDIF

IF (HEmploye = Employ) OR (HDirctr = Yes) THEN

HEmpStat

Are/Were/Will you/name (Head of Household) *be* a ...READ OUT...

  1 manager,
  2 foreman or supervisor,
  3 or other employee?

HNEmplee

Including *yourself/name* (Head of Household), about how many people *are/were/will be* employed at the place where *you/name usually work(s)/usually worked/will work*?

  1 1 or 2
  2 3-24
  3 25-499
  4 500+

ELSEIF (HEmploye = SelfEmp) AND (HDirctr = No) THEN

HSNEmple

Do/Did/Will you/name (Head of Household) have any employees?

  1 None
  2 1-24
  3 25-499
  4 500+

ENDIF

IF (HEmploye = Employ) THEN

HInd

What does/did your/HoH's employer make or do at the place where *you/name* (Head of Household) *(usually work/usually worked/will work)*?

    Text: Maximum 100 characters

ELSEIF (HEmploye = SelfEmp) THEN

HSIfWtMa

What *do/did/will you/name* (Head of Household) make or do in your business?

    Text: Maximum 100 characters

ENDIF
ENDIF

NOFAd
Number of adults
  Range: 0..14

NOFCh
Number of children.
  Range: 0..14

NOFInf
Number of infants.
  Range: 0..14

The Health Survey for England – 1998 – Household Questionnaire

NofIQ
Number of individual sessions.
   Range: 0..7

HoHAct
Head of Household working at Activ
   1 Yes
   2 No

INTERVIEWER CODING FROM OBSERVATION

AreaType
TYPE OF AREA
   1 Inner city
   2 Other dense urban/town centre
   3 Suburban residential (city/large town outskirts)
   4 Rural residential/village centre
   5 Rural agricultural with isolated dwellings or small hamlets

BldType
PREDOMINANT RESIDENTIAL BUILDING TYPE
   1 Terraced houses
   2 Semi-detached houses
   3 Detached houses
   4 Mixed houses
   5 Low rise flats (5 storey blocks or less)
   6 High rise flats (blocks over 5 storeys)
   7 Flats with commercial (flats/maisonettes over parades of shops)
   8 Flats mixed (high and low rise)
   9 Mixed houses and flats

TypDwell
HOUSEHOLD DWELLING TYPE
   1 Detached whole house or bungalow
   2 Semi-detached whole house or bungalow
   3 Terraced/end of terrace whole house or bungalow
   4 Flat or maisonette in a purpose built block: basement to 3rd floor
   5 Flat or maisonette in a purpose built block: 4th floor or higher
   6 Flat or maisonette in a converted house or some other kind of building
   7 Caravan, mobile home or houseboat
   8 Some other kind of accommodation

IF TypDwell = Other THEN
   TypDwOth
   PLEASE SPECIFY OTHER DWELLING TYPE.
      Text: Maximum 40 characters.
ENDIF

EthMix
ETHNIC MIX OF AREA
   1 Predominantly white
   2 Predominantly black/brown
   3 Mixed

National Centre for Social Research

Formerly SCPR

Charity No. 258538

Head Office
35 Northampton Square
London EC1V 0AX
Telephone 0171 250 1866
Fax 0171 250 1524

Operations Department
100 Kings Road, Brentwood
Essex CM14 4LX
Telephone 01277 200 600
Fax 01277 214 117

P1727

The Health Survey for England 1998

Program Documentation

Individual Questionnaire

Introduction

ALL

AllocP

PLEASE CHOOSE THE *(first/second/third/fourth)* PERSON YOU WISH TO INTERVIEW IN THIS QUESTIONNAIRE FROM THE LIST BELOW. YOU CAN INTERVIEW AT THE MOST 4 PERSONS IN THE SAME QUESTIONNAIRE.

(List of household members)

IF AgeP=2-12 THEN
  AdResp
  WHO IS ANSWERING ON BEHALF OF *(Name of selected child aged <13)*?
  (List of adult household members)
ENDIF

ALL

PersDisp

INTERVIEWER: FOR YOUR INFORMATION... the person(s) now allocated to this interview are:
(List of allocated household members)

OwnDoB

Can I just check, what is your date of birth?
ENTER DAY OF MONTH IN NUMBERS, NAME OF MONTH IN **WORDS** (FIRST THREE LETTERS), YEAR IN NUMBERS.
IF *(Name)* DOES NOT KNOW HIS/HER DATE OF BIRTH, PLEASE GET AN ESTIMATE.

IF OwnDoB=Response THEN
  OwnAge
  Can I just check, your age is *(computed age)*?
    1 Yes
    2 No
ENDIF

IF OwnDoB=Not known/Refused THEN
  OwnAgeE
  Can you tell me your age last birthday?
  IF NECESSARY: What do you estimate your age to be?
  Range: 1..120

IF OwnAgeE=Not known/Refused THEN
  IF Estimated age from household grid <16 THEN
    AgeCEst
    INTERVIEWER: ESTIMATE NEAREST AGE:
      3 3 years
      5 5 years
      7 7 years
      9 9 years
     11 11 years
     13 13 years
     15 15 years

  ELSE IF Estimated age from household grid >=16 THEN
    AgeAEst
    INTERVIEWER: ESTIMATE NEAREST AGE:
     18 (ie between 16 - 19)
     25 (ie between 20 - 29)
     35 (ie between 30 - 39)
     45 (ie between 40 - 49)
     55 (ie between 50 - 59)
     65 (ie between 60 - 69)
     75 (ie between 70 - 79)
     85 (ie 80+)
    ENDIF
  ENDIF
ENDIF

General health module

ASK ALL
GenHelf
How is your health in general? Would you say it was ...READ OUT...
1   ...very good,
2   good,
3   fair,
4   bad, or
5   very bad?

LongIll
Do you have any long-standing illness, disability or infirmity? By long-standing I mean anything that has troubled you over a period of time, or that is likely to affect you over a period of time?
1   Yes
2   No

IF LongIll=Yes THEN
FOR I=1 to 6 DO
  IF (i = 1) OR (More[i - 1] = Yes) THEN
    Records up to six long-standing illnesses
    IllsM[i]
    What *(else)* is the matter with you?
    INTERVIEWER: RECORD FULLY. PROBE FOR DETAIL.
    IF MORE THAN ONE MENTIONED, ENTER ONE HERE ONLY.
    Text: Maximum 60 characters
    Variable names for text are Illtxt01-Illtxt06

    IF (i < 6) THEN
      More[i]
      (Can I check) do you have any other long-standing illness, disability or infirmity?
      1   Yes
      2   No
    ENDIF
  ENDIF
ENDDO

LimitAct
Does this illness or disability *(do any of these illnesses or disabilities)* limit your activities in any way?
1   Yes
2   No
ENDIF

ASK ALL
LastFort
Now I'd like you to think about the **two weeks** ending yesterday. During those two weeks did you have to cut down on any of the **things** you **usually** do about the house or at *(school/work)* or in your free time because of *(a condition you have just told me about or some other)* illness or injury?
1   Yes
2   No

IF Lastfort = Yes THEN
DaysCut
How many days was this in all during these 2 weeks, including Saturdays and Sundays?
Range: 1..14
ENDIF

IF Age of Respondent is 16 or over THEN
NDocTalk
During the two weeks ending yesterday, apart from any visit to a hospital, did you talk to a doctor for any reason at all, either in person or by telephone? *(Please exclude any consultations made on behalf of children under 16)*
EXCLUDE CONSULTATIONS MADE ON BEHALF OF PERSONS OUTSIDE THE HOUSEHOLD
1   Yes
2   No

IF NDocTalk = Yes THEN
Nchats
How many times did you talk to a doctor in these two weeks?
Range: 1..9

IF Nchats IN [1..9] THEN
  FOR Indx:=1 TO 9 DO
    IF Nchats >= Indx THEN
      Repeat WhsBhlf to Presc for each consultation: QuServs[1-9]
      WhsBhlf
      (Thinking of the last time you talked to a doctor/Thinking now about the consultation before that) On whose behalf was this consultation made?
      1   Respondent
      2   Other member of household aged 16 or over

      IF WhsBhlf=Other THEN
        ForPer
        INTERVIEWER: ENTER PERSON NUMBER OF HOUSEHOLD MEMBER ON WHOSE BEHALF RESPONDENT TALKED TO A DOCTOR.
        (List of adults aged 16+ displayed)
        Range: 1..14
      ENDIF

      NHS
      (Still thinking of the last time you talked to a doctor) Was this consultation... READ OUT..
      1   ...under the National Health Service,
      2   or paid for privately?

      GP
      Was the doctor... READ OUT..
      1   ... a GP (i.e. a family doctor).
      2   or a specialist,
      3   or some other kind of doctor?

      DocWher
      Did you talk to the doctor... READ OUT..
      1   ... by telephone,
      2   at your home,
      3   in the doctor's surgery,
      4   at a health centre,
      5   or elsewhere?

      Presc
      Did the doctor give *(or send)* you a prescription?
      1   Yes
      2   No
    ENDIF
  ENDDO
ENDIF
ENDIF
ENDIF

IF NDocTalk=No OR (NDocTalk=Yes AND ALL(QuServs[1-9],WhsBhlf<>Self)) THEN

WhenDoc

Apart from any visit to a hospital, when was the last time you talked to a doctor on your own behalf?

1 2 weeks ago but less than a month ago
2 1 month ago but less than 3 months ago
3 3 months ago but less than 6 months ago
4 6 months ago but less than a year ago
5 A year or more ago
6 Never consulted a doctor

ENDIF
ENDIF

IF Age of Respondent is 2-15 years THEN

CDocTalk

And during the two weeks ending yesterday, apart from any visit to a hospital, did you talk to a doctor for any reason at all, or did any other member of the household talk to a doctor on your behalf?
INCLUDE TELEPHONE CONSULTATIONS

1 Yes
2 No

IF CDocTalk = Yes THEN

CNchats

How many times did you talk to the doctor, or did any other member of the household consult the doctor on your behalf in those two weeks?
Range: 1..4

IF CNchats IN [1..4] THEN
FOR Indx:=1 TO 4 DO
IF CNchats >= Indx THEN
Repeat CNHS to CPresc for each consultation: QuServs[1-4]

CNHS

(Thinking of the last time you talked to the doctor or any other member of the household consulted the doctor on your behalf/Thinking now about the consultation before that) Was this consultation....READ OUT.

1 ...under the National Health Service,
2 or paid for privately?

CGP

Was the doctor... READ OUT..

1 ... a GP (i.e. a family doctor),
2 or a specialist,
3 or some other kind of doctor?

CDrWher

Did you talk to the doctor... READ OUT..

1 ... by telephone,
2 at your home,
3 in the doctor's surgery,
4 at a health centre,
5 or elsewhere?

CPresc

Did the doctor give (or send) you a prescription?

1 Yes
2 No

ENDIF
ENDDO
ENDIF
ENDIF
ENDIF

IF Age of Respondent is 16 or over THEN

NOutPat

During the last 12 months, that is since *(date)* did you attend as a patient the casualty or outpatient department of a hospital *(apart from straightforward ante- or post-natal visits)*?

1 Yes
2 No

IF NOutPat = YES THEN

OutPatmt

During the months of *(last three months)* did you attend as a patient the casualty or outpatient department of a hospital *(apart from straightforward ante- or post-natal visits)*?

1 Yes
2 No

IF Outpatnt=Yes THEN

Ntimes1

How many times did you attend in *(third to last month)*?
Range: 0..31

Ntimes2

How many times did you attend in *(second to last month)*?
Range: 0..31

Ntimes3

How many times did you attend in *(last month)*?
Range: 0..31

ENDIF
ENDIF
ENDIF

IF Age of Respondent is 2-15 years THEN

COutPat

During the months of *(last three months)* did you attend as a patient the casualty or outpatient department of a hospital?

1 Yes
2 No

IF COutPat=Yes THEN

CNtimes1

How many times did you attend in *(third to last month)*?
Range: 0..31

CNtimes2

How many times did attend in *(second to last month)*?
Range: 0..31

CNtimes3

How many times did you attend in *(last month)*?
Range: 0..31

ENDIF
ENDIF

IF Age of Respondent is 16 or over THEN

DayPatnt

During the last year, that is since *(date 1 year ago)* have you been in hospital for treatment as a day patient, that is admitted to a hospital bed or day ward, but not required to remain overnight?

1 Yes
2 No

IF CNstays IN [1..97] THEN
  FOR Indx:=1 TO 6 DO
    IF (CNstays >=Indx AND CNstays <=97) THEN
      Repeat for up to last 6 inpatient experiences
      Cnights
      (Thinking of the last time you stayed in hospital as an inpatient/Thinking now about the stay before that) How many nights altogether were you in hospital?
        Range: 1..97
    ENDIF
  ENDDO
ENDIF
ENDIF
ENDIF

IF DayPatnt=Yes THEN
  NHSPDays
  How many separate days in hospital have you had as a day patient since *(date 1 year ago)*?
    Range: 1..97
ENDIF

IF Age of Respondent is 2-15 years THEN
  CDayPat
  During the last year, that is since *(date 1 year ago)* have you been in hospital for treatment as a day patient, that is admitted to a hospital bed or day ward, but not required to remain in hospital overnight?
    1 Yes
    2 No

IF CDayPat=Yes THEN
  CNHSPDay
  How many separate days in hospital have you had as a day patient since *(date 1 year ago)*?
    Range: 1..97
ENDIF
ENDIF

IF Age of Respondent is 16 or over THEN
  InPatnt
  During the last year, that is since *(date 1 year ago)* have you been in hospital as an inpatient, overnight or longer?
    1 Yes
    2 No

IF InPatnt=Yes THEN
  Nstays
  How many separate stays in hospital as an inpatient have you had since *(date 1 year ago)*?
    Range: 1..97

IF Nstays IN [1..97] THEN
  FOR Indx:=1 TO 6 DO
    IF Nstays >=Indx THEN
      Repeat for up to last 6 inpatient experiences
      Nights
      (Thinking of the last time you stayed in hospital as an inpatient/Thinking now about the time before that) How many nights altogether were you in hospital?
        Range: 1..97
    ENDIF
  ENDDO
ENDIF
ENDIF
ENDIF

IF Age of Respondent is 2-15 years THEN
  CInPat
  During the last year, that is, since *(date 1 year ago)* have you been in hospital as an inpatient, overnight or longer?
    1 Yes
    2 No

IF CInPat=Yes THEN
  CNstays
  How many separate stays in hospital as an inpatient have you had since *(date 1 year ago)*?
    Range: 1..97

Cardiovascular disease module (16+)

ASK ALL AGE 16+
Chest
I am now going to ask you some questions mainly about symptoms of the chest. Have you ever had any pain or discomfort in your chest?
1 Yes
2 No

IF Chest = Yes THEN
UpHill
Do you get it when you walk uphill or hurry?
1 Yes
2 No
3 Sometimes/ Occasionally
4 Never walks uphill or hurries
5 (Cannot walk)

IF Uphill = Sometimes/Occasionally THEN
Most1
Does this happen on most occasions?
1 Yes
2 No
ENDIF

IF Uphill = Yes, Sometimes/Occasionally or Never walks uphill or hurries THEN
OrdPace
Do you get it when you walk at an ordinary pace on the level?
1 Yes
2 No
3 Sometimes/Occasionally
4 Never walks at an ordinary pace on the level

IF OrdPace = Sometimes/Occasionally THEN
Most2
Does this happen on most occasions?
1 Yes
2 No
ENDIF
ENDIF

IF (Uphill=Yes) OR (OrdPace=Yes) OR (Most1=Yes) OR (Most2=Yes) THEN
WalkDo
What do you do if you get it while you are walking? Do you stop, slow down or carry on?
IF RESPONDENT UNSURE, PROBE: What do you do on most occasions?
1 Stop
2 Slow down
3 Carry on

IF Walkdo = Stop or SlowDown THEN
PainAway
If you stand still does the pain go away or not?
IF RESPONDENT UNSURE, PROBE: What happens to the pain on most occasions?
1 Pain goes away
2 Pain doesn't go away

IF PainAway = Pain goes away THEN
SoonAway
How soon does the pain go away? does it go in ...READ OUT...
1 ...10 minutes or less,
2 or more than 10 minutes?

IF SoonAway = 10 minutes or less THEN
ShowPain
Will you show me where you get this pain or discomfort?
INTERVIEWER: USE CARD F TO HELP CODE POSITION OF PAIN OR DISCOMFORT CODE ALL THAT APPLY. PROBE: Where else?
1 Sternum (upper or middle)
2 Sternum lower
3 Left anterior chest
4 Left arm
5 Right anterior chest
6 Right arm
7 (Somewhere else)
ENDIF
ENDIF
ENDIF

SevPain
Have you ever had a severe pain across the front of your chest lasting for half an hour or more?
1 Yes
2 No

IF SevPain=Yes THEN
DocSee
Did you see a doctor because of this pain?
1 Yes
2 No

IF DocSee = Yes THEN
DocWhat
What did the doctor say it was?
CODE ALL THAT APPLY
1 Angina
2 Heart attack
3 Did not say
4 Other
ENDIF
ENDIF

ASK ALL AGE 16+
ECGEver
Have you ever had an electrical recording of your heart (ECG) performed?
1 Yes
2 No

IF ECGEver = Yes THEN
WhereECG
Where did you have it?
CODE ALL THAT APPLY. PROBE: Where else?
1 Hospital (inpatient)
2 Hospital (outpatient)
3 GP Surgery
4 Other

WhenECG
How long ago was this?
TYPE IN NUMBER OF YEARS AGO. IF MORE THAN ONE, TAKE LAST OCCASION.
LESS THAN ONE YEAR = 0
Range: 0..110
ENDIF

ASK ALL AGE 16+
Flegm
Do you **usually** bring up any phlegm from your chest, first thing in the morning in winter?
1 Yes
2 No

IF Flegm = No or Don't know THEN
FleDa
Do you **usually** bring up any phlegm from your chest, during the day or at night in the winter?
1 Yes
2 No
ENDIF

IF Flegm=Yes OR FleDa=Yes THEN
FreFl
Do you bring up phlegm like this on most days for as much as three months each year?
1 Yes
2 No
ENDIF

IF Uphill <>Cannot walk THEN
SoBUp
Are you troubled by shortness of breath when hurrying on level ground or walking up a slight hill?
1 Yes
2 No
3 Never walks uphill or hurries
4 Cannot walk

IF SoBUp = Yes, Never walks uphill or hurries or Don't know THEN
SoBAg
Do you get short of breath walking with other people of your own age on level ground?
1 Yes
2 No
3 Never walks with people of own age on level ground

IF SoBAg = Yes or No THEN
SoLev
Do you have to stop for breath when walking at your own pace on level ground?
1 Yes
2 No
ENDIF
ENDIF

ASK ALL AGE 16+
Wheeze
Have you had attacks of wheezing or whistling in your chest at any time in the last 12 months?
1 Yes
2 No

ShBrth
Have you at any time in the past 12 months been woken at night by an attack of shortness of breath?
1 Yes
2 No

WhzAttk
Have you ever had attacks of shortness of breath with wheezing?
1 Yes
2 No

IF Whzattk=Yes THEN
Normal
Is/Was your breathing absolutely normal between attacks?
1 Yes
2 No
ENDIF

ASK ALL AGE 16+
IntroCVD
INTERVIEWER READ OUT: You have already talked to me about your health, and now I would like to go on and talk in more detail about some particular conditions. (They may include some of the things you have already mentioned.)

CVD1
Do you now have, or have you ever had...READ OUT ...high blood pressure (sometimes called hypertension)?
1 Yes
2 No

CVD2
Have you ever had angina?
1 Yes
2 No

CVD3
Have you ever had a heart attack (including myocardial infarction or coronary thrombosis)?
1 Yes
2 No

CVD4
And do you now have, or have you ever had...READ OUT ...a heart murmur?
1 Yes
2 No

CVD5
...abnormal heart rhythm?
1 Yes
2 No

CVD6
...any other heart trouble?
1 Yes
2 No

IF CVD6 = Yes THEN
CVDOth
What is that condition? INTERVIEWER: RECORD FULLY. PROBE FOR DETAIL.
Text: Maximum 50 characters
ENDIF

ASK ALL AGE 16+
CVD7
Have you ever had a stroke?
1 Yes
2 No

CVD8

Do you now have, or have you ever had diabetes?

  1 Yes
  2 No

IF CVD2 = Yes THEN

  DocTold2

  You said that you had Angina. Were you told by a doctor that you had angina?

    1 Yes
    2 No

  IF DocTold2 = Yes THEN

    AgeTold2

    Approximately how old were you when you were first told by a doctor that you had angina?
    TYPE IN AGE IN YEARS
    Range: 0..110

    PastYr2

    Have you had angina during the past 12 months?

      1 Yes
      2 No

    ENDIF

ENDIF

IF CVD3 = Yes THEN

  DocTold3

  Were you told by a doctor that you had a heart attack (including myocardial infarction or coronary thrombosis)?

    1 Yes
    2 No

  IF DocTold3 = Yes THEN

    AgeTold3

    Approximately how old were you when you were first told by a doctor that you had a **heart attack** (including myocardial infarction and coronary thrombosis)? TYPE IN AGE IN YEARS
    Range: 0..110

    PastYr3

    Have you had a heart attack (including myocardial infarction and coronary thrombosis) during the past 12 months?

      1 Yes
      2 No

    ENDIF

ENDIF

IF CVD5 = Yes THEN

  DocTold5

  Were you told by a doctor that you had abnormal heart rhythm?

    1 Yes
    2 No

  IF DocTold5 = Yes THEN

    AgeTold5

    Approximately how old were you when you were first told by a doctor that you had abnormal heart rhythm?
    TYPE IN AGE IN YEARS, IF BORN WITH IT, CODE 0
    Range: 0..110

    PastYr5

    Have you had abnormal heart rhythm during the past 12 months?

      1 Yes
      2 No

    ENDIF

ENDIF

IF CVD6 = Yes THEN

  DocTold6

  Were you told by a doctor that you had *(name of 'other heart condition')*?

    1 Yes
    2 No

  IF DocTold6 = Yes THEN

    AgeTold6

    Approximately how old were you when you were first told by a doctor that you had *(name of 'other heart condition')*?
    TYPE IN AGE IN YEARS, IF BORN WITH IT, CODE 0
    Range: 0..110

    PastYr6

    Have you had *(name of 'other heart condition')* during the past 12 months?

      1 Yes
      2 No

    ENDIF

ENDIF

IF CVD7 = Yes THEN

  DocTold7

  Were you told by a doctor that you had a stroke?

    1 Yes
    2 No

  IF DocTold7 = Yes THEN

    AgeTold7

    Approximately how old were you when you were first told by a doctor that you had a stroke?
    TYPE IN AGE IN YEARS
    Range: 0..110

    PastYr7

    Have you had a stroke during the past 12 months?

      1 Yes
      2 No

    ENDIF

ENDIF

IF (CVD2 = Yes) OR (CVD3 = Yes) OR (CVD5 = Yes) OR (CVD6 = Yes) OR (CVD7 = Yes) THEN

  Medicin

  Are you currently taking any medicines, tablets or pills because of your *(heart condition or stroke)*?

    1 Yes
    2 No

IF (CVD2 = Yes) OR (CVD3 = Yes) OR (CVD5 = Yes) OR (CVD6 = Yes) THEN

  Surgery

  Have you ever undergone any surgery or operation because of your heart condition?

    1 Yes
    2 No

IF (DocBP = Yes) AND (OthBP <> No) THEN

AgeBP

(Apart from when you were pregnant, approximately/Approximately) how old were you when you were first told by a (doctor/nurse) that you had high blood pressure? ENTER AGE IN YEARS

Range: 0..110

MedBP

Are you currently taking any medicines, tablets or pills for high blood pressure?

1 Yes
2 No

IF MedBP = No, Don't know or refused THEN

BPStill

ASK OR RECORD: Do you still have high blood pressure?

1 Yes
2 No

EverMed

Have you **ever** taken medicines, tablets, or pills for high blood pressure in the past?

1 Yes
2 No

IF EverMed = Yes THEN

StopMed

Why did you stop taking (medicines/tablets/pills) for high blood pressure? PROBE: What other reason? TAKE LAST OCCASION, CODE ALL THAT APPLY

1 **Doctor advised me to stop due to:** improvement
2 lack of improvement
3 other problem
4 **Respondent decided to stop:** because felt better
5 ... for other reason
6 **Other reason**

ENDIF
ENDIF

OthAdv

Are you receiving any *(other)* treatment or advice because of your high blood pressure? INCLUDE REGULAR CHECK-UPS

1 Yes
2 No

IF OthAdv = Yes THEN

WhatTrt

What other treatment or advice are you currently receiving because of your high blood pressure? PROBE: What else? CODE ALL THAT APPLY

1 Blood pressure monitored by GP/nurse
2 Advice or treatment to lose weight
3 Blood tests
4 Change diet
5 Stop smoking
6 Reduce stress
7 Other (RECORD AT NEXT QUESTION)

IF WhatTrt = Other THEN

WhatTSp

PLEASE SPECIFY...

Text: Maximum 50 characters

ENDIF
ENDIF
ENDIF

IF (Surgery = Yes) THEN

WhenSur

How long ago was this?
TYPE IN NUMBER OF YEARS AGO. IF MORE THAN ONE OPERATION, TAKE LAST OCCASION. LESS THAN ONE YEAR = 0

Range: 0..110

ENDIF

Waiting

Can I just check, are you currently on a waiting list for any such surgery or operation?

1 Yes
2 No

ENDIF

OthTrt

Are you currently receiving any *(other)* treatment or advice because of your *(heart condition or stroke)*? INCLUDE REGULAR CHECK-UPS

1 Yes
2 No

IF OthTrt = Yes THEN

WhatOth

What *(other)* treatment or advice are you currently receiving because of your *(heart condition or stroke)*? PROBE: What else? CODE ALL THAT APPLY

1 Special diet
2 Regular check-up with GP/hospital/clinic
3 Taking medication
4 Other (RECORD AT NEXT QUESTION)

IF WhatOth = Other THEN

WhatOSp

PLEASE SPECIFY...

Text: Maximum 60 characters

ENDIF
ENDIF

IF CVD1 = Yes THEN

DocBP

You mentioned that you have had high blood pressure. Were you told **by a doctor or nurse** that you had high blood pressure?

1 Yes
2 No

IF (DocBP = Yes) AND (Sex = Female) THEN

PregBP

Can I just check, were you pregnant when you were told that you had high blood pressure?

1 Yes
2 No

IF PregBP = Yes THEN

OthBP

Have you ever had high blood pressure apart from when you were pregnant?

1 Yes
2 No

ENDIF
ENDIF
ENDIF

IF CVD8 = Yes THEN

Diabetes

Were you told by a doctor that you had diabetes?
1　Yes
2　No

IF (Diabetes = Yes) AND (Sex = Female) THEN

DiPreg

Can I just check, were you pregnant when you were told that you had diabetes?
1　Yes
2　No

IF DiPreg = Yes THEN

DiOth

Have you ever had diabetes apart from when you were pregnant?
1　Yes
2　No

ENDIF
ENDIF

IF (Diabetes = Yes) AND (DiOth <> No) THEN

DiAge

(Apart from when you were pregnant, approximately/Approximately) how old were you when you were first told by a doctor that you had diabetes? ENTER AGE IN YEARS
Range:　0..110

Insulin

Do you currently inject insulin for diabetes?
1　Yes
2　No

DiMed

Are you currently taking any medicines, tablets or pills *(other than insulin injections)* for diabetes?
1　Yes
2　No

OthDi

Are you currently receiving any *(other)* treatment or advice for diabetes? INCLUDE REGULAR
CHECK-UPS.
1　Yes
2　No

IF (OthDi = Yes) THEN

OtherDi

What *(other)* treatment or advice are you currently receiving for diabetes?
PROBE: What else? CODE ALL THAT APPLY
1　Special diet
2　Regular check-up with GP/hospital/clinic
3　Other (RECORD AT NEXT QUESTION)

IF OtherDi = Other THEN

WhatDSp

PLEASE SPECIFY...
Text: Maximum 50 characters

ENDIF
ENDIF
ENDIF

IF CVD4 = Yes THEN

Murmur

You mentioned that you have had a heart murmur. Were you told by a **doctor** that you had a heart murmur?
1　Yes
2　No

IF (Murmur = Yes) AND (Sex = Female) THEN

PregMur

Can I just check, were you pregnant when you were told that you had a heart murmur?
1　Yes
2　No

IF PregMur = Yes THEN

NoPregM

Have you ever had a heart murmur apart from when you were pregnant?
1　Yes
2　No

ENDIF
ENDIF

IF (Murmur = Yes) AND (NoPregM <> No) THEN

AgeMur

(Apart from when you were pregnant, approximately/Approximately) how old were you when you were first told by a doctor that you had a heart murmur?
ENTER AGE IN YEARS. IF BORN WITH IT ENTER 0
Range:　0..110

MurYr

Have you had a heart murmur during the past twelve months?
1　Yes
2　No

MedMur

Are you currently taking any medicines, tablets or pills because of your heart murmur?
1　Yes
2　No

SurgMur

Have you ever undergone any surgery or operation because of your heart murmur?
1　Yes
2　No

IF SurgMur = Yes THEN

LongMur

How long ago was this?
ENTER NUMBER OF YEARS AGO. IF MORE THAN ONE OPERATION, TAKE LAST OCCASION.
LESS THAN ONE YEAR AGO = 0
Range:　0..110

ENDIF

WaitMur

Can I just check, are you currently on a waiting list for any such surgery or operation?
1　Yes
2　No

OthMur

Are you currently receiving any *(other)* treatment or advice because of your heart murmur?
INCLUDE REGULAR CHECK-UPS
2　No

IF OthMur = Yes THEN
MurOth
What other treatment or advice are you currently receiving because of your heart murmur?
INTERVIEWER: RECORD FULLY. PROBE FOR DETAIL.
Text: Maximum 50 characters
ENDIF
ENDIF

IF Yes at any of CVD1 – CVD8 THEN
LastDoc
Apart from any visit to a hospital, when was the last time you talked to a doctor on your own behalf about your (name of heart condition)? PROMPT IF NECESSARY
1   Less than 2 weeks ago
2   2 weeks ago but less than a month ago
3   1 month ago but less than 3 months ago
4   3 months ago but less than 6 months ago
5   6 months ago but less than 1 year ago
6   1 year or more ago
7   Never consulted a doctor

IF (LastDoc <> Never consulted a doctor) AND (More than one coded Yes at CVD1 – CVD8) THEN
ConCons
Which condition was the consultation about? CODE ALL THAT APPLY
1   high blood pressure
2   angina
3   heart attack
4   heart murmur
5   abnormal heart rhythm
6   other heart trouble
7   stroke
8   diabetes
ENDIF
ENDIF

IF (OutPatN=Yes OR NOutPat=Yes OR DayPatn=Yes) AND Yes at any of CVD1 – CVD8 THEN
NWhyOutP
Earlier you told me that, during the last year, you had attended hospital *(as an out-patient and/or as a day patient and/or casualty.)* Was this visit *(were any of these visits)* because of your *(name of heart condition(s))*?
1   Yes
2   No
ENDIF

IF (InPatnt=Yes) AND Yes at any of CVD1 – CVD8 THEN
NWhyInP
Earlier you told me that, during the last year, you had been in hospital as an inpatient, overnight or longer. *(Was this stay/Were any of these stays)* because of your *(name of heart condition)*?
1   Yes
2   No
ENDIF

ASK ALL AGE 16+
BPMeas
May I just check, have you ever had your blood pressure measured by a doctor or nurse?
1   Yes
2   No

IF BPMeas = Yes THEN
LastBP
When was the last time your blood pressure was measured by a doctor or nurse? Was it ...READ OUT.
1   ...during the last 12 months,
2   at least a year but less than 3 years ago,
3   at least 3 years but less than 5 years ago,
4   or 5 years ago or more?

NormBP
Thinking about the last time your blood pressure was measured, were you told it was ... READ OUT ...
INTERVIEWER: CODES 1,2,3 = TOLD WITH OR WITHOUT RESPONDENT ASKING
1   normal (alright/fine).
2   higher than normal,
3   lower than normal,
4   or were you not told anything?

IF (NormBP = High) AND CVD1 <> Yes) THEN
OnlyHi
Is this the only time your blood pressure has been higher than normal or has it been higher than normal a number of times?
1   Only time
2   A number of times
ENDIF
ENDIF

ASK ALL AGE 16+
CHMeas
Have you ever had your blood cholesterol level measured by a doctor or nurse?
1   Yes
2   No

IF CHMeas = Yes THEN
LastCH
When was the last time your blood cholesterol level was measured by a doctor or nurse? Was it ... READ OUT ...
1   ...during the last 12 months,
2   at least a year but less than 3 years ago,
3   at least 3 years but less than 5 years ago
4   or five years ago or more?

NormCH
Thinking about the last time your blood cholesterol level was measured, were you told it was...
READ OUT.....INTERVIEWER: CODES 1,2,3 = TOLD WITH OR WITHOUT RESPONDENT ASKING.
1   normal (alright/fine),
2   higher than normal,
3   lower than normal,
4   or were you not told anything?
ENDIF

The Health Survey for England – 1998 – Individual Questionnaire

Child physical activity module (2-15)

IF Age of Respondent is 4 years THEN
ChSch
Can I just check, is *(name of child)* at school in reception class yet?
1 Yes
2 No
ENDIF

ASK ALL AGE 2-15
Wlk5Ch
Now I'd like to ask you about some of the things you have done **in the last week**. By last week I mean in the seven days up to yesterday. In the last week have you done a **continuous** walk that lasted **at least** 5 minutes *(not counting things done as part of school lessons)?*
1 Yes
2 No

IF Wlk5Ch = Yes THEN
DaysWlk
On how many **days** in the last week did you do a continuous walk that lasted at least 5 minutes *(not counting things done as part of school lessons)?*
1 One day
2 Two days
3 Three days
4 Four days
5 Five days
6 Six days
7 Every day

DayWlkT
SHOW CARD G
On each **day** that you did a walk like this for at least 5 minutes, how long did you spend walking altogether? Please give an answer from this card
INTERVIEWER NOTE: COUNT TOTAL TIME SPENT WALKING. SO TWO WALKS OF 10 MINUTES EACH = 20 MINUTES WALKING
2 5 minutes, less than 15 minutes
3 15 minutes, less than 30 minutes
4 30 minutes, less than 1 hour
5 1 hour, less than 1½ hours
6 1½ hours, less than 2 hours
7 2 hours, less than 2½ hours
8 2½ hours, less than 3 hours
9 3 hours, less than 3½ hours
10 3½ hours, less than 4 hours
11 4 hours or more (please specify how long)

IF DayWlkT = 4 hours or more THEN
WlkHrs
How long did you spend walking on each day?
RECORD HOURS SPENT BELOW. RECORD MINUTES AT NEXT QUESTION
Range: 4.12

WlkMin
RECORD HERE MINUTES SPENT WALKING.
Range: 0.59

WlkTot
Computed total time from WlkHrs and WlkMin; Range: 0..9997
ENDIF

The Health Survey for England – 1998 – Individual Questionnaire

IF Age of Respondent is 13-15 years THEN
ChPace
Which of the following describes your usual walking pace ... READ OUT ...
1 ... a slow pace,
2 ... a steady average pace,
3 ... a fairly brisk pace,
4 ... or, a fast pace - at least 4 mph?
5 None of these
ENDIF
ENDIF

IF Age of Respondent is 8-15 years THEN
HWkCh
In the last week have you done any housework or gardening which involved pulling or pushing, like hoovering, cleaning a car, mowing grass or sweeping up leaves for at least 15 minutes a time?
1 Yes
2 No

IF HWkCh = Yes THEN
DHWkCh
On how many **days** in the last week have you done any housework or gardening of this type for at least 15 minutes a time?
1 One day
2 Two days
3 Three days
4 Four days
5 Five days
6 Six days
7 Every day

THwk
SHOW CARD G
On each **day** that you did any housework or gardening of this type for at least 15 minutes a time, how long did you spend?
Please give an answer from this card.
3 15 minutes, less than 30 minutes
4 30 minutes, less than 1 hour
5 1 hour, less than 1½ hours
6 1½ hours, less than 2 hours
7 2 hours, less than 2½ hours
8 2½ hours, less than 3 hours
9 3 hours, less than 3½ hours
10 3½ hours, less than 4 hours
11 4 hours or more (please specify how long)

IF THWk = 4 hours or more THEN
HWkHrs
How long did you spend doing housework or gardening on each day?
RECORD HOURS SPEND BELOW. RECORD MINUTES AT NEXT QUESTION.
Range: 4.12

HWkMin
RECORD HERE MINUTES SPENT DOING HOUSEWORK/GARDENING.
Range: 0.59

HWKTot
Computed total time from HWkHrs and HwkMin; Range: 0..9997
ENDIF
ENDIF
ENDIF

ASK ALL AGE 2-15
SPORT
I would now like to ask you about any sports or exercise activities that you have done. I will then go on to ask about other active things you may have done like running about, riding a bike, kicking a ball around and things like that. For the following questions please *(include any activities done at a nursery or playgroup/don't count any activities done as part of school lessons)*.

SportDo
SHOW CARD H
In the last week, that is last *(day)* up to yesterday, have you done any sports or exercise activities *(not counting things done as part of school lessons)*? This card shows some of the things you might have done; please also include any other sports or exercise activities like these.
INTERVIEWER: DO NOT COUNT ANYTHING DONE TODAY.
1 Yes
2 No

IF SportDo = Yes THEN
WESpDo
Did you do any of these sports or exercise activities at the weekend, that is last Saturday and Sunday *(yesterday and last Sunday)*?
1 Yes
2 No

IF WESpDo = Yes THEN
DWESp
Was that on Saturday or Sunday or on both days?
1 Saturday only
2 Sunday only
3 Both Saturday and Sunday

WeSpor
SHOW CARD G
On *(Saturday/Sunday/Saturday and Sunday)* when you did these sports or exercise activities, how long did you spend *(on each day)*? Please give an answer from this card.
INTERVIEWER: IF IT VARIED, TAKE AVERAGE
1 Less than 5 minutes
2 5 minutes, less than 15 minutes
3 15 minutes, less than 30 minutes
4 30 minutes, less than 1 hour
5 1 hour, less than 1½ hours
6 1½ hours, less than 2 hours
7 2 hours, less than 2½ hours
8 2½ hours, less than 3 hours
9 3 hours, less than 3½ hours
10 3½ hours, less than 4 hours
11 4 hours or more (please specify how long)

IF WeSpor = 4 hours or more THEN
WeSpH
How long did you spend doing these sports or exercise activities, how long did you spend *(on each day)*?
RECORD HOURS SPENT BELOW. RECORD MINUTES AT NEXT QUESTION.
Range: 4..12

WeSpM
RECORD HERE MINUTES SPEND DOING SPORTS OR EXERCISE ACTIVITIES.
Range: 0..59

WeSpT
Computed total time from WeSpH and WeSpM
Range: *0..9997*
ENDIF
ENDIF

DaySp
Still thinking about last week. On how many of the **weekdays** did you do any of these sports or exercise activities? *(Please remember not to count things done as part of school lessons)*
0 None in last week
1 1 day
2 2 days
3 3 days
4 4 days
5 5 days

IF DaySp = 1 day to 5 days THEN
WkSpor
SHOW CARD G
On each weekday that you did these sports or exercise activities, how long did you spend? Please give an answer from this card.
1 Less than 5 minutes
2 5 minutes, less than 15 minutes
3 15 minutes, less than 30 minutes
4 30 minutes, less than 1 hour
5 1 hour, less than 1½ hours
6 1½ hours, less than 2 hours
7 2 hours, less than 2½ hours
8 2½ hours, less than 3 hours
9 3 hours, less than 3½ hours
10 3½ hours, less than 4 hours
11 4 hours or more (please specify how long)

IF WkSpor = 4 hours or more THEN
WkSpH
How long did you spend doing these sports or exercise activities on each weekday?
RECORD HOURS SPENT BELOW. RECORD MINUTES AT NEXT QUESTION
Range: 4..12

WkSpM
RECORD HERE MINUTES SPENT DOING SPORTS OR EXERCISE ACTIVITIES
Range: 0..59

WkSpT
Computed total time from WkSpH and WkSpM; Range: *0..9997*
ENDIF
ENDIF

ASK ALL AGE 2-15
WEActDo
SHOW CARD I
Now I would like to know about when you do active things, like the things on this card or other activities like these. Did you do any active things like these at the weekend, that is last Saturday and Sunday *(yesterday and last Sunday)*?
INTERVIEWER NOTE: DO NOT INCLUDE ANY ACTIVITIES ALREADY COVERED UNDER SPORTS AND EXERCISE ACTIVITIES
1 Yes
2 No

IF WEActDo = Yes THEN
DWEAct
Was that on Saturday or Sunday or on both days?
1 Saturday only
2 Sunday only
3 Both Saturday and Sunday

WeAct
SHOW CARD G
On *(Saturday/Sunday/Saturday and Sunday)* when you did active things like these, how long did you spend *(on each day)*? Please give an answer from this card.
INTERVIEWER: IF IT VARIED, TAKE AVERAGE
1 Less than 5 minutes
2 5 minutes, less than 15 minutes
3 15 minutes, less than 30 minutes
4 30 minutes, less than 1 hour
5 1 hour, less than 1½ hours
6 1½ hours, less than 2 hours
7 2 hours, less than 2½ hours
8 2½ hours, less than 3 hours
9 3 hours, less than 3½ hours
10 3½ hours, less than 4 hours
11 4 hours or more (please specify how long)

IF WeAct= 4 hours or more THEN
WeActH
How long did you spend doing active things like these?
RECORD HOURS SPENT BELOW RECORD MINUTES AT NEXT QUESTION.
Range: 4..12

WeActM
RECORD HERE MINUTES SPENT DOING ACTIVE THINGS LIKE THESE
Range: 0.59

WeActT
Computed total time from WeActH and WeActM; Range: 0..9997
ENDIF

ASK ALL AGE 2-15
WkActDo
SHOW CARD I
Still thinking about last week. On how many of the **weekdays** did you do active things like these, like **the things on** this card or other activities like these *(not counting things done as part of school lessons)*?
INTERVIEWER NOTE: DO NOT INCLUDE ANY ACTIVITIES ALREADY COVERED UNDER SPORTS AND EXERCISE ACTIVITIES
0 None in last week
1 1 day
2 2 days
3 3 days
4 4 days
5 5 days

IF WkActDo = 1 day to 5 days THEN
WkAct
SHOW CARD G
On each **weekday** that you did active things like these, how long did you spend? Please give an answer from this card.
INTERVIEWER: IF IT VARIED, TAKE AVERAGE
1 Less than 5 minutes
2 5 minutes, less than 15 minutes
3 15 minutes, less than 30 minutes
4 30 minutes, less than 1 hour
5 1 hour, less than 1½ hours
6 1½ hours, less than 2 hours
7 2 hours, less than 2½ hours
8 2½ hours, less than 3 hours
9 3 hours, less than 3½ hours
10 3½ hours, less than 4 hours
11 4 hours or more (please specify how long)

IF WkAct = 4 hours or more THEN
WkActH
How long did you spend doing active things like these on each weekday?
RECORD HOURS SPENT BELOW RECORD MINUTES AT NEXT QUESTION
Range: 4..12

WkActM
RECORD HERE MINUTES SPENT DOING ACTIVE THINGS LIKE THESE.
Range: 0..59

WkActT
Computed total time from WkActH and WkActM; Range: 0..9997
ENDIF
ENDIF

ASK ALL AGE 2-15
DaysTot
Now thinking about all the activities during the past week you have just told me about including any walking, *(gardening, housework,)* sports or other active things. On how many **days** in the last week **in total** did you do any of these activities *(not counting things done as part of school lessons)*?
0 None
1 One day
2 Two days
3 Three days
4 Four days
5 Five days
6 Six days
7 Every day

WESitDo
SHOW CARD J
Now I'd like to know about when you spend time sitting down doing things like these the ones on this card. Did you spend time sitting down doing any things like these for at least 5 minutes a time at the weekend, that is last Saturday and Sunday *(yesterday and last Sunday)*?
1 Yes
2 No

IF WESitDo = Yes THEN
DSitWE
Was that on Saturday or Sunday or on both days?
1 Saturday only
2 Sunday only
3 Both Saturday and Sunday

SitWE
SHOW CARD G
On *(Saturday/Sunday/Saturday and Sunday)* when you spent time sitting down doing things like these, how long did you spend *(on each day)*? Please give an answer from this card.
INTERVIEWER: IF IT VARIED, TAKE AVERAGE
2 5 minutes, less than 15 minutes
3 15 minutes, less than 30 minutes
4 30 minutes, less than 1 hour
5 1 hour, less than 1½ hours
6 1½ hours, less than 2 hours
7 2 hours, less than 2½ hours
8 2½ hours, less than 3 hours
9 3 hours, less than 3½ hours
10 3½ hours, less than 4 hours
11 4 hours or more (please specify how long)

IF SitWE = 4 hours or more THEN
WeSitH
How long did you spend sitting down doing things like these?
RECORD HOURS SPENT BELOW RECORD MINUTES AT NEXT QUESTION.
Range 4..12

WeSitM
RECORD HERE MINUTES SPENT SITTING DOWN DOING THINGS LIKE THESE.
Range: 0..59

WeSitT Computed total time from WeSitH and WeSiiM; Range: *0..9997*
ENDIF
ENDIF

ASK ALL AGE 2-15
WkSitDo
SHOW CARD J
On how many **weekdays** last week did you spend time sitting down doing things like the ones on this card for at least 5 minutes a time, *(not counting things you did as part of school lessons)?*
0 None in last week
1 1 day
2 2 days
3 3 days
4 4 days
5 5 days

IF WkSitDo = 1 day to 5 days THEN
WkSitHrs
SHOW CARD G
On each **weekday** that you spent time sitting down doing things like these, how long did you spend?
Please give an answer from this card.
2 5 minutes, less than 15 minutes
3 15 minutes, less than 30 minutes
4 30 minutes, less than 1 hour
5 1 hour, less than 1½ hours
6 1½ hours, less than 2 hours
7 2 hours, less than 2½ hours
8 2½ hours, less than 3 hours
9 3 hours, less than 3½ hours
10 3½ hours, less than 4 hours
11 4 hours or more (please specify how long)

IF **WkSitHrs**=4 hours or more THEN
WkSitH
How long did you spend sitting down doing things like these?
RECORD HOURS SPENT BELOW RECORD MINUTES AT NEXT QUESTION.
Range: 4..12

WkSitM
RECORD HERE MINUTES SPENT SITTING DOWN DOING THINGS LIKE THESE.
Range: 0..59

WkSitT Computed total time from WkSitH and WkSitM; Range: *0..9997*
ENDIF

ASK ALL AGE 2-15
Usual
Were the activities you did last week different from what you would usually do for any reason?
IF YES PROBE: Would you usually do more physical activity or less?
1 NO - same as usual
2 YES DIFFERENT - usually do MORE
3 YES DIFFERENT - usually do LESS

Adult physical activity module (16+)

ASK ALL AGE 16+
Work
I'd like to ask you about some of the things you have done in the past four weeks that involve physical activity, this could be at work (*school/college*) or in your free time. (Can I just check) were you in paid employment or self-employed in the past four weeks?
1 Yes
2 No

IF Work = Yes THEN
Active
Thinking about your job in general would you say that you are ...READ OUT...
1 ...very physically active,
2 ...fairly physically active,
3 ...not very physically active,
4 ...or, not at all physically active in your job?

SitWork
When you're at work are you mainly sitting down, standing up or walking about?
1 Sitting down
2 Standing up
3 Walking about

ClimbWrk
Do you do any climbing in the course of your work (ladders, scaffolding etc)? EXCLUDE CLIMBING STAIRS.
1 Yes
2 No

LiftWrk
Do you usually have to lift or carry things at work which you find heavy? IF YES, PROMPT: Is that just lifting or lifting and carrying?
1 Yes - lift heavy loads
2 Yes - lift and carry heavy loads
3 No
ENDIF

ASK ALL AGE 16+
Housewrk
I'd like you to think about the physical activities you have done in the last few weeks (*when you were not doing your paid job.*) Have you done any housework in the past four weeks, that is from (*date four weeks ago*) up to yesterday?
1 Yes
2 No

IF Housewrk = Yes THEN
HWrkList
SHOW CARD K
Have you done any housework listed on this card?
1 Yes
2 No

HevyHWrk
SHOW CARD L
Some kinds of housework are heavier than others. This card gives some examples of heavy housework. It does not include everything, these are just examples. Was any of the housework you did in the last four weeks this kind of heavy housework?
1 Yes
2 No

ASK ALL AGE 16+
Wlk5Int

I'd like you to think about **all** the **walking** you have done in the past 4 weeks either locally or away from here. Please include any country walks, walking to and from work and any other walks that you have done. In the past four weeks, **that** is since *(date four weeks ago)*, have you done a **continuous** walk that lasted **at least 5 minutes?**

    1 Yes
    2 No
    3 Can't walk at all

IF Wlk5Int = Yes THEN
Wlk15M

In the past four weeks, have you done a **continuous** walk that lasted **at least** 15 minutes? (That is since *(date four weeks ago)*)

    1 Yes
    2 No

IF Wlk15M = Yes THEN
DayWlk

During the past four weeks, on how **many days** did you do a walk of at least 15 minutes? (That is since *(date four weeks ago)*)
    Range: 1..28

Day1Wlk

On that day *(any of those days)* did you do **more than one** walk lasting at least 15 minutes?
    1 Yes, more than one walk of 15+ mins (on at least one day)
    2 No, only one walk of 15+ mins a day

IF (DayWlk in [2..28]) AND (Day1Wlk = Yes) THEN
Day2Wlk

On how many days in the last four weeks did you do more than one walk that lasted at least 15 minutes?
    Range: 1..28
ENDIF

IF Wlk15M = Yes THEN
HrsWlk

How long did you usually spend walking each time you did a walk for 15 minutes or more?
IF VERY DIFFERENT LENGTHS, PROBE FOR MOST REGULAR. RECORD HOURS SPENT BELOW. ENTER 0 IF LESS THAN 1 HOUR. RECORD MINUTES AT NEXT QUESTION.
    Range: 0..12

MinWlk

RECORD HERE MINUTES SPENT WALKING.
    Range: 0..59

TotTim
Computed total time from HrsWlk and MinWlk.
    Range: *0..779*
ENDIF
ENDIF

WalkPace

Which of the following best describes your **usual** walking pace ...READ OUT...
    1 ...a slow pace,
    2 ...a steady average pace,
    3 ...a fairly brisk pace,
    4 ...or, a fast pace - at least 4 mph?
    5 (none of these)
ENDIF

IF HevyHWrk = Yes THEN
HeavyDay

During the past four weeks on how many **days** have you done this kind of **heavy** housework?
    Range: 1..28

HrsHHW

On the days you did heavy housework, how long did you usually spend?
RECORD HOURS SPENT BELOW. ENTER 0 IF LESS THAN 1 HOUR. RECORD MINUTES AT NEXT QUESTION.
    Range: 0..12

MinHHW

RECORD MINUTES SPENT ON HEAVY HOUSEWORK.
    Range: 0..59

HWTim
Computed total time from HRSHHW and MINHHW.
    Range: *0..779*
ENDIF

ASK ALL AGE 16+
Garden

Have you done any gardening, DIY or building work in the past four weeks, that is since *(date four weeks ago)*?
    1 Yes
    2 No

IF Garden = Yes THEN
GardList
SHOW CARD M

Have you done any gardening, DIY or building work listed on this card?
    1 Yes
    2 No

ManWork
SHOW CARD N

Have you done any gardening, DIY or building work from this other card, or any similar **heavy manual** work?
    1 Yes
    2 No

IF ManWork = Yes THEN
ManDays

During the past 4 weeks on how many **days** have you done this kind of **heavy** manual gardening or DIY?
    Range: 1..28

HrsDIY

On the days you did heavy manual gardening or DIY, how long did you usually spend?
RECORD HOURS SPENT BELOW. ENTER 0 IF LESS THAN 1 HOUR. RECORD MINUTES AT NEXT QUESTION.
    Range: 0..12

MinDIY

RECORD MINUTES SPENT ON GARDENING OR DIY.
    Range: 0..59

DIYTim
Computed total time from HrsDIY and MinDIY.
    Range: *0..779*
ENDIF
ENDIF

ASK ALL AGE 16+

ActPhy

SHOW CARD O

Can you tell me if you have done any activities on this card during the last 4 weeks, that is since *(date four weeks ago)*? Include teaching, coaching, training and practice sessions.

1 Yes
2 No

IF ActPhy = Yes THEN

WhtAct

Which have you done in the last four weeks? PROBE: Any others? CODE ALL THAT APPLY.

1 Swimming,
2 Cycling,
3 Workout at a gym/Exercise bike/ Weight training
4 Aerobics/Keep fit/Gymnastics/ Dance for fitness
5 Any other type of dancing
6 Running/jogging
7 Football/rugby
8 Badminton/tennis
9 Squash
10 Exercises (e.g. press-ups, sit ups)

ENDIF

Repeat for up to 6 additional sports:

FOR ActVar := 11 TO 16 DO
IF (ActVar = 11) OR (OActQ[ActVar - 1] = Yes) THEN

OactQ[i]

Have you done any other sport or exercise not listed on the card?
ARRAY[11..16] OF Yes, No

IF (OActQ = Yes) THEN

OthAct[i]

PROBE FOR NAME OF SPORT OR EXERCISE. WRITE IN.
ARRAY[11..16] OF STRING[20]

Actvs[ActVar] := OthAct[ActVar]

ENDIF
ENDIF
ENDDO

DayExc to ExcSwt repeated for each sport/exercise coded at WhtAct or mentioned at OthAct

FOR ActVar := 1 TO 16 DO
IF ((ActVar in [1..10]) AND (ActVar IN WhtAct)) OR ((ActVar in [11..16]) AND (OActQ[ActVar] = Yes)) THEN

DayExc

Can you tell me on how many separate days did you do *(name of activity)* for at least 15 minutes a time during the past four weeks, that is since *(date four weeks ago)*? IF ONLY DONE FOR LESS THAN 15 MINUTES ENTER 0.
Range: 0..28

IF DayExc ≥ 1 THEN

ExcHrs

How much time did you usually spend doing *(name of activity)* on each day? (Only count times you did it for at least 15 minutes.)
RECORD HOURS SPENT BELOW. ENTER 0 IF LESS THAN 1 HOUR. RECORD MINUTES AT NEXT QUESTION.
Range: 0..12

ExcMin

RECORD MINUTES HERE.
Range: 0..59

ExcTim

Computed total time from ExcHrs and ExcMin.
Range: 0..779

ExcSwt

During the past four weeks, was the effort of *(name of activity)* usually enough to make you out of breath or sweaty?

1 Yes
2 No

ENDIF
ENDIF
ENDDO

Eating habits module (16+)

ASK ALL AGE 16+

BreadA

What kind of bread do you usually eat? Is it ...READ OUT...

CODE ONE ONLY.

  1 white (INCL CHOLLAH),

  2 brown, granary, wheatmeal, (INCL WHEATGERM, SOFTGRAIN, RYE, GERMAN),

  3 wholemeal (INCL HIGHBRAN),

  4 or, some other kind of bread?

SPONTANEOUS:

  5 Does not have a usual type

  9 Does not eat any type of bread

IF BROWN, CHECK IF WHOLEMEAL OR SOME OTHER SORT OF BROWN BREAD.

IF PITTA/NAN/SODA BREAD ETC, CHECK IF WHITE OR WHOLEMEAL.

IF BreadA = OTHER THEN

OBread

Please specify other kind of bread.

    Text: Maximum 20 characters

ENDIF

IF (Breda IN [White..UnUse]) THEN

BreadQua

How many rolls or pieces of bread do you eat each day, on average?

Is it... READ OUT...

  1 Less than 1 a day,

  2 1 or 2 a day,

  3 3 or 4 a day,

  4 or 5 or more a day?

ENDIF

ASK ALL AGE 16+

NSpread

What type of margarine, butter or other spread do you usually use, for example on bread, sandwiches, toast, potatoes or vegetables?

CODE ONE ONLY. REFER TO CODING LIST A.

  1 Butter or margarine

  2 Low fat or reduced fat spread, or half-fat butter

  3 Spread not on coding list

SPONTANEOUS:

  4 Does not have usual type

  5 Does not use fat spread

IF NSpread = OTHER THEN

OthSprd

INTERVIEWER: SPECIFY NAME OF SPREAD.

    Text: Maximum 40 characters

ENDIF

IF (NSpread IN [Butter..NoType]) THEN

SprdQua

How many pats or rounded teaspoons of margarine, butter or other spread do you use each day on average, for example on bread, sandwiches, toast, potatoes or vegetables?

    Range: 0..99

ENDIF

ASK ALL AGE 16+

Milk

What kind of milk do you **usually** use for drinks, in tea or coffee and on cereals? Is it ...READ OUT...

  1 whole milk,

  2 semi-skimmed (INCL DRIED SEMI-SKIMMED),

  3 skimmed (INCL DRIED SKIMMED, BOOTS DRIED POWDER, CO-OP POWDER),

  4 or, some other kind of milk?

SPONTANEOUS:

  5 Does not have usual type

  6 Does not drink milk

IF Milk = OTHER THEN

OMilk

Please specify other kind of milk.

    Text: Maximum 20 characters

ENDIF

IF (Milk IN [Whole..NoType]) THEN

MilkQua

About how much milk do you yourself use each day, on average (for drinks, in tea and coffee, on cereals etc)?

Is it ...READ OUT...

  1 less than a quarter of a pint,

  2 about a quarter of a pint,

  3 about half a pint,

  4 or, one pint or more?

ENDIF

ASK ALL AGE 16+

TabSalt

At the table do you ...READ OUT...

CODE ONE ONLY. TREAT LOSALT AS SALT.

  1 generally add salt to your food without tasting it first,

  2 taste the food, but then generally add salt,

  3 taste the food, but only occasionally add salt,

  4 rarely, or never, add salt at the table?

NCereal

Which type of breakfast cereal do you usually eat?

CODE ONE ONLY. USE CODING LIST B FOR QUERIES

  1 Bran cereal on coding list (e.g. AllBran, Branflakes, Sultana Bran)

  2 Oat or wheat cereal on coding list (e.g. Shredded Wheat, Muesli, porridge, Weetabix)

  3 Bran, oat or wheat cereal not on coding list

  4 Others (e.g. Cornflakes, Rice Krispies, Special K, Sugar Puffs, Honey Smacks)

SPONTANEOUS:

  5 Does not have usual type

  6 Does not eat breakfast cereal

IF NCereal = Bran, oat or wheat cereal not on coding list THEN

OthCer

INTERVIEWER: SPECIFY NAME OF BRAN, OAT OR WHEAT CEREAL.

    Text: Maximum 40 characters

ENDIF

IF (NCereal IN [Bran..NoType]) THEN

CerQua

SHOW CARD P

About how many times a week do you have a bowl of breakfast cereal or porridge?

1 6 or more times a week
2 3-5 times a week
3 1-2 times a week
4 Less than once a week
5 Rarely or never

ENDIF

ASK ALL AGE 16+

PstRePot

SHOW CARD P

I would like to ask you about some foods which you may eat. Can you tell me how often on average do you eat a serving of these foods by choosing your answer from this card. How often, on average, do you eat a serving of pasta, rice or potatoes?

1 6 or more times a week
2 3-5 times a week
3 1-2 times a week
4 Less than once a week
5 Rarely or never

NBeans

SHOW CARD P

How often on average do you eat a serving of peas, lentils or beans including baked beans?

1 6 or more times a week
2 3-5 times a week
3 1-2 times a week
4 Less than once a week
5 Rarely or never

NVeges

SHOW CARD P

How often on average do you eat a serving of other types of vegetables (raw or cooked)?

1 6 or more times a week
2 3-5 times a week
3 1-2 times a week
4 Less than once a week
5 Rarely or never

NFruit

SHOW CARD P

How often on average do you eat a serving of fruit, including fresh, tinned or frozen?

1 6 or more times a week
2 3-5 times a week
3 1-2 times a week
4 Less than once a week
5 Rarely or never

Cheese

SHOW CARD P

How often on average does you eat a serving of any type of cheese, except cottage cheese?

1 6 or more times a week
2 3-5 times a week
3 1-2 times a week
4 Less than once a week
5 Rarely or never

RedMeat

SHOW CARD P

How often on average do you eat a serving of beef, pork or lamb, including beefburgers, sausages, bacon, meat pies and processed meat?

1 6 or more times a week
2 3-5 times a week
3 1-2 times a week
4 Less than once a week
5 Rarely or never

WhitMeat

SHOW CARD P

How often on average do you eat a serving of chicken or turkey (including processed chicken or turkey)?

1 6 or more times a week
2 3-5 times a week
3 1-2 times a week
4 Less than once a week
5 Rarely or never

FriedFd

SHOW CARD P

How often on average do you eat a serving of **any** fried food, including fried fish, chips, cooked breakfast, samosas?

1 6 or more times a week
2 3-5 times a week
3 1-2 times a week
4 Less than once a week
5 Rarely or never

Fish

SHOW CARD P

Apart from fried fish, how often on average do you eat a serving of fish?

1 6 or more times a week
2 3-5 times a week
3 1-2 times a week
4 Less than once a week
5 Rarely or never

ChocCrBs

SHOW CARD P

How often on average do you eat chocolate, crisps or biscuits, including savoury biscuits such as cream crackers?

1 6 or more times a week
2 3-5 times a week
3 1-2 times a week
4 Less than once a week
5 Rarely or never

NCakes

SHOW CARD P

How often on average do you eat a serving of cakes, pies, puddings or pastries?

1 6 or more times a week
2 3-5 times a week
3 1-2 times a week
4 Less than once a week
5 Rarely or never

Smoking module

IF Age of Respondent is 18 or 19 years THEN
BookChe
INTERVIEWER CHECK: *(Name of respondent)* IS AGED *(age of respondent)*. RESPONDENT TO BE...
  1 Asked Smoking/Drinking questions
  2 Given ORANGE SELF-COMPLETION BOOKLET FOR YOUNG ADULTS
ENDIF

IF (Age of Respondent is 20 years or over) OR (BookChe = Asked) THEN
SmokEver
May I just check, have you ever smoked a cigarette, a cigar or a pipe?
  1 Yes
  2 No

IF SmokEver = Yes THEN
SmokeNow
Do you smoke cigarettes at all nowadays?
  1 Yes
  2 No

IF SmokeNow = Yes THEN
DlySmoke
About how many cigarettes a day do you usually smoke on weekdays?
INTERVIEWER: IF LESS THAN ONE A DAY, ENTER 0. IF RANGE GIVEN AND CAN'T ESTIMATE, ENTER MID POINT. IF RESPONDENT SMOKES ROLL UPS AND CANNOT GIVE NUMBER OF CIGARETTES, CODE 97.
  Range: 0..97.

IF DlySmoke = 97 THEN
DlyEst
INTERVIEWER: ASK RESPONDENT FOR AN ESTIMATED CONSUMPTION OF TOBACCO ON WEEKDAYS. WILL IT BE GIVEN IN GRAMS OR IN OUNCES?
  1 Grams
  2 Ounces

IF DlyEst = grams THEN
Dlyg
PLEASE RECORD ESTIMATED CONSUMPTION OF TOBACCO ON WEEKDAYS IN GRAMS.
  Range: 1..67

ELSEIF DlyEst = ounces THEN
Dlyoz
PLEASE RECORD ESTIMATED CONSUMPTION OF TOBACCO ON WEEKDAYS IN OUNCES. FOR FRACTIONS OF OUNCES RECORD:
1/4 (a quarter) oz as .25
1/3 (a third) oz as .33
1/2 (half) oz as .5
2/3 (two thirds) oz as .66
3/4 (three quarters) oz as .75
  Range: 0.01..2.40
ENDIF

RolDly
Computed: estimated tobacco consumption in ounces.
  Range: 1..97
ENDIF

For analysis purposes ounces or grams of tobacco are converted to number of cigarettes and stored in the variable DlySmoke.

WkndSmok
And about how many cigarettes a day do you usually smoke at weekends?
INTERVIEWER: IF RANGE GIVEN AND CAN'T ESTIMATE, ENTER MID POINT. IF RESPONDENT SMOKES ROLL UPS AND CANNOT GIVE NUMBER OF CIGARETTES, CODE 97.
  Range: 0..97

IF WkndSmok = 97 THEN
WkndEst
INTERVIEWER: ASK RESPONDENT FOR AN ESTIMATED CONSUMPTION OF TOBACCO AT WEEKENDS. WILL IT BE GIVEN IN GRAMS OR IN OUNCES?
  1 Grams
  2 Ounces

IF WkndEst = grams THEN
Wkndg
PLEASE RECORD ESTIMATED CONSUMPTION OF TOBACCO AT WEEKENDS IN GRAMS.
  Range: 1..67

ELSEIF WkndEst = ounces THEN
Wkndoz
PLEASE RECORD ESTIMATED CONSUMPTION OF TOBACCO AT WEEKENDS IN OUNCES. FOR FRACTIONS OF OUNCES RECORD:
1/4 (a quarter) oz as .25
1/3 (a third) oz as .33
1/2 (half) oz as .5
2/3 (two thirds) oz as .66
3/4 (three quarters) oz as .75
  Range: 0.01..2.40
ENDIF

RolWknd
Computed: estimated tobacco consumption in ounces.
  Range: 1..97
ENDIF

For analysis purposes ounces or grams of tobacco are converted to number of cigarettes and stored in the variable WkndSmoke.

CigType
Do you mainly smoke ...READ OUT...
  1 ...filter-tipped cigarettes,
  2 plain or untipped cigarettes,
  3 or hand-rolled cigarettes?

IF CigType = filter-tipped cigarettes OR plain or untipped cigarettes THEN
CigBrand
Which brand of cigarette do you usually smoke?
ASIGN 3-DIGIT CODE FROM CODING CARD C. IF NOT ON LIST, CODE AS 997.
  Range: 1..997

IF CigBrand=997 THEN
Tar
INTERVIEWER: ASK TO SEE PACKET AND CODE TAR LEVEL (not nicotine content) OF USUAL BRAND OF CIGARETTES, IN MG. THIS IS USUALLY PRINTED ON THE SIDE OF THE PACKET. IF NO PACKET AVAILABLE, ASK RESPONDENT TO ESTIMATE.
  Range: 0..25

IF Tar=Response THEN
  TarEst
  INTERVIEWER CODE:
    1 Tar level obtained by looking at packet
    2 Respondent estimated tar level
  ENDIF
ENDIF

ELSE (*Smokes, but not nowadays*)
  SmokeCig
  Have you ever smoked cigarettes?
    1 Yes
    2 No

IF SmokeCig = Yes THEN
  SmokeReg
  Did you smoke cigarettes regularly, that is at least one cigarette a day, or did you smoke them only occasionally?
    1 Smoked cigarettes regularly, at least 1 per day
    2 Smoked them only occasionally
    3 SPONTANEOUS: Never really smoked cigarettes, just tried them once or twice

IF SmokeReg = Smoked cigarettes regularly THEN
  NumSmok
  About how many cigarettes did you smoke in a day?
  INTERVIEWER: IF RANGE GIVEN AND CAN'T ESTIMATE, ENTER MID POINT. IF RESPONDENT SMOKES ROLL UPS AND CANNOT GIVE NUMBER OF CIGARETTES, CODE 97.
  Range: 0..97

IF NumSmok = 97 THEN
  NumEst
  INTERVIEWER: ASK RESPONDENT FOR AN ESTIMATED CONSUMPTION OF TOBACCO. WILL IT BE GIVEN IN GRAMS OR IN OUNCES?
    1 Grams
    2 Ounces

IF NumEst = grams THEN
  Numg
  PLEASE RECORD ESTIMATED DAILY CONSUMPTION OF TOBACCO IN GRAMS.
  Range: 1..67

ELSEIF NumEst = ounces THEN
  Numoz
  PLEASE RECORD ESTIMATED DAILY CONSUMPTION OF TOBACCO IN OUNCES. FOR FRACTIONS OF OUNCES RECORD:
  1/4 (a quarter) oz as .25
  1/3 (a third) oz as .33
  1/2 (half) oz as .5
  2/3 (two thirds) oz as .66
  3/4 (three quarters) oz as .75
  Range: 0.01..2.40
ENDIF

RolNum
Computed: estimated tobacco consumption in ounces.
Range: 1..97

ENDIF
For analysis purposes ounces or grams of tobacco are converted to number of cigarettes and stored in the variable NumSmoke.

SmokYrs
And for approximately how many years did you smoke cigarettes regularly?
INTERVIEWER: IF LESS THAN ONE YEAR, CODE 0.
  Range: 0..97
ENDIF

IF SmokeReg = Smoked cigarettes regularly OR Smoked them only occasionally THEN
  EndSmoke
  How long ago did you stop smoking cigarettes?
  INTERVIEWER: IF LESS THAN ONE YEAR AGO, CODE 0.
  Range: 0..97

IF EndSmoke = 0 THEN
  LongEnd
  How many months ago was that?
    1 Less than six months ago
    2 Six months, but less than one year
ENDIF

IF (EndSmoke <> EMPTY) AND (EndSmoke < 2) THEN
  Nicot
  Did you use any nicotine products, such as nicotine patches, chewing gum, lozenges or other similar products at all to help you give up?
  INTERVIEWER: IF RESPONDENT HAS GIVEN UP MORE THAN ONCE, ASK ABOUT MOST RECENT OCCASION.
    1 Yes
    2 No
  ENDIF
ENDIF
ENDIF

IF (SmokeNow = Yes) OR (SmokeReg = Smoked cigarettes regularly) THEN
  StartSmk
  How old were you when you started to smoke cigarettes regularly?
  INTERVIEWER: IF Never smoked regularly CODE 97
  Range: 1..97
ENDIF

IF (Sex = Female) AND (Age of Respondent is 18 to 49 years THEN
IF (EndSmoke <> EMPTY) AND (EndSmoke < 2) THEN
  IsPreg
  Can I check, are you pregnant now?
    1 Yes
    2 No

IF IsPreg = Yes THEN
  SmokePrg
  Have you smoked at all since you've known you've been pregnant?
  IF YES, PROBE: All the time or just some of the time?
    1 Yes, all the time
    2 Yes, some of the time
    3 No, not at all

IF SmokePrg = Yes, some of the time OR No, not at all THEN
  StopPreg
  Did you stop smoking specifically because of your pregnancy, or for some other reason?
    1 Because of pregnancy
    2 For some other reason
  ENDIF
ENDIF

IF (IsPreg = No) OR (IsPreg = DONTKNOW) OR (IsPreg = REFUSAL) OR (SmokeNow = Yes) THEN
  PregRec
  Can I check, have you been pregnant in the last twelve months?
    1 Currently pregnant
    2 Was pregnant in last twelve months but not now
    3 Not pregnant in last twelve months

  IF PregRec = Was pregnant in last twelve months but not now THEN
    PregSmok
    Did you smoke at all during pregnancy? (I.E. DURING TIME WHEN KNEW SHE WAS PREGNANT) IF YES, PROBE:All the time or just some of the time?
      1 Yes, all the time
      2 Yes, some of the time
      3 No, not at all

    IF PregSmok = Yes, some of the time OR No, not at all THEN
      PregStop
      Did you stop smoking specifically because of your pregnancy, or for some other reason?
        1 Because of pregnancy
        2 For some other reason
      ENDIF
    ENDIF
  ENDIF

IF (SmokeNow = Yes) OR (SmokeReg = Smoked cigarettes regularly OR Smoked them only occasionally) THEN
  SmokeTry
  (*Apart from any attempts during this/that pregnancy,*) have (*did*) you ever tried (*try*) to give up smoking because of a particular health condition you had at the time?
    1 Yes
    2 No

  DrSmoke
  Has (*did*) a medical person, for example a doctor or nurse ever advised (*advise*) you to stop smoking altogether because of your health?
    1 Yes
    2 No

  IF DrSmoke = Yes THEN
    DrSmoke1
    How long ago was that?
      1 Within the last twelve months
      2 Over twelve months ago
    ENDIF
  ENDIF

CigarNow
Do you smoke cigars at all nowadays?
  1 Yes
  2 No

IF CigarNow = Yes THEN
  CigarReg
  Do you smoke cigars regularly, that is at least one cigar a month, or do you smoke them only occasionally?
    1 Smoke at least one cigar a month
    2 Smoke them only occasionally
ENDIF

IF Sex = Male THEN
  PipeNowA
  Do you smoke a pipe at all nowadays?
    1 Yes
    2 No
  ENDIF
ENDIF

ASK ALL.
IF Age of Respondent is13 years or over THEN
  ExpSm
  Now, in most weeks, how many hours a week are you exposed to other people's tobacco smoke?
    Range: 0..97

ELSEIF Age of Respondent is 2 to 12 years THEN
  ChExpSm
  Is (*Name of child*) looked after for more than two hours per week by anyone who smokes while looking after (*him/her*)?
    1 Yes
    2 No
ENDIF

IF (Age of Respondent is 20 years or over) OR (BookChc = Asked) THEN
  FathSm
  Did your father ever smoke regularly when you were a child?
    1 Yes
    2 No

  MothSm
  Did your mother ever smoke regularly when you were a child?
    1 Yes
    2 No
ENDIF

Drinking module (16+)

IF (Age of Respondent is 20 years or over) OR (BookChc = Asked)
Jump7
INTERVIEWER: NOW FOLLOWS THE DRINKING MODULE.

Drink
I am now going to ask you a few questions about what you drink - that is if you drink. Do you ever drink alcohol nowadays, including drinks you brew or make at home?
1 Yes
2 No

IF Drink = No THEN
DrinkAny
Could I just check, does that mean you never have an alcoholic drink nowadays, or do you have an alcoholic drink very occasionally, perhaps for medicinal purposes or on special occasions like Christmas and New Year?
1 Very occasionally
2 Never
ENDIF

IF (Drink = Yes) OR (DrinkAny = Very occasionally) THEN
Intro
INTERVIEWER - READ OUT: I'd like to ask you (all) whether you have drunk different types of alcoholic drink in the last 12 months. I do not need to know about non-alcoholic or low alcohol drinks.

NBeer
SHOW CARD Q
I'd like to ask you first about normal strength beer or cider which has less than 6% alcohol. How often have you had a drink of normal strength BEER, LAGER, STOUT, CIDER or SHANDY (excluding cans and bottles of shandy) during the last 12 months? (NORMAL = less than 6% Alcohol by volume)
INTERVIEWER: IF RESPONDENT DOES NOT KNOW WHETHER BEER ETC DRUNK IS STRONG OR NORMAL, INCLUDE HERE AS NORMAL.
1 Almost every day
2 Five or six days a week
3 Three or four days a week
4 Once or twice a week
5 Once or twice a month
6 Once every couple of months
7 Once or twice a year
8 Not at all in the last 12 months

IF Nbeer IN [Almost every day...Once or twice a year] THEN
NBeerM
How much NORMAL STRENGTH BEER, LAGER, STOUT, CIDER or SHANDY (excluding cans and bottles of shandy) have you usually drunk on any one day?
INTERVIEWER: CODE MEASURES THAT YOU ARE GOING TO USE.
1 Half pints
2 Small cans
3 Large cans
4 Bottles

IF NbeerM = Half pints THEN
NBeerQ[1]
ASK OR CODE: How many half pints of NORMAL STRENGTH BEER, LAGER, STOUT, CIDER OR SHANDY (excluding cans and bottles of shandy) have you usually drunk on any one day?
ARRAY[1..4] OF
Range: 1..97
ENDIF

IF NbeerM = Small cans THEN
NBeerQ[2]
ASK OR CODE: How many small cans of NORMAL STRENGTH BEER, LAGER, STOUT or CIDER have you usually drunk on any one day?
ARRAY[1..4] OF
Range: 1..97
ENDIF

IF NbeerM = Large cans THEN
NBeerQ[3]
ASK OR CODE: How many large cans of NORMAL STRENGTH BEER, LAGER, STOUT or CIDER have you usually drunk on any one day?
ARRAY[1..4] OF
Range: 1..97
ENDIF

IF NbeerM = Bottles THEN
NBeerQ[4]
ASK OR CODE: How many bottles of NORMAL STRENGTH BEER, LAGER, STOUT or CIDER have you usually drunk on any one day?
ARRAY[1..4] OF
Range: 1..97

NBottle
ASK OR CODE: What make of NORMAL STRENGTH BEER, LAGER, STOUT or CIDER do you usually drink from bottles?
INTERVIEWER: IF RESPONDENT DOES NOT KNOW WHAT MAKE, OR RESPONDENT DRINKS DIFFERENT MAKES OF NORMAL STRENGTH BEER, LAGER, STOUT OR CIDER,
PROBE: What make have you drunk most frequently or most recently?
Text: Maximum 21 characters

NCodeEq
Computed: Pint Equivalent of Bottles
ENDIF
ENDIF

SBeer
SHOW CARD Q
Now I'd like to ask you about strong beer or cider which has 6% or more alcohol (e.g. Tennants Extra, Special Brew, Diamond White). How often have you had a drink of strong BEER, LAGER, STOUT or CIDER during the last 12 months? (STRONG=6% and over Alcohol by volume)
INTERVIEWER: IF RESPONDENT DOES NOT KNOW WHETHER BEER ETC DRUNK IS STRONG OR NORMAL, INCLUDE AS NORMAL STRENGTH AT NBeer ABOVE.
1 Almost every day
2 Five or six days a week
3 Three or four days a week
4 Once or twice a week
5 Once or twice a month
6 Once every couple of months
7 Once or twice a year
8 Not at all in the last 12 months

Spirits

SHOW CARD Q

How often have you had a drink of spirits or liqueurs, such as gin, whisky, brandy, rum, vodka, advocaat or cocktails during the last 12 months?

1 Almost every day
2 Five or six days a week
3 Three or four days a week
4 Once or twice a week
5 Once or twice a month
6 Once every couple of months
7 Once or twice a year
8 Not at all in the last 12 months

IF Spirits IN [Almost every day...Once or twice a year] THEN
SpiritsQ
How much spirits or liqueurs (such as gin, whisky, brandy, rum, vodka, advocaat or cocktails) have you usually drunk on any one day?
CODE THE NUMBER OF SINGLES - COUNT DOUBLES AS TWO SINGLES.
Range: 1..97
ENDIF

Sherry

SHOW CARD Q

How often have you had a drink of sherry or martini including port, vermouth, Cinzano and Dubonnet, during the last 12 months?

1 Almost every day
2 Five or six days a week
3 Three or four days a week
4 Once or twice a week
5 Once or twice a month
6 Once every couple of months
7 Once or twice a year
8 Not at all in the last 12 months

IF Sherry IN [Almost every day...Once or twice a year] THEN
SherryQ
How much sherry or martini, including port, vermouth, Cinzano and Dubonnet have you usually drunk on any one day?
CODE THE NUMBER OF GLASSES
Range: 1..97
ENDIF

Wine

SHOW CARD Q

How often have you had a drink of wine, including Babycham and champagne, during the last 12 months?

1 Almost every day
2 Five or six days a week
3 Three or four days a week
4 Once or twice a week
5 Once or twice a month
6 Once every couple of months
7 Once or twice a year
8 Not at all in the last 12 months

IF Wine IN [Almost every day...Once or twice a year] THEN
WineQ
How much wine, including Babycham and champagne, have you usually drunk on any one day?
CODE THE NUMBER OF GLASSES. 1 BOTTLE = 6 GLASSES. 1 LITRE = 8 GLASSES
Range: 1..97
ENDIF

IF SBeer IN [Almost every day...Once or twice a year] THEN
SBeerM
How much STRONG BEER, LAGER, STOUT or CIDER have you usually drunk on any one day?
INTERVIEWER: CODE MEASURES THAT YOU ARE GOING TO USE.

1 Half pints
2 Small cans
3 Large cans
4 Bottles

IF SbeerM = Half pints THEN
SBeerQ[1]
ASK OR CODE: How many half pints of STRONG BEER, LAGER, STOUT or CIDER have you usually drunk on any one day?
ARRAY[1..4] OF
Range: 1..97
ENDIF

IF SbeerM = Small cans THEN
SBeerQ[2]
ASK OR CODE: How many small cans of STRONG BEER, LAGER, STOUT or CIDER have you usually drunk on any one day?
ARRAY[1..4] OF
Range: 1..97
ENDIF

IF SbeerM = Large cans THEN
SBeerQ[3]
ASK OR CODE: How many large cans of STRONG BEER, LAGER, STOUT or CIDER have you usually drunk on any one day?
ARRAY[1..4] OF
Range: 1..97
ENDIF

IF SbeerM = Bottles THEN
SBeerQ[4]
ASK OR CODE: How many bottles of STRONG BEER, LAGER, STOUT or CIDER have you usually drunk on any one day?
ARRAY[1..4] OF
Range: 1..97

SBottle
ASK OR CODE: What make of STRONG BEER, LAGER, STOUT or CIDER do you usually drink from bottles?
INTERVIEWER. IF RESPONDENT DOES KNOW MAKE, OR RESPONDENT DRINKS DIFFERENT MAKES OF STRONG BEER, LAGER, STOUT OR CIDER.
PROBE: What make have you drunk most frequently or most recently?
Text: Maximum 21 characters

SCodeEq
Computed: Pint equivalent of bottles

ENDIF
ENDIF

Pops
SHOW CARD Q
How often have you had a drink of alcoholic soft drink ('alcopop'), such as Hooch, Two Dogs or Alcola, in the last 12 months?

1 Almost every day
2 Five or six days a week
3 Three or four days a week
4 Once or twice a week
5 Once or twice a month
6 Once every couple of months
7 Once or twice a year
8 Not at all in the last 12 months

IF Pops IN [Almost every day...Once or twice a year] THEN
  PopsM
  How much alcoholic soft drink ('alcopop') have you usually drunk on any one day?
  INTERVIEWER CODE THE MEASURE(S) THAT YOU ARE GOING TO USE.

  1 Small cans
  2 Bottles

  IF PopsM = Small cans THEN
    PopsQl[1]
    ASK OR CODE: How many small cans of alcoholic soft drink ('alcopop') have you usually drunk on any one day?
    ARRAY[1..2] OF
    Range: 1..97
  ENDIF

  IF PopsM = Bottles THEN
    PopsQl[2]
    ASK OR CODE: How many bottles of alcoholic soft drink ('alcopop') have you usually drunk on any one day?
    ARRAY[1..2] OF
    Range: 1..97
  ENDIF
ENDIF

AlcotA
Have you drunk any other types of alcoholic drink in the last 12 months?
1 Yes
2 No

IF AlcotA = Yes THEN
  OthDrnkA
  What other type of alcoholic drink have you drunk in the last 12 months?
  CODE FIRST MENTIONED ONLY.
    Text: Maximun 30 characters

FreqA
SHOW CARD Q
How often have you had a drink of (name of 'other' alcoholic drink) in the last 12 months?

1 Almost every day
2 Five or six days a week
3 Three or four days a week
4 Once or twice a week
5 Once or twice a month
6 Once every couple of months
7 Once or twice a year
8 Not at all in the last 12 months

IF FreqA IN [Almost every day...Once or twice a year] THEN
  OthQMA
  How much (name of 'other' alcoholic drink) have you usually drunk on any one day?
  INTERVIEWER: CODE MEASURES THAT YOU ARE GOING TO USE.

  1 Half pints
  2 Singles
  3 Glasses
  4 Bottles
  5 Other

  IF OthQMA = Other THEN
    OthQOA
    WHAT OTHER MEASURE?
      Text: Maximum 12 characters
  ENDIF

  OthQA
  ASK OR CODE: How many (half pints/singles/glasses/bottles/ other measures) of (name of 'other' alcoholic drink) have you usually drunk on any one day?
    Range: 0..97
ENDIF
ENDIF

Note: All drinks recorded under OthDrnkA backcoded into Nbeer-Wine

AlcotB
Have you drunk any other types of alcoholic drink in the last 12 months?
1 Yes
2 No

IF AlcotB = Yes THEN
  OthDrnkB
  What other type of alcoholic drink have you drunk in the last 12 months?
  CODE FIRST MENTIONED ONLY.
    Text: Maximum 30 characters

FreqB
SHOW CARD Q
How often have you had a drink of (name of 'other' alcoholic drink) in the last 12 months?

1 Almost every day
2 Five or six days a week
3 Three or four days a week
4 Once or twice a week
5 Once or twice a month
6 Once every couple of months
7 Once or twice a year
8 Not at all in the last 12 months

IF FreqB IN [Amost every day...Once or twice a year] THEN
  OthQMB
  How much (name of 'other' alcoholic drink) have you usually drunk on any one day?
  INTERVIEWER: CODE MEASURES THAT YOU ARE GOING TO USE.

  1 Half pints
  2 Singles
  3 Glasses
  4 Bottles
  5 Other

DrinkOft
SHOW CARD Q
Thinking now about all kinds of drinks, how often have you had an alcoholic drink of any kind during the last 12 months?
 1   Almost every day
 2   Five or six days a week
 3   Three or four days a week
 4   Once or twice a week
 5   Once or twice a month
 6   Once every couple of months
 7   Once or twice a year
 8   Not at all in the last 12 months

IF DrinkOft <> NotYr THEN
DrinkL7
You have told me what you have drunk over the last 12 months, but we know that what people drink can vary a lot from week to week, so I'd like to ask you a few questions about last week. Did you have an alcoholic drink in the seven days ending yesterday?
 1   Yes
 2   No

IF DrinkL7=Yes THEN
DrnkDay
On how many days out of the last seven did you have an alcoholic drink?
 Range: 1..7

IF DrnkDay = 2 to 7 days THEN
DrnkSame
Did you drink more on one of the days (some days than others), or did you drink about the same on both (each of those) days?
 1   Drank more on one/some day(s) than other(s)
 2   Same each day
ENDIF

WhichDay
Which day (last week) did you (last have an alcoholic drink) have the most to drink)?
 1   Sunday
 2   Monday
 3   Tuesday
 4   Wednesday
 5   Thursday
 6   Friday
 7   Saturday

DrnkType
SHOW CARD R
Thinking about last (answer to WhichDay), what types of drink did you have that day? CODE ALL THAT APPLY.
 1   Normal strength beer/lager/cider/shandy
 2   Strong beer/lager/cider
 3   Spirits or liqueurs
 4   Sherry or martini
 5   Wine
 6   Alcoholic lemonades/colas
 7   Other alcoholic drinks
 8   Low alcohol drinks only

IF OthQMB = Other THEN
OthQOB
WHAT OTHER MEASURE?
 Text: Maximum 12 characters
ENDIF

OthQB
ASK OR CODE: How many (half pints/singles/glasses/bottles/'other' measure) of (name of 'other' alcoholic drink) have you usually drunk on any one day?
 Range: 0..97
ENDIF
ENDIF

Note: All drinks recorded under OthDrnkB backcoded into Nbeer-Wine

AlcotC
Have you drunk any other types of alcoholic drink in the last 12 months?
 1   Yes
 2   No

IF AlcotC = Yes THEN
OthDrnkC
What other type of alcoholic drink have you drunk in the last 12 months?
 CODE FIRST MENTIONED ONLY.
 Text: Maximum 30 characters

FreqC
SHOW CARD Q
How often have you had a drink of (name of 'other' alcoholic drink) in the last 12 months?
 1   Almost every day
 2   Five or six days a week
 3   Three or four days a week
 4   Once or twice a week
 5   Once or twice a month
 6   Once every couple of months
 7   Once or twice a year
 8   Not at all in the last 12 months

IF FreqC IN [Almost every day...Once or twice a year] THEN
OthQMC
How much (name of 'other' alcoholic drink) have you usually drunk on any one day?
 INTERVIEWER: CODE MEASURES THAT YOU ARE GOING TO USE.
 1   Half pints
 2   Singles
 3   Glasses
 4   Bottles
 5   Other

IF OthQMC = Other THEN
OthQOC
WHAT OTHER MEASURE?
 Text: Maximum 12 characters
ENDIF

OthQC
ASK OR CODE: How many (half pints/singles/glasses/bottles/'other' measures) of (name of 'other' alcoholic drink) have you usually drunk on any one day?
 Range: 0..97
ENDIF
ENDIF

Note: All drinks recorded under OthDrnkC backcoded into Nbeer-Wine

IF DrnkType=Normal strength beer/lager/cider/shandy THEN
NBrL7
Still thinking about last *(answer to WhichDay)*, how much NORMAL STRENGTH BEER, LAGER, STOUT, CIDER or SHANDY (excluding cans and bottles of shandy) did you drink that day?
INTERVIEWER: CODE MEASURES THAT YOU ARE GOING TO USE.
1   Half pints
2   Small cans
3   Large cans
4   Bottles

IF NBrL7=Half pints THEN
NBrL7Q[1]
ASK OR CODE: How many half pints of NORMAL STRENGTH BEER, LAGER, STOUT, CIDER or SHANDY (excluding cans and bottles of shandy) did you drink that day?
ARRAY[1..4] OF
Range: 1..97
ENDIF

IF NBrL7=Small cans THEN
NBrL7Q[2]
ASK OR CODE: How many small cans of NORMAL STRENGTH BEER, LAGER, STOUT or CIDER did you drink that day?
ARRAY[1..4] OF
Range: 1..97
ENDIF

IF NBrL7=Large cans THEN
NBrL7Q[3]
ASK OR CODE: How many large cans of NORMAL STRENGTH BEER, LAGER, STOUT or CIDER did you drink that day?
ARRAY[1..4] OF
Range: 1..97
ENDIF

IF NBrL7=Bottles THEN
NBrL7Q[4]
ASK OR CODE: How many bottles of NORMAL STRENGTH BEER, LAGER, STOUT or CIDER did you drink that day?
ARRAY[1..4] OF
Range: 1..97

NBotL7
ASK OR CODE: What make of NORMAL STRENGTH BEER, LAGER, STOUT or CIDER did you drink from bottles on that day?
INTERVIEWER: IF RESPONDENT DRANK DIFFERENT MAKES CODE WHICH THEY DRANK MOST.
Text: Maximum 21 characters
ENDIF
ENDIF

IF DrnkType=Strong beer/lager/cider THEN
SBrL7
Still thinking about last *(answer to WhichDay)*, how much STRONG BEER, LAGER, STOUT or CIDER did you drink that day?
INTERVIEWER: CODE MEASURES THAT YOU ARE GOING TO USE.
1   Half pints
2   Small cans
3   Large cans
4   Bottles

IF SBrL7=Half pints THEN
SBrL7Q[1]
ASK OR CODE: How many half pints of STRONG BEER, LAGER, STOUT or CIDER did you drink on that day?
ARRAY[1..4] OF
Range: 1..97
ENDIF

IF SBrL7=Small cans THEN
SBrL7Q[2]
ASK OR CODE: How many small cans of STRONG BEER, LAGER, STOUT or CIDER did you drink on that day?
ARRAY[1..4] OF
Range: 1..97
ENDIF

IF SBrL7=Large cans THEN
SBrL7Q[3]
ASK OR CODE: How many large cans of STRONG BEER, LAGER, STOUT or CIDER did you drink on that day?
ARRAY[1..4] OF
Range: 1..97
ENDIF

IF SBrL7=Bottles THEN
SBrL7Q[4]
ASK OR CODE: How many bottles of STRONG BEER, LAGER, STOUT or CIDER did you drink on that day?
ARRAY[1..4] OF
Range: 1..97
ENDIF

SBotL7
ASK OR CODE: What make of STRONG BEER, LAGER, STOUT or CIDER did you drink from bottles on that day?
INTERVIEWER: IF RESPONDENT DRANK DIFFERENT MAKES CODE WHICH THEY DRANK MOST.
Text: Maximum 21 characters
ENDIF

IF DrnkType=Spirits THEN
SpirL7
Still thinking about last *(answer to WhichDay)*, how much spirits or liqueurs (such as gin, whisky, brandy, rum, vodka, advocaat or cocktails) did you drink on that day?
CODE THE NUMBER OF SINGLES - COUNT DOUBLES AS TWO SINGLES.
Range: 1..97
ENDIF

IF DrnkType=Sherry THEN
ShryL7
Still thinking about last *(answer to WhichDay)*, how much sherry or martini, including port, vermouth, Cinzano and Dubonnet did you drink on that day?
CODE THE NUMBER OF GLASSES.
Range: 1..97
ENDIF

IF DrnkType=Wine THEN
WineL7
Still thinking about last *(answer to WhichDay)*, how much wine, including Babycham and champagne, did you drink on that day?
CODE THE NUMBER OF GLASSES 1 BOTTLE = 6 GLASSES. 1 LITRE = 8 GLASSES.
Range: 1..97
ENDIF

IF DrnkType=Alcoholic lemonades/colas THEN
PopsL7
Still thinking about last *(answer to Which Day)*, how much ALCOHOLIC SOFT DRINK ('alcopop') did you drink on that day?
INTERVIEWER: CODE MEASURES THAT YOU ARE GOING TO USE.
1 Small cans
2 Bottles

IF PopsL7=Small cans THEN
PopsL7Q[1]
ASK OR CODE: How many small cans of ALCOHOLIC SOFT DRINK ('alcopop') did you drink on that day?
ARRAY[1..2] OF
Range: 1..97
ENDIF

IF PopsL7=Bottles THEN
PopsL7Q[2]
ASK OR CODE: How many bottles of ALCOHOLIC SOFT DRINK ('alcopop') did you drink on that day?
ARRAY[1..2] OF
Range: 1..97
ENDIF

IF DrnkType=Other THEN
OthL7TA
Still thinking about last *(answer to WhichDay)*, what other type of alcoholic drink did you drink on that day?
CODE FIRST MENTIONED ONLY
Text: Maximum 30 characters

OthL7QA
How much *(name of 'other' alcoholic drink)* did you drink on that day?
WRITE IN HOW MUCH. REMEMBER TO SPECIFY HALF PINTS/ SINGLES/ GLASSES/ BOTTLES.
Text: Maximum 30 characters

OthL7B
Did you drink any other type of alcoholic drink on that day?
1 Yes
2 No

IF OthL7B=Yes THEN
OthL7TB
Still thinking about last *(answer to WhichDay)*, what other type of alcoholic drink did you drink on that day?
CODE FIRST MENTIONED ONLY.
Text: Maximum 30 characters

OthL7QB
How much *(name of 'other' alcoholic drink)* did you drink on that day?
WRITE IN HOW MUCH. REMEMBER TO SPECIFY HALF PINTS/SINGLES/ GLASSES/ BOTTLES.
Text: Maximum 30 characters

OthL7C
Did you drink any other type of alcoholic drink on that day?
1 Yes
2 No

IF OthL7C=Yes THEN
OthL7TC
Still thinking about last *(answer to WhichDay)*, what other type of alcoholic drink did you drink on that day?
CODE FIRST MENTIONED ONLY.
Text: Maximum 30 characters

OthL7QC
How much *(name of 'other' alcoholic drink)* did you drink on that day?
WRITE IN HOW MUCH. REMEMBER TO SPECIFY HALF PINTS/ SINGLES/GLASSES/ BOTTLES.
Text: Maximum 30 characters
ENDIF
ENDIF
ENDIF

DrAmount
Compared to five years ago, would you say that on the whole you drink more, about the same or less nowadays?
1 More nowadays
2 About the same
3 Less nowadays
ENDIF

IF DrinkAny = Never THEN
AlwaysTT
Have you always been a non-drinker or did you stop drinking for some reason?
1 Always a non-drinker
2 Used to drink but stopped

IF AlwaysTT = Used to drink but stopped THEN
WhyTT
Did you stop drinking because of a particular health condition that you had at the time?
INTERVIEWER: IF RESPONDENT SAYS PREGNANCY, CODE YES.
1 Yes
2 No
ENDIF
ENDIF
ENDIF

Classification module

IF RESPONDENT AGED 16+ AND NOT HEAD OF HOUSEHOLD or IF RESPONDENT IS HEAD OF HOUSEHOLD BUT DID NOT ANSWER HOUSEHOLD QUESTIONNAIRE
(IF ((Age of Respondent is 16 to 120 years) AND (DMHoH <> PerNum)) OR (DMHoH = PerNum AND DMHoH <> DMHHResp))

NActiv
SHOW CARD E
Which of these descriptions applies to what you were doing last week, that is in the seven days ending *(date last Sunday)*?
CODE FIRST TO APPLY

1 Going to school or college full-time (including on vacation)
2 In paid employment or self-employment (or away temporarily)
3 On a Government scheme for employment training
4 Doing unpaid work for a business that you own, or that a relative owns
5 Waiting to take up paid work already obtained
6 Looking for paid work or a Government training scheme
7 Intending to look for work but prevented by temporary sickness or injury (CHECK 28 DAYS OR LESS)
8 Permanently unable to work because of long-term sickness or disability (USE ONLY FOR MEN AGED 16-64 OR WOMEN AGED 16-59)
9 Retired from paid work
10 Looking after the home or family
11 Doing something else (SPECIFY)

IF NActiv=Doing something else THEN
 NActivO
 OTHER: PLEASE SPECIFY
  Text: Maximum 60 characters
ENDIF

IF NActiv=Going to school or college full-time THEN
 StWork
 Did you do any paid work in the seven days ending *(date last Sunday)*, either as an employee or self-employed?
  1 Yes
  2 No
ENDIF

IF ((NActiv=Intending to look for work but prevented by temporary sickness or injury, Retired from paid work, Looking after the home or family or Doing something else OR StWork=No) AND (Age of Respondent is 16 to 64years AND Sex=Male) OR (Age of Respondent is 16 to 59 years AND Sex=Female)) THEN
 4WkLook
 Thinking now of the four weeks ending *(date last Sunday)*. Were you looking for any paid work or Government training scheme at any time in those four weeks?
  1 Yes
  2 No
ENDIF

IF NActiv=Looking for paid work or a government training scheme OR 4WkLook=Yes THEN
 2WkStrt
 If a job or a place on a Government training scheme had been available in the *(7 days/four weeks)* ending *(date last Sunday)*, would you have been able to start within two weeks?
  1 Yes
  2 No
ENDIF

IF (NActiv IN [Looking for paid work or a Government training scheme...Doing something else] OR StWork=No) THEN
 EverJob
 Have you ever been in paid employment or self-employed?
  1 Yes
  2 No
ENDIF

IF NActiv=Waiting to take up paid work already obtained THEN
 OthPaid
 Apart from the job you are waiting to take up, have you ever been in paid employment or self-employed?
  1 Yes
  2 No
ENDIF

IF (EverJob = Yes) OR (NActiv IN [In paid employment or self-employment...Waiting to take up paid work already obtained] OR (StWork = Yes) THEN
 JobTitle
 I'd like to ask you some details about the job you were doing last week *(your most recent job/the main job you had/the job you are waiting to take up)*. What is *(was/will be)* the name or title of the job?
  Text: Maximum 60 characters

 FtPTime
 Are you *(were you/will you be)* working full-time or part-time?
 (FULL-TIME = MORE THAN 30 HOURSPART-TIME = 30 HOURS OR LESS)
  1 Full-time
  2 Part-time

 WtWork
 What kind of work do *(did/will)* you do most of the time?
  Text: Maximum 50 characters

 MatUsed
 IF RELEVANT: What materials or machinery do *(did/will)* you use?
 IF NONE USED, WRITE IN 'NONE'.
  Text: Maximum 50 characters

 SkilNee
 What skills or qualifications are *(were)* needed for the job?
  Text: Maximum 120 characters

 Employe
 Are you *(were you/will you be)* ...READ OUT...
  1 an employee,
  2 or, self-employed
  IF IN DOUBT, CHECK HOW THIS EMPLOYMENT IS TREATED FOR TAX & NI PURPOSES.

 IF Employe = Self-employed THEN
  Dirctr
  Can I just check, in this job are you *(were you/will you be)* a Director of a limited company?
   1 Yes
   2 No
 ENDIF

IF Employee=an employee OR Dirctr=Yes THEN
EmpStat
Are you *(were you/will you be)* a ...READ OUT...
1 manager,
2 foreman or supervisor,
3 or other employee?

NEmplee
Including yourself, about how many people are *(were)* employed at the place where you usually work *(usually worked/will work)*?
1 1 or 2
2 3-24
3 25-499
4 500+

ELSEIF Employe=Self-employed AND Dirctr=No THEN
SNEmplee
Do *(did/will)* you have any employees?
1 None
2 1-24
3 25-499
4 500+
ENDIF

IF Employe=Employee THEN
Ind
What does *(did)* your employer make or do at the place where you usually work *(usually worked/will work)*?
Text: Maximum 100 characters

ELSEIF Employe=Self-employed THEN
SIfWtMad
What do *(did/will)* you make or do in your business?
Text: Maximum 100 characters
ENDIF

OEmpStat
Derived employment status.
Range: 0..8

SOC, SocCls, SEG, SIC Coded during edit stage
ENDIF
ENDIF

ASK ALL
Jump8
INTERVIEWER: NOW FOLLOWS THE REST OF THE CLASSIFICATION QUESTIONS.

IF Age of Respondent is 16 to 120 years THEN
EducEnd
At what age did you finish your continuous full-time education at school or college?
1 Not yet finished
2 Never went to school
3 14 or under
4 15
5 16
6 17
7 18
8 19 or over

Qual
SHOW CARD S
Do you have any of the qualifications listed on this card? Please look down the whole list before telling me.
1 Yes
2 No

IF Qual = Yes THEN
QualA
Which of the qualifications on this card do you have? Just tell me the number written beside each one.
RECORD ALL THAT APPLY. PROBE: Any others?
1 Degree/degree level qualification (including higher degree)
2 Teaching qualification
3 Nursing qualifications SRN, SCM, SEN, RGN, RM, RHV, Midwife
4 HNC/HND, BEC/TEC Higher, BTEC Higher/SCOTECH Higher
5 ONC/OND/BEC/TEC/BTEC not higher
6 City and Guilds Full Technological Certificate
7 City and Guilds Advanced/Final Level
8 City and Guilds Craft/Ordinary Level
9 A-levels/Higher School Certificate
10 AS level
11 SLC/SCE/SUPE at Higher Grade or Certificate of Sixth Year Studies
12 O-level passes taken in 1975 or earlier
13 O-level passes taken after 1975 GRADES A-C
14 O-level passes taken after 1975 GRADES D-E
15 GCSE GRADES A-C
16 GCSE GRADES D-G
17 CSE GRADE 1/SCE BANDS A-C/Standard Grade LEVEL 1-3
18 CSE GRADES 2-5/SCE Ordinary BANDS D-E
19 CSE Ungraded
20 SLC Lower
21 SUPE Lower or Ordinary
22 School Certificate or Matric
23 NVQ Level 5
24 NVQ Level 4
25 NVQ Level 3/Advanced level GNVQ
26 NVQ Level 2/Intermediate level GNVQ
27 NVQ Level 1/Foundation level GNVQ
28 Recognised Trade Apprenticeship completed
29 Clerical or Commercial Qualification (e.g. typing/book-keeping/commerce)
ENDIF

IF NOT (Degree IN QualA) THEN
OthQual
Do you have any qualifications not listed on this card?
1 Yes
2 No

IF OthQual = Yes THEN
QualB
What qualifications are these?
RECORD ALL OTHER QUALIFICATIONS IN FULL. PROBE: Any others?
Text: Maximum 60 characters
ENDIF
ENDIF
ENDIF

ASK ALL
PoB
In which country were you born?
1 England
2 Scotland
3 Wales
4 Northern Ireland
5 Republic of Ireland
6 Elsewhere outside of UK

NEthnic
SHOW CARD T
To which of these groups do you consider you belong?
1 White
2 Black - Caribbean
3 Black - African
4 Black - Other Black Groups
5 Indian
6 Pakistani
7 Bangladeshi
8 Chinese
9 None of these

IF Age of Respondent is 16 years or over THEN
MaInHH
I would like to ask you some questions about your parents in order to compare health across generations of families. INTERVIEWER CODE
1 Mother is in household
2 Mother NOT in household

IF MaInHH=Mother is in household THEN
NatMaB
May I just check, is she your natural mother?
1 Yes
2 No
ENDIF

IF MaInHH<>Mother is in household OR NatMaB=No THEN
LiveMaB
Is your natural mother still alive?
1 Yes
2 No

IF LiveMaB=Yes THEN
AgeMA
How old is your natural mother?
Range: 1..120

ELSEIF LiveMaB=No THEN
ConsMaB
SHOW CARD U
Did your mother die from any of the conditions on the card?
CODE ONE ONLY
1 High blood pressure (sometimes called hypertension)
2 Angina
3 Heart attack (including myocardial infarction and coronary thrombosis)
4 Stroke
5 Other heart trouble (incl. heart murmur, damaged heart valves, trachycardia or rapid heart)
6 Diabetes
7 None of the above conditions

AgeMaB
How old was your mother when she died?
Range: 1..120
ENDIF
ENDIF

PaInHH
INTERVIEWER CODE:
1 Father is in household
2 Father NOT in household

IF PaInHH=Father is in household THEN
NatPaB
May I just check, is he your natural father?
1 Yes
2 No
ENDIF

IF PaInHH<>Father is in household OR NatPaB=No THEN
LivePaB
Is your natural father still alive?
1 Yes
2 No

IF LivePaB=Yes THEN
AgePa
How old is your natural father?
Range: 1..120

ELSEIF LivePaB=No THEN
ConsPaB
SHOW CARD U
Did your father die from any of the conditions on the card?
CODE ONE ONLY
1 High blood pressure (sometimes called hypertension)
2 Angina
3 Heart attack (including myocardial infarction and coronary thrombosis)
4 Stroke
5 Other heart trouble (incl. heart murmur, damaged heart valves, trachycardia or rapid heart)
6 Diabetes
7 None of the above conditions

AgePaB
How old was your father when he died?
Range: 1..120
ENDIF
ENDIF
ENDIF

Self-completion booklets

Jump9
INTERVIEWER: NOW FOLLOWS THE PRESENTATION OF THE SELF-COMPLETION BOOKLETS:

IF Age of Respondent is13 years or over THEN
SCIntro
PREPARE *(BLUE/WHITE/GREEN)* SELF-COMPLETION BOOKLET BY ENTERING SERIAL NUMBERS.CHECK YOU HAVE CORRECT PERSON NUMBER.

ELSEIF Age of Respondent is 8 to 12 years THEN
SCIntCh
Here is a little booklet which I would like to ask *(name of child)* to complete for *(him/herself)*. It asks children if they have ever tried cigarettes or alcohol, and about cycling. May I explain it to him/her?
IF ASKED, SHOW PINK BOOKLET TO PARENT(S). IF AGREES, PREPARE PINK BOOKLET. SEE CHILD.
EXPLAIN HOW TO COMPLETE.REMEMBER TO USE A BLACK PEN.
ENDIF

IF Age of Respondent is 13 to 120 years THEN
IF (DrinkAny = Never) OR (DrinkOft=Once or twice a year OR Not at all in the last twelve months) THEN
PagEx
INTERVIEWER NOTE: This respondent does not drink (or drinks once or twice a year or less). Cross out the Drinking Experiences questions before handing over the self-completion booklet.
ENDIF

SComp2
I would now like you to answer some questions by completing this booklet on your own. The questions cover *(smoking, (and) drinking (and some about your) general health)*.
EXPLAIN HOW TO COMPLETE BOOKLET. REMEMBER TO USE A BLACK PEN:
ENDIF

SCCheck
INTERVIEWER: WAIT UNTIL RESPONDENT(S) HAVE FINISHED AND THEN CHECK EACH BOOKLET COMPLETED. IF NOT, ASK IF QUESTIONS MISSED IN ERROR. IF IN ERROR, ASK RESPONDENT TO COMPLETE.

IF Age of respondent is 8 years or over THEN
SComp3
INTERVIEWER CHECK: WAS THE *(PINK/GREEN/BLUE/WHITE)* BOOKLET *(8-12/13-15)* COMPLETED?
1   Fully completed
2   Partially completed
3   Not completed

IF SComp3=Fully completed or Partially completed THEN
SC3Acc
Was it completed without assistance?:
1   Completed independently
2   *(Assistance from other children)*
3   Assistance from other household member *(Assistance from adult(s) (not interviewer)*
4   Assistance from interviewer
5   Interviewer
ENDIF

IF SComp3=Partially completed OR Not completed THEN
SComp6
INTERVIEWER: RECORD WHY BOOKLET NOT COMPLETED / PARTIALLY COMPLETED. CODE ALL THAT APPLY
1   Child away from home during fieldwork period
2   Eyesight problems
3   Language problems
4   Reading/writing/comprehension problems
5   Respondent bored/fed up/tired
6   Questions too sensitive/invasion of privacy
7   Too long/too busy/taken long enough already
8   Refused to complete booklet (no other reason given)
9   Other (SPECIFY)

IF SComp6=Other THEN
SComp6O
PLEASE SPECIFY OTHER REASON:
Text: Maximum 60 characters
ENDIF
ENDIF

IF SComp3=Fully completed OR Partially completed THEN
SComp5A
INTERVIEWER: CODE WHO WAS PRESENT IN ROOM WHILE *(name of respondent)* COMPLETED SELF-COMPLETION. INCLUDE YOURSELF, ANYONE INTERVIEWED AT THE SAME TIME AS RESPONDENT, PARENT ANSWERING ON BEHALF OF 8-12 YEAR OLDS OR OTHERS IN THE ROOM.CODE ALL THAT APPLY.
1   Spouse / partner
2   Parent(s) (incl step-/foster-)
3   Brother(s)/Sister(s)
4   Own/Related child(ren)(incl step-/ foster-/ partner's)
5   Other relative(s)
6   Unrelated adult(s)
7   Unrelated child(ren)
8   Interviewer
9   No-one else present
ENDIF
ENDIF

Measurements module

Jump10
INTERVIEWER: NOW FOLLOWS THE MEASUREMENTS MODULE

Intro
PREAMBLE: I would now like to measure height and weight. There is interest in how people's weight, given their height, is associated with their health. MAKE OUT GREY COLOURED MRC FOR EACH PERSON:

RespHts
MEASURE HEIGHT AND CODE. INCLUDE 'DISGUISED' REFUSALS SUCH AS 'IT WILL TAKE TOO LONG', 'I HAVE TO GO OUT ETC. AT CODE 2: Height refused.
1 Height measured
2 Height refused
3 Height attempted, not obtained
4 Height not attempted

IF RespHts = Height measured THEN
Height
ENTER HEIGHT.
Range: 60.0..244.0

RelHiteB
INTERVIEWER CODE ONE ONLY
1 No problems experienced reliable height measurement obtained
Problems experienced - measurement likely to be:
2 Reliable
3 Unreliable

IF RelHiteB = Unreliable THEN
HiNRel
WHAT CAUSED THE HEIGHT MEASUREMENT TO BE UNRELIABLE?
1 Hairstyle or wig
2 Turban or other religious headgear
3 Respondent stooped
4 Child respondent refused stretching
5 Respondent would not stand still
6 Respondent wore shoes
7 Other, please specify
8 *Difficulty standing*

IF HiNRel = Other THEN
OHiNRel
PLEASE SPECIFY WHAT CAUSED UNRELIABLE HEIGHT MEASUREMENT.
Text: Maximum 49 characters
ENDIF
ENDIF

MBookHt
INTERVIEWER: CHECK HEIGHT RECORDED ON MEASUREMENT RECORD CARD.
HEIGHT: (x) cm OR (x) feet (x) inches.

ELSEIF RespHts = Height refused THEN
ResNHi
GIVE REASONS FOR REFUSAL.
1 Cannot see point/Height already known/Doctor has measurement
2 Too busy/Taken too long already/ No time
3 Respondent too ill/frail/tired
4 Considered intrusive information
5 Respondent too anxious/nervous/ shy/embarrassed
6 Refused (no other reason given)
7 Other

ELSEIF RespHts = Height attempted, not obtained OR Height not attempted THEN
NoHitM
CODE REASON FOR NOT OBTAINING HEIGHT CODE ALL THAT APPLY.
1 Child: away from home during fieldwork period (specify in a Note)
2 Respondent is unsteady on feet
3 Respondent cannot stand upright/too stooped
4 Respondent is chairbound
5 Child: subject would not stand still
6 Ill or in pain
7 Stadiometer faulty or not available
8 Other - specify

IF (OTHER IN NoHitM) THEN
NoHitMO
PLEASE SPECIFY OTHER REASON.
Text: Maximum 60 characters
ENDIF
ENDIF

IF RespHts=Height refused, Height attempted, not obtained OR Height not attempted THEN
EHtCh
INTERVIEWER: ASK *(respondent)* FOR AN ESTIMATED HEIGHT. WILL IT BE GIVEN IN METRES OR IN FEET AND INCHES?
1 Metres
2 Feet and inches

IF EHtCh = Metres THEN
EHtm
PLEASE RECORD ESTIMATED HEIGHT IN METRES.
Range: 0.01..2.44

ELSEIF EHtCh = Feet and inches THEN
EHtFt
PLEASE RECORD ESTIMATED HEIGHT. ENTER FEET.
Range: 0..7

EHtIn
PLEASE RECORD ESTIMATED HEIGHT. ENTER INCHES.
Range: 0..11
ENDIF
ENDIF

EMHeight *Final measured or estimated height (cm), to be fed into household admin.*
IF (Sex = Female) AND (Age of Respondent is 16 to 49) THEN
PregNowB
May I check, are you pregnant now?
1 Yes
2 No
ENDIF

IF PregNowB <> Yes THEN
RespWts
MEASURE WEIGHT AND CODE. *(INTERVIEWER: IF RESPONDENT WEIGHS MORE THAN 130KG (20 ½ STONES) DO NOT WEIGH. CODE AS 'WEIGHT NOT OBTAINED').* INCLUDE 'DISGUISED' REFUSALS SUCH AS 'IT WILL TAKE TOO LONG', 'I HAVE TO GO OUT' ETC. AT CODE 2: Weight refused.
0 *If Age 2-5 years: Weight obtained (child held by adult)/If Age over 5 years: DO NOT USE THIS CODE*
1 Weight obtained (subject on own)
2 Weight refused
3 Weight attempted, not obtained
4 Weight not attempted

IF RespWtsMeas=Weight obtained (subject on own) OR Weight obtained (child held by adult) THEN
IF RespWts = Weight obtained (subject on own) THEN
Weight
RECORD WEIGHT.
Range: 10.0..130.0

ELSEIF RespWts = Weight obtained (child held by adult) THEN
WtAdult
ENTER WEIGHT OF ADULT ON HIS/HER OWN.
Range: 15.0..130.0

WtChAd
ENTER WEIGHT OF ADULT HOLDING CHILD.
Range: 15.0..130.0
ENDIF

FWeight *Measured weight, either Weight or WtChAd - WtAdult*
Range: 0.0..140.0

FloorM
SCALES PLACED ON?
1 Uneven floor
2 Carpet
3 Neither

RelWaitB
INTERVIEWER CODE ONE ONLY.
1 No problems experienced, reliable weight measurement obtained
   Problems experienced - measurement likely to be:
2 Reliable
3 Unreliable
ENDIF

MBookWt
INTERVIEWER: CHECK WEIGHT RECORDED ON MEASUREMENT RECORD CARD. WEIGHT: (x) kg OR (x) stones (x) pounds. IF WEIGHT LOOKS WRONG, GO BACK TO 'Weight' AND REWEIGH.
ENDIF

IF RespWts = Weight refused, Weight attempted, not obtained OR Weight not attempted THEN
IF RespWts = Weight refused THEN
ResNWt
GIVE REASONS FOR REFUSAL.
1 Cannot see point/Weight already known/Doctor has measurement
2 Too busy/Taken long enough already/No time
3 Respondent too ill/frail/tired
4 Considered intrusive information
5 Respondent too anxious/nervous/shy/embarrassed
6 Child refused to be held by parent
7 Parent refused to hold child
8 Refused (no other reason given)
9 Other

ELSEIF RespWts = Weight attempted, not obtained OR Weight not attempted THEN
NoWaitM
CODE REASON FOR NOT OBTAINING WEIGHT CODE ALL THAT APPLY.
1 Child: away from home during fieldwork period (specify in a Note)
2 Respondent is unsteady on feet
3 Respondent cannot stand upright
4 Respondent is chairbound
5 Respondent weighs more than 130 kg
6 Ill or in pain
7 Scales not working
8 Parent unable to hold child
9 Other - specify

IF NoWaitM = Other THEN
NoWaitMO
PLEASE SPECIFY OTHER REASON.
Text: Maximum 60 characters
ENDIF

EWtCh
INTERVIEWER: ASK *(respondent)* FOR AN ESTIMATED WEIGHT. WILL IT BE GIVEN IN KILOGRAMS OR IN STONES AND POUNDS
1 Kilograms
2 Stones and pounds

IF EWtCh = Kilograms THEN
EWtkg
PLEASE RECORD ESTIMATED WEIGHT IN KILOGRAMS.
Range: 1.0..210.0

ELSEIF EWtCh = Stones and pounds THEN
EWtSt
PLEASE RECORD ESTIMATED WEIGHT. ENTER STONES.
Range: 1..32

EWtL
PLEASE RECORD ESTIMATED WEIGHT. ENTER POUNDS.
Range: 0..13
ENDIF
ENDIF

EMWeight *Final measured or estimated weight (kg), computed*

ENDIF

Consents module

IF (Age of Respondent is 2-15 years) AND (No parent in household) THEN
NurseA
In order for the nurse to take any of *(name of child's)* measurements we have to have the permission of *(his/her)* parents or the person who has legal parental responsibility. As there is no-one in your household who I can ask, I won't be making an appointment for *(name of child)*:
  1 Kilograms
  2 Pounds and ounces

ELSEIF NOT (AWAY IN NoH(tM)) THEN
Nurse
There are two parts to this survey. You have just helped us with the first part. We hope you will also help us with the second part, which is a visit by a qualified nurse to collect more medical information and carry out some measurements. I would like to make an appointment for the nurse to come round and explain some more about what is required. May I suggest some dates and times and see when you are free? IF ASKED FOR DETAILS: for example, to make some general measurements *(and take his/her blood pressure (and take a small blood sample))*
  1 Agreed nurse could contact
  2 Refused nurse contact

IF Nurse = Refused nurse contact THEN
NurseRef
RECORD REASON WHY RESPONDENT REFUSED NURSE CONTACT. CODE BELOW AND RECORD AT Q 15 ON A.R.F.
  1 Own doctor already has information
  2 Given enough time already to this survey/expecting too much
  3 Too busy, cannot spare the time (if Code 1 does not apply)
  4 Had enough of medical tests/medical profession at present time
  5 Worried about what nurse may find out/'might tempt fate'
  6 Scared of medical profession/ particular medical procedures (e.g. blood sample)
  7 Not interested/Can't be bothered/No particular reason
  8 Other reason (specify)

IF NurseRef = Other reason THEN
NrsRefO
PLEASE SPECIFY OTHER REASON FOR REFUSAL. CODE BELOW AND RECORD AT Q 15 ON A.R.F.
  Text: Maximum 60 characters
ENDIF
ENDIF
ENDIF

ASK ALL
NHSCR
The National Health Service has a central register which records information on important diseases and causes of death. May we have your permission to pass your name, address, and date of birth to this register?
  1 Permission given
  2 Refused

ReInter
If at some future date we wanted to talk to you further about your health, may we contact you to see if you are willing to help us again?
  1 Yes
  2 No

IF RESPONDENT IS MOTHER OF CHILD IN HOUSEHOLD THEN
Birth[1]
We are interested in the birthweight of children taking part in this survey. Can you tell me, what was *(name of child's)* weight at birth?
INTERVIEWER: IS WEIGHT GIVEN IN KILOGRAMS OR IN POUNDS AND OUNCES?:
  1 Kilograms
  2 Pounds and ounces

IF Birth[1] = Kilograms THEN
Birthkg[1]
PLEASE RECORD *(name of child's)* BIRTHWEIGHT IN KILOGRAMS.
  Range: 1.00..6.75

ELSEIF Birth[1] = Pounds and ounces THEN
BirthL[1]
PLEASE RECORD *(name of child's)* BIRTHWEIGHT. ENTER POUNDS.
  Range: 2..15

BirthO[1]
PLEASE RECORD *(name of child's)* BIRTHWEIGHT. ENTER OUNCES.
  Range: 0..15
ENDIF

BirthWt[1] *Given birthweight (kg), computed*

IF BirthWt[1] = between 0.1kg and 2.5kg THEN
Prmature[1]
Was *(name of child)* born prematurely?
  1 Yes
  2 No

IF Prmature[1] = Yes THEN
PrWeeks[1]
How many weeks early was *(name of child)* born?
ENTER NUMBER OF WEEKS, ROUNDED TO NEAREST WEEK. IF LESS THAN FOUR DAYS, ENTER '0'.
  Range: 0..20
ENDIF
ENDIF

Birth to PRWeeks repeated for each child of respondent.

IF Age of Respondent is 13+ THEN

InTog

INTERVIEWER: RECORD WHO ELSE WAS INTERVIEWED WITH *(Name of respondent)*.

CODE ALL THAT APPLY.

1 Interviewed alone
2 Spouse/Partner
3 Parent(s) (incl step-/foster-)
4 Brother(s)/Sister(s)
5 Own/Related child(ren)(incl step-/foster-/partner's)
6 Other relative(s)
7 Unrelated adult(s)
8 Unrelated child(ren)

ENDIF

ASK ALL

FstNm

INTERVIEWER - AT THE HOUSEHOLD GRID YOU RECORDED THE FIRST NAME OF THIS

PERSON AS: *(Name from household grid)*

IS THIS CORRECT (IE NOT INITIALS, NOT ABBREVIATED, NOT A NICKNAME)?

IF NAME NOT SPELT CORRECTLY, CODE 'NO'.

1 Yes, name correct
2 No, name not correct

IF FstNm = No THEN

NewNm

PLEASE TYPE IN THE CORRECT FIRST NAME OF THIS PERSON.

ENDIF

TPhone

IINTERVIEWER NOTE: YOU ARE NOW IN THE ADMIN FILE, NOT THE QUESTIONNAIRE FILE.

Some interviews in a survey are checked to make sure that people like yourself are satisfied with the way

the interview was carried out. Just in case yours is one of the interviews that is checked, it would be helpful

if we could have your telephone number.

1 Number given
2 Number refused
3 No telephone

HSE 98

CARD B

1   Own it outright

2   Buying it with the help of a mortgage or loan

3   Pay part rent and part mortgage (shared ownership)

4   Rent it

5   Live rent-free (include rent-free in relative's/friend property but not squatting)

6   Squatting

HSE 98

CARD A

<u>RELATIONSHIP</u>

1   Husband / Wife
2   Partner / Cohabitee

3   Natural son / daughter
4   Adopted son / daughter
5   Foster son / daughter
6   Stepson / Stepdaughter / Child of partner
7   Son-in-law / Daughter-in-law

8   Natural parent
9   Adoptive parent
10   Foster parent
11   Step-parent
12   Parent-in-law

13   Natural brother / Natural sister (ie. both natural parents the same)
14   Half-brother / Half-sister (ie. one natural parent the same)
15   Step-brother / Step-sister (ie. no natural parents the same)
16   Adopted brother / Adopted sister
17   Foster brother / Foster sister
18   Brother-in-law / Sister-in-law

19   Grandchild
20   Grandparent

21   Other relative
22   Other non-relative

CARD C

1 Earnings from employment or self-employment

2 State retirement pension

3 Pension from former employer

4 Child Benefit

5 Job-Seekers Allowance

6 Income Support

7 Family Credit

8 Housing Benefit

9 Other State Benefits

10 Interest from savings and investments (eg. stocks and shares)

11 Other kinds of regular allowance from outside your household (eg. maintenance, student grants, rent)

12 No source of income

CARD D

GROSS INCOME FROM ALL SOURCES
(before any deductions for tax, national insurance, etc.)

WEEKLY	or	MONTHLY	or	ANNUAL
Less than £10 ... 1		Less than £40 ... 1		Less than £520 ... 1
£10 less than £30 ... 2		£40 less than £130 ... 2		£520 less than £1,600 ... 2
£30 less than £50 ... 3		£130 less than £220 ... 3		£1,600 less than £2,600 ... 3
£50 less than £70 ... 4		£220 less than £300 ... 4		£2,600 less than £3,600 ... 4
£70 less than £100 ... 5		£300 less than £430 ... 5		£3,600 less than £5,200 ... 5
£100 less than £150 ... 6		£430 less than £650 ... 6		£5,200 less than £7,800 ... 6
£150 less than £200 ... 7		£650 less than £870 ... 7		£7,800 less than £10,400 ... 7
£200 less than £250 ... 8		£870 less than £1,100 ... 8		£10,400 less than £13,000 ... 8
£250 less than £300 ... 9		£1,100 less than £1,300 ... 9		£13,000 less than £15,600 ... 9
£300 less than £350 ... 10		£1,300 less than £1,500 ... 10		£15,600 less than £18,200 ... 10
£350 less than £400 ... 11		£1,500 less than £1,700 ... 11		£18,200 less than £20,800 ... 11
£400 less than £450 ... 12		£1,700 less than £2,000 ... 12		£20,800 less than £23,400 ... 12
£450 less than £500 ... 13		£2,000 less than £2,200 ... 13		£23,400 less than £26,000 ... 13
£500 less than £550 ... 14		£2,200 less than £2,400 ... 14		£26,000 less than £28,600 ... 14
£550 less than £600 ... 15		£2,400 less than £2,600 ... 15		£28,600 less than £31,200 ... 15
£600 less than £650 ... 16		£2,600 less than £2,800 ... 16		£31,200 less than £33,800 ... 16
£650 less than £700 ... 17		£2,800 less than £3,000 ... 17		£33,800 less than £36,400 ... 17
£700 less than £800 ... 18		£3,000 less than £3,500 ... 18		£36,400 less than £41,600 ... 18
£800 less than £900 ... 19		£3,500 less than £3,900 ... 19		£41,600 less than £46,800 ... 19
£900 less than £1,000 ... 20		£3,900 less than £4,300 ... 20		£46,800 less than £52,000 ... 20
£1,000 less than £1,150 ... 21		£4,300 less than £5,000 ... 21		£52,000 less than £60,000 ... 21
£1,150 less than £1,350 ... 22		£5,000 less than £5,800 ... 22		£60,000 less than £70,000 ... 22
£1,350 less than £1,550 ... 23		£5,800 less than £6,700 ... 23		£70,000 less than £80,000 ... 23
£1,550 less than £1,750 ... 24		£6,700 less than £7,500 ... 24		£80,000 less than £90,000 ... 24
£1,750 less than £1,900 ... 25		£7,500 less than £8,300 ... 25		£90,000 less than £100,000 ... 25
£1,900 less than £2,100 ... 26		£8,300 less than £9,200 ... 26		£100,000 less than £110,000 ... 26
£2,100 less than £2,300 ... 27		£9,200 less than £10,000 ... 27		£110,000 less than £120,000 ... 27
£2,300 less than £2,500 ... 28		£10,000 less than £10,800 ... 28		£120,000 less than £130,000 ... 28
£2,500 less than £2,700 ... 29		£10,800 less than £11,700 ... 29		£130,000 less than £140,000 ... 29
£2,700 less than £2,900 ... 30		£11,700 less than £12,500 ... 30		£140,000 less than £150,000 ... 30
£2,900 or more ... 31		£12,500 or more ... 31		£150,000 or more ... 31

CARD F

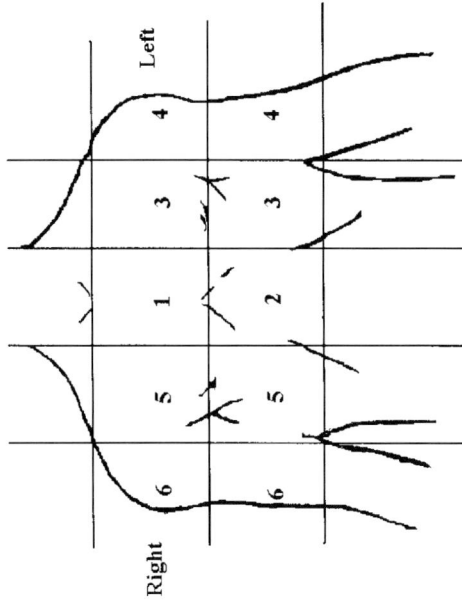

CARD E

1 Going to school or college full-time (including on vacation)

2 In paid employment or self-employment (or away temporarily)

3 On a Government scheme for employment training

4 Doing unpaid work for a business that you own, or that a relative owns

5 Waiting to take up paid work already obtained

6 Looking for paid work or a Government training scheme

7 Intending to look for work but prevented by temporary sickness or injury

8 Permanently unable to work because of long-term sickness or disability

9 Retired from paid work

10 Looking after the home or family

11 Doing something else (PLEASE SAY WHAT)

CARD G

Less than 5 minutes

5 minutes, less than 15 minutes

15 minutes, less than 30 minutes

30 minutes, less than 1 hour

1 hour, less than 1 ½ hours

1 ½ hours, less than 2 hours

2 hours, less than 2 ½ hours

2 ½ hours, less than 3 hours

3 hours, less than 3 ½ hours

3 ½ hours, less than 4 hours

4 hours or more (please say how long)

CARD H

SPORTS AND EXERCISE ACTIVITIES

INCLUDE any sports and exercise activities like:

Playing football, rugby or netball in a team, or any other organised team games

Playing tennis, squash or badminton

include playing in:
a practice session
a match
a club
out-of-school lesson

Going swimming or swimming lessons

Gymnastics (include Toddler Gym, Tumble Tots etc)

Dance lessons, ballet lessons, ice skating

Horse riding

Disco dancing

Any other organised sports, team sports or exercise activities

CARD I

Other active things like:

Ride a bike

Kick a ball around

Run about (outdoors or indoors)

Play active games

Jump around

Any other things like these

CARD J

Sitting down doing things like :

Watching television

Reading (or being read to)

Doing homework

Listening to music

Talking to friends

Playing computer games

Playing boardgames

Drawing

Playing quietly

Sitting in a car

Sitting in a pushchair

Any other things like these

CARD L

HEAVY HOUSEWORK

Moving heavy furniture

Spring cleaning

Walking with heavy shopping
(for more than 5 minutes)

Cleaning windows

Scrubbing floors with a scrubbing brush

CARD K

HOUSEWORK

Hoovering

Dusting

Ironing

General tidying

Washing floors and paint work

HSE 98

CARD N

HEAVY MANUAL WORK

Digging, clearing rough ground

Building in stone/bricklaying

Mowing large areas with a hand mower

Felling trees, chopping wood

Mixing/laying concrete

Moving heavy loads

Refitting a kitchen or bathroom

HSE 98

CARD M

GARDENING, DIY AND BUILDING WORK

Hoeing, weeding, pruning

Mowing with a power mower

Planting flowers/seeds

Decorating

Minor household repairs

Car washing and polishing

Car repairs and maintenance

HSE 98

CARD P

1   6 or more times a week

2   3-5 times a week

3   1-2 times a week

4   Less than once a week

5   Rarely or never

HSE 98

CARD O

1   Swimming

2   Cycling

3   Workout at a gym / Exercise bike / Weight training

4   Aerobics / Keep fit / Gymnastics / Dance for fitness

5   Any other type of dancing

6   Running / Jogging

7   Football / Rugby

8   Badminton / Tennis

9   Squash

10 Exercises (e.g. press-ups, sit-ups)

Please also include teaching, coaching and training/practice sessions

CARD Q

1   Almost every day

2   Five or six days a week

3   Three or four days a week

4   Once or twice a week

5   Once or twice a month

6   Once every couple of months

7   Once or twice a year

8   Not at all in the last twelve months

CARD R

1. Normal strength (less than 6 % alcohol) beer, lager, stout, cider, or shandy (excluding cans or bottles of shandy)

2. Strong beer, lager, stout or cider (6% alcohol or more) (eg. Tennants Extra, Special Brew, Diamond White)

3. Spirits or Liqueurs (e.g. Gin, Whiskey, Brandy, Rum, Vodka, Advocaat, Cocktails)

4. Sherry or Martini (including Port, Vermouth, Cinzano and Dubonnet)

5. Wine (including Babycham and Champagne)

6. Alcoholic soft drinks or 'alcopops' (such as Hooch, Two Dogs, Alcola)

7. Other alcoholic drinks

8. Low alcohol drinks only

HSE 98

CARD T

White

Black - Caribbean

Black - African

Black - Other Black Groups

Indian

Pakistani

Bangladeshi

Chinese

None of these

HSE 98

CARD S

1 Degree or degree level qualification (including higher degree)
2 Teaching qualification
3 Nursing qualifications SRN, SCM, SEN, RGN, RM, RHV, Midwife
4 HNC/HND, BEC/TEC Higher, BTEC Higher/SCOTECH Higher
5 ONC/OND, BEC/TEC/BTEC **not** higher
6 City and Guilds Full Technological Certificate
7 City and Guilds Advanced/Final Level
8 City and Guilds Craft/Ordinary Level
9 A-levels/Higher School Certificate
10 AS level
11 SLC/SCE/SUPE at Higher Grade or Certificate of Sixth Year Studies
12 O-level passes taken in 1975 or earlier
13 O-level passes taken after 1975 GRADES A-C
14 O-level passes taken after 1975 GRADES D-E
15 GCSE GRADES A-C
16 GCSE GRADES D-G
17 CSE GRADE 1/SCE BANDS A-C/Standard Grade LEVEL 1-3
18 CSE GRADES 2-5/SCE Ordinary BANDS D-E
19 CSE Ungraded
20 SLC Lower
21 SUPE Lower or Ordinary
22 School Certificate or Matric
23 NVQ Level 5
24 NVQ Level 4
25 NVQ Level 3/Advanced level GNVQ
26 NVQ Level 2/Intermediate level GNVQ
27 NVQ Level 1/Foundation level GNVQ
28 Recognised Trade Apprenticeship completed
29 Clerical or Commercial Qualification (eg typing/bookkeeping/commerce)

HSE 98

CARD U

1. High Blood Pressure

2. Angina

3. Heart Attack

4. Stroke

5. Other Heart Trouble

6. Diabetes

HSE 98

CARD T

White

Black - Caribbean

Black - African

Black - Other Black Groups

Indian

Pakistani

Bangladeshi

Chinese

None of these

THE HEALTH SURVEY FOR ENGLAND

On behalf of the Department of Health

SCPR
SOCIAL & COMMUNITY
PLANNING RESEARCH

MEDICAL SCHOOL (UCL)

P1727   IN CONFIDENCE

Health Survey for England: 1998

BOOKLET FOR 8-12 YEAR-OLDS

Survey Month: _____

POINT (1-3)

ADDRESS (4-5)

HHLD (6)

CKL (7-8)

PERSON No (from HH Grid)

Spare (9-11)

OUO (12-13) 3 4

Card (14)

Spare

First name: _____

Here are some questions for you to answer on your own.

We are interested in your honest answers. We will not tell anyone what your answers are.

Look at the instructions on the next page and read what to do. Ask the interviewer for help if you do not understand a question or you are not sure what to do.

Thank you for taking part in this survey.

INSTRUCTIONS

Please read each question carefully.

Most of the questions can be answered by putting a tick in the box next to the answer that best describes you.

Example:

(✓)

Yes [✓] 1

No   [ ] 2

Sometimes you are asked to write a number instead.

Example:

I was [1 0] years old

write in

Cigarette Smoking

1. Have you ever tried smoking a cigarette, even if it was only a puff or two?

(✓)

No ☐ 2

Yes ☐ 1 →

How old were you when you first tried smoking a cigarette, even if it was only a puff or two?

I was ☐ **years old**

write in

15

16-17

2. Now read all the following sentences carefully and tick the box next to the one which best describes you.

(✓)

I have never smoked ☐ 1

I have only smoked once or twice ☐ 2

I used to smoke sometimes, but I never smoke a cigarette now ☐ 3

I sometimes smoke, but I don't smoke every week ☐ 4

I smoke between one and six cigarettes a week ☐ 5

I smoke more than six cigarettes a week ☐ 6

18

3. Did you smoke any cigarettes last week?

(✓)

No ☐ 2

Yes ☐ 1 →

How many cigarettes did you smoke last week?

I smoked ☐ **cigarettes**

write in

19

20-21

Drinking

4. Have you ever had a proper alcoholic drink - a whole drink, not just a sip? **Please don't count drinks labelled low alcohol.**

(✓)

Yes ☐ 1 → **GO TO Q5**

No ☐ 2 → **GO TO Q8 on the next page**

5. How old were you the first time you had a proper alcoholic drink?

I was ☐ **years old**

write in

6. How often do you usually have an alcoholic drink?

(✓)

Almost every day ☐ 1

About twice a week ☐ 2

About once a week ☐ 3

About once a fortnight ☐ 4

About once a month ☐ 5

Only a few times a year ☐ 6

I never drink alcohol now ☐ 7

7. When did you **last** have an alcoholic drink?

(✓)

Today ☐ 1

Yesterday ☐ 2

Some other time during the last week ☐ 3

1 week, but less than 2 weeks ago ☐ 4

2 weeks, but less than 4 weeks ago ☐ 5

1 month, but less than 6 months ago ☐ 6

6 months ago or more ☐ 7

Your weight

Everyone answer

8. Given your age and height, would you say
that you are ...

	(✓)
About the right weight	1
too heavy	2
or, too light?	3
Not sure	8

27

9. At the present time, are you trying to **lose** weight,
trying to **gain** weight, or are you **not trying** to change
your weight?

	(✓)
Trying to lose weight	1
Trying to gain weight	2
Not trying to change weight	3

28

Cycling

10. Do you have a bicycle?

	(✓)
Yes	1
No	2

29

11. Do you wear a bicycle helmet
when you ride a bike?

	(✓)
I always wear a helmet when I ride a bike	1
I sometimes wear a helmet when I ride a bike	2
I never wear a helmet when I ride a bike	3
I never ride a bike	4

30

12. What do you think about bicycle helmets?

**PLEASE TICK ALL THE BOXES THAT
YOU AGREE WITH**

	(✓)
Wearing a helmet makes me feel safer when I ride a bike	1
I sometimes forget to put my helmet on	2
Bicycle helmets cost too much money	3
Helmets look good	4
It is difficult to get helmets to fit	5
Helmets can protect you if you have an accident	6
Wearing a helmet makes me feel like a proper cyclist	7

31-37

Thank you for answering these questions.

Now please give the booklet back to the interviewer

THE HEALTH SURVEY FOR ENGLAND

On behalf of the Department of Health

SCPR
SOCIAL & COMMUNITY PLANNING RESEARCH

P1727

IN CONFIDENCE

Health Survey for England: 1998

BOOKLET FOR 13-15 YEAR OLDS

Survey Month: [ ]

(1-3) [ ] [ ]

POINT   (4-5) [ ][ ]   **ADDRESS**   (6) [ ]   **HHLD**   [ ]   **CKL**   (7-8) [ ][ ]   **PERSON No (from HH Grid)**   (9-11) [ ] Spare

First name: [ ]

DUO (12-13) [3] [3]

Card (14-20) [3] Spare

Here are some questions for you to answer on your own.

We are interested in your honest answers. We will not tell anyone what your answers are.

Look at the instructions on the next page and read what to do. Ask the interviewer for help if you do not understand a question or you are not sure what to do.

Thank you for taking part in this survey.

Instructions

Please read each question carefully.

Most of the questions can be answered by ticking the box next to the answer that applies to you.

Example:

(tick **one** box)

Yes [✓]₁

No [ ]₂

Sometimes you are asked to write a number inside a box instead.

Example:

Write in no. [6] → GO TO Q5

Next to the boxes there are arrows and instructions. They tell you which question to answer next. If there are no special instructions, you should answer the next question.

Example:

(tick **one** box)

Yes [✓]₁ → GO TO Q4

No [ ]₂ → GO TO Q5

Cigarette smoking

1. Have you ever tried smoking a cigarette, even if it was only a puff or two?

(tick **one** box)

- Yes ☐ 1
- No ☐ 2

21

2. Now read all the following sentences carefully and tick the box next to the one which best describes you.

(tick **one** box)

- I have never smoked ☐ 1 → **GO TO THE DRINKING SECTION ON PAGE 4**
- I have only smoked once or twice ☐ 2
- I used to smoke sometimes, but I never smoke a cigarette now ☐ 3
- I sometimes smoke, but I don't smoke every week ☐ 4
- I smoke between one and six cigarettes a week ☐ 5
- I smoke more than six cigarettes a week ☐ 6

→ **GO TO Q3**

22

3. How old were you when you first tried smoking a cigarette, even if it was only a puff or two?

Write how old you were then ☐

23-24

4. Did you smoke any cigarettes last week?

(tick **one** box)

- No ☐ 2
- Yes ☐ 1 → **How many cigarettes did you smoke last week?**

25

I smoked ☐ cigarettes
write in

26-27

Drinking

Everyone answer

5. Have you ever had a proper alcoholic drink - a whole drink, not just a sip? **Please don't count drinks labelled low alcohol.**

(tick **one** box)

- Yes ☐ 1 → **GO TO Q6**
- No ☐ 2 → **GO TO Q15 on page 7**

28

6. How old were you the first time you had a proper alcoholic drink?

I was ☐ **years old**
write in

29-30

7. How often do you usually have an alcoholic drink?

(tick **one** box)

- Almost every day ☐ 1
- About twice a week ☐ 2
- About once a week ☐ 3
- About once a fortnight ☐ 4
- About once a month ☐ 5
- Only a few times a year ☐ 6
- I never drink alcohol now ☐ 7

31

8. When did you **last** have an alcoholic drink?

(tick **one** box)

- Today ☐ 1
- Yesterday ☐ 2 → **GO TO Q9**
- Some other time during the last week ☐ 3
- 1 week, but less than 2 weeks ago ☐ 4
- 2 weeks, but less than 4 weeks ago ☐ 5
- 1 month, but less than 6 months ago ☐ 6 → **GO TO Q15 on page 7**
- 6 months ago or more ☐ 7

32

9. Which, if any, of the drinks shown below, have you drunk in the last 7 days?
Please tick (✓) either yes or no for each kind of drink.
For each kind of drink, write in the box how much you drank in the last 7 days.

Beer, lager, cider or shandy (exclude bottles or cans of shandy)

Have you drunk this in _the last 7 days?_

(tick **one** box)

No   2   → GO TO Q10

Yes   1

33

How much did you drink in the last 7 days?

Write in:

Pints (if ½ pint, write in ½)   34-37

AND/OR   Large cans or bottles   38-39

AND/OR   Small cans or bottles   40-41

10. **Spirits or liqueurs, such as gin, vodka, whisky, rum, brandy, or cocktails**

Have you drunk this in _the last 7 days?_

(tick **one** box)

No   2   → GO TO Q11

Yes   1

42

How much did you drink in the last 7 days?

Write in: Glasses (count doubles as two singles)   43-44

11. **Sherry or martini (including port, vermouth, cinzano, dubonnet)**

Have you drunk this in _the last 7 days?_

(tick **one** box)

No   2   → GO TO Q12

Yes   1

45

How much did you drink in the last 7 days?

Write in: Glasses (count doubles as two singles)   46-47

12. **Wine (incl. babycham & champagne)**

Have you drunk this in _the last 7 days?_

(tick **one** box)

No   2   → GO TO Q13

Yes   1

48

How much did you drink in the last 7 days?

Write in: Glasses   49-50

13. **Alcoholic soft drinks or 'alcopops' (such as Hooch, Two Dogs, Alcola)**

Have you drunk this in _the last 7 days?_

(tick **one** box)

No   2   → GO TO Q14

Yes   1

51

How much did you drink in the last 7 days?

Write in: Large cans or bottles   52-53

AND/OR   Small cans or bottles   54-55

14. **Other kinds of alcoholic drink**

Have you drunk this in _the last 7 days?_

(tick **one** box)

No   2   → GO TO Q15 on next page

Yes   1   → COMPLETE DETAILS BELOW

56

How much did you drink in the last 7 days?

WRITE IN NAME OF DRINK   WRITE IN

57-66

67

68-77

78

79-88

Spare 89-100

Your weight

Everyone answer

15. Given your age and height, would you say that you are …

(tick **one** box)

About the right weight,	1
too heavy,	2
or, too light?	3
Not sure	8

101

16. At the present time, are you trying to **lose** weight, trying to **gain** weight, or are you **not trying** to change your weight?

(tick **one** box)

Trying to lose weight	1
Trying to gain weight	2
Not trying to change weight	3

102

General health over the last few weeks

Please read this carefully:

We should like to know how your health has been in general, **over the past few weeks.**
Please answer ALL the questions by putting a tick in the box under the answer which you think most applies to you.

HAVE YOU RECENTLY:

17. been able to concentrate on whatever you're doing?

(tick **one** box)

Better than usual	Same as usual	Less than usual	Much less than usual
☐	☐	☐	☐

103

18. lost much sleep over worry?

(tick **one** box)

Not at all	No more than usual	Rather more than usual	Much more than usual
☐	☐	☐	☐

104

19. felt you were playing a useful part in things?

(tick **one** box)

More so than usual	Same as usual	Less useful than usual	Much less useful
☐	☐	☐	☐

105

20. felt capable of making decisions about things?

(tick **one** box)

More so than usual	Same as usual	Less so than usual	Much less capable
☐	☐	☐	☐

106

21. felt constantly under strain?

(tick **one** box)

Not at all	No more than usual	Rather more than usual	Much more than usual
☐	☐	☐	☐

107

22. felt you couldn't overcome your difficulties?

(tick **one** box)

Not at all	No more than usual	Rather more than usual	Much more than usual
☐	☐	☐	☐
1	2	3	4

108

THE HEALTH SURVEY FOR ENGLAND
On behalf of the Department of Health

IN CONFIDENCE

P1727

Health Survey for England: 1998

BOOKLET FOR YOUNG ADULTS

Survey Month: _____

POINT (1-3) | ADDRESS (4-5) | HHLD (6) | CKL | PERSON No (from HH Grid) (7-8) | Spare (9-11)

First name: _____

OFFICE USE (12-13): 3 2

Card (14-20): 2

Spare

Please read this before completing:

A. Some questions on the following pages can be answered simply by ticking the box below the answer that applies to you.

Example:

Do you feel that you lead a ...

Very healthy life	Fairly healthy life	Not very healthy life	An unhealthy life
1	2 ✓	3	4

(tick one box)

B. Sometimes you are asked to write in a number or the answer in your own words. Please enter numbers as figures rather than words.

Example:

Write in no. [6]

C. On most pages you should answer ALL the questions but sometimes you will find the box you have ticked has an arrow next to it with an instruction to go to another question.

Example:

(tick one box)

Yes........... 1 → GO TO Q4

No........... 2 ✓ → GO TO Q3

HAVE YOU RECENTLY:

23. been able to enjoy your normal day-to-day activities?

More so than usual	Same as usual	Less so than usual	Much less than usual

(tick one box)   109

24. been able to face up to your problems?

More so than usual	Same as usual	Less able than usual	Much less able

(tick one box)   110

25. been feeling unhappy and depressed?

Not at all	No more than usual	Rather more than usual	Much more than usual

(tick one box)   111

26. been losing confidence in yourself?

Not at all	No more than usual	Rather more than usual	Much more than usual

(tick one box)   112

27. been thinking of yourself as a worthless person?

Not at all	No more than usual	Rather more than usual	Much more than usual

(tick one box)   113

28. been feeling reasonably happy, all things considered?

More so than usual	About same as usual	Less so than usual	Much less than usual
1	2	3	4

(tick one box)   114

Thank you for answering these questions.

Please give the booklet back to the interviewer.

IN CONFIDENCE

Smoking

1. Have you ever smoked a cigarette, a cigar or a pipe?

(tick one box)

Yes............ ☐ 1 → **GO TO Q2**

No............ ☐ 2 → **GO TO Q10**

21

2. Have you ever smoked a cigarette?

(tick one box)

Yes............ ☐ 1 → **GO TO Q3**

No............ ☐ 2 → **GO TO Q10**

22

3. How old were you when you first tried smoking a cigarette, even if it was only a puff or two?

Write in how old you were then ...... ☐

23-24

4. Do you smoke cigarettes at all nowadays?

(tick one box)

Yes............ ☐ 1 → **GO TO Q6**

No............ ☐ 2 → **GO TO Q5**

25

5. Did you smoke cigarettes regularly or occasionally?

(tick one box)

Regularly, that is at least one cigarette a day ...... ☐ 1

Occasionally............ ☐ 2 } → **GO TO Q10**

I never really smoked cigarettes, just tried them once or twice ...... ☐ 3

26

CURRENT SMOKERS

6. About how many cigarettes a day do you usually smoke on <u>weekdays?</u>

Write in no. smoked a day ...... ☐

27-28

7. And about how many cigarettes a day do you usually smoke at <u>weekends?</u>

Write in no. smoked a day ...... ☐

29-30

8. Do you <u>mainly</u> smoke...

(tick one box)

.... filter-tipped cigarettes, ☐ 1 → **GO TO Q9**

plain or untipped cigarettes, ☐ 2 → **GO TO Q9**

or hand-rolled cigarettes? ☐ 3 → **GO TO Q10**

31

9. Which brand of cigarette do you <u>usually</u> smoke?

WRITE IN

Brand: _____

32-34

TYPE (eg Superkings) _____

35-36

TAR LEVEL
(check side of packet) ☐ mg

EVERYONE PLEASE ANSWER

10. Did your father ever smoke regularly when you were a child?

(tick one box)

Yes............ ☐ 1

No............ ☐ 2

Don't know ...... ☐ 8

37

11. Did your mother ever smoke regularly when you were a child?

(tick one box)

Yes............ ☐ 1

No............ ☐ 2

Don't know...... ☐ 8

38

Drinking

16. The next few questions are concerned with different types of alcoholic drink. Please tick the box underneath the answer that best describes how often you usually drank each of them in the last 12 months. For the ones you drank, write in how much you usually drank on any one day. **EXCLUDE ANY NON-ALCOHOLIC OR LOW-ALCOHOL DRINKS, EXCEPT SHANDY.**

EXAMPLE:

A. How often have you had this type of drink in the past year?
TICK ONE BOX

Almost every day	Five or six days a week	Three or four days a week	Once or twice a week	Once or twice a month	Once every couple of months	Once or twice in last 12 months	Never in last 12 months
1	2	3	✓ 4	5	6	7	8 → GO TO B

How much did you usually drink on any one day? (**WRITE IN NUMBER**):

½ Pints

AND/OR [ ] Large cans or bottles

AND/OR 2 Small cans or bottles

NOW PLEASE ANSWER A-H

A. Normal strength beer, lager, stout, cider or shandy (less than 6% alcohol) - exclude bottles/cans of shandy.

How often have you had this type of drink in the past year?
TICK ONE BOX

Almost every day	Five or six days a week	Three or four days a week	Once or twice a week	Once or twice a month	Once every couple of months	Once or twice in last 12 months	Never in last 12 months
1	2	3	4	5	6	7	8 → GO TO B.

How much did you usually drink on any one day? (**WRITE IN NUMBER**):

[ ] Pints

AND/OR [ ] Large cans or bottles

AND/OR [ ] Small cans or bottles

44
45-52

---

12. Do you ever drink alcohol nowadays, including drinks you brew or make at home?

(tick one box)

Yes........... 1 → GO TO Q15

No............ 2 → GO TO Q13

39

13. Just to check, does that mean you never have an alcoholic drink nowadays, or do you have an alcoholic drink very occasionally, perhaps for medicinal purposes or on special occasions like Christmas and New Year?

(tick one box)

Very occasionally........... 1 → GO TO Q15

Never .... 2 → GO TO Q14

40

14. Have you always been a non-drinker or did you stop drinking for some reason?

(tick one box)

Always a non-drinker........... 1 } → GO TO Q30 ON PAGE 13

Used to drink but stopped........... 2 }

41

15. How old were you the first time you ever had a proper alcoholic drink?

Write in how old you were then ..... [ ] → GO TO Q16 ON NEXT PAGE

42-43

B. Strong beer, lager, stout, cider (6% alcohol or more, such as Tennants Extra, Special Brew, Diamond White)

How often have you had this type of drink in the past year?
TICK ONE BOX

Almost every day	Five or six days a week	Three or four days a week	Once or twice a week	Once or twice a month	Once every couple of months	Once or twice in last 12 months	Never in last 12 months
1	2	3	4	5	6	7	8

GO TO C.

53

How much did you usually drink on any one day? (**WRITE IN NUMBER**):

Pints

AND/OR   Large cans or bottles

AND/OR   Small cans or bottles

54-61

C. Spirits or liqueurs, such as gin, whisky, rum, brandy, vodka, or cocktails

How often have you had this type of drink in the past year?
TICK ONE BOX

Almost every day	Five or six days a week	Three or four days a week	Once or twice a week	Once or twice a month	Once every couple of months	Once or twice in last 12 months	Never in last 12 months
1	2	3	4	5	6	7	8

GO TO D.

62

How much did you usually drink on any one day? (**WRITE IN NUMBER**):

Glasses (count doubles as 2 singles)

63-64

D. Sherry or martini (including port, vermouth, cinzano, dubonnet)

How often have you had this type of drink in the past year?
TICK ONE BOX

Almost every day	Five or six days a week	Three or four days a week	Once or twice a week	Once or twice a month	Once every couple of months	Once or twice in last 12 months	Never in last 12 months
1	2	3	4	5	6	7	8

GO TO E.

65

How much did you usually drink on any one day? (**WRITE IN NUMBER**):

Glasses (count doubles as 2 singles)

66-67

E. Wine (including babycham and champagne)

How often have you had this type of drink in the past year?
TICK ONE BOX

Almost every day	Five or six days a week	Three or four days a week	Once or twice a week	Once or twice a month	Once every couple of months	Once or twice in last 12 months	Never in last 12 months
1	2	3	4	5	6	7	8

GO TO F.

68

How much did you usually drink on any one day? (**WRITE IN NUMBER**):

Glasses

69-70

F. Alcoholic soft drinks or 'alcopops' (such as Hooch, Two Dogs, Alcola)

How often have you had this type of drink in the past year?
TICK ONE BOX

Almost every day	Five or six days a week	Three or four days a week	Once or twice a week	Once or twice a month	Once every couple of months	Once or twice in last 12 months	Never in last 12 months
☐ 1	☐ 2	☐ 3	☐ 4	☐ 5	☐ 6	☐ 7	☐ 8 → GO TO G.

How much did you usually drink on any one day? (**WRITE IN NUMBER**): ☐
Small cans or bottles

G. Have you had any other kinds of alcoholic drink in the last 12 months?

No ☐ 2 → **GO TO Q17**
Yes ☐ 1

WRITE IN NAME OF DRINK:

How often have you had this type of drink in the past year?
TICK ONE BOX

Almost every day	Five or six days a week	Three or four days a week	Once or twice a week	Once or twice a month	Once every couple of months	Once or twice in last 12 months
☐ 1	☐ 2	☐ 3	☐ 4	☐ 5	☐ 6	☐ 7

How much did you usually drink on any one day? (**WRITE IN NUMBER**):

☐	Glasses (count doubles as 2 singles)
AND/OR ☐	Pints
AND/OR ☐	Large cans or bottles
AND/OR ☐	Small cans or bottles

H. Have you had any other kinds of alcoholic drink in the last 12 months?

No ☐ 2 → **GO TO Q17**
Yes ☐ 1

WRITE IN NAME OF DRINK:

How often have you had this type of drink in the past year?
TICK ONE BOX

Almost every day	Five or six days a week	Three or four days a week	Once or twice a week	Once or twice a month	Once every couple of months	Once or twice in last 12 months
☐ 1	☐ 2	☐ 3	☐ 4	☐ 5	☐ 6	☐ 7

How much did you usually drink on any one day? (**WRITE IN NUMBER**):

☐	Glasses (count doubles as 2 singles)
AND/OR ☐	Pints
AND/OR ☐	Large cans or bottles
AND/OR ☐	Small cans or bottles

17. Thinking now about all kinds of drinks, how often have you had an alcoholic drink of any kind during the last 12 months?

(tick **one** box)

Almost every day......... 01
Five or six days a week......... 02
Three or four days a week......... 03
Once or twice a week......... 04
Once or twice a month......... 05
Once every couple of months......... 06
Once or twice a year......... 07
Not at all in the last 12 months......... 08

102-103

18. Did you have an alcoholic drink in the seven days ending yesterday?

(tick **one** box)

Yes......... 1 → GO TO Q19

No......... 2 → GO TO Q21 ON PAGE 12

104

19. On how many days out of the last seven did you have an alcoholic drink?

(tick **one** box)

One......... 1
Two......... 2
Three......... 3
Four......... 4
Five......... 5
Six......... 6
Seven......... 7

105

20. Please think about the day in the last week on which you drank the most. (If you drank the same amount on more than one day, please answer about the most recent of those days.)

From this list, please tick all the types of alcoholic drink which you drank on that day. For the ones you drank, write in how much you drank on that day. EXCLUDE NON-ALCOHOLIC OR LOW-ALCOHOL DRINKS, EXCEPT SHANDY.

WRITE IN HOW MUCH DRUNK ON THAT DAY

TICK **ALL** DRINKS DRUNK ON THAT DAY		Glasses (count doubles as 2 singles)	Pints	Large cans or bottles	Small cans or bottles
Normal strength beer, lager, stout, cider or shandy (less than 6% alcohol - exclude bottles or cans of shandy)	106-121 01				122-129
Strong beer, lager, stout or cider (6% alcohol or more, such as Tennants Extra, Special Brew, Diamond White)	02				130-137
Spirits or liqueurs, such as gin, whisky, rum, brandy, vodka or cocktails	03				138-139
Sherry or martini (including port, vermouth, cinzano, dubonnet)	04				140-141
Wine (including babycham and champagne)	05				142-143
Alcoholic soft drinks or 'alcopops' (such as Hooch, Two Dogs, Alcola)	06				144-145
Other kinds of alcoholic drink WRITE IN NAME OF DRINK 1.	07				146-155
2.	08				156-165

Drinking Experiences

PLEASE READ THIS CAREFULLY
Please read each statement. Thinking about the last three months only, if you have had the experience tick the box next to the word "Yes". If you have not had the experience in the last three months, tick the box next to the word "No".

21. I have felt that I ought to cut down on my drinking
Yes......... 1
No......... 2

22. I have felt ashamed or guilty about my drinking
Yes......... 1
No......... 2

23. People have annoyed me by criticising my drinking
Yes......... 1
No......... 2

24. I have found that my hands were shaking in the morning after drinking the previous night
Yes......... 1
No......... 2

25. I have had a drink first thing in the morning to steady my nerves or get rid of a hangover
Yes......... 1
No......... 2

26. There have been occasions when I felt that I was unable to stop drinking
Yes......... 1
No......... 2

27. I have been drunk at least once a week, on average, in the last three months
Yes......... 1 → GO TO Q30
No......... 2 → GO TO Q28

28. Drinking has made me slightly (or very) drunk in the last three months
Yes .... 1 → GO TO Q29
No .... 2 → GO TO Q30

29. If yes, please tick one of the boxes to show how many times in the last 3 months

(tick one box)

Once	Twice	Three times	Four or more times
1	2	3	4

NOW PLEASE GO TO Q30

Your Weight

EVERYONE ANSWER

30. Given your age and height, would you say that you are ...

(tick one box)

About the right weight,......... 1
too heavy,......... 2
or, too light?......... 3
Not sure 4

31. At the present time, are you trying to **lose** weight, trying to **gain** weight, or are you **not trying** to change your weight?

(tick one box)

Trying to lose weight......... 1
Trying to gain weight......... 2
Not trying to change weight 3

Health over the last 12 months

32. Over the last twelve months, would you say your health has on the whole been...

(tick one box)

... good,......... 1
fairly good,......... 2
or, not good?......... 3

General health over the last few weeks

Please read this carefully:

We should like to know how your health has been in general, **over the past few weeks.** Please answer ALL the questions by putting a tick in the box under the answer which you think most applies to you.

HAVE YOU RECENTLY:

(tick one box)

	Better than usual	Same as usual	Less than usual	Much less than usual
33. been able to concentrate on whatever you're doing?	☐	☐	☐	☐ 178

	Not at all	No more than usual	Rather more than usual	Much more than usual
34. lost much sleep over worry?	☐	☐	☐	☐ 179

	More so than usual	Same as usual	Less useful than usual	Much less useful
35. felt you were playing a useful part in things?	☐	☐	☐	☐ 180

	More so than usual	Same as usual	Less so than usual	Much less capable
36. felt capable of making decisions about things?	☐	☐	☐	☐ 181

	Not at all	No more than usual	Rather more than usual	Much more than usual
37. felt constantly under strain?	☐	☐	☐	☐ 182

	Not at all	No more than usual	Rather more than usual	Much more than usual
38. felt you couldn't overcome your difficulties?	☐	☐	☐	☐ 183

1	2	3	4

HAVE YOU RECENTLY:

(tick one box)

	More so than usual	Same as usual	Less so than usual	Much less than usual
39. been able to enjoy your normal day-to-day activities?	☐	☐	☐	☐ 184

	More so than usual	Same as usual	Less able than usual	Much less able
40. been able to face up to your problems?	☐	☐	☐	☐ 185

	Not at all	No more than usual	Rather more than usual	Much more than usual
41. been feeling unhappy and depressed?	☐	☐	☐	☐ 186

	Not at all	No more than usual	Rather more than usual	Much more than usual
42. been losing confidence in yourself?	☐	☐	☐	☐ 187

	Not at all	No more than usual	Rather more than usual	Much more than usual
43. been thinking of yourself as a worthless person?	☐	☐	☐	☐ 188

	More so than usual	About same as usual	Less so than usual	Much less than usual
44. been feeling reasonably happy, all things considered?	☐	☐	☐	☐ 189

1	2	3	4

45. We would now like you to think about your family and friends. By 'family' we mean those who live with you as well as those elsewhere.

Here are some comments people have made about their family and friends. We would like you to say how far each statement is true for you.

Please answer ALL the questions, ticking the box which you think most applies to you.

A. There are people I know - amongst my family or friends - who do things to make me happy.

*(tick **one** box)*

Not true .... ☐ 1
Partly true .... ☐ 2
Certainly true .... ☐ 3

190

B. There are people I know - amongst my family or friends - who make me feel loved.

*(tick **one** box)*

Not true .... ☐ 1
Partly true .... ☐ 2
Certainly true .... ☐ 3

191

C. There are people I know - amongst my family or friends - who can be relied on no matter what happens.

*(tick **one** box)*

Not true .... ☐ 1
Partly true .... ☐ 2
Certainly true .... ☐ 3

192

D. There are people I know - amongst my family or friends - who would see that I am taken care of if I needed to be.

*(tick **one** box)*

Not true .... ☐ 1
Partly true .... ☐ 2
Certainly true .... ☐ 3

{ GO TO E
ON THE
NEXT PAGE

193

E. There are people I know - amongst my family or friends - who accept me just as I am.

*(tick **one** box)*

Not true .... ☐ 1
Partly true .... ☐ 2
Certainly true .... ☐ 3

194

F. There are people I know - amongst my family or friends - who make me feel an important part of their lives.

*(tick **one** box)*

Not true .... ☐ 1
Partly true .... ☐ 2
Certainly true .... ☐ 3

195

G. There are people I know - amongst my family or friends - who would give me support and encouragement.

*(tick **one** box)*

Not true .... ☐ 1
Partly true .... ☐ 2
Certainly true .... ☐ 3

196

IF YOU ARE A WOMAN, PLEASE GO TO Q46
IF YOU ARE A MAN, PLEASE GIVE THE BOOKLET BACK TO THE INTERVIEWER.

UCL MEDICAL SCHOOL

SCPR
SOCIAL & COMMUNITY PLANNING RESEARCH

THE HEALTH SURVEY FOR ENGLAND

On behalf of the Department of Health

IN CONFIDENCE

P1727   **Health Survey for England: 1998**

BOOKLET FOR ADULTS

Survey Month
(1-3)

POINT | ADDRESS | HHLD | CKL
(4-5) | (6) |

First name

(7-8)   (9-11) Spare

PERSON No
(from HH Grid)

(12-13)   O.U.O   3 | 1

Card (14-20) Spare

Please read this before completing:

A. Most questions on the following pages can be answered simply by ticking the box below or alongside the answer that applies to you.

Example:

Do you feel that you lead a...

(tick one box)

Very healthy life	Fairly healthy life	Not very healthy life	An unhealthy life
1	2 ✓	3	4

B. On most pages you should answer ALL the questions but sometimes you will find the box you have ticked has an arrow next to it with an instruction to go to another question.

Example:

(tick one box)

Yes [✓] 1 → GO TO Q4

No [ ] 2 → GO TO Q3

By following the arrows carefully you will miss out questions which do not apply to you.

Women only please answer

46. Are you currently taking the contraceptive pill or having a contraceptive injection or implant?

(tick one box)

Yes .... 1 → GO TO Q47

No .... 2 → GO TO Q49

197

47. What is the brand name of your contraceptive?
Please write in name below:

[   ]

198-203

48. What kind of contraceptive is this?

(tick one box)

Injection 1

Mini pill (progestogen only) 2

Combined pill 3

Implant (Norplant) 4

Not sure 8

204

49. THANK YOU FOR ANSWERING THESE QUESTIONS. PLEASE GIVE THE BOOKLET BACK TO THE INTERVIEWER.

DRINKING EXPERIENCES

Please read this carefully:

Please read each statement. Thinking about the last three months only, if you have had the experience tick the box next to the word 'Yes'. If you have not had the experience in the last three months, tick the box next to the word 'No'.

(tick **one** box)

1. I have felt that I ought to cut down on my drinking

Yes ☐ 1
No ☐ 2

21

2. I have felt ashamed or guilty about my drinking

(tick **one** box)

Yes ☐ 1
No ☐ 2

22

3. People have annoyed me by criticising my drinking

(tick **one** box)

Yes ☐ 1
No ☐ 2

23

4. I have found that my hands were shaking in the morning after drinking the previous night

(tick **one** box)

Yes ☐ 1
No ☐ 2

24

5. I have had a drink first thing in the morning to steady my nerves or get rid of a hangover

(tick **one** box)

Yes ☐ 1
No ☐ 2

25

6. There have been occasions when I felt that I was unable to stop drinking

(tick **one** box)

Yes ☐ 1
No ☐ 2

26

7. I have been drunk at least once a week, on average, in the last three months

(tick **one** box)

Yes ☐ 1 → **GO TO Q10 on the next page**
No ☐ 2 → **GO TO Q8**

27

8. Drinking has made me slightly (or very) drunk in the last three months

(tick **one** box)

Yes ☐ 1 → **GO TO Q9**
No ☐ 2 → **GO TO Q10 on the next page**

28

9. If yes please tick one box to show how many times in the last 3 months.

Once	Twice	Three times	Four or more times
☐ 1	☐ 2	☐ 3	☐ 4

29

NOW PLEASE GO TO Q10.

YOUR WEIGHT

10. Given your age and height, would you say that you are ...

(tick **one** box)

About the right weight ☐ 1
too heavy ☐ 2
or, too light? ☐ 3
Not sure ☐ 8

30

11. At the present time, are you trying to **lose** weight, trying to **gain** weight, or are you **not trying** to change your weight?

(tick **one** box)

Trying to lose weight ☐ 1
Trying to gain weight ☐ 2
Not trying to change weight ☐ 3

31

HEALTH OVER THE LAST TWELVE MONTHS

12. Over the last twelve months would you say your health has on the whole been ...

(tick **one** box)

Good ☐ 1
Fairly good ☐ 2
Not good ☐ 3

32

GENERAL HEALTH OVER THE LAST FEW WEEKS

Please read this carefully:

We should like to know how your health has been in general **over the past few weeks.** Please answer ALL the questions by ticking the box below the answer which you think most applies to you.

HAVE YOU RECENTLY: *(tick one box)*

13.	been able to concentrate on whatever you're doing?	Better than usual ☐	Same as usual ☐	Less than usual ☐	Much less than usual ☐	33
14.	lost much sleep over worry?	Not at all ☐	No more than usual ☐	Rather more than usual ☐	Much more than usual ☐	34
15.	felt you were playing a useful part in things?	More so than usual ☐	Same as usual ☐	Less useful than usual ☐	Much less useful ☐	35
16.	felt capable of making decisions about things?	More so than usual ☐	Same as usual ☐	Less so than usual ☐	Much less capable ☐	36
17.	felt constantly under strain?	Not at all ☐	No more than usual ☐	Rather more than usual ☐	Much more than usual ☐	37
18.	felt you couldn't overcome your difficulties?	Not at all ☐	No more than usual ☐	Rather more than usual ☐	Much more than usual ☐	38

1   2   3   4

HAVE YOU RECENTLY: *(tick one box)*

19.	been able to enjoy your normal day-to-day activities?	More so than usual ☐	Same as usual ☐	Less so than usual ☐	Much less than usual ☐	39
20.	been able to face up to your problems?	More so than usual ☐	Same as usual ☐	Less able than usual ☐	Much less able ☐	40
21.	been feeling unhappy and depressed?	Not at all ☐	No more than usual ☐	Rather more than usual ☐	Much more than usual ☐	41
22.	been losing confidence in yourself?	Not at all ☐	No more than usual ☐	Rather more than usual ☐	Much more than usual ☐	42
23.	been thinking of yourself as a worthless person?	Not at all ☐	No more than usual ☐	Rather more than usual ☐	Much more than usual ☐	43
24.	been feeling reasonably happy, all things considered?	More so than usual ☐	About same as usual ☐	Less so than usual ☐	Much less than usual ☐	44

1   2   3   4

25. We would now like you to think about your family and friends.
By family we mean those who live with you as well as those elsewhere.

Here are some comments people have made about their family and friends.
We would like you to say how far each statement is true for you.

Please answer ALL the questions, ticking the box which you
think most applies to you.

A. There are people I know - amongst my family or friends -
who do things to make me happy.

(tick **one** box)

Not true	☐ 1
Partly true	☐ 2
Certainly true	☐ 3

45

B. There are people I know - amongst my family or friends -
who make me feel loved.

(tick **one** box)

Not true	☐ 1
Partly true	☐ 2
Certainly true	☐ 3

46

C. There are people I know - amongst my family or friends -
who can be relied on no matter what happens.

(tick **one** box)

Not true	☐ 1
Partly true	☐ 2
Certainly true	☐ 3

47

D. There are people I know - amongst my family or friends -
who would see that I am taken care of if I needed to be.

(tick **one** box)

Not true	☐ 1
Partly true	☐ 2
Certainly true	☐ 3

48

E. There are people I know - amongst my family or friends -
who accept me just as I am.

(tick **one** box)

Not true	☐ 1
Partly true	☐ 2
Certainly true	☐ 3

49

F. There are people I know - amongst my family or friends -
who make me feel an important part of their lives.

(tick **one** box)

Not true	☐ 1
Partly true	☐ 2
Certainly true	☐ 3

50

G. There are people I know - amongst my family or friends -
who give me support and encouragement.

(tick **one** box)

Not true	☐ 1
Partly true	☐ 2
Certainly true	☐ 3

51

> IF YOU ARE A WOMAN, PLEASE GO TO Q26
>
> IF YOU ARE A MAN, PLEASE GIVE THE BOOKLET BACK TO THE INTERVIEWER

WOMEN ONLY PLEASE ANSWER

26. Have you ever taken the contraceptive pill or had a contraceptive injection or implant?

(tick **one** box)

Yes	☐	1 →	**GO TO Q27**
No	☐	2 →	**GO TO Q30**

52

27. Are you currently taking the contraceptive pill or having a contraceptive injection or implant?

(tick **one** box)

Yes	☐	1 →	**GO TO Q28**
No	☐	2 →	**GO TO Q30**

53

28. What is the brand name of your contraceptive?
Please write in name below:

54-59

29. What kind of contraceptive is this?

(tick **one** box)

Injection	☐	1
Mini pill (progestogen only)	☐	2
Combined pill	☐	3
Implant (Norplant)	☐	4
Not sure	☐	8

60

30. Are you still having periods (menstruating)?

(tick **one** box)

Yes	☐	1 →	**GO TO Q33**
No	☐	2 →	**GO TO Q31**

61

31. Did your periods stop as a result of an operation?

(tick **one** box)

Yes	☐	1 →	**GO TO Q32**
No	☐	2 →	**GO TO Q33**

62

32. Have you had any ovaries removed?

(tick **one** box)

Yes	☐	1 →	**GO TO Q33**
No	☐	2 →	

63

33. Have you ever been on Hormone Replacement Therapy (HRT)?

(tick **one** box)

Yes	☐	1 →	**GO TO Q34**
No	☐	2 →	**GO TO Q37**

64

34. At what age did you start Hormone Replacement Therapy?
WRITE IN AGE

☐ YEARS OLD → **GO TO Q35**

65-66

35. Are you still on Hormone Replacement Therapy?

(tick **one** box)

Yes	☐	1 →	**GO TO Q37**
No	☐	2 →	**GO TO Q36**

67

36. At what age did you stop Hormone Replacement Therapy?
WRITE IN AGE

☐ YEARS OLD

68-69

37. Thank you for answering these questions. Please give the booklet back to the interviewer.

National Centre *for* **Social Research**

Formerly SCPR
Charity No. 238638

Head Office
35 Northampton Square
London EC1V 0AX
Telephone 0171 250 1866
Fax 0171 250 1524

Operations Department
100 Kings Road, Brentwood
Essex CM14 4LX
Telephone 01277 200 600
Fax 01277 214 117

P1727

The Health Survey for England 1998

Program Documentation

Nurse Schedule

Household grid

PERSON to NATPS2 are usually transmitted directly from the interview data to the nurse CAPI program. There is also a facility for nurses to key this information directly from the Nurse Record Form, for example if the nurse visit follows too quickly from the interview to allow the automatic transmission to take place.

Person
Person number of person who was interviewed
Range 01..12

Name
Name of person who was interviewed

Sex
Sex of person who was interviewed
1   Male
2   Female

Age
Age of person who was interviewed
Range 2..120

OC
Interview outcome of person who was interviewed
1   Agreed Nurse Visit
2   Refused Nurse Visit
3   No outcome yet

IF (AGE IN [2..15]) THEN
P1
Person number of child's Parent 1
Range 01..12

NatPs1
Parent type of Parent 1
1   Parent
2   Legal parental responsibility

P2
Person number of child's Parent 2
(code 97=no Parent 2 in household)
Range 01..97

IF (P2 IN [01..12]) THEN
NatPs2
Parent type of Parent 2
1   Parent
2   Legal parental responsibility
ENDIF
ENDIF

AdrField
PLEASE ENTER THE FIRST TEN CHARACTERS OF THE FIRST LINE OF THE ADDRESS TAKEN FROM N.R.F. ADDRESS LABEL.
MAKE SURE TO TYPE IT EXACTLY AS IT IS PRINTED.:
STRING[10]

HHDate
NURSE: ENTER THE DATE OF THE ORIGINAL HOUSEHOLD INTERVIEW FROM Q2 ON THE NRF (OR INTERIM APPOINTMENT RECORD).
ENTER DAY OF MONTH IN NUMBER, NAME OF MONTH IN WORDS (FIRST THREE LETTERS) AND YEAR IN NUMBERS, EG 2 JAN 97.

OpenDisp
HERE ARE THE PEOPLE AT THIS HOUSEHOLD WHO HAVE BEEN SEEN BY THE INTERVIEWER (NB. N/Y UNDER Nurse MEANS 'Not yet' or 'Not ever'.)
No Name Sex Age Nurse Par1 NatPs1 Par2 NatPs2
PRESS 1 AND <Enter> TO SEE WHICH NURSE SCHEDULE TO SELECT FOR EACH PERSON.

SchDisp
TO INTERVIEW EACH PERSON, PRESS <Ctrl+Enter> AND SELECT THE CORRESPONDING NURSE SCHEDULE AS LISTED BELOW.
No Name Sex Age Nurse Nurse Schedule

PRESS <Ctrl+Enter> TO SELECT A NURSE SCHEDULE FOR THE PERSON YOU WANT TO INTERVIEW, OR TO EXIT.

Introduction

IF OC = 1 THEN

Info

You are in the Nurse Schedule for:

Person Number:
Name:
Age:
Sex:

Can you interview this person? TO LEAVE THIS SCHEDULE FOR NOW, PRESS <Ctrl Enter>

  1 Yes, I will do the interview now
  2 No, I will not be able to do this interview

ELSEIF OC=2 OR 3 THEN

RefInfo

NURSE: *(Name of respondent)* IS RECORDED AS HAVING REFUSED A NURSE VISIT. HAS *(he/she)* CHANGED *(his/her)* MIND?!

NURSE: THERE IS NO INFORMATION YET FROM THE INTERVIEWER WHETHER *(Name of respondent)* HAS AGREED TO A NURSE VISIT. IF YOU ARE SURE THAT *(he/she)* HAS COMPLETED AN INTERVIEW AND HAS AGREED TO SEE YOU, CODE 1 FOR "Yes" HERE. ELSE CODE 2 FOR "No"

  1 Yes, *(now/this person)* agrees nurse visit
  2 No, *(still refuses/this person will not have a)* nurse visit

ENDIF

ALL WITH A NURSE VISIT (Info = Yes OR RefInfo = Yes, agrees nurse visit)

NurDate

NURSE: ENTER THE DATE OF THIS INTERVIEW. ENTER DAY OF MONTH IN NUMBERS, NAME OF MONTH IN WORDS (FIRST THREE LETTERS), YEAR IN NUMBERS, EG 2Jan72.

NDoB

Can I just check your date of birth?

ENTER RESPONDENT'S DATE OF BIRTH. ENTER DAY OF MONTH IN NUMBERS, NAME OF MONTH IN WORDS (FIRST THREE LETTERS), YEAR IN NUMBERS, EG 2Jan72

ConfAge

Age of respondent based on Nurse entered date of birth and date at time of household interview.

Range: 0..120

DispAge

CHECK WITH RESPONDENT: So you are *(computed age)* years old?

  1 Yes
  2 No

IF (Age IN [2..15]) THEN

CParInt

NURSE: A child can be interviewed only with the permission of, and in the presence of, their parent or person who has (permanent) legal parental responsibility, ('parent'). No measurements should be carried out without the agreement of both parent and the child.

ENTER '1' TO CONTINUE

CParNo

NURSE CHECK: WHICH PARENT (OR 'PARENT') IS GIVING PERMISSION FOR MEASUREMENTS TO BE TAKEN AND ANSWERING QUESTIONS FOR THIS CHILD?

  A *(Name of Parent 1)*
  B *(Name of Parent 2)*

ENDIF

IF (Age of respondent is 16 to 49 years) AND (Sex = Female) THEN

PregNTJ

Can I check, are you pregnant at the moment?

  1 Yes
  2 No

ENDIF

Prescribed medicines and drug coding

ALL WITH A NURSE VISIT

MedCNJD

Are you taking or using any medicines, pills, syrups, ointments, puffers or injections prescribed for you by a doctor?

  1 Yes
  2 No

IF MedCNJD = Yes THEN

MedIntro

Could I take down the names of the medicines, including pills, syrups, ointments, puffers or injections, prescribed for you by a doctor?

  1 Continue

Collect details of up to 22 prescribed medicines

FOR i:= 1 TO 22 DO

  IF (i = 1) OR (MedBIC[i-1] = Yes) THEN

    MedBI[i]

    NURSE: ENTER NAME OF DRUG NO. *(1,2,3, etc.)* ASK IF YOU CAN SEE THE CONTAINERS FOR ALL PRESCRIBED MEDICINES CURRENTLY BEING TAKEN IF ASPIRIN, RECORD DOSAGE AS WELL AS NAME.

    Text: Maximum 30 characters

    MedBIA[i]

    Have you taken/used *(name of medicine)* in the last 7 days?

      1 Yes
      2 No

    MedBIC[i]

    NURSE CHECK: Any more drugs to enter?

      1 Yes
      2 No

  ENDIF

ENDDO

DrCod1

NURSE: To do the drug coding now, press <Ctrl + Enter>, select **DrugCode[schedule no]** with the highlight bar and press <Enter>.

Else, enter '1' to continue.

  1 Continue

ENDIF

Vitamin supplements/Nicotine replacements

ALL WITH A NURSE VISIT

Vitamin

At present, are you taking any vitamin or mineral supplements or anything else to supplement your diet or improve your health, other than those prescribed by your doctor?

1 Yes
2 No

IF (Sex = Female) AND (Age of Respondent is 10 to 15 years) THEN

UPreg

NURSE: HAS THE RESPONDENT (OR HER PARENT/"PARENT") TOLD YOU THAT SHE IS PREGNANT? DO NOT ASK FOR THIS INFORMATION - ONLY CODE WHETHER OR NOT IT HAS BEEN VOLUNTEERED.

1 Yes, told me she is pregnant
2 No, not told me she is pregnant

ENDIF

IF Age of Respondent is over 15 years THEN

Smoke

Can I ask, do you smoke cigarettes, cigars or a pipe at all these days?
CODE ALL THAT APPLY.
IF RESPONDENT USED TO SMOKE BUT DOES NOT ANY MORE, CODE 'NO'.

1 Yes, cigarettes
2 Yes, cigars
3 Yes, pipe
4 No

IF (Smoke = Yes, cigarettes) OR (Smoke = Yes, cigars) OR (Smoke = Yes, pipe) THEN

LastSmok

How long is it since you last smoked a (cigarette, (and/or a) cigar, (and/or a) pipe)?

1 Within the last 30 minutes
2 Within the last 31-60 minutes
3 Over an hour ago, but within the last 2 hours
4 Over two hours ago, but within the last 24 hours
5 More than 24 hours ago

ENDIF

UseGum

We are also interested in whether people use any of the nicotine replacement products that are now available, such as nicotine chewing gum or patches. First, in the last seven days have you used any nicotine chewing gum?

1 Yes
2 No

IF UseGum=Yes THEN

GumMG

What strength is the nicotine chewing gum you are using - is it 2mg or 4mg?
CODE ONE ONLY . IF BOTH - WHICH MOST RECENTLY? IF CAN'T SAY - ASK TO SEE PACKET

1 2mg
2 4mg
3 Can't say (and no packet available)

ENDIF

UsePat

In the last seven days have you used nicotine patches that you stick on your skin?

1 Yes
2 No

IF MedCNJD = Yes THEN

Drug coding block

DIntro

NURSE: PLEASE COMPLETE DRUG CODING FOR Person (person no.) (person name).
PRESS 1 AND <Enter> TO CONTINUE.

1 Continue

Repeat for up to 22 drugs coded

FOR j:= 1 TO (Number of drugs recorded) DO

DrC1

NURSE: ENTER CODE FOR (name of drug) ENTER 999999 IF UNABLE TO CODE
Text: Maximum 6 characters

IF (Age of Respondent is over 15 years) AND (Drug code begins 02) THEN

YTake1

Do you take (name of drug) because of a heart problem, high blood pressure or for some other reason?

1 Heart problem
2 High blood pressure
3 Other reason

IF YTake1 = Other THEN

TakeOth1

NURSE: GIVE FULL DETAILS OF REASON(S) FOR TAKING (name of drug):
Text: Maximum 255 characters

ENDIF
ENDIF
ENDDO
ENDIF

Upper arm circumference

IF (Age of Respondent is less than 16 years) AND (UPreg <> Pregnant) THEN

UAIntro
ENTER '1' TO CONTINUE.

MUACInt
(As I mentioned earlier,) I would like to measure your *(name of child's)* upper arm circumference.
IF ASKED: This gives us information about the distribution of fat.
1 Respondent agrees to have upper arm circumference measured
2 Respondent refuses to have upper arm circumference measured
3 Unable to measure upper arm circumference for reason other than refusal

Mid-upper arm circumference measurement repeated up to 3 times.
Third measurement taken only if first two measurements differ by more than 1.5cm.

IF MUACInt=Agrees THEN
FOR Loop:= 1 TO 3 DO
IF (Loop IN [1,2]) OR ((Loop = 3) AND (Measure[1].CUpArm <> 99.9) AND (Measure[2].CUpArm <> 99.9) AND (ABS(Measure[1].CUpArm - Measure[2].CUpArm) > 1.5)) THEN

CUpArm[i]
MEASURE CIRCUMFERENCE OF LEFT ARM AND RECORD IN CENTIMETRES. IF MEASUREMENT NOT OBTAINED, ENTER '99.9'
Range: 10.0..100.0

IF CUpArm IN [10.0..99.8] THEN
CUpRel[i]
Is the *(first/second/third)* measurement reliable?
1 Yes
2 No
ENDIF
ENDIF
ENDDO

IF NO MEASUREMENT OBTAINED (CupArm1 = 99.9 AND CUpArm2 = 99.9) THEN
CRespUp
NURSE CHECK:
1 Both measurements refused
2 Attempted not obtained
3 Measurement not attempted
ENDIF

IF AT LEAST ONE MEASUREMENT OBTAINED (CupArm1 <> 99.9 OR CUpArm2 <> 99.9) THEN
CUpMeas
NURSE CHECK: Arm circumference measured with respondent:
1 Standing
2 Sitting
3 Lying down
4 Measured on right arm as left arm unsuitable
ENDIF
ENDIF

IF UsePat=Yes THEN
NicPats
Can you tell me which brand and strength of nicotine patches you use?
CODE ONE ONLY. DO NOT PROMPT.
IF MORE THAN ONE TYPE - WHICH MOST RECENTLY? IF NOT SURE - ASK TO SEE PACKET
1 Niconil: 11mg
2 Niconil: 22mg
3 Nicorette: 5mg
4 Nicorette: 10mg
5 Nicorette: 15mg
6 Nicotinell TTS: 10 (7mg)
7 Nicotinell TTS: 20 (14mg)
8 Nicotinell TTS: 30 (21mg)
9 Other (SPECIFY AT NEXT QUESTION)
10 Can't say (and no packet available)

IF NicPats=Other THEN
OthNic
STATE NAME AND STRENGTH OF NICOTINE PATCHES
Text: Maximum 140 characters
ENDIF
ENDIF

UseNas
In the last seven days, have you used nicotine nasal spray or a nicotine inhaler?
1 Yes
2 No
ENDIF

IF NO OR ONE MEASUREMENT OBTAINED (MUACInt=Refuses OR Unable OR CUpArm1 = 99.9 OR CUpArm2 = 99.9) THEN
NoCUpArm
GIVE REASON(S) FOR *(ONLY OBTAINING ONE MEASUREMENT/REFUSAL/NOT OBTAINING MEASUREMENT/MEASUREMENT NOT BEING ATTEMPTED)*
Text: Maximum 140 characters
ENDIF

IF MEASUREMENT OBTAINED (CUpArm1 IN [10.0..99.8] OR CUpArm2 IN [10.0..99.8]) THEN
ArmRes
OFFER TO WRITE RESULTS OF ARM CIRCUMFERENCE MEASUREMENT ON RESPONDENT'S MEASUREMENT RECORD CARD. COMPLETE NEW CARD IF REQUIRED
Upper arm circumference: *(First measurement)*
                            (Second measurement)

ENTER '1' TO CONTINUE
ENDIF
ENDIF

Blood pressure

IF **Age of Respondent is 2 to 4 years** THEN
NoBP
NO BLOOD PRESSURE READING TO BE DONE. ENTER '1' TO CONTINUE.
1   Continue
ENDIF

IF **(PregNTJ = Yes) OR (UPreg = Pregnant)** THEN
PregMes
RESPONDENT IS PREGNANT. NO MEASUREMENTS TO BE DONE. ENTER '1' TO CONTINUE.
1   Continue
ENDIF

ALL AGED OVER 4 YEARS (EXCEPT PREGNANT WOMEN)
BPMod
NURSE: NOW FOLLOWS THE BLOOD PRESSURE MODULE. ENTER '1' TO CONTINUE:
1   Continue

IF **Age of Respondent is over 15 years** THEN
BPIntro
(As I mentioned earlier) We would like to measure your blood pressure. The analysis of blood pressure readings will tell us a lot about the health of the population.
ENTER '1' TO CONTINUE
1   Continue

ELSE *(Respondent aged 5-15)*
BPBlurb
READ OUT TO PARENT/PARENTS: (As I mentioned earlier) we would like to measure *(name of child's)* blood pressure. If you wish, I will write the results on *(his/her)* Measurement Record Card. I will not, however, be able to tell you what the results mean. This has to be calculated using *(his/her)* age, sex and height. Also blood pressure can vary from day to day and throughout the day, so one high reading would not necessarily mean that your child has a high blood pressure. However if you would like us to, we will send your results to your GP who is better placed to interpret them. In the unlikely event that your child should be found to have a high blood pressure for *(his/her)* age and height, we shall advise *(his/her)* GP (with your permission) that *(name of child's)* blood pressure should be measured again.
ENTER '1' TO CONTINUE.
1   Continue
ENDIF

BPConst
NURSE: Does respondent agree to blood pressure measurement?
1   Yes, agrees
2   No, refuses
3   Unable to measure BP for reason other than refusal

IF **BPConst = Yes, agrees** THEN
IF **Age of Respondent is 13 years or over** THEN
ConSubX
May I just check, have you eaten, smoked, drunk alcohol or done any vigorous exercise in the past 30 minutes?
CODE ALL THAT APPLY.
1   Eaten
2   Smoked
3   Drunk alcohol
4   Done vigorous exercise
5   (None of these)

ELSEIF (Age of Respondent is 5 to 12 years AND BPConst = Yes, agrees) THEN

ConSubX2

May I just check, has *(name of child)* eaten, or done any vigorous exercise, in the past 30 minutes?

CODE ALL THAT APPLY.

1 Eaten
2 Done vigorous exercise
3 Neither

ENDIF

DINNo

RECORD DINAMAP SERIAL NUMBER:

Range: 001..999

CufSize

SELECT CUFF AND ASK RESPONDENT TO SIT STILL FOR FIVE MINUTES. RECORD CUFF SIZE CHOSEN.

1 Child (12-19 cm)
2 Small adult (17-25 cm)
3 Adult (23-33 cm)
4 Large adult (31-40 cm)
5 Extra large adult (38-50 cm)

AirTemp

ENTER AMBIENT AIR TEMPERATURE IN CELSIUS.

Range: 00.0..40.0

Map to Dias repeated for up to 3 blood pressure measurements

FOR I:= 1 TO 3 DO

Map[i]

TAKE THREE MEASUREMENTS FROM RIGHT ARM.

ENTER *(FIRST/SECOND/THIRD)* MAP READING (mmHg).

IF READING NOT OBTAINED, ENTER 999.

IF YOU ARE NOT GOING TO GET ANY BP READINGS AT ALL, ENTER "996".

Range: 001..999

Pulse[i]

ENTER *(FIRST/SECOND/THIRD)* PULSE READING (bpm).

IF READING NOT OBTAINED, ENTER 999.

Range: 001..999

Sys[i]

ENTER *(FIRST/SECOND/THIRD)* SYSTOLIC READING (mmHg).

IF READING NOT OBTAINED, ENTER 999.

Range: 001..999

Dias[i]

ENTER *(FIRST/SECOND/THIRD)* DIASTOLIC READING (mmHg).

IF READING NOT OBTAINED, ENTER 999.": 001..999

ENDDO

IF NO FULL MEASUREMENT OBTAINED (at least one '999' reading in all 3 sets of 4 readings) THEN

YNoBP

ENTER REASON FOR NOT RECORDING ANY FULL BP READINGS

1 Blood pressure measurement attempted but not obtained
2 Blood pressure measurement not attempted
3 Blood pressure measurement refused

ENDIF

IF BLOOD PRESSURE MEASUREMENT REFSED OR NOT ATTEMPTED, OR FEWER THAN THREE FULL READINGS OBTAINED THEN

NAttBP

RECORD WHY *(ONLY TWO READINGS OBTAINED/ONLY ONE READING OBTAINED/READING NOT OBTAINED/READING NOT ATTEMPTED/READING REFUSED/UNABLE TO TAKE READING).*

CODE ALL THAT APPLY.

1 Respondent upset/anxious/nervous
2 Error 844' reading
3 *(IF AGED UNDER 16: Too shy)*
4 *(IF AGED UNDER 16: Child would not sit still long enough)*
5 Other reason(s) (SPECIFY AT NEXT QUESTION)

ENDIF

IF NattBP = Other THEN

OthNBP

ENTER FULL DETAILS OF OTHER REASON(S) FOR NOT OBTAINING/ATTEMPTING THREE BP READINGS:

Text: Maximum 140 characters

ENDIF

IF ONE, TWO OR THREE FULL BLOOD PRESSURE READINGS OBTAINED THEN

DifBP

RECORD ANY PROBLEMS TAKING READINGS. CODE ALL THAT APPLY.

1 No problems taking blood pressure
2 Reading taken on left arm because right arm not suitable
3 Respondent was upset/anxious/nervous
4 Other problems (SPECIFY AT NEXT QUESTION)

ENDIF

IF DifBP=Other THEN

OthDifBP

NURSE: RECORD FULL DETAILS OF OTHER PROBLEM(S) TAKING READINGS.

Text: Maximum 140 characters

ENDIF

IF ONE, TWO OR THREE FULL BLOOD PRESSURE READINGS OBTAINED THEN

GPRegB

Are you registered with a GP?

1 Yes
2 No

IF GPRegB = Yes THEN

GPSend

May we send your blood pressure readings to your GP?

1 Yes
2 No

IF GPSend = No THEN

GPRefM

SPECIFY REASON(S) FOR REFUSAL TO ALLOW BP READINGS TO BE SENT TO GP. CODE ALL THAT APPLY.

1 Hardly/Never sees GP
2 GP knows respondent's BP level
3 Does not want to bother GP
4 Other (SPECIFY AT NEXT QUESTION)

Demispan

IF Age of Respondent is over 64 THEN
SpanIntro
NURSE: NOW FOLLOWS THE MEASUREMENT OF DEMI-SPAN. ENTER '1' TO CONTINUE.
  1 Continue

SpanInt
I would now like to measure the length of your arm. Like height, it is an indicator of size.
  1 Respondent agrees to have demispan measured
  2 Respondent refuses to have demispan measured
  3 Unable to measure demispan for reason other than refusal

Repeat for up to three demispan measurements.
Third measurement taken only if first two differ by more than 3cm.

IF SpanInt=Agrees THEN
FOR Loop:= 1 TO 3 DO
IF (Loop IN [1..2]) OR ((Loop = 3) AND (Span1 <> 999.9) AND (Span2 <> 999.9) AND (ABS(Span1 - Span2) > 3)) THEN
Span[j]
ENTER (FIRST/SECOND/THIRD) MEASUREMENT IN CENTIMETRES.
IF MEASUREMENT NOT OBTAINED, ENTER '999.9'.
Range: 45.0..1000.0

IF Span <> 999.9 THEN
SpanRel[j]
Is the (First/Second/Third) measurement reliable?
  1 Yes
  2 No
ENDIF
ENDIF
ENDDO

IF (Span1 = 999.9) AND (Span2 = 999.9) THEN
YNoSpan
NURSE: GIVE REASON FOR NOT OBTAINING AT LEAST ONE DEMI-SPAN MEASUREMENT.
  1 Both measurements refused
  2 Attempted but not obtained
  3 Measurement not attempted
ENDIF
ENDIF

IF NO MEASUREMENT OBTAINED (SpanInt=Refuse OR SpanInt=Unable OR (Span1=999.9 AND Span2=999.9) THEN
NotAttM
NURSE: GIVE REASON FOR (REFUSAL/NOT OBTAINING MEASUREMENT/MEASUREMENT NOT BEING ATTEMPTED):
  1 Cannot straighten arms
  2 Other

IF NotAttM = Other THEN
OthAttM
NURSE: GIVE FULL DETAILS OF OTHER REASON FOR (REFUSAL/NOT OBTAINING MEASUREMENT/MEASUREMENT NOT BEING ATTEMPTED)
Text: Maximum 140 characters
ENDIF

ENDIF

IF GPRefM = Other THEN
OthRefM
NURSE: GIVE FULL DETAILS OF REASON(S) FOR REFUSAL.
Text: Maximum 140 characters
ENDIF
ENDIF

IF (GPRegB <> Yes) OR (GPSend = No) THEN
Code022
CIRCLE CONSENT CODE 02 ON FRONT OF CONSENT BOOKLET.
ENTER '1' TO CONTINUE
  1 Continue

ELSEIF GPSend = Yes THEN
ConsFrm1
a) COMPLETE 'BLOOD PRESSURE TO GP CONSENT FORM (CHILD UNDER 16: FORM BP (C)/ADULT 16+: FORM BP (A))
b) ASK (RESPONDENT/RESPONDENT'S PARENT/'PARENT') TO READ, SIGN AND DATE IT.
c) CHECK GP NAME, ADDRESS AND PHONE NO. ARE RECORDED ON CONSENT FORM.
d) CHECK NAME BY WHICH GP KNOWS RESPONDENT.
e) CIRCLE CONSENT CODE 01 ON FRONT OF CONSENT BOOKLET.
ENTER '1' TO CONTINUE.
  1 Continue

ENDIF

BPOffer
OFFER BLOOD PRESSURE RESULTS TO (RESPONDENT/PARENT/'PARENT')

Pulse	Systolic	Diastolic
i) (First Pulse reading)	(First Systolic reading)	(First Diastolic reading)
ii) (Second Pulse reading)	(Second Systolic reading)	(Second Diastolic reading)
iii) (Third Pulse reading)	(Third Systolic reading)	(Third Diastolic reading)

ENTER ON THEIR MEASUREMENT RECORD CARD (COMPLETE NEW RECORD CARD IF REQUIRED).

ADVICE TO RESPONDENTS ON BLOOD PRESSURE READING (AGE 16+ ONLY)

IF Systolic reading >179 OR Diastolic reading >114 THEN
TICK THE CONSIDERABLY RAISED BOX AND READ OUT TO RESPONDENT: Your blood pressure is high today. Blood pressure can vary from day to day and throughout the day so that one high reading does not necessarily mean that you suffer from high blood pressure. You are strongly advised to visit your GP within 5 days to have a further blood pressure reading to see whether this is a once-off finding or not.
NURSE: IF RESPONDENT IS ELDERLY, ADVISE HIM/HER TO CONTACT GP WITHIN NEXT 7-10 DAYS.

IF Systolic reading 160-179 OR Diastolic reading 100-114 (Men aged 16-49 OR Women aged 16+)
OR IF Systolic reading 170-179 OR Diastolic reading 105-114 (Men aged 50+) THEN
TICK THE MODERATELY RAISED BOX AND READ OUT TO RESPONDENT: Your blood pressure is a bit high today. Blood pressure can vary from day to day and throughout the day so that one high reading does not necessarily mean that you suffer from high blood pressure. You are advised to visit your GP within 2-3 weeks to have a further blood pressure reading to see whether this is a once-off finding or not.

IF Systolic reading 140-159 OR Diastolic reading 85-99 (Men aged 16-49 OR Women aged 16+)
OR IF Systolic reading 160-169 OR Diastolic reading 96-104 (Men aged 50+) THEN
TICK THE MILDLY RAISED BOX AND READ OUT TO RESPONDENT: Your blood pressure is a bit high today. Blood pressure can vary from day to day and throughout the day so that one high reading does not necessarily mean that you suffer from high blood pressure. You are advised to visit your GP within 3 months to have a further blood pressure reading to see whether this is a once-off finding or not.

IF Systolic reading <140 AND Diastolic reading <85 (Men aged 16-49 OR Women aged 16+)
OR IF Systolic reading <160 AND Diastolic reading <95 (Men aged 50+) THEN
TICK THE NORMAL BOX AND READ OUT TO RESPONDENT: Your blood pressure is normal.

ENDIF
ENDIF

The Health Survey for England – 1998 – Nurse Schedule

ELSE (If at least one measurement obtained)

SpnM

NURSE CHECK: Demi-span was measured with the respondent: CODE ALL THAT APPLY.

1 Standing against the wall
2 Standing not against the wall
3 Sitting
4 Lying down
5 Demi-span measured on left arm due to unsuitable right arm

DSCard

WRITE RESULTS OF DEMI-SPAN MEASUREMENT ON RESPONDENT'S MEASUREMENT RECORD
CARD. Demi-span : *(Measurement 1 and 2 displayed)*
ENTER '1' TO CONTINUE.
1 Continue

ENDIF
ENDIF

The Health Survey for England – 1998 – Nurse Schedule

Waist and hip circumference

ALL AGED OVER 15 YEARS (EXCEPT PREGNANT WOMEN)

WHMod

NURSE: NOW FOLLOWS THE WAIST AND HIP CIRCUMFERENCE MEASUREMENT.
ENTER '1' TO CONTINUE
1 Continue

WHIntro

I would now like to measure your waist and hips. The waist relative to hip measurement is very useful for assessing the distribution of weight over the body.

1 Respondent agrees to have waist/hip ratio measured
2 Respondent refuses to have waist/hip ratio measured
3 Unable to measure waist/hip ratio for reason other than refusal

IF (WHIntro=Agree) THEN

Repeat for up to three waist-hip measurements.
Third measurement taken only if difference between first two measurements is greater than 3cm.
FOR Loop:= 1 TO 3 DO
IF (Loop IN [1..2]) OR ((Loop = 3) AND (Measure[1].Waist <> 999.9) AND (Measure[2].Waist <> 999.9) AND (ABS(Measure[1].Waist - Measure[2].Waist) > 3)) THEN

Waist

NURSE: MEASURE THE WAIST AND HIP CIRCUMFERENCES TO THE NEAREST MM.
ENTER *(FIRST/SECOND/THIRD)* WAIST MEASUREMENT IN CENTIMETRES (Remember to include the decimal point).
IF MEASUREMENT NOT OBTAINED, ENTER '999.9'.
    Range: 45.0..1000.0
ENDIF

IF (Loop IN [1..2]) OR ((Loop = 3) AND (Measure[1].Hip <> 999.9) AND (Measure[2].Hip <> 999.9) AND (ABS(Measure[1].Hip - Measure[2].Hip) > 3)) THEN

Hip

NURSE: MEASURE THE WAIST AND HIP CIRCUMFERENCES TO THE NEAREST MM.
ENTER *(FIRST/SECOND/THIRD)* MEASUREMENT OF HIP CIRCUMFERENCE IN CENTIMETRES (Remember to include the decimal point).
IF MEASUREMENT NOT OBTAINED, ENTER '999.9'.
    Range: 75.0..1000.0
ENDIF
ENDDO

IF (Waist1 = 999.9) OR (Waist2 = 999.9) OR (Hip1 = 999.9) OR (Hip2 = 999.9) THEN

YNoWH

ENTER REASON FOR NOT GETTING BOTH MEASUREMENTS
1 Both measurements refused
2 Attempted but not obtained
3 Measurement not attempted
ENDIF
ENDIF

IF NO OR ONE MEASUREMENT OBTAINED ((WHIntro=Refuse OR Unable) OR Only one **waist/hip** measurement obtained) THEN

WHPNABM

GIVE REASON(S) *(FOR REFUSAL/WHY UNABLE/FOR NOT OBTAINING MEASUREMENT/FOR NOT ATTEMPTING/WHY ONLY ONE MEASUREMENT OBTAINED),CODE ALL THAT APPLY.*
1 Respondent is chairbound
2 Other (SPECIFY AT NEXT QUESTION)

IF WHPNABM = Other THEN
OthWH
GIVE FULL DETAILS OF 'OTHER' REASON(S) FOR NOT GETTING FULL WAIST/HIP MEASUREMENT:
Text: Maximum 140 characters
ENDIF

IF AT LEAST ONE WAIST MEASUREMENT OBTAINED (IF (Waist1 <> 999.9 AND Waist1 <> EMPTY) OR (Waist2 <> 999.9 AND Waist2 <> EMPTY)) THEN
WJRel
RECORD ANY PROBLEMS WITH WAIST MEASUREMENT:
1 No problems experienced, RELIABLE waist measurement
2 Problems experienced - waist measurement likely to be RELIABLE
3 Problems experienced - waist measurement likely to be SLIGHTLY UNRELIABLE
4 Problems experienced - waist measurement likely to be UNRELIABLE

IF WJRel = Problems experienced THEN
ProbWJ
RECORD WHETHER PROBLEMS EXPERIENCED ARE LIKELY TO INCREASE OR DECREASE THE WAIST MEASUREMENT.
1 Increases measurement
2 Decreases measurement
ENDIF
ENDIF

IF AT LEAST ONE HIP MEASUREMENT OBTAINED (IF (Hip1 <> 999.9 AND Hip1 <> EMPTY) OR (Hip2 <> 999.9 AND Hip2 <> EMPTY)) THEN
HJRel
RECORD ANY PROBLEMS WITH HIP MEASUREMENT:
1 No problems experienced, RELIABLE hip measurement
2 Problems experienced - hip measurement likely to be RELIABLE
3 Problems experienced - hip measurement likely to be SLIGHTLY UNRELIABLE
4 Problems experienced - hip measurement likely to be UNRELIABLE

IF HJRel = Problems experienced THEN
ProbHJ
RECORD WHETHER PROBLEMS EXPERIENCED ARE LIKELY TO INCREASE OR DECREASE THE HIP MEASUREMENT.
1 Increases measurement
2 Decreases measurement
ENDIF
ENDIF

IF ONE OR TWO WAIST/HIP MEASUREMENTS OBTAINED THEN
WHRes
OFFER TO WRITE RESULTS OF WAIST AND HIP MEASUREMENTS, WHERE APPLICABLE, ONTO RESPONDENT'S MEASUREMENT RECORD CARD.
Waist: *(Write in waist measurements 1 and 2)*
Hip: *(Write in hip measurements 1 and 2)*
ENTER '1' TO CONTINUE.
ENDIF

Blood sample

ALL AGED 11+ (EXCEPT PREGNANT WOMEN)

BlIntro
NURSE: NOW FOLLOWS THE BLOOD SAMPLE MODULE. ENTER '1' TO CONTINUE.
1 Continue

IF Age of Respondent is 16 or 17 years THEN
NCGuard
NURSE CHECK:
1 Respondent lives with parent or person with legal responsibility ('Parent')
2 Does NOT live with parent or person with legal responsibility ('Parent')
ENDIF

IF (Age of Respondent is 11 to 15 years) OR (Age of Respondent is over 17 years) OR (NCGuard = Parent) THEN
ClotB
EXPLAIN PURPOSE AND PROCEDURE FOR TAKING BLOOD. May I just check, do you have a clotting or bleeding disorder or are you currently on anti-coagulant drugs such as Warfarin? (NB ASPIRIN THERAPY IS NOT A CONTRAINDICATION FOR BLOOD SAMPLE.)
1 Yes
2 No

IF ClotB = No THEN
Fit
May I just check, have you ever had a fit (including epileptic fit, convulsion, convulsion associated with high fever)?
1 Yes
2 No
ENDIF
ENDIF

IF Fit = No THEN
IF Age of Respondent is 11 to 17 years THEN
EMLA
Explain that there is the option of using EMLA cream, but that a sample can be given without EMLA. Give parent/respondent the EMLA information sheet and allow them time to read it.
ENTER '1' TO CONTINUE.
1 Continue

IF Age of Respondent is 11 to 15 years THEN
CBSConst
ASK PARENT/'PARENT': Are you willing for your child to have a blood sample taken?
1 Yes
2 No
ENDIF
ENDIF

IF (Fit = No) AND (CBSConst <> No) THEN
BSWill
Would you be willing to have a blood sample taken?
1 Yes
2 No

IF Age of Respondent is 11 to 17years AND BSWill = Yes THEN

EMLAUse
Do you want EMLA cream to be used?
1 Yes
2 No

IF EMLAuse = Yes THEN

Allergy
Have you ever had a bad reaction to a local or general anaesthetic bought over the counter at a chemist, or given at the doctor, the dentist or in hospital?
1 Yes
2 No

IF Allergy = Yes THEN

NoEMLA
EMLA CREAM CANNOT BE USED. IS RESPONDENT WILLING TO GIVE BLOOD SAMPLE WITHOUT EMLA CREAM?
Code 1 if yes, willing to give blood sample without EMLA cream Code 2 if no, not willing to give blood sample without EMLA.
1 Yes, willing
2 No, no blood sample

ELSEIF Allergy = No THEN

EMLANow
NURSE CODE: ARE YOU GOING TO APPLY EMLA DURING THE FIRST VISIT, OR RETURN FOR A SECOND VISIT?
1 During the first visit
2 Return for a second visit

IF EMLANow = Return for a second visit THEN

Later
NURSE: CODE 1 TO CONTINUE WITH REST OF SCHEDULE ON THE FIRST VISIT. CODE 2 IF THIS IS THE RETURN VISIT.
1 Finish rest of schedule now (ONLY APPLIES TO FIRST VISIT)
2 This is the return visit and ready to take blood sample
ENDIF
ENDIF
ENDIF

IF (BSWill = No OR CBSConst = No) THEN

RefBS
RECORD WHY BLOOD SAMPLE REFUSED. CODE ALL THAT APPLY.
1 Previous difficulties with venepuncture
2 Dislike/fear of needles
3 Respondent recently had blood test/health check
4 Refused because of current illness
5 Worried about HIV or AIDS
6 Other

IF RefBS = Other THEN

OthRefBS
GIVE FULL DETAILS OF OTHER REASON(S) FOR REFUSING BLOOD SAMPLE.
Text: Maximum 135 characters
ENDIF

ELSEIF BSWill = Yes THEN

IF (Age of Respondent is 11 to 17 years) AND (EMLAUse = No OR EMLANow = Now OR Later = Return OR NoEMLA = Yes) THEN

BSConsC
EXPLAIN NEED FOR WRITTEN CONSENT *(FROM PARENT/"PARENT")*: Before 1 can take any blood, I have to obtain *(written consent from you/the written consent of both parent and child)*.
ENTER '1' TO CONTINUE.
1 Continue

IF NCGuard = Parent THEN

GuardCon
CHECK: Is a parent or person with legal responsibility willing to give consent?
1 Yes
2 No

IF GuardCon = No THEN

Ignore
RECORD DETAILS OF WHY CONSENT REFUSED:
STRING[140]
ENDIF
ENDIF
ENDIF

IF (Age of respondent is [2 to 15 years OR 18+ years] OR GuardCon = Yes] AND NoEMLA <> No THEN

BSCons
FILL IN *(RESPONDENT'S/CHILD'S)* NAME AND YOUR NAME AT TOP OF FORM*(BS(C) CHILD AGED 11-17/BS(A) ADULT AGED 18+)* IN CONSENT BOOKLET.
(If aged 11-17. TICK THE BOX: (With the use of EMLA/Without the use of EMLA)).
ASK *(RESPONDENT/CHILD AND PARENT/"PARENT")* TO READ, SIGN AND DATE PART 1 OF BLOOD SAMPLE CONSENT FORM.
CIRCLE CONSENT CODE 05 ON THE FRONT OF THE CONSENT BOOKLET.
ENTER '1' TO CONTINUE.
1 Continue
ENDIF

IF (NoEMLA <> No) AND (Later <> Now) THEN
IF (BSWill = Yes) AND ((Age of Respondent is 16 or 17 years AND GuardCon = Yes) OR (Age of Respondent is 2 to 15 years AND CBSConst = Yes) OR (Ageof respondent is 18+ years)) THEN
IF (GPRegB (blood pressure module) not answered) THEN

GPSam
NURSE CHECK:
1 Respondent registered with GP
2 Respondent not registered with GP
ENDIF

IF (GPRegB = Yes OR GPSam = GP) THEN

SendSam
May we send the results of your blood sample analysis to your GP?
1 Yes
2 No

IF SendSam = Yes THEN

BSSign
OBTAIN *(SIGNATURES OF RESPONDENT AND PARENT/"PARENT"/PARENT'/SIGNATURE)* FOR PART II OF BLOOD SAMPLE CONSENT FORM.
CHECK NAME BY WHICH GP KNOWS RESPONDENT. CHECK GP NAME, ADDRESS AND PHONE NO. ARE RECORDED ON FRONT OF CONSENT BOOKLET.
CIRCLE CONSENT CODE 07 ON FRONT OF CONSENT BOOKLET.
ENTER '1' TO CONTINUE.
1 Continue

ELSEIF SendSam = No THEN

SenSam

Why do you not want your blood sample results sent to your GP?

1 Hardly/never sees GP
2 GP recently took blood sample
3 Does not want to bother GP
4 Other

  IF SenSam=Other THEN

  OthSam

  GIVE FULL DETAILS OF REASON(S) FOR NOT WANTING RESULTS SENT TO GP.

  Text: Maximum 140 characters

  ENDIF

ENDIF

IF (GPSam = NoGP OR SendSam = No) THEN

Code08

CIRCLE CONSENT CODE 08 ON FRONT OF CONSENT BOOKLET.
ENTER '1' TO CONTINUE.

1 Continue

ENDIF

ConStorB

ASK *(PARENT'/PARENT'/RESPONDENT)*: May we have your consent to store any remaining blood for future analysis?

1 Storage consent given
2 Consent refused

IF ConStorB = Yes THEN

Code09

OBTAIN *(SIGNATURES OF RESPONDENT AND PARENT'/PARENT'/SIGNATURE OF RESPONDENT)* AT PART III OF BLOOD SAMPLE CONSENT FORM.
CIRCLE CONSENT CODE 09 ON FRONT OF CONSENT BOOKLET.
ENTER '1' TO CONTINUE.

1 Continue

ELSEIF ConStorB = No THEN

Code10

CIRCLE CONSENT CODE 10 ON FRONT OF CONSENT BOOKLET.
ENTER '1' TO CONTINUE.

1 Continue

ENDIF

IF (EMLAuse = Yes AND NoEMLA <> Yes) THEN

DoEMLA

CHECK YOU HAVE ALL APPLICABLE SIGNATURES.
APPLY EMLA CREAM FOLLOWING INSTRUCTIONS.
WAIT AT LEAST ONE HOUR BEFORE ATTEMPTING BLOOD SAMPLE.
ENTER '1' TO COMPLETE REST OF SCHEDULE OR OTHER SCHEDULES WHILE WAITING.
ENTER '2' WHEN THE HOUR HAS PASSED TO TAKE BLOOD SAMPLE.

1 Complete rest of schedule
2 The hour has passed, ready to take blood sample

ENDIF

IF (DoEMLA <> Rest) THEN

TakeSam

CHECK YOU HAVE ALL APPLICABLE SIGNATURES.
TAKE BLOOD SAMPLES: FILL *(1 Plain (red) tube and 1 EDTA (purple) tube/1 Plain (red) tube, 1 EDTA (purple) tube and 1 citrate (blue) tube)* (in this order).
WRITE THE SERIAL NUMBER AND DATE OF BIRTH ONTO THE GREEN LABEL USING A BLUE BIRO. DO ONE LABEL PER TUBE.

Serial number: *(displays serial number)*
Date of birth: *(displays date of birth)*

CHECK THE DATE OF BIRTH AGAIN WITH THE RESPONDENT. STICK THE GREEN LABEL OVER THE LABEL WHICH IS ALREADY ON THE TUBE.
ENTER '1' TO CONTINUE.

1 Continue

SampF1

CODE IF PLAIN RED TUBE FILLED (INCLUDE PARTIALLY FILLED TUBE)

1 Yes
2 No

SampF2

CODE IF EDTA PURPLE TUBE FILLED (INCLUDE PARTIALLY FILLED TUBE):

1 Yes
2 No

IF Age of Respondent is 16 years or over THEN

SampF3

CODE IF CITRATE (BLUE) TUBE FILLED (INCLUDE PARTIALLY-FILLED TUBE):

1 Yes
2 No

ENDIF

IF SampF1=Yes OR SampF2=Yes OR SampF3 = Yes THEN

SampArm

RECORD WHICH ARM BLOOD TAKEN FROM:

1 Right
2 Left
3 Both

SamDif

RECORD ANY PROBLEMS IN TAKING BLOOD SAMPLE.
CODE ALL THAT APPLY

1 No problem
2 Incomplete sample
3 Collapsing/poor veins
4 Second attempt necessary
5 Some blood obtained, but respondent felt faint/fainted
6 Unable to use tourniquet
7 Other (SPECIFY AT NEXT QUESTION)

IF SamDif = Other THEN

OthBDif

GIVE FULL DETAILS OF OTHER PROBLEM(S) IN TAKING BLOOD SAMPLE.

Text: Maximum 140 characters

ENDIF

SnDrSam

Would you like to be sent the results of your blood sample analysis?

1 Yes
2 No

Saliva sample

ALL AGED 4+ (EXCEPT PREGNANT WOMEN)

SalInt1
NURSE: NOW FOLLOWS THE SALIVARY SAMPLE.
ENTER '1' TO CONTINUE.
  1 Continue

SalIntr1
NURSE: IF YOU HAVE NOT ALREADY DONE SO, ASK RESPONDENT FOR A SALIVA SAMPLE.
READ OUT: I would like to take a sample of saliva (spit). This simply involves *(dribbling saliva down a straw into a tube/keeping a dental roll in your mouth for a few minutes)* The sample will be analysed for cotinine, which is related to the intake of tobacco smoke and is of particular interest to see if non-smokers may have raised levels as a result of 'passive' smoking
  1 Respondent agrees to give saliva sample
  2 Respondent refuses to give saliva sample
  3 Unable to obtain saliva sample for reason other than refusal

IF SalIntr1=Agree THEN

SalInst
(ASK CHILD TO DRIBBLE THROUGH STRAW INTO TUBE/ASK RESPONDENT TO INSERT DENTAL ROLL IN MOUTH AND PROVIDE SALIVA SAMPLE)
ENTER '1' TO CONTINUE.
  1 Continue

SalObt1
NURSE CHECK
  1 Saliva sample obtained
  2 Saliva sample refused
  3 Saliva sample not attempted
  4 Attempted but not obtained

ENDIF

IF (SalObt1=Refused, Not attempted or Attempted, not obtained) OR (SalIntr1=Unable) THEN

SalNObt
RECORD WHY SALIVA SAMPLE NOT OBTAINED.
CODE ALL THAT APPLY.
  1 Parent/'Parent' refused
  2 Respondent refused
  3 Respondent not able to produce any saliva
  4 Other (SPECIFY AT NEXT QUESTION)

IF SalNObt = Other THEN

OthNObt
GIVE FULL DETAILS OF REASON(S) WHY SALIVA SAMPLE NOT OBTAINED.
    Text: Maximum 140 characters

ENDIF
ENDIF
ENDIF

AllCheck
CHECK BEFORE LEAVING RESPONDENT:
• THAT ALL *(CHILDREN AGED 2-15/RESPONDENTS)* HAVE A CONSENT BOOKLET.
• THAT FULL GP DETAILS ARE ENTERED ON FRONT OF CONSENT BOOKLET.
• THE NAME BY WHICH GP KNOWS RESPONDENT.
• THAT ALL DETAILS ARE COMPLETED ON FRONT OF CONSENT BOOKLET.
• THAT ALL NECESSARY SIGNATURES HAVE BEEN COLLECTED.
• THAT THERE ARE FIVE APPROPRIATE CONSENT CODES RINGED ON FRONT OF CONSENT BOOKLET.
  1 Continue

Thank
NURSE: END OF QUESTIONNAIRE REACHED. THANK RESPONDENTS FOR THEIR CO-OPERATION.
THEN ENTER '1' TO FINISH.

IF SnDrSam = Yes THEN

Code11
CIRCLE CONSENT CODE 11 ON FRONT OF CONSENT BOOKLET.
ENTER '1' TO CONTINUE.
  1 Continue

ELSEIF SnDrSam = No THEN

Code12
CIRCLE CONSENT CODE 12 ON FRONT OF CONSENT BOOKLET.
ENTER '1' TO CONTINUE.
  1 Continue

ENDIF

ELSEIF SampF1<>Yes AND SampF2<>Yes AND SampF3<>Yes THEN

NoBSM
CODE REASON(S) NO BLOOD OBTAINED.
CODE ALL THAT APPLY.
  1 No suitable or no palpable vein/collapsed veins
  2 Respondent was too anxious/nervous
  3 Respondent felt faint/fainted
  4 Other

IF NoBSM = Other THEN

OthNoBSM
GIVE FULL DETAILS OF REASON(S) NO BLOOD OBTAINED.
    Text: Maximum 140 characters

ENDIF

Code12
CROSS OUT CONSENT CODES 05, 07, AND 09 IF ALREADY CIRCLED ON FRONT OF CONSENT BOOKLET.
REPLACE WITH CONSENT CODES 06, 08, 10 AND 12 ON FRONT OF CONSENT BOOKLET.
ENTER '1' TO CONTINUE.
  1 Continue

ENDIF
ENDIF
ENDIF
ENDIF

IF (Age of Respondent less than 11 years) OR (Age of Respondent is 11 to 17 years AND ChBlood = No) OR (NCGuard = NoParent) OR (ClotB = Yes) OR (ClotB = NONRESPONSE) OR (Fit = Yes) OR (Fit = NONRESPONSE) OR (CBSConst = No) OR (BSWill = No) OR (GuardCon = No) OR (NoEMLA = No) THEN

NoCodes
CIRCLE CONSENT CODES 06, 08, 10 AND 12 ON FRONT OF CONSENT BOOKLET.
ENTER '1' TO CONTINUE.
  1 Continue.

ENDIF

BLOOD PRESSURE TO GP CONSENT FORM

(ADULT 16+)

I, (name) _____

consent to the SCPR/UCL Joint Health Surveys Unit informing my General Practitioner (GP) of my blood pressure results. *I am aware that the results of my blood pressure measurement may be used by my GP to help monitor my health and that my GP may wish to include the results in any future report about me.*

Signed _____

Date _____

UCL MEDICAL SCHOOL

THE HEALTH SURVEY FOR ENGLAND

On behalf of the Department of Health

SCPR — SOCIAL & COMMUNITY PLANNING RESEARCH

P1727

Health Survey for England: 1998
CONSENT BOOKLET/V2

Please use capital letters and write in ink

ADDRESS

Survey month: _____

POINT HHLD CKL ADDRESS PERSON

1. Nurse number

2. Date schedule completed — DAY MONTH YEAR

3. Full name (of person tested)

Name by which GP knows person (if different)

4. Sex Male 1 Female 2

5. Date of birth: — DAY MONTH YEAR

6. Full name of parent/guardian (*if person under 18*)

7. **GP NAME AND ADDRESS**

Dr: ....

Practice Name: ....

Address: ....

Town: ....

County: ....

Postcode: ....

Telephone no: ....

8. **NURSE USE ONLY**

GP address complete	1
GP address incomplete	2
No GP	3

9. **SUMMARY OF CONSENTS** - RING CODE FOR EACH ITEM

	YES	NO
a) Blood pressure to GP	01	02
b) Sample of blood to be taken	05	06
c) Blood sample result to **GP**	07	08
d) Blood sample for **storage**	09	10
e) Blood sample result to **respondent**	11	12

BLOOD PRESSURE TO GP CONSENT FORM

(CHILD UNDER 16)

I, (name) _____

am the parent/guardian of

(child's name) _____

and I consent to the SCPR/UCL Joint Health Surveys Unit informing his/her General Practitioner (GP) of his/her blood pressure results. I am aware that the results of his/her blood pressure measurement may be used by his/her GP to help monitor his/her health and that his/her GP may wish to include the results in any future report about him/her.

Signed _____

Date _____

BLOOD SAMPLE CONSENT FORM   BS (A)

ADULT AGED 18+

I, (name) _____

I. Consent to _____ (qualified nurse) taking a sample of my blood on behalf of the SCPR/UCL Joint Health Surveys Unit. This blood sample will not be used to test for viruses (eg HIV test). The sample will be tested for: total cholesterol, HDL cholesterol, haemoglobin, ferritin, C-reactive protein and fibrinogen.

The purpose and procedure have been explained to me by the nurse and I have had an opportunity to discuss this with him/her. I have received a written explanation of these matters.

Signed _____   Date _____

II. I consent to the SCPR/UCL Joint Health Surveys Unit informing my General Practitioner (GP) of the blood sample analysis results for total cholesterol, HDL cholesterol, haemoglobin, ferritin, C-reactive protein and fibrinogen. I am aware that the results of my blood sample analysis may be used by my GP to help him/her monitor my health and that my GP may wish to include the results in any future report about me.

Signed _____   Date _____

III. I consent to any remaining blood being stored for future analysis. The sample will not be used to test for viruses (eg HIV test).

Signed _____   Date _____

BLOOD SAMPLE CONSENT FORM

BS (C)

CHILD AGED 11-17

I, (name) _____

I. Consent to _____ (qualified nurse) taking a
    sample of my blood on behalf of the SCPR/UCL Joint Health Surveys Unit.
    This blood sample will not be used to test for viruses (eg HIV test). The
    sample will be tested for: total cholesterol, HDL cholesterol, haemoglobin
    and ferritin. For respondents aged 16 and over it will also be tested for C-
    reactive protein and fibrinogen.

    The purpose and procedure, and possible use of EMLA cream, have been
    explained to me by the nurse and I have had an opportunity to discuss this
    with him/her. I have received a written explanation of these matters.

    I consent to the sample being taken......**tick one box:**

    With the use of EMLA cream   ☐

    Without EMLA cream   ☐

    Signed _____   Date _____

    Countersigned by Parent or Person with legal parental responsibility:

    Signed _____   Date _____

II. I consent to the SCPR/UCL Joint Health Surveys Unit informing my
    General Practitioner (GP) of the blood sample analysis results for total
    cholesterol, HDL cholesterol, haemoglobin, ferritin, (and if age 16 and
    over) C-reactive protein and fibrinogen. I am aware that the results of my
    blood sample analysis may be used by my GP to help him/her monitor my
    health and that my GP may wish to include the results in any future report
    about me.

    Signed _____   Date _____

    Countersigned by Parent or Person with legal parental responsibility

    Signed _____   Date _____

III. I consent to any remaining blood being stored for future analysis. The
     sample will not be used to test for viruses (eg HIV test).

    Signed _____   Date _____

    Countersigned by Parent or Person with legal parental responsibility

    Signed _____   Date _____

Appendix B: Measurement protocols

1 Height and weight measurements

1.1 Eligibility

You should be able to measure the height and weight of most of the informants. However, in some cases it may not be possible or appropriate to do so. Do not force the informant to be measured if it is clear that the measurement will be far from reliable but whenever you think a reasonable measurement can be taken do so. Examples of people who should not be measured are:

- Chairbound informants should not have their height and weight taken.

- If after discussion with an informant it becomes clear that they are too unsteady on their feet for these measurements, do not attempt to take them.

- If the informant finds it painful to stand or stand straight, do not attempt to measure height.

- Pregnant women are not eligible for weight as this is clearly affected by their condition.

- For small children, there is an option to weigh them held by an adult. In this case, you weigh the adult on his/her own first and then the adult and the child. The computer will calculate the child's weight.

1.2 Site

It is strongly preferable to measure height and weight on a floor which is level and not carpeted. If all the household is carpeted, choose a floor with the thinnest and hardest carpet (usually the kitchen or bathroom).

1.3 Height measurements

The equipment

Portable stadiometer – a collapsible device with a sliding head plate, a base plate and three contacting rods marked with a measuring scale.

Frankfort plane card

The protocol - adults (aged 16 and over)

1. Ask the informant to remove their shoes in order to obtain a measurement that is as accurate as possible.

2. Assemble the stadiometer and raise the headplate to allow sufficient room for the informant to stand underneath it. Double check that you have assembled the stadiometer correctly.

3. The informant should stand with their feet flat on the centre of the base plate, feet together and heels against the rod. The informant's back should be as straight as possible, preferably against the rod but not leaning on it. They should have their arms hanging loosely by their sides. They should be facing forwards.

4. Move the informant's head so that the Frankfort Plane is in a horizontal position (ie parallel to the floor). The Frankfort Plane is an imaginary line passing through the external ear canal and across the top of the lower bone of the eye socket, immediately

under the eye. This position is important if an accurate reading is to be obtained. An additional check is to ensure that the measuring arm rests on the crown of the head, ie the top back half.

To make sure that the Frankfort Plane is horizontal, you can use the Frankfort Plane Card to line up the bottom of the eye socket with the flap of skin on the ear. The Frankfort Plane is horizontal when the card is parallel to the stadiometer arm.

5. Instruct the informant to keep their eyes focused on a point straight ahead, to breath in deeply and to stretch to their fullest height. If after stretching up the informant's head is no longer horizontal, repeat the procedure. It can be difficult to determine whether the stadiometer headplate is resting on the informant's head. If so, ask the informant to tell you when s/he feels it touching their head.

6. Ask the informant to step forwards. If the measurement has been done correctly the informant will be able to step off the stadiometer without ducking their head. Make sure that the head plate does not move when the informant does this.

7. Look at the bottom edge of the head plate cuff. There is a green arrowhead pointing to the measuring scale. Take the reading from this point and record the informant's height in centimetres and millimetres, that is in the form 123.4, at *Height* in the Questionnaire. You may at this time record the informant's height onto their Measurement Record Card and at the question *MbookHt* you will be asked to check that you have done so. At that point the computer will display the recorded height in both centimetres and in feet and inches. At *RelHiteB* you will be asked to code whether the measurement you obtained was reliable or unreliable.

8. Height must be recorded in centimetres and millimetres, eg 176.5 cms. If a measurement falls between two millimetres, it should be recorded to the nearest even millimetre. eg if an informant's height is between 176.4 and 176.5 cms, you should round it down to 176.4. Likewise, if the informant's height is between 176.5 and 176.6 cms, you should round it up to 176.6 cms.

9. Push the head plate high enough to avoid any member of the household hitting their head against it when getting ready to be measured.

The Protocol - children (age 2-15)

The protocol for measuring children differs slightly to that for adults. You must get the co-operation of an adult household member. You will need their assistance in order to carry out the protocol, and children are much more likely to be co-operative themselves if another household member is involved in the measurement. If possible measure children last so that they can see what is going on before they are measured themselves.

Children's bodies are much more elastic than those of adults. Unlike adults they will need your help in order to stretch to their fullest height. This is done by stretching them. This is essential in order to get an accurate measurement. It causes no pain and simply helps support the child while they stretch to their tallest height.

It is important that you practice these measurement techniques on any young children among your family or friends. The more practice you get before going into the field the better your technique will be.

1. In addition to removing their shoes, children should remove their socks as well. This is not because the socks affect the measurement. It is so that you can make sure that children don't lift their heels off of the base plate. (See 3 below).

2. Assemble the stadiometer and raise the head plate to allow sufficient room for the child to stand underneath it.

3. The child should stand with their feet flat on the centre of the base plate, feet together and heels against the rod. The child's back should be as straight as possible, preferably against the rod, and their arms hanging loosely by their sides. They should be facing forwards.

4. Place the measuring arm just above the child's head.

5. Move the child's head so that the Frankfort Plane is in a horizontal position. This position is as important when measuring children as it is when measuring adults if the

measurements are to be accurate. To make sure that the Frankfort Plane is horizontal, you can use the Frankfort Plane Card to line up the bottom of the eye socket with the flap of skin on the ear. The Frankfort Plane is horizontal when the card is parallel to the stadiometer arm.

6. Cup the child's head in you hands, placing the heals of your palms either side of the chin. Your fingers should come to rest just under the ears.

7. Firmly but gently, apply upward pressure lifting the child's head upwards towards the stadiometer headplate and thus stretching the child to their maximum height. Avoid jerky movements, perform the procedure smoothly and take care not to tilt the head at an angle: you must keep it in the Frankfort plane. Explain what you are doing and tell the child that you want them to stand up straight and tall but not to move their head or stand on their tip-toes.

8. Ask the household member who is helping you to lower the headplate down gently onto the child's head. Make sure that the plate touches the skull and that it is not pressing down too hard.

9. Still holding the child's head, relieve traction and allow the child to stand relaxed. If the measurement has been done properly the child should be able to step off the stadiometer without ducking their head. Make sure that the child does not knock the head plate as they step off.

10. Read the height value in metric units to the nearest millimetre and enter the reading into the computer at Height. At *MbookHt* you will be asked to check that you have entered the child's height onto their Measurement Record Card. At that point the computer will display the recorded height in both centimetres and in feet and inches.

11. Push the head plate high enough to avoid any member of the household hitting their head against it when getting ready to be measured.

Additional points - all informants

1. If the informant cannot stand upright with their back against the stadiometer and have their heels against the rod (eg those with protruding bottoms) then give priority to standing upright.

2. If the informant has a hair style which stands well above the top of their head, (or is wearing a turban), bring the headplate down until it touches the hair/turban. With some hairstyles you can compress the hair to touch the head. If you can not lower the headplate to touch the head, and think that this will lead to an unreliable measure, record this at question *RelHiteB*. If it is a hairstyle that can be altered, eg a bun, if possible ask the informant to change/undo it.

3. If the informant is tall, it can be difficult to line up the Frankfort Plane in the way described. When you think that the plane is horizontal, take one step back to check from a short distance that this is the case.

1.4 Weight measurments

The equipment

Soehnle electronic bathroom scales

The scales have an inbuilt memory which stores the weight for 10 minutes. If during this time you weigh another object that differs in weight by less than 500 grams (about 1lb), the stored weight will be displayed and not the weight that is being measured. This means that if you weigh someone else during this time, you could be given the wrong reading for the second person.

So if you get an identical reading for a second person, make sure that the memory has been cleared. Clear the memory from the last reading by weighing an object that is more than 500 grams lighter (eg a pile of books, your briefcase or even the stadiometer). You will then get the correct weight when you weigh the second informant.

You will only need to clear the memory in this way if:

a) You have to have a second or subsequent attempt at measuring the same person

b) Two informants appear to be of a very similar weight

c) Your reading for an informant in a household is identical to the reading for another informant in the household whom you have just weighed.

The protocol

1. Turn the display on by pressing firmly with your hand or foot on the top of the scales (the scales will turn themselves off after a short while). The readout should display 888.8 momentarily as a check for the operation – if this is not displayed check the batteries, if this is not the cause you may need to report the problem to SCPR. While the scales read 888.8 do not attempt to weigh anyone.

2. Ask the informant to remove shoes, heavy outer garments such as jackets and cardigans, heavy jewellery, loose change and keys.

3. Turn the scales on with your foot again. Wait for a display of 0.0 before the informant stands on the scales.

4. Ask the informant to stand with their feet together in the centre and their heels against the back edge of the scales. Arms should be hanging loosely at their sides and head facing forward. Ensure that they keep looking ahead – it may be tempting for the informant to look down at their weight reading. Ask them not to do this and assure them that you will tell them their weight afterwards if they want to know.

   The posture of the informant is important. If they stand to one side, look down, or do not otherwise have their weight evenly spread, it can affect the reading.

5. The scales will take a short while to stabilize and will read 'C' until they have done so. If the informant moves excessively while the scales are stabilizing you may get a false reading. If you think this is the case reweigh, but first ensure that you have erased the memory.

6. The Soehnle scales have been calibrated in kilograms and 100 gram units (0.1 kg). Record the reading into the computer at the question Weight before the informant steps off the scales. *At MBookWt* you will be asked to check that you have entered the informant's weight onto their Measurement Record Card. At that point the computer will display the measured weight in both kilos and in stones and pounds.

WARNING

The maximum weight registering accurately on the scales is 130kg (20½ stone). If you think the informant exceeds this limit code them as 'Weight not attempted' at *WtResp*. The computer will display a question asking them for an estimate. Do not attempt to weigh them.

Weighing children

You must get the co-operation of an adult household member. This will help the child to relax and children, especially small children are much more likely to be co-operative themselves if an adult known to them is involved in the procedure.

Children wearing nappies should be wearing a dry disposable. If the nappy is wet, please ask the parent to change it for a dry one and explain that the wetness of the nappy will affect the weight measurement.

In most cases it will be possible to measure children's weight following the protocol set out for adults. However, if accurate readings are to be obtained, it is very important that informants stand still. Ask the child to stand perfectly still – 'Be a statue.î If small children find this difficult you will need to alter the protocol and first weigh an adult then weigh that adult holding the child as follows:

a) Code as 'Weight obtained (child held by adult)' at *RespWts*

b) Weigh the adult as normal following the protocol as set out above. Enter this weight into the computer at *WtAdult*.

c) Weigh the adult and child together and enter this into the computer at *WtChAd*.

The computer will then calculate the weight of the child and you will be asked to check that you have recorded the weight onto the child's Measurement Record Card at *MBookWt*. Again the computer will give the weight in both kilos and in stones and pounds.

2 Measurement of mid upper arm circumference

2.1 Purpose

The mid upper arm circumference is a key indicator of the nutritional status of children, being reduced substantially in the undernourished and being substantially increased in children who are overweight.

2.2 Eligibility

All informants from age two to age fifteen inclusive are to be measured. Exclude any child who is known to be pregnant.

2.3 Equipment

You will be provided with a short tape. One end of this tape is broad and on it you will see the words READ HERE, with a small arrow. This is the start of the tape. You will first use this tape to measure the length of the arm and then, having found the mid point of the arm, you will measure the circumference of the arm.

When measuring the circumference of the arm, the tape is threaded as indicated in the illustration below. Pull the tapered end up through slot 1, down through slot 2 and up through slot 3.

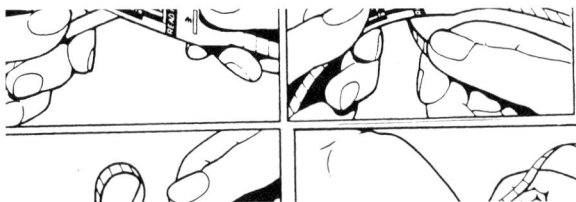

2.4 Procedure

The child must have a bare arm and shoulder for this measurement. The interviewer will have asked the child to wear a sleeveless garment for your visit. Explain to the child and parent the importance of the accuracy of the measurement and that clothing can substantially affect the reading. If the child is wearing a sleeved garment ask her/him to slip their arm out of the garment or to change into a suitable garment.

Where possible the left arm should always be used. If the left arm cannot be used eg because it is in plaster then carry out the measurement on the right arm and record that you have done so in the Nurse Questionnaire at *CupMeas*.

Measuring the length of the informant's upper arm

1. The informant should be standing with their left arm across their body and held at a right angle at the elbow.

2. Using the skin marker pen, mark the process of the acromium; this is the bony tip of the shoulder.

3. Mark the process of the olecranon of the child, this is the bony tip of the elbow.

4. Using the paper tape, measure the distance between the two points marked. Divide this measurement in half. This will be the mid point of the upper arm. Mark this using the skin marker pen.

Measuring the arm circumference

5. Now let the arm hang loosely by the side, just away from the body. Thread the tape through and slip it up the child's arm to the mid-point you have marked. The tape should be centred on the mid-point mark ie it should lie on top of the mark. Check that the tape is passing horizontally about the arm (not sloping) and that it is in continuous

contact with the skin. It should not be loose, but neither should it be puckering the skin. Read off the measurement where the 'READ HERE' arrow appears on the tape.

6. Record the measurement on the Nurse Questionnaire in centimetres and millimetres eg 20.3cm. Should the measurement lie between two millimetres, then round it to the nearest even millimetre. For example if the measurement is half way between 20.3 and 20.4 round up to 20.4. If the measurement is between 20.8 and 20.9 round down to 20.8.

7. Repeat all the above procedure (points 1 to 6) to obtain a second measurement and record this in the Nurse Questionnaire. Do not re-measure the circumference using the original marks – remark the positions.

8. Indicate on the Questionnaire the position of the child when the measurement was taken. Also give reasons why if it was not possible to take a measurement or if only one measurement was obtained.

3 Recording Ambient Air Temperature

3.1 The thermometer

You have been provided with a digital thermometer and probe. This instrument is very sensitive to minor changes in temperature. It is therefore important that you record temperature at the appropriate time in your routine. It can also take a few minutes to settle down to a final reading if it is experiencing a large change in temperature (eg coming into a warm house from a cold outside).

Immediately after you have settled the informant down to rest for five minutes prior to taking their blood pressure set up the thermometer to take a reading. Just prior to recording the blood pressure note the temperature and record it in the appropriate part of the Nurse Questionnaire. Always switch it off after taking a reading, to avoid battery problems. The thermometer automatically switches off if you have left it on for more than 7 minutes.

Place the thermometer on a surface near the Dinamap. Do not let the probe touch anything – you can for example let it hang over the edge of a table. Do not put it on top of the Dinamap as it will be warm.

3.2 Instructions for using the thermometer

1. The probe plug fits into the socket at the top of the instrument.

2. Press the completely white circle to turn the instrument on. To turn off, press the white ring.

3. Before taking a reading off the display, ensure that the reading has stabilised.

4. Be careful of the probe – it is quite fragile.

5. When 'LO BAT' is shown on the display the battery needs replacing, take no further readings.

6. The battery in your thermometer is a long-life battery and should last at least one year. However, should it run low please purchase a new battery. Take the old one with you to ensure it is the same type.

7. To remove old battery and insert a new one, unscrew the screw on the back of the thermometer.

4 Blood pressure measurement and heart rate readings

4.2 Purpose

High blood pressure is an important risk factor for cardiovascular disease. It is important that we look at the blood pressure of everyone in the survey using a standard method so we can see the distribution of blood pressure across the population. This is vital for monitoring change over time, and monitoring progress towards lower blood pressure targets set in the Health of the Nation.

4.3 Eligibility

All children aged 5 and over are eligible for this measurement. The technique is exactly the same as with adults. The survey equipment is not suitable for taking the blood pressure of younger children.

The only people not eligible for blood pressure measurement are those who are pregnant. However, if a pregnant woman wishes to have her blood pressure measured, you may do so, but do not record the readings in the Nurse Questionnaire.

4.3 Equipment

Dinamap 8100 blood pressure monitor
Blue pneumatic hose
Power Cord
Cuffs: Child cuff (12-19cm)
        Small adult cuff (17-25 cm)
        Standard adult cuff (23-33 cm)
        Large adult cuff (31-40 cm)

Extra large cuffs are also available from your Nurse Supervisor, should you require one.

The Dinamap 8100 blood pressure monitor is an automated machine. It is designed to measure systolic blood pressure, diastolic blood pressure, mean arterial pressure (MAP) and pulse rate automatically at pre-selected time intervals. On this survey three readings are collected at one minute intervals.

> The Dinamap is equipped with a rechargeable battery, which can run for a minimum of six hours when fully charged. It is essential to keep the battery charged as fully as possible. A yellow battery light will flash as a warning sign on the monitor to alert the user when the charge has fallen below 10%. To recharge the battery, connect the monitor to the mains and press the rear panel AC power switch to the ON ('I') position. The green MAINS AC light will indicate that the battery is charging. An overnight charge (eight hours) will provide about four hours of operation.
>
> ### !!PLEASE REMEMBER TO CHARGE THE BATTERY!!

When the Dinamap is switched on the monitor momentarily displays eights (888s) in all the digital displays and all indicators will flash as a check for the operation of all LEDs. The audio alarm is also sounded as a check for its operation. If on turning on the monitor any of the displays fail to show the 888s, contact the nurse supervisor immediately and inform them that there is a problem with the monitor.

4.4 Preparing the informant

The informant should not have eaten, smoked, drunk alcohol or taken vigorous exercise during the 30 minutes preceding the blood pressure measurement. If possible, arrange the timing of the measurements to ensure that this is the case.

Ask the informant to remove outer garments (eg jumper, cardigan, jacket) and expose the right upper arm. The sleeve should be rolled or slid up to allow sufficient room to place the cuff. If the sleeve constricts the arm, restricting the circulation of blood, ask the informant if they would mind taking their arm out of the sleeve for the measurement.

As with adults, a child's blood pressure reading on a single occasion is not enough to define whether a child's blood pressure is normal or abnormal. In addition the level at which a child's blood pressure is considered to be abnormal will be dependant on that child's age, height and sex. Because of this, unlike the adult situation, you will not be given statements to read out regarding blood pressure for children. Instead we wish you to explain to the parents in advance of the measurement, what the measurement will mean. The Nurse Questionnaire contains a detailed statement at *BPBlurb* which you should read out to all parents **before** taking a child's blood pressure. This procedure must always be followed. Otherwise, the parent may feel you are withholding information later because a child has an unsatisfactory result.

4.5 Selecting the correct cuff

Adults aged 16+

Do **not** measure the upper arm circumference. Instead, choose the correct cuff size based on the acceptable range which is marked on the inside of the cuff. You will note that there is some overlap between the cuffs. If the informant falls within this overlap range then use the **standard** cuff where possible.

Children aged 5-15

It is important to select the correct cuff size. The appropriate cuff is the largest cuff which fits between the axilla (underarm) and the antecubital fossa (front of elbow) without obscuring the brachial pulse and so that the index line is within the range marked on the inside of the cuff

You will be provided with a child's cuff as well as the other adult cuffs. Many children will not need the children's cuff and instead will require a small adult cuff or a standard adult cuff. You should choose the cuff that is appropriate to the circumference of the arm.

Adults and children

The appropriate cuff should be connected via the blue pneumatic hose to the two cuff connectors at the bottom of the display. It is important to ensure these screw connectors are properly connected to avoid any air leak. However **do not overtighten**. The pneumatic seal is not made by tightening the connector.

4.6 The Procedure

Wrap the correct sized cuff round the upper **right** arm and check that the index line falls within the range lines. Use the left arm only if it is impossible to use the right. If the left arm is used, record this in the Nurse Questionnaire. Locate the brachial pulse just medial to the biceps tendon and position the arrow on the cuff over the brachial artery. The lower edge should be about 2 cm above the cubital fossa (elbow crease).

Do not put the cuff on too tightly as bruising may occur on inflation. Ideally, it should be possible to insert two fingers between cuff and arm. However the cuff should not be applied too loosely, as this will result in an inaccurate measurement.

The informant should be sitting in a comfortable chair with a suitable support so that the right arm will be resting at a level to bring the antecubital fossa (elbow) to approximately heart level. If a child is being measured beside a low table it may be necessary to use cushions or a pillow under the arm. They should be seated in a comfortable position with cuff applied, legs uncrossed and feet flat on the floor.

Explain to the informant that before the blood pressure measurement we need them to sit quietly for five minutes to rest. They should not smoke, eat, drink or read during this time. Explain that during the measurement the cuff will inflate three times and they will feel some pressure on their arm during the procedure.

It is important that children as well as adults rest for five minutes before the measurement is taken. However, making children sit still for five minutes can be unrealistic. It is allowable for them to move around a little. They should not be running or taking vigorous exercise. As with adults, they should not eat or drink during this time.

After five minutes explain you are starting the measurement. Ask the informant to relax and not to speak until the measurement is completed as this may affect their reading.

1. Switch the monitor **'ON'**.

2. Press the SILENCE button until the yellow triangle above it lights up.

3. Press the AUTO/MANUAL button until the green triangle above it lights up. The cuff will now start to inflate and take the first measurement.

4. Press the cycle SET button until the number 1 lights up in the minutes box. Blood pressure will then be recorded at one minute intervals thereafter. After each interval record the reading on the Questionnaire.

5. It is possible to retrieve any of the three readings if they need to be checked or if you didn't record them for any reason. To do this wait until the three readings have been

taken then press the **AUTO/MANUAL** button followed by the **PRIOR DATA** button. This will display the previous reading ie the second blood pressure. Press the **PRIOR DATA** button again to display the first blood pressure reading, and once again to return to the final reading. The minutes display indicates how long ago the measurement was taken. **It is not possible** to retrieve the readings once the monitor has been switched off.

6. After the three measurements are complete and recorded in the Nurse Questionnaire switch the monitor **'OFF'** and remove the cuff.

If there are any problems during the blood pressure measurements or the measurement is disturbed for any reason, press the red cancel button or the power OFF button and start the procedure again. If the informant has to get up to do something, then ask them to sit and rest for five minutes again. Do not carry out more than three measurements.

Error readings

The most common error reading is 844. This is displayed if one measurement exceeds 120 seconds. This is usually caused by the informant moving during the measurement. Ask the informant to sit as still as possible and take the measurement again. **Do not palpate the pulse** and **do not tell the informant that their pulse is erratic**. If you still get another 844 error reading, record that it wasn't possible to get a reading and explain to the informant that this sometimes happens.

Other error readings are detailed on the side of the Dinamap itself.

Do not carry out more than three measurements.

4.7 **Informing informants of their blood pressure readings**

If the informant/parent wishes, record details of the three readings on their Measurement Record Card. If the informant is an adult, record what advice you have given them.

a) Child informants (age 5 to 15)

We do **not** wish you to comment on the child's blood pressure readings to the parents. If they seek comment, reiterate what you have already said about not being able to interpret a single blood pressure measurement without checking to see whether it is normal for the child's age and height. Reassure them that if it is found to be abnormal and if they have given consent for the results to go to the GP, then the GP will get in touch to have the measurement repeated. This rule applies for **all** readings you obtain.

b) Adult informants (aged 16+)

In answering queries about an adults blood pressure it is very **important** to remember that it is not the purpose of the survey to provide informants with medical advice, nor are you in a position to do so as you do not have the informant's full medical history. But you will need to say something. What you say in each situation has been agreed with the Department of Health. It is very important that **you make all the points relevant to the particular situation and that you do not provide a more detailed interpretation as this could be misleading**. Read the instructions below very carefully and make sure you always follow these guidelines.

Base your comments on the last two of the three readings. The computer will disregard the first reading when working out which advice to display. If the first reading is higher than the other two, explain that the first reading can be high because people are nervous of having their pressure taken.

Definitions of raised blood pressure differ slightly. The Department of Health have decided to adopt the ones given below for this survey. It is important that you adhere to these definitions, so that all informants are treated in an identical manner. These are shown below.

Adults Only

Survey definition of blood pressure ratings

For men aged less than 50 and all women

Rating	Systolic		Diastolic
Normal	< 140	and	< 85
Mildly raised	140 - 159	or	85 - 99
Moderately raised	160 - 179	or	100 - 114
Considerably raised	180 or more	or	115 or more

Men aged 50 or over

Rating	Systolic		Diastolic
Normal	< 160	and	< 95
Mildly raised	160 - 169	or	96 - 104
Moderately raised	170 - 179	or	105 - 114
Considerably raised	180 or more	or	115 or more

NB: < less than

Points to make to the informant about their blood pressure (given on screen)

Normal:

'Your blood pressure is normal'

Mildly raised:

'Your blood pressure is a *bit high* today.'

'Blood pressure can vary from day to day and throughout the day so that one high reading does not necessarily mean that you suffer from high blood pressure.'

'You are advised to visit your GP *within 3 months* to have a further blood pressure reading to see whether this is a once-off finding or not.'

Moderately raised:

'Your blood pressure is a *bit high* today.'

'Blood pressure can vary from day to day and throughout the day so that one high reading does not necessarily mean that you suffer from high blood pressure.'

'You are advised to visit your GP *within 2-3 weeks* to have a further blood pressure reading to see whether this is a once-off finding or not.'

Considerably raised:

'Your blood pressure is *high* today.'

'Blood pressure can vary from day to day and throughout the day so that one high reading does not necessarily mean that you suffer from high blood pressure.'

'You are *strongly* advised to visit your GP *within 5 days* to have a further blood pressure reading to see whether this is a once-off finding or not.'

Note: If the informant is elderly and has severely raised blood pressure, amend your advice so that they are advised to contact their GP within the next week or so about this reading. This is because in many cases the GP will be well aware of their high blood pressure and we do not want to worry the informant unduly. It is however important that they do contact their GP about the reading within 7 to 10 days. In the meantime, we will have informed the GP of their result (providing the informant has given their permission).

4.8   Action to be taken by the nurse after the visit

The action you should take **after** the visit in respect of raised blood pressure readings, differs for children and adults. If you need to contact the Survey Doctor, do not do this from the informant's home – you will cause unnecessary distress.

Pulse – for all informants the survey doctor routinely checks fast and slow pulse rates so no further action is necessary.

a) Children

No further action is required after taking blood pressure readings on children. All high readings are viewed routinely by the Survey Doctor. However, in the rare event that you encounter a child with a very high blood pressure, ie systolic 160 or above or diastolic 100 or above please call the Survey Doctor.

b) Adults

The chart below summarises what action you should take as a result of the knowledge you have gained from taking an adult's blood pressure readings. **For this purpose you should only take into account the last two readings** as the first reading from the Dinamap is prone to error for the reason stated above.

Blood pressure	Action
Normal/mild/moderate bp Systolic < 180 mmHg and diastolic < 115 mmHg	No further action necessary. If you feel that the circumstances demand further action, inform the Survey Doctor who will then inform the informant's GP immediately if she deems it necessary.**
Considerably raised bp Systolic ≥180 mmHg or diastolic ≥115 mmHg	Contact the Survey Doctor at the earliest opportunity and she will inform the informant's GP.** If the informant has any symptoms of a hypertensive crisis* contact the survey doctor immediately or call an ambulance. The Survey Doctor must be informed as soon as possible.**

* A hypertensive crisis is an extremely rare complication of high blood pressure. Its signs and symptoms include diastolic bp > 135 mmHg, headache, confusion, sleepiness, stupor, visual loss, seizures, coma, cardiac failure, oliguria, nausea & vomiting.

** You must still contact the Survey Doctor even if informants tell you that their GP knows about their raised BP.

All high or unusual readings will be looked at by the Survey Doctor when they reach the office. If the reading is high, then the Survey Doctor will contact the informant's GP. If the informant is not registered with a GP, or has refused consent for us to contact their GP, the informant will be contacted directly.

5 Measurement of demi-span

5.1 Purpose

When the interviewer visits the informant s/he attempts to measure the informant's height and weight. However, measuring height can be quite difficult if the informant cannot stand straight or is unsteady on their feet. This can occur with some elderly people, and with people who have particular disabilities. Additionally, height decreases with age. This decrease varies from person to person, and may be considerable.

Prior to the 1991 Health Survey there had been no attempt to measure the height of informants older than 64 years. However, it is becoming more important to have information about the health of the elderly. Therefore an alternative measure of skeletal size, the demi-span, was developed which can be measured easily and does not cause unnecessary discomfort or distress to the elderly or disabled.

The demi-span measurement is the distance between the sternal notch and the finger roots with arm out-stretched laterally.

5.2 Eligibility

Only those aged 65 or over are eligible for the demi-span measurement.

Informants aged 65 or over who cannot straighten either arm, should not have this measurement taken and this reason should be recorded at *SpanInt* and *NotAttM*.

5.3 Equipment

A thin retractable demi-span tape calibrated in cm and mm

A skin marker pencil

A hook is attached to the tape and this is anchored between the middle and ring fingers at the finger roots. The tape is then extended horizontally to the sternal notch (see illustration below).

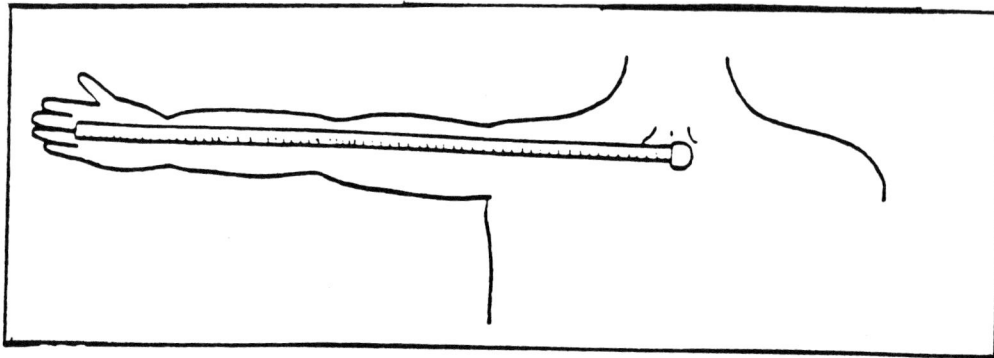

5.4 Preparing the informant

The measurement is made on the right arm unless this arm cannot be fully stretched. In which case the left arm may be used and this should be recorded in the Nurse Questionnaire at *SpnM*.

Although the measurement requires minimal undressing, certain items that might distort the measurement will need to be removed. These include:

Ties

Jackets and thick garments such as jumpers

Jewellery items such as chunky necklaces/bracelets

Shoulder pads

High heeled shoes

Shirts should be unbuttoned at the neck.

If the informant does not wish to remove any item that you think might affect the measurement, you should record this in the Nurse Questionnaire at *SpanRel* but still take the measurement.

5.5 Procedure

1. Locate a wall where there is room for the informant to stretch his/her arm. They should stand with their back to the wall but not support themselves on it. Ask the informant to stand about 3 inches (7cm) away from it.

2. Ask the informant to stand with weight evenly distributed on both feet, head facing forward.

3. Ask the informant to raise their right arm until it is horizontal. The right wrist should be in neutral rotation and neutral inflexion. Rest your left arm against the wall allowing the informant's right wrist to rest on your left wrist.

4. When the informant is standing in the correct position **mark the skin at the centre of the sternal notch** using the skin marker pencil (explain to the informant that this mark will wash off afterwards). It is important to mark the sternal notch while the informant is standing in the correct position.

   If the sternal notch is obscured by clothing, use a piece of tape (eg Sellotape or masking tape) on the clothing. Note this in the Nurse Questionnaire. Use tape that will not mark the clothing.

   If the informant will not allow use of either the marker pencil or the tape, proceed with the measurement but record in the Nurse Questionnaire that you were not able to mark the skin.

5. Ask the informant to relax while you get the demi-span tape.

6. Place the hook between the middle and ring fingers so that the tape runs smoothly along the arm.

7. Ask the informant to raise their arm. Check they are in the correct position, the arm horizontal, the wrist in neutral flexion and rotation.

8. Extend the tape to the sternal notch. If no mark was made, feel the correct position and extend the tape to this position.

9. When ready to record the measurement ask the informant to stretch his/her arm.

   Check that:

   - the informant is in the right position; no extension or flexion at the wrist or at the shoulders;

   - the hook has not slipped forward and the zero remains anchored at the finger roots;

   - the informant is not leaning against the wall.

10. Record the measurement in cms and to the nearest mm at *Span* in the Nurse Questionnaire. If the length lies half-way between two millimetres, then round to the nearest **even** millimetre. For example, if the measurement is halfway between 68.3 and 68.4, round up to 68.4. And if the measurement is halfway between 68.8 and 68.9, round down to 68.8. Please note that you must enter the measurement to one decimal place - do not round it to the nearest centimetre. For example, enter '70.2', not just '70'. If you do not enter a decimal point, the computer will give you a warning. If the measurement is exactly, say, 70cm, then all you need to do is suppress the warning and it will automatically fill in the '.0' for you. Otherwise, you must go back and amend your answer. As a further check, the computer will ask you to confirm that a measurement ending in '.0' is correct.

11. Ask the informant to relax and loosen up the right arm by shaking it.

12. Repeat the measurement from steps 4-11.

If the two measurements are more than 3cm apart, the computer will give you a warning. If you have made a mistake when entering the figures (eg typed 78.2 instead of 68.2), you should type over the mistake. If it was not a mistake, you should suppress the warning and take a third measurement.

5.6 Using the tape

The tape is fairly fragile. It can be easily damaged and will dent or snap, if bent or pressed too firmly against the informant's skin. Also the ring connecting the hook to the tape is a relatively weak point. Avoid putting more strain on this ring than necessary to make the measurements.

When extending the tape, hold the tape case rather than the tape itself as this puts less strain on the hook and tape.

When holding the tape to the sternal notch, do not press into the sternal notch so much that the tape kinks.

5.7 Points to watch

Make sure that the informant does not flex their wrist or move their trunk or shoulder when stretching their arm.

Be careful that the corner of the hook acting as the zero point does not move away from the finger root so affecting the point from which the measurement is taken.

5.8 Seated and lying measurements

If the informant is unable to stand in the correct position, or finds it difficult to stand steadily, ask them to sit for the measurement. Use an upright chair and position it close to a wall. Still try to support the arm if possible. You may need to sit or kneel to take the reading.

If the informant is much taller than you, take the measurement with the informant sitting.

If the informant finds both standing and sitting in the correct position difficult, the measurement can be taken lying down.

If the informant's arm is much longer than yours, support the arm close to the elbow rather than wrist level. Your arm must not be between the elbow and shoulder as this will not provide sufficient support.

6 Measurement of waist and hip circumferences

6.1 Purpose

There has been increasing interest in the distribution of body fat as an important indicator of increased risk of cardiovascular disease. The waist-to-hip ratio is a measure of distribution of body fat (both subcutaneous and intra-abdominal). Analyses suggest that this ratio is a predictor of health risk like the body mass index (weight relative to height).

6.2 Eligibility

The informant is ineligible for the waist and hip measurement if:

a) Pregnant

b) Chairbound

c) Has a colostomy/ileostomy.

If any of the above apply, record this in the Nurse Questionnaire at *WHPNABM*. If there are any other reasons why the measurement was not taken, record this at *OthWH*.

6.3 Equipment

Insertion tape calibrated in mm, with a metal buckle at one end.

The tape is passed around the circumference and the end of the tape is inserted through the metal buckle at the other end of the tape.

6.4 Preparing the informant

The interviewer will have asked the informant to wear light clothing for your visit. Explain to the informant the importance of this measurement and that clothing can substantially affect the reading.

If possible, without embarrassing you or the informant, ensure that the following items of clothing are removed:

All outer layers of clothing, such as jackets, heavy or baggy jumpers, cardigans and waistcoats

Shoes with heels

Tight garments intended to alter the shape of the body, such as corsets, lycra body suits and support tights

If the informant is wearing a belt, ask them if it would be possible to remove it or loosen it for the measurement.

Pockets should be emptied.

If the informant is not willing to remove bulky outer garments or tight garments and you are of the opinion that this will significantly affect the measurement, record this in the Nurse Questionnaire at *WJRel* and/or *HJRel...*

If possible, ask the informant to empty their bladder before taking the measurement.

6.5 Using the insertion tape

All measurements should be taken to the nearest millimetre. If the length lies half-way between two millimetres, then round to the nearest even millimetre. For example, if the measurement is halfway between 68.3 and 68.4, round up to 68.4. And if the measurement is halfway between 68.8 and 68.9, round down to 68.8.

Ensure the informant is standing erect in a relaxed manner and breathing normally. Weight should be evenly balanced on both feet and the feet should be about 25-30cm (1 foot) apart.

The arms should be hanging loosely at their sides.

If possible, kneel or sit on a chair to the side of the informant.

Pass the tape around the body of the informant and insert the plain end of the tape through the metal ring at the other end of the tape.

To check the tape is horizontal you have to position the tape on the right flank and peer round the participant's back from his/her left flank to check that it is level. This will be easier if you are kneeling or sitting on a chair to the side of the informant.

Hold the buckle flat against the body and flatten the end of the tape to read the measurement from the outer edge of the buckle. Do not pull the tape towards you, as this will lift away from the informant's body, affecting the measurement.

6.6 Measuring waist circumference

1. The waist is defined as the point midway between the iliac crest and the costal margin (lower rib). To locate the levels of the costal margin and the iliac crest use the fingers of the right hand held straight and pointing in front of the participant to slide upward over the iliac crest. Men's waists tend to be above the top of their trousers whereas women's waists are often under the waistband of their trousers or skirts.

2. Do not try to avoid the effects of waistbands by measuring the circumference at a different position or by lifting or lowering clothing items. For example, if the informant has a waistband at the correct level of the waist (midway between the lower rib margin and the iliac crest) measure the waist circumference over the waistband.

3. Ensure the tape is horizontal. Ask the participant to breathe out gently and to look straight ahead (to prevent the informant from contracting their muscles or holding their breath). Take the measurement at the end of a normal expiration. Measure to the nearest millimetre and record this in the Nurse Questionnaire.

4. Repeat this measurement again.

5. If you are of the opinion that clothing, posture or any other factor is significantly affecting the waist measurement, record this in the Nurse Questionnaire.

6.7 Measuring hip circumference

1. The hip circumference is defined as being the widest circumference over the buttocks and below the iliac crest. To obtain an accurate measurement you should measure the circumference at several positions and record the widest circumference.

2. Check the tape is horizontal and the informant is not contracting the gluteal muscles. Pull the tape, allowing it to maintain its position but not to cause indentation. Record the measurement on the Questionnaire to the nearest millimetre, eg 095.3.

3. If clothing is significantly affecting the measurement, record this on the Questionnaire.

4. Repeat this measurement again.

6.8 General points

The tape should be tight enough so that it doesn't slip but not tight enough to indent clothing. If clothing is baggy, it should be folded before the measure is taken.

If the informant is large, ask him/her to pass the tape around rather than having to 'hug' them. Remember though to check that the tape is correctly placed for the measurement being taken and that the tape is horizontal all the way around.

If the measurement falls between two millimetres, the measurement should be recorded to the nearest even millimetre

If your second waist or hip measurement differs by 3cm or more from the first, then take another measurement to work out which is more correct. If an incorrect measurement has been entered in the Questionnaire, go back and amend it.

6.9 Measuring the waist circumference

If you have problems palpating the rib, ask the informant to breathe in very deeply. Locate the rib and as the informant breathes out, follow the rib as it moves down with your finger.

If your informant has a bow at the back of her skirt, this should be untied as it may add a substantial amount to the waist circumference.

Female informants wearing jeans may present a problem if the waistband of the jeans is on the waist at the back but dips down at the front. It is essential that the waist measurement is taken midway between the iliac crest and the lower rib and that the tape is horizontal. Therefore in this circumstance the waist measurement would be taken on the waist band at the back and off the waist band at the front. Only if the waistband is over the waist all the way around can the measurement be taken on the waistband. If there are belt loops, the tape should be threaded through these so they don't add to the measurement.

6.10 Recording problems

We only want to record problems that will affect the measurement by more than would be expected when measuring over light clothing. As a rough guide only record a problem if you feel it affected the measurements by more than 0.5cm. We particularly want to know if waist and hip are affected differently.

7 Saliva sample collection

7.1 Purpose

We wish to obtain a measure of exposure to passive smoking. This can be detected by measuring the level of cotinine in saliva. Cotinine is a derivative of nicotine and shows recent exposure to tobacco smoke, either because the individual is a smoker or because they have been exposed to other people's tobacco smoke. Cotinine can also be detected in serum, and this method was used in 1997 for those aged 16-24 while collecting salivary cotinine for children. For 1998, it has been decided to obtain a saliva sample from adults as well as children. Note that respondents' cotinine analysis results will not be sent to them or their GP.

7.2 Eligibility

A saliva sample should be obtained from all informants aged 4 and over.

7.3 Equipment

For adults (aged 16+):
Plain 5 ml tube
Dental roll
Kitchen paper

For children (aged 4-15):
Plain 5 ml tube
Short wide bore straw.
Kitchen paper

The straw makes it easier for children to direct their saliva sample into the tube. Its use will also minimise the amount of other items that are included in saliva, such as crumbs, which might enter the tube.

7.4 Procedure

The aim is to get as much saliva as possible into the tube.

For adults:

The procedure is very simple, but it is crucial to make sure that an adequate amount of saliva is collected.

1. Instruct the informant to take the dental roll from the tube, insert it in his/her mouth and leave it there until soaked. The aim is to get the dental roll saturated with saliva.

2. Moving the dental roll about the mouth, without chewing, helps to ensure thorough wetting. For most people, 3 minutes will be ample to ensure thorough wetting.

3. If the informant complains of a dry mouth, and you think you will have difficulties in filling the roll, you can ask them to drink some water before starting the procedure. Wait for a few minutes to ensure that no water is retained when they provide the saliva sample.

4. When the informant has finished, ask her/him to remove the dental roll from her/his mouth and place it in the plain tube.

5. Check that the roll is well soaked. The tube should feel noticeably heavier than an unused one. If the dental roll rattles around in the tube like a pea, it is not sufficiently wet, and you should ask the informant to put it back in her/his mouth for a further period.

6. Record on the computer that you have taken the sample, and mention any problems you might have encountered.

For children:

1. Remove the cap from the plain tube.

2. Give the straw to the child. Explain that you want him/her to gather up their saliva (spit) in their mouth and then let it dribble through the straw into the tube. Make sure that you are not getting sputum i.e. that the child is not clearing their chest for the spit.

3. Allow the child about three minutes to do this. Collect as much as you can in this time. The saliva will be frothy, so it is easy to think you have collected more than you actually have, so do not give up too soon.

4. If children find it difficult to use the straw they may dribble into the tube directly. This is acceptable, but encourage them to use the straw where possible.

5. If the child's mouth is excessively dry and they can not produce saliva allow them to have a drink of plain water. Wait for a few minutes to ensure that no water is retained when they provide the saliva sample.

6. Record on the computer that you have taken the sample along with any problems you may have encountered.

7.5 **Packaging the saliva sample**

1. Make sure that the lid of the salivary tube is secure.

2. Label the tube (using the green labels provided for blood samples). Enter the respondent's serial number and date of birth on the label.

3. Wrap the tube with kitchen towel and put into a resealable plastic bag. Pack this bag into the envelope, either together with that respondent's blood container (if blood was obtained), or on its own.

4. Put the despatch note in the envelope.

5. If you have 'saliva-only' samples from the **same** household, they should be separately wrapped in kitchen towel and put into a resealable plastic bag as above. They should then all be packed in the same envelope, up to a maximum of four per envelope. Put the relevant number of despatch notes loose into the envelope. **NB this only applies to informants for whom a blood sample was not collected**. If there are more than four 'saliva only' samples in a household, you will need to use more than one envelope.

8 Blood sample collection

8.1 Purpose

Different analytes will be carried out for children and adults.

For Children age 11 to 15 years inclusive, the blood will be analysed for total cholesterol, HDL cholesterol, haemoglobin, ferritin.

For Adults aged 16 and over, the blood will be analysed for total cholesterol, HDL cholesterol, haemoglobin, ferritin, fibrinogen and C-reactive protein.

Haemoglobin and ferritin are being measured because they are indicators of nutritional status, being reduced if there is an inadequate iron supply in the diet. Frequently, an inadequate iron supply can imply a more general nutritional problem.

Total cholesterol and fibrinogen are being measured because raised levels are associated with higher risks of heart attacks, while HDL cholesterol has a protective role.

The level of C-reactive protein in the blood gives information on inflammatory activity in the body, and it is also associated with risk of heart disease.

The blood will not be tested for any viruses, such as HIV (AIDS).

8.2 **Eligibility**

All persons aged 11 and over, with the following exceptions, are eligible to give blood:

a) Pregnant
b) Have a clotting or bleeding disorder
c) People who have ever had a fit
d) Aged 11 -17 and do **not** live with a parent or guardian
e) Not willing to give their consent in writing and/or parent or guardian not willing
f) People who are currently on anticoagulant drugs, eg Warfarin therapy

8.3 **Equipment**

Tourniquet	Vacutainer holder
Alcohol swabs	Vacutainer needles 21G (green)
Dental rolls	Butterfly needles 23G
Rubber gloves	Needle disposal box
Adhesive dressing	Vacutainer plain red tubes
Plastic postal containers	Vacutainer EDTA purple tubes
Padded envelopes	Vacutainer citrate blue tubes
Sealable plastic bags	Vacutainer needles 22G (black)
Kitchen roll	Set of labels for blood sample tubes
Micropore tape	EMLA cream tubes and Tegaderm dressings

8.4 **Blood Tubes**

For adults aged 16 and over **three** tubes need to be filled. They should be filled in the following order so that, if a situation arises where there will be insufficient blood to fill all the tubes, the analyses with the highest priority can still be undertaken.

1. Plain (red, large) tube. Only use tubes with white inset in lid.
2. EDTA (purple, small) tube.
3. Citrate (blue, small) tube.

For children aged 11-15 **two** tubes need to be filled. They should be filled in the following order so that, if a situation arises where there will be insufficient blood to fill all the tubes, the analyses with the highest priority can still be undertaken.

1. Plain (red, large) tube. Only use tubes with white inset in lid.
2. EDTA (purple, small) tube.

8.5 **Obtaining consent**

Before taking blood from 11 to 17 year olds, you must make sure that you always obtain both the informant's own signature and the signature of their parent or person who has legal parental responsibility. Remember that even if 16/17 year old informants are married and not living with their parent or person who has legal parental responsibility, you cannot take blood until you have their parent's consent.

It is not sufficient to simply have one signature at items I-III on the BS page of the Consent Booklet. You must make sure that you have **all** relevant signatures.

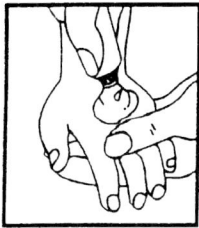

1. Squeeze ½ a tube in a mound on the area to anaesthetised. **Do not rub in.**

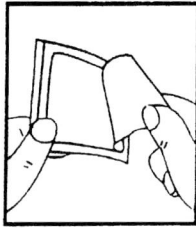

2. Peel the beige coloured 'centre cut-out' from the dressing.

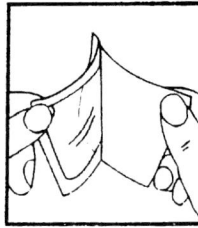

3. Peel the paper layer marked 3M Tegaderm from the dressing.

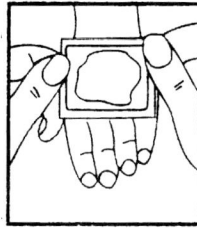

4. Apply the adhesive dressing with its paper frame to cover the EMLA. **Do not spread the cream.**

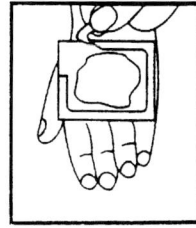

5. Remove the paper frame using the cut mark. Smooth down the edges of the dressing carefully and leave in place for at least an hour. The time of application can be written on the occlusive dressing.

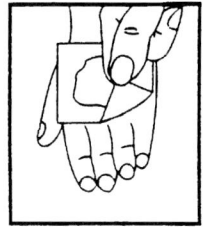

6. After 60 minutes (max. 5hrs), remove the dressing. Wipe off the EMLA. Clean entire area with alcohol and begin procedure.

8.6 EMLA cream

All informants aged 11 to 17 who consent to give a blood sample must be offered EMLA cream. The parent and young person should be given the information sheet about EMLA and allowed time to read it.

EMLA cream may also be used with informants aged 18 and over who request it, but should not specifically be offered to older informants. This may arise for example if a child in a household has been offered EMLA and an older household member also requests EMLA.

EMLA should never be offered in a household where no person aged under 18 is eligible for phlebotomy.

Informants who have had a reaction to any anaesthetic (local or general) are not eligible to have EMLA cream. This means that you may not take a blood sample from these informants, unless they consent to give a sample without using EMLA.

8.7 Applying EMLA Cream

EMLA cream must only be applied to healthy skin; therefore it must not be applied to sore or broken skin (eg eczema or cuts). Make sure the EMLA cream is kept away from eyes or ears.

If the young person requires EMLA to be applied prior to venepuncture, inspect the antecubital fossae and decide which arm you will use for blood-taking. If both arms are suitable, use the left arm.

EMLA cream must be applied to **one** arm only. This means that, if you encounter problems during blood-taking (eg collapsing vein), **no attempt** can be made to take blood from the other arm.

Apply EMLA cream over the antecubital fossa. Cover with a Tegaderm dressing (a vapour permeable and self-sticking film dressing) to keep the EMLA in place. See details about how to apply EMLA below. **Please note the illustration shows EMLA being used on the hand. SCPR policy is to only take blood samples from the arm**.

As you may well be aware, removing the Tegaderm is sometimes painful so take care on hairy arms!

It is very important that the used tubes of EMLA should not be left lying around. Make sure you have removed them from the household on completion of the phlebotomy.

Use the EMLA record sheet to record the informant's serial number and the date EMLA cream was used. Return this sheet with any unused tubes of EMLA cream to the Brentwood office.

8.8 Preparing the informant

Ask the informant if they have had any problems having blood taken before.

1. Explain the procedure to the informant (and parent if informant aged under 18). The informant should be seated comfortably in a chair, or if they wish, lying down on a bed or sofa.

2. **If no EMLA Cream has been used:** Ask the informant to roll up their left sleeve and rest their arm on a suitable surface. Ask them to remove their jacket or any thick clothing, if it is difficult to roll up their sleeve.

   The antecubital fossae may then be inspected. It may be necessary to inspect both arms for a suitable choice to be made, and the informant may have to be repositioned accordingly.

   If EMLA Cream has been used: Remove the Tegaderm dressing and wipe away excess EMLA cream.

3. Do **not** ask the informant to clench his/her fist.

   Select a suitable vein and apply the tourniquet around the informant's arm. However, it is desirable to use the tourniquet applying minimal pressure and for the shortest duration of time. Do not leave the tourniquet in place for longer than 2 minutes.

   Ask the informant to keep his/her arm as still as possible during the procedure.

4. Put on your rubber gloves at this point.

   Clean the venepuncture site gently with an alcohol swab. Allow the area to dry completely before the sample is drawn.

8.9 Taking the sample

Venepuncture is performed with a green 21 gauge Vacutainer needle or butterfly.

For children you have the option of using a black 22 gauge Vacutainer needle if it is more appropriate.

Grasp the informant's arm firmly at the elbow to control the natural tendency for the informant to pull the arm away when the skin is punctured. Place your thumb an inch or two below the vein and pull gently to make the skin a little taut. This will anchor the vein and make it more visible. Ensuring that the needle is bevelled upwards, enter the vein in a smooth continuous motion.

Remember to take the tubes in the correct order. The first tube should always be the large plain tube with the red cap followed by the EDTA tube and then (if informant aged 16 or older) the blue citrate tube. The vacutainers should be filled to capacity in turn and inverted gently on removal to ensure complete mixing of blood and preservative.

Release the tourniquet (if not already loosened) as the blood starts to be drawn into the tube. Remove the needle and place a dental roll firmly over the venepuncture site. Ask the informant to hold the pad firmly for three minutes to prevent haematoma formation.

For Adults (aged 18+) and Older Teenagers (aged 16-17):

If no EMLA cream has been used: if venepuncture is unsuccessful on the first attempt, make a second attempt on the other arm. If a second attempt is unsuccessful, do not attempt to try again. Record the number of attempts within CAPI.

If EMLA cream has been used: you must only make one attempt at venepuncture. If venepuncture is unsuccessful at the first attempt, **do not** attempt to try again.

For Children (aged 11-15):

Whether or not EMLA cream was used: you must only make one attempt at venepuncture. If venepuncture is unsuccessful at the first attempt, **do not** attempt to try again.

For both Adults and Children: Record which arm the sample was drawn from.

Remove the needle from the Vacutainer holder by inserting it into the slot at the top of the needle disposal box. Push it towards the narrow end of the slot until the hub fins are engaged. Twist the holder anti-clockwise to unthread the needle. Then slide the holder towards the centre of the slot, allowing the needle to drop into the container.

IMPORTANT WARNING

Never re-sheath the needle after use.

Do not allow the disposal box to become overfull as this can present a potential hazard.

Check on the venepuncture site and affix an adhesive dressing, if the informant is not allergic to them. If they are allergic, use a dental roll secured with micropore.

8.10   Fainting informants

If the informant looks or feels faint during the procedure, it should be discontinued. The informant should be asked to place their head between their knees. They should subsequently be asked to lie down.

If the informant is happy for the test to be continued after a suitable length of time, it should be done so with the informant supine and the circumstances should be recorded. The informant may wish to discontinue the procedure at this point, but be willing to give the blood sample at a later time.

8.11   Disposal of needles and other materials

Place the used cotton wool balls in the sharps box and put gloves etc. in the self-seal disposal bag. The needle disposable box should be taken to your local hospital for incineration. Telephone them beforehand, if you are not sure where to go. If you come across any problems with the disposal, contact the Survey Doctor who will contact your local hospital. The sealed bag can be disposed of with household waste as long as it does not have any items in it that are contaminated by blood.

8.12   Needle stick injuries

Any nurse who sustains such an injury should seek immediate advice from their GP. The nurse should inform his/her nurse supervisor of the incident, and the nurse supervisor should inform the Survey Doctor at UCL.

8.13   Informants who are HIV or Hepatitis B positive

If an informant **volunteers** that they are HIV or Hepatitis B positive, **do not** take a blood sample. Record this as the reason in the Nurse Questionnaire. You should never, of course, seek this information.

8.14   Sending blood samples to the laboratory

The blood samples are sent to the Royal Victoria Infirmary Laboratory in Newcastle upon Tyne. It is important that the blood is sent properly labelled and safely packaged and that it is despatched immediately after it has been taken.

Labelling the Blood Tubes

Label the tubes as you take the blood. It is **vital** that you do not confuse blood tubes within a household.

Use the set of serial number and date of birth labels (blue) to label the vacutainer tubes. Attach a serial number label to every tube that you send to the lab. Enter the serial number and date of birth very clearly on each label. Make sure you use blue biro - it will not run if it gets damp. Check the Date of Birth with the informant again verbally.

Stick blue label over the label already on the tube. The laboratory need to be able to see on receipt how much blood there is in the tube.

We cannot stress too much the importance of ensuring that you label each tube with the correct serial number for the person from whom the blood was obtained. Apart from the risk of matching up the blood analyses to the wrong person's data, we will be sending the GP the wrong results. Imagine if we detect an abnormality and you have attached the wrong label to the tube!

Packaging the blood samples

Pack the tubes for each informant separately from those of other members of the household. All the tubes from one person can be packed together in one container.

The following procedures are designed to minimise accidental damage and, should there be any damage, any blood spillage.

1. You are supplied with plastic containers designed to take tubes. Place the filled tubes in a container. Enclose the informant's salivary tube in the central compartment of the plastic container if saliva was also taken. Press the two halves of the container firmly together.

2. Wrap a piece of kitchen towelling paper around the plastic container.

3. Place the wrapped container into the resealable plastic bag (in your supplies), with the opening of the bag covering the hinged part of the plastic container. Ensure that the bag is sealed.

4. Place the wrapped container into the pre-addressed envelope, inserting it so that the opening of the plastic bag goes in first (ie away from the entrance to the envelope).

5. Put the Blood Sample Despatch Note in the envelope.

6. Fold over the end of the envelope, and seal firmly with **sellotape.** Wrap the tape right round the envelope.

   Never use staples to seal the envelope

   Staples can cut post office workers' hands. When blood is transported this can be dangerous.

7. Post the envelope immediately. It will go special delivery. This ensures that it arrives the next day.

   If you do your interview too late to catch the last post, post it to catch the next post. If you miss the Saturday post collection, take the envelope to a box that has a **Sunday collection**. The blood should not be refrigerated.

8. When you have posted the blood samples, fill in the time and date of posting on the office copy of the Blood Sample Despatch Note.

Completing the Blood Despatch Note (Despatch 1)

The Consent Booklet contains a Despatch Note that should be filled in and sent to the laboratory with the blood sample.

- Enter the informant's serial number very carefully. This should both correspond to your entry on page 1 of the Consent Booklet and to the serial numbers you have recorded on the tubes.

- Complete items 2, 3 and 4. Check that the date of birth is correct and consistent with entry on nurse Questionnaire and tube label. Do not forget to code which age group category the informant belongs to.

- Complete item 5.

- At Item 6 ring a code to tell the laboratory whether or not permission has been obtained to store part of the blood. Your entry here should correspond to your entry at Item 9e on the front page of the booklet.

- At Item 7 enter your SCPR Nurse Number.

Tear off this despatch note and send with the blood samples to the laboratory.

Complete the Office **Despatch Note (Despatch 2)** on the last page of the Consent Booklet. This tells us the date you sent the samples to the lab and indicates what we should expect back from the laboratory.

If you have only achieved an incomplete blood sample (eg have only filled one tube), please state this clearly on both copies of the despatch note and give the reason.

Appendix C: Coding frame for medicines

The codes given below are the BNF section numbers for the class of medications listed. These numbers, with leading zeros, form the first four digits of the six digit drug code. For example, diuretics are coded on the dataset as 020201-020208. The last 2 digits of the six digit code indicate the BNF subsection where the specific drug is listed.

(British National Formulary classifications from BNF No. 34 September 1997)

1 Gastro-intestinal system

1.1 Antacids
1.2 Antispasmodics and other drugs altering gut motility
1.3 Ulcer-healing drugs
1.4 Antidiarrhoeal drugs
1.5 Treatment of chronic diarrhoeas
1.6 Laxatives
1.7 Preparations for haemorrhoids
1.8 Stoma care
1.9 Drugs affecting intestinal secretions

2 Cardiovascular system

2.1 Positive inotropic drugs
2.2 Diuretics
2.3 Anti-arrhythmic drugs
2.4 Beta-adrenoceptor blocking drugs
2.5 Drugs affecting the renin-angiotensin system and some other antihypertensive drugs
2.6 Nitrates, calcium-channel blockers, and potassium-channel activators
2.7 Sympathomimetics
2.8 Anticoagulants and protamine
2.9 Antiplatelet drugs
2.10 Myocardial infarction and fibrinolysis
2.11 Antifibrinolytic drugs and haemostatics
2.12 Lipid-lowering drugs
2.13 Local sclerosants

3 Respiratory system

3.1 Bronchodilators
3.2 Corticosteroids
3.3 Cromoglycate and related therapy
3.4 Antihistamines, hyposensitisation, and allergic emergencies
3.5 Respiratory stimulants and pulmonary surfactants
3.6 Oxygen
3.7 Mucolytics
3.8 Aromatic inhalations
3.9 Cough preparations
3.10 Systemic nasal decongestants

4 Central nervous system

4.1   Hypnotics and anxiolytics
4.2   Drugs used in psychoses and related disorders
4.3   Antidepressant drugs
4.4   Central nervous system stimulants
4.5   Appetite suppressants
4.6   Drugs used in nausea and vertigo
4.7   Analgesics
4.8   Antiepileptics
4.9   Drugs used in parkinsonism and related disorders
4.10 Drugs used in substance dependence
4.11 Drugs for dementia

5 Infections

5.1   Antibacterial drugs
5.2   Antifungal drugs
5.3   Antiviral drugs
5.4   Antiprotozoal drugs
5.5   Anthelmintics

6 Endocrine system

6.1   Drugs used in diabetes
6.2   Thyroid and antithyroid drugs
6.3   Corticosteroids
6.4   Sex hormones
6.5   Hypothalamic and pituitary hormones and anti-oestrogens
6.6   Drugs affecting bone metabolism
6.7   Other endocrine drugs

7 Obstetrics, gynaecology, and urinary-tract disorders

7.1   Drugs used in obstetrics
7.2   Treatment of vaginal and vulval conditions
7.3   Contraceptives
7.4   Drugs for genito-urinary disorders

8 Malignant disease and immunosuppression

8.1   Cytotoxic drugs
8.2   Drugs affecting the immune response
8.3   Sex hormones and antagonists in malignant disease

9 Nutrition and blood

9.1   Anaemias and some other blood disorders
9.2   Fluids and electrolytes
9.3   Intravenous nutrition
9.4   Oral nutrition
9.5   Minerals
9.6   Vitamins
9.7   Bitters and tonics
9.8   Metabolic disorders

10 Musculoskeletal and joint diseases

10.1 Drugs used in rheumatic diseases and gout
10.2 Drugs used in neuromuscular disorders
10.3 Drugs for the relief of soft-tissue inflammation

11 Eye

11.1 Administration of drugs to the eye
11.2 Control of microbial contamination
11.3 Anti-infective eye preparations
11.4 Corticosteroids and other anti-inflammatory preparations
11.5 Mydriatics and cycloplegics
11.6 Treatment of glaucoma
11.7 Local anaesthetics
11.8 Miscellaneous ophthalmic preparations
11.9 Contact lenses

12 Ear, nose, and oropharynx

12.1 Drugs acting on the ear
12.2 Drugs acting on the nose
12.3 Drugs acting on the oropharynx

13 Skin

13.1 Vehicles
13.2 Emollient and barrier preparations
13.3 Topical local anaesthetics and antipruritics
13.4 Topical corticosteroids
13.5 Preparations for eczema and psoriasis
13.6 Acne and rosacea
13.7 Preparations for warts and calluses
13.8 Sunscreens and camouflagers
13.9 Shampoos and some other scalp preparations
13.10 Anti-infective skin preparations
13.11 Disinfectants and cleansers
13.12 Antiperspirants
13.13 Wound management products
13.14 Topical circulatory preparations

14 Immunological products and vaccines

14.1 Active immunity
14.2 Passive immunity
14.3 Storage and use
14.4 Vaccines and antisera
14.5 Immunoglobulins
14.6 International travel

15 Anaesthesia

15.1 General anaesthesia
15.2 Local anaesthesia

Appendix D: Regional map

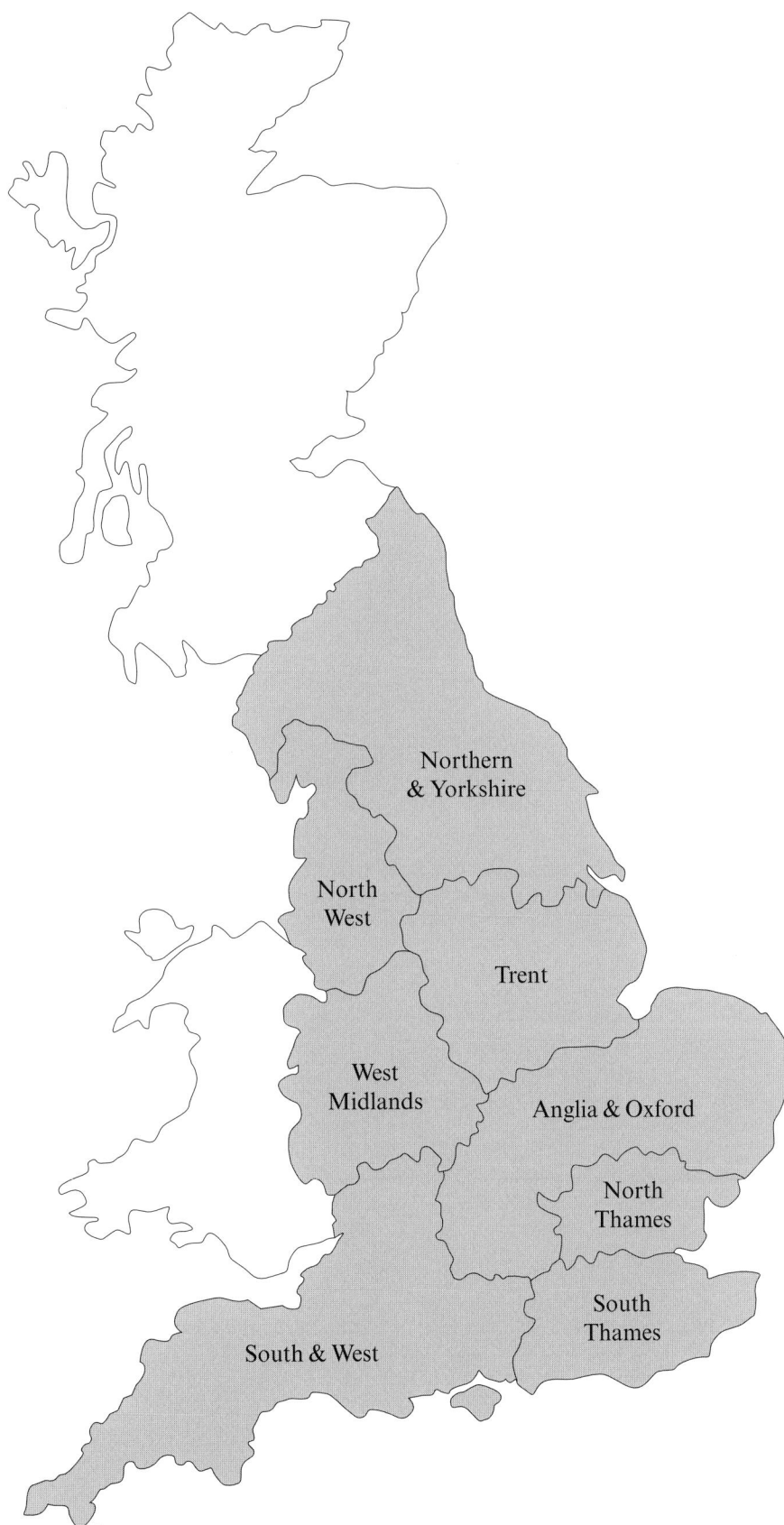

Northern
& Yorkshire

North
West

Trent

West
Midlands

Anglia & Oxford

North
Thames

South
Thames

South & West

Appendix E: Glossary

This glossary explains terms used in the report, other than those fully described in particular chapters.

Acute sickness An illness or injury which caused the informant to cut down on any of the things he or she usually does about the house, at work or school or in his or her free time (in the two weeks prior to the interview).

Age standardisation Age standardisation has been extensively used in this report in order to enable groups to be compared after adjusting for the effects of any differences in their age distributions. Age standardisation has not been used, however, in the child tables posted on the Department of Health website (see Volume I Chapter 1 *Introduction,* Section 1.6.6).

When proportions are compared across different sub-groups in respect of a variable on which age has an important influence, any differences in age distributions between these sub-groups are likely to affect the observed differences in the proportions of interest. The objective of the direct age standardisation procedure used in this report was to enable proportions to be presented across sub-groups after adjustment for the effects of age. Direct standardisation estimates the values of the proportions of interest in the case where the compared sub-groups have the same age distribution. However, it should be stressed that age-standardised proportions provide only a summary reflecting the average relationship between the variables across all age bands and that age standardisation adjusts only for age and not for other factors that may affect the variable of interest.

Age standardisation was carried out (separately for men and women) by ten-year age groups. The standard population to which the age distribution of sub-groups was adjusted was the mid-1997 population estimates for England. The age-standardised proportion p' was calculated as follows, where p_i is the age specific proportion in age group i and N_i is the standard population size in age group i:

$$p' = \frac{\sum_i N_i p_i}{\sum_i N_i}$$

Therefore p' can be viewed as a weighted mean of p_i using the weights N_i. Age standardisation was carried out using the age groups: 16-24, 25-34, 35-44, 45-54, 55-64, 65-74 and 75 and over. The variance of the standardised proportion can be estimated by:

$$var(p') = \frac{\sum_i (N_i^2 p_i q_i / n_i)}{(\sum_i N_i)^2}$$

Where $q_i = 1 - p_i$.

Anthropometric measurements See **Body mass index (BMI)**, **Demi-span, Mid-upper arm circumference** and **Waist-hip ratio**.

Blood analytes See **Cholesterol, HDL-cholesterol, Ferritin, Fibrinogen, C-reactive protein, Haemoglobin**.

Blood pressure	Systolic (SBP) and diastolic (DBP) blood pressure were measured in informants aged 5 and above using a standard method (see Appendix B for measurement protocol). In adults, high blood pressure is presented according to two definitions: SBP≥160 mmHg or DBP≥95 mmHg or on antihypertensive drugs ('old' definition) and SBP≥140 mmHg or DBP≥90 mmHg or on antihypertensive drugs ('new' definition).
Body mass index	Weight in kg divided by the square of height in metres. In adults, if the resulting value is more than 25.0 but no greater than 30.0, the condition is defined as 'overweight'. If it exceeds 30.0, the condition is defined as 'obese'. If it exceeds 40.0, the condition is defined as 'morbid obesity'.
Breathlessness	See **MRC Respiratory Questionnaire**
Cardiovascular disease	Informants were classified as having cardiovascular (CVD) disease if they reported ever having any of the following conditions diagnosed by a doctor (or a nurse in case of blood pressure): angina, heart attack, stroke, heart murmur, irregular heart rhythm, 'other heart trouble', high blood pressure or diabetes.
Cholesterol (total and HDL)	An important component of blood lipids transported in plasma. For the purpose of this survey total cholesterol was considered to be raised at a level of 6.5 mmol/l or over. In a normal individual, high density lipoprotein (HDL) constitutes approximately 20% of total plasma cholesterol. HDL-cholesterol was considered low at a level of 0.9 mmol/l or less.
Cotinine	Cotinine is a metabolite of nicotine. It is one of several biological markers that are indicators of smoking (others include carbon monoxide and thiocyanate), and is generally considered the most useful. It can be measured in, among other things, saliva and serum. It has a half-life in the body of between 16 and 20 hours, which means that it will detect regular smoking but may not detect occasional smoking if the last occasion was several days ago. Saliva and serum yield different estimates of cotinine levels, but they are very highly correlated and experiments have enabled serum values to be converted to equivalents of saliva values, so that they can be aggregated in analysis. Using saliva values, anyone with a level of 15 nanograms per millilitre or more is highly likely to be a smoker.
C-reactive protein	C-reactive protein is the major protein indicating inflammation activity in acute illness in humans. It is also a marker of cardiovascular risk. No recommendations for C-reactive protein thresholds appear in the literature so quintile distributions have been presented in this report. The categories of CRP defined on the basis of the quintile distribution, separately for men and women, are:

mg/l	Men	Women
Bottom quintile	≤0.5	≤0.5
2nd quintile	0.6-1.0	0.6-1.2
3rd quintile	1.1-1.9	1.3-2.4
4th quintile	2.0-3.7	2.5-4.9
Top quintile	>3.7	>4.9

Demi-span	Demi-span is an alternative to height as a measure of skeletal size in elderly people. It is defined as the distance between the mid-point of the sternal notch and the finger roots with the arm outstretched laterally.
Educational qualifications	Educational qualifications were coded according to the highest level of qualifications obtained into the following categories: Degree/NVQ5; A level/NVQ3/4; O Level (A-C)/GCSE(A-C)/NVQ1/2; No qualifications.
Equivalised household income	Income was not included in the Health Survey series until 1997. Making precise estimates of household income, as is done for example in the Family Resources Survey, requires far more interview time than was

available in the Health Survey. Household income was thus established by means of a card (see Appendix A) on which banded incomes were presented. Information was obtained from the head of the household or their partner. Initially they were asked to state their own (head and partner) aggregate gross income, and were then asked to estimate the total household income including that of any other persons in the household. Household income can be used as an analysis variable, but there has been increasing interest recently in using measures of equivalised income that adjust income to take account of the number of persons in the household. Methods of doing this vary in detail: the starting point is usually an exact estimate of net income, rather than the banded estimate of gross income obtained in the Health Survey. The method used in the present report was as follows. It utilises the widely used McClements scoring system, described below.

1. A score was allocated to each household member, and these were added together to produce an overall household McClements score. Household members were given scores as follows.

First adult (head)	0.61
Spouse/partner of head	0.39
Other second adult	0.46
Third adult	0.42
Subsequent adults	0.36
Dependent aged 0-1	0.09
Dependent aged 2-4	0.18
Dependent aged 5-7	0.21
Dependent aged 8-10	0.23
Dependent aged 11-12	0.25
Dependent aged 13-15	0.27
Dependent aged 16+	0.36

2. The equivalised income was derived as the annual household income divided by the McClements score.

3. This equivalised annual household income was attributed to all members of the household, including children.

4. Households were ranked by equivalised income, and quintiles q1, q2... were identified. Because income was obtained in banded form, there were clumps of households with the same income spanning the quintiles. It was decided not to split clumps but to define the quintiles as 'households with equivalised income up to q1', 'over q1 up to q2' etc.

5. All individuals in each household were allocated to the equivalised household income quintile to which their household had been allocated. Insofar as the mean number of persons per household may vary between quintiles, the numbers in the quintiles will be unequal. Inequalities in numbers are also introduced by the clumping referred to above, and by the fact that in any sub-group analysed the proportionate distribution across quintiles will differ from that of the total sample.

Ferritin Ferritin is the main form in which iron is stored in the liver, spleen and bone marrow. A small fraction of ferritin circulates in the bloodstream and this fraction correlates well with body iron status.

Fibrinogen Fibrinogen is a soluble protein involved in the blood clotting mechanism. Prospective population studies have established that fibrinogen is an independent predictor for ischaemic heart disease and stroke.

Reference: Maresca G, Di Blasio A. Marchioli R, Di Minno G. *Measuring plasma fibrinogen to predict stroke and myocardial infarction.* Arterioscler Thromb Vasc Biol 1999; **19**:1368-1377.

Geometric mean   The geometric mean is a measure of central tendency. It is sometimes preferable to the arithmetic mean, since it takes account of positive skewness in a distribution. The geometric of a continuous variable is calculated by taking the antilog of the mean of the logged values.

GHQ12   The General Health Questionnaire (GHQ12) is a scale designed to detect possible psychiatric morbidity in the general population. The questionnaire contains 12 questions about the informant's general level of happiness, depression, anxiety and sleep disturbance over the past four weeks.

Reference: Goldberg D, Williams PA. *User's Guide to the General Health Questionnaire.* NFER-NELSON, 1988.

Haemoglobin   The iron-containing molecule in red blood cells. Low haemoglobin (anaemia) is most commonly caused by iron deficiency.

HDL-cholesterol   See **Cholesterol**.

Head of household   The head of household was defined as the household member who owned or rented the property, or was a man married to or cohabiting with a woman who was the owner/renter (ie husband/male partner took precedence). If there was equal claim to be head of household, male took precedence over female and, where they were of the same sex, older took precedence over younger.

Height standardisation   For variables that are associated with height, comparisons between groups have been 'height standardised' in some of the child tables posted on the Department of Health website (see Volume I Chapter 1 *Introduction,* Section 1.6.6). The height standardised mean, $\bar{x}_{(st)h}$, within sub-group h was calculated as

$$\bar{x}_{(st)h} = \sum_{q=1}^{5} \bar{x}_{qh}$$

where $q = 1$ represents those respondents whose height is less than or equal to the first quintile for height; $q = 2$ represents those respondents whose height is greater than the first height quintile but less than or equal to the second quintile, and so on; and where $\bar{x}_{qh}$ is the mean of x for respondents within quintile q. The values of the quintiles are calculated from the total survey population of interest.

High blood pressure   See **Blood pressure.**

Hormone replacement therapy (HRT)   The treatment of women with pharmacological doses of oral oestrogen taken alone or with an oral progestogen to alleviate menopause symptoms. Most women on HRT are postmenopausal (ie stopped menstruating) or perimenopausal (in transition). Younger women (before age 45) may also be prescribed HRT following a hysterectomy, also termed surgical menopause, or because of an early natural menopause.

Household   A household was defined as one person or a group of people who have the accommodation as their only or main residence and who either share at least one meal a day or share the living accommodation.

Income   See **Equivalised household income.**

Ischaemic heart disease   Informants were classified as having ischaemic heart disease (IHD) if they reported ever having angina or a heart attack diagnosed by a doctor.

Logistic regression   Logistic regression was used to investigate the effect of two or more independent or predictor variables on a two-category (binary) outcome variable. The independent variables can be continuous or categorical (grouped) variables. The parameter estimates from a logistic regression model for each independent variable give an estimate of the effect of that variable on the outcome variable, adjusted for all other independent variables in the model.

Logistic regression models the log 'odds' of a binary outcome variable. The 'odds' of an outcome is the ratio of the probability of its occurring to the probability of its not occurring. The parameter estimates obtained from a logistic regression model have been presented as odds ratios for ease of interpretation.

For *continuous* independent variables, the odds ratio gives the change in the odds of the outcome occurring for a one unit change in the value of the predictor variable.

Parameter estimates for *categorical* independent variables have been presented in two ways. In some cases, one category of the categorical variable has been selected as a baseline or reference category, with all other categories compared to it. Therefore there is no parameter estimate for the reference category and odds ratios for all other categories are the ratio of the odds of the outcome occurring between each category and the reference category, adjusted for all other variables in the model. In other cases, where there is no obvious reference category, the odds ratios for a given category of a categorical independent variable gives the change in the odds of the outcome occurring compared to the overall odds ('to average').

The statistical significance of independent variables in models was assessed by the likelihood ratio test and its associated p value. 95% confidence intervals were also calculated for the odds ratios. These can be interpreted as meaning that there is a 95% chance that the given interval for the sample will contain the true population parameter of interest. In logistic regression a 95% confidence interval which does not include 1.0 indicates the given parameter estimate is statistically significant.

References: Norusis MJ. SPSS for Windows: *Advanced statistics release 6.0.* SPSS Inc, Chicago, 1993.

Hosmer DW Jr. and Lemeshow. *Applied logistic regression.* John Wiley & Sons, New York, 1989.

Mean   Unless otherwise specified, means in this report are arithmetic means (the sum of the values for cases divided by the number of cases).

Median   The value of a distribution which divides it into two equal parts such that half the cases have values below the median and half the cases have values above the median.

Mid-upper arm circumference   The circumference taken at the mid-point between the shoulder and elbow of the child's bare left arm using an insertion tape, as described in Appendix B.

Morbid obesity   See **Body mass index**.

MRC Respiratory Questionnaire   The MRC Respiratory Questionnaire was designed as a simple device to measure chronic bronchitis and other diseases of chronic airways limitation, based on the prevalence of cough, sputum and breathlessness as predictors of chronic respiratory disability.

Obesity   See **Body mass index.**

Odds ratio   See **Logistic regression.**

Ordinal regression   Ordinal regression has been used to investigate the effect of two or more independent variables on a three or more category ordinal dependent variables. In logistic regression, the odds of being in category 1 of a binary variable are modelled. Ordinal regression is a variation of logistic regression that accommodates an ordinal rather than a binary dependent variable. The odds being modelled are the odds of the case being in category j if it is within the group of categories 1,...j. In algebraic terms the ordinal regression model is represented by:

$$\ln\left(\frac{\pi_j(z)}{1-\gamma_j(z)}\right) = \alpha + \theta_j + \beta z \qquad j = 1,\dots,c-1$$

where $\pi_j(z)$ is the probability of an individual with covariate z being in Category j, j=1,..,c, and $\gamma_j(z)= \pi_1(z)+...+\pi_j(z)$. The interpretation of the ordinal regression model is similar to that for the logistic regression model, the coefficients for the covariates representing the change in the odds of being in each category associated with an increase of one in the value of the covariate.

Overweight See **Body mass index**.

Percentile The value of a distribution which partitions the cases into groups of a specified size. For example, the 20th percentile is the value of the distribution where 20 percent of the cases have values below the 20th percentile and 80 percent have values above it. The 50th percentile is the median.

p value A p value is the probability of the observed result occurring due to chance alone. A p value of less than 5% is conventionally taken to indicate a statistically significant result ($p<0.05$). It should be noted that the p value is dependent on the sample size, so that with large samples differences or associations which are very small may still be statistically significant. Results should therefore be assessed on the magnitude of the differences or associations as well as on the p value itself. The p values given in this report are based on the assumption of a simple random sample and do not take into account the clustered sampling design of the survey.

Quintile Quintiles are percentiles which divide a distribution into fifths ie the 20th, 40th, 60th and 80th percentiles.

Region Regional analyses in this report are based on the eight areas covered by the regional offices of the NHS Executive: Northern & Yorkshire; North West; West Midlands; Trent; Anglia & Oxford; North Thames; South Thames; and South & West, as constituted at the time of the fieldwork (1998) (see map in Appendix D). The four southern regions were reorganised in 1999.

Sensitivity The proportion of actual cases of a given condition that are correctly identified by a test designed to identify that condition. A test has high sensitivity if there are few false negatives. See also **Specificity.**

Social class of head of household A social class was assigned on the basis of the occupation of the head of household using the Registrar General's Standard Occupational Classification. Occupations are assigned to six social class categories:

Social Class	Occupations
I	Professional occupations
II	Managerial and technical occupations
III	Skilled occupations
(IIINM)	(non-manual)
(IIIM)	(manual)
IV	Partly skilled occupations
V	Unskilled occupations

In some analyses Classes I and II and Classes IV and V have been combined. In others, I, II and IIINM have been combined under the heading of 'non-manual', while IIIM, IV and V have been combined under the heading of 'manual'.

In households where the head of household was not interviewed the social class of the head of household was derived from information obtained from their spouse or partner. Heads of households who were in the armed forces, whose occupation was not adequately described or who were full-time students were not allocated a social class and are not shown separately in the tables. They are, however, included in the total column.

Social support The perceived social support scale, originally used in the Health and Lifestyle Survey, was based on seven questions about physical and emotional aspects of social support. Informants were asked about the amount of support and encouragement they received from family friends. These questions were combined into a single scale categorising informants as having 'a severe lack', 'some lack' or 'no lack' of social support.

Reference: Cox BD et al. *The Health and Lifestyles Survey*. The Health Promotion Research Trust, London, 1987.

Specificity The proportion of cases that do not have a given condition that are correctly identified by that test as not having the condition. A test has high specificity if there are few false positives. See also **Sensitivity**.

Standard Occupational Classification The Registrar General's Standard Occupational Classification (SOC) classifies occupations in terms of the type and level of skill required to carry out the main work activity. There are several hundred Occupational Unit Groups. These are grouped at successive higher levels of aggregation, culminating in the nine Major Groups:

1. Managers and Administrators
2. Professional Occupations
3. Associate Professional and Technical Occupations
4. Clerical and Secretarial Occupations
5. Craft and Related Occupations
6. Personal and Protective Service Occupations
7. Sales Occupations
8. Plant and Machine Operatives
9. Other Occupations

Reference: Volume 3 *Standard Occupational Classification*. OPCS, HMSO, London, 1991.

Tertiles Tertiles are percentiles which divide a distribution into thirds.

Unit of alcohol A unit of alcohol is 8 gms. of ethanol, and is the amount contained in half a pint of ordinary beer or lager, or in a small glass of wine, or in a measure of spirits.

Waist-hip ratio Waist-hip ratio (WHR) was defined as the waist circumference divided by the hip circumference, ie waist girth (m)/ hip girth (m). WHR is a measure of deposition of abdominal fat ie central obesity. Unlike BMI there is no consensus to define a cut-off point for WHR and several were proposed in a recent review. For consistency the same cut-off values as in the 1994 report have been used. A raised WHR has been taken to be 0.95 or more in men and 0.85 or more in women.

Reference: Molarius A, Seidell JC. *Selection of anthropometric indicators for classification of abdominal fatness - a critical review*. Int J Obes 1998; **22**:719-727.

Health Survey for England

Cardiovascular Disease

'98

Summary of Key Findings

Joint Health Surveys Unit
National Centre for Social Research
Department of Epidemiology and Public Health at the Royal Free and
University College Medical School

Health Survey for England: Cardiovascular Disease '98

The Health Survey for England is a series of annual surveys about the health of people living in private households in England. It was commissioned by the Department of Health to provide better and more reliable information about various aspects of people's health, and to monitor selected health targets.

The survey combines questionnaire-based interviews with physical measurements and the analysis of blood samples. Blood pressure, height and weight, smoking, drinking and general health are covered every year. Each year's survey also has a particular focus on a disease or condition or population group. The 1998 survey focused on cardiovascular disease and related conditions.

Summary of Key Findings

Background

The 1998 survey

The main focus of the 1998 survey was on cardiovascular disease (CVD) and CVD risk factors, including alcohol consumption, cigarette smoking, eating habits, physical activity, blood pressure and obesity. The Medical Research Council (MRC) respiratory questionnaire formed a module within the main questionnaire. The survey also included questions about people's perceptions of their health, and about their use of health services and medication (including contraception and Hormone Replacement Therapy (HRT)).

This booklet is a summary of the 1998 Health Survey, and presents a selection of survey findings relating to adults. The full results are available in a separate report published by the Stationery Office, and also in an anonymised data file that will be lodged with the Data Archive at the University of Essex. Reports and data files from earlier surveys in the series are similarly available. Tables containing additional data, including tables presenting 1998 survey results for children, together with selected trends for both children and adults, will be found on the Department of Health website. (See page 20 for references and addresses.)

The survey components

All adults (aged 16 and over) and all children aged 2-15 in sampled households were eligible for interview, except that if there were three or more children, two were selected at random to take part in the survey.

After the interviewer had completed the interview, a nurse called to take blood pressure and make other body measurements such as waist and hip circumference. Informants aged 18 and over and (in the second half of the survey year) those aged 11 to 17 were asked to provide a small sample of blood by venepuncture. A saliva sample was requested from those aged 4 and over.

Response to the survey

13,680 addresses were sampled for the survey, and 9,208 private households co-operated (74% of sampled eligible households). In these co-operating households there were 17,240 adults aged 16 and over.

Of adults in co-operating households, 92% were successfully interviewed, 79% were visited by a nurse, 77% had their blood pressure taken, 77% gave a saliva sample and 62% gave a blood sample.

Topics covered in the survey

Interviewer administered

General health, longstanding illness and acute sickness
Use of health services
Respiratory problems
Cardiovascular disease and related conditions
Physical activity
Eating habits
Smoking and drinking
Psychosocial health (GHQ12)
Social support
Use of contraceptive pill
Use of HRT
Family history of cardiovascular disease
Demographic and socio-economic information
Height and weight measurements

Nurse administered

Prescribed medication and vitamin supplements
Upper arm circumference
Waist/hip circumference
Blood pressure
Demi-span
Saliva sample for analyte:
 Cotinine
Blood sample for analytes:
 Total cholesterol
 HDL-cholesterol
 Haemoglobin
 Ferritin
 Fibrinogen
 C-reactive protein

Cardiovascular disease

The chart shows the proportion of men and women with any CVD condition, using two alternative definitions. Included in the first definition are those who reported that a doctor had diagnosed angina, heart attack, stroke, heart murmur, abnormal heart rhythm, 'other heart trouble' or diabetes. In the second definition, high blood pressure (confirmed by a doctor or a nurse) is also included.

The inclusion of high blood pressure almost doubled the proportion with a CVD condition. The proportion of men with a CVD condition was 28% if blood pressure is included, 16% if it is excluded. Comparable figures for women were 28% and 14%.

The age pattern shown was broadly similar on either definition. Under the age of 45, the proportion with a CVD condition was relatively low (below 20% including high blood pressure, below 10% excluding it), and differences between men and women were small.

The gradual increase with age observed in these younger groups accelerated from age 45 onwards, and some differences appeared in the age/sex pattern shown by each definition. Among those aged 65 and over, when high blood pressure was included, the proportion with a CVD condition was higher for women than men. When it was excluded, the

Proportion with CVD condition
by age

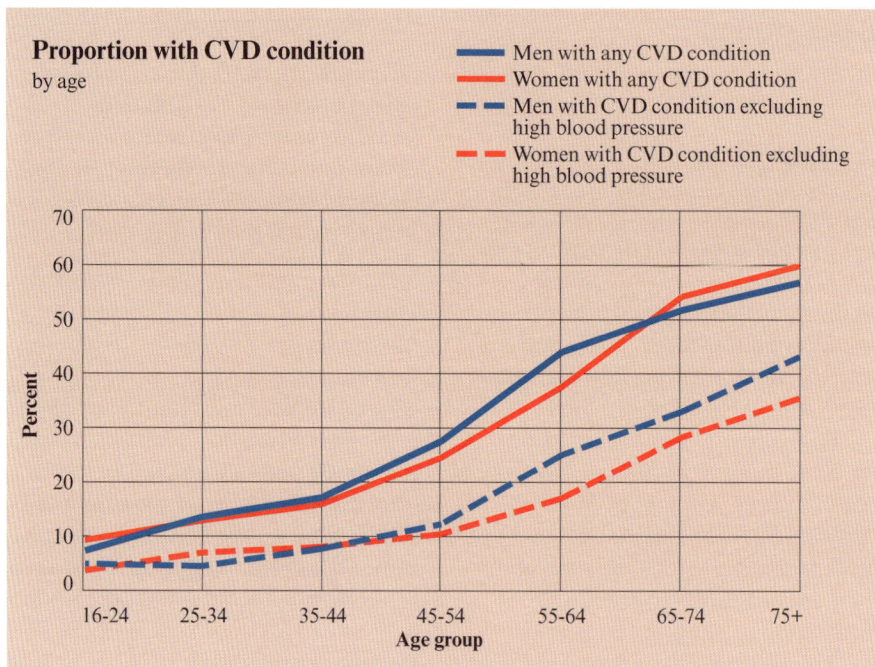

Proportion with CVD (excluding high BP) and IHD or stroke
by survey year

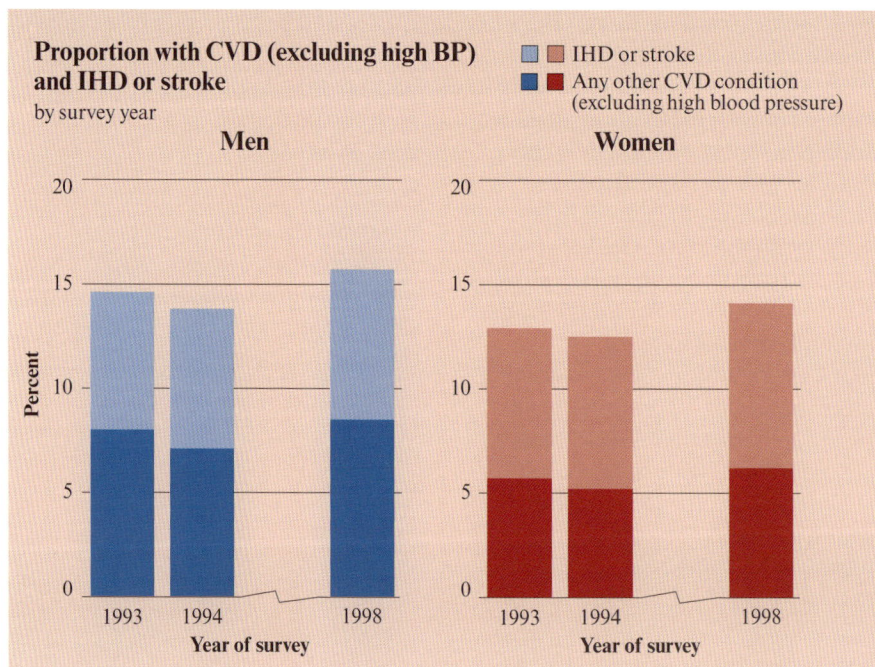

proportion was higher for men than women.

The chart at the bottom of the opposite page shows the prevalence of CVD conditions (excluding high blood pressure) and of ischaemic heart disease (IHD, ie angina or heart attack) or stroke in 1993, 1994 and 1998. Observed prevalence decreased between 1993 and 1994, and then increased again in 1998. A longer time series is required to establish whether there is any trend underlying these fluctuations.

The overall prevalence in 1998 of IHD or stroke was 8.5% in men and 6.2% in women. A socio-economic gradient in CVD morbidity and mortality has been repeatedly demonstrated. The two charts show the prevalence of IHD or stroke by social class and by equivalised household income, but only among informants aged 35 and over because of the low prevalence of these conditions in younger people. A social class gradient in prevalence was observed in both sexes. After adjusting for the effects of age, the prevalence of IHD or stroke among women was highest in Social Classes IV and V. Among men, it was lowest in Social Classes I and II.

Among men, the prevalence of IHD or stroke (adjusted for age) decreased with increasing equivalised household income. A similar but less marked decrease was seen among women.

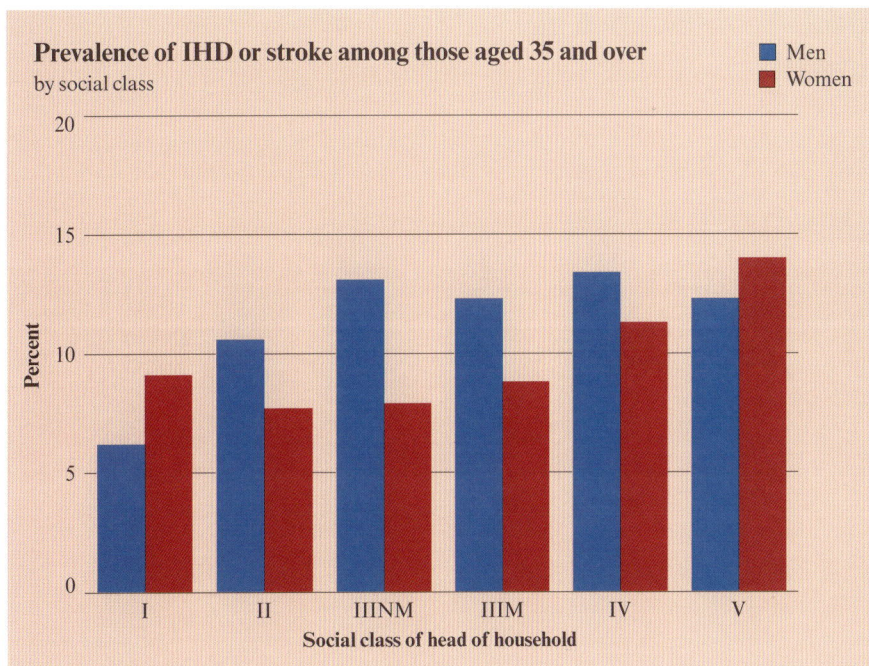

Prevalence of IHD or stroke among those aged 35 and over
by social class

Percent

■ Men
■ Women

Social class of head of household

Age standardised

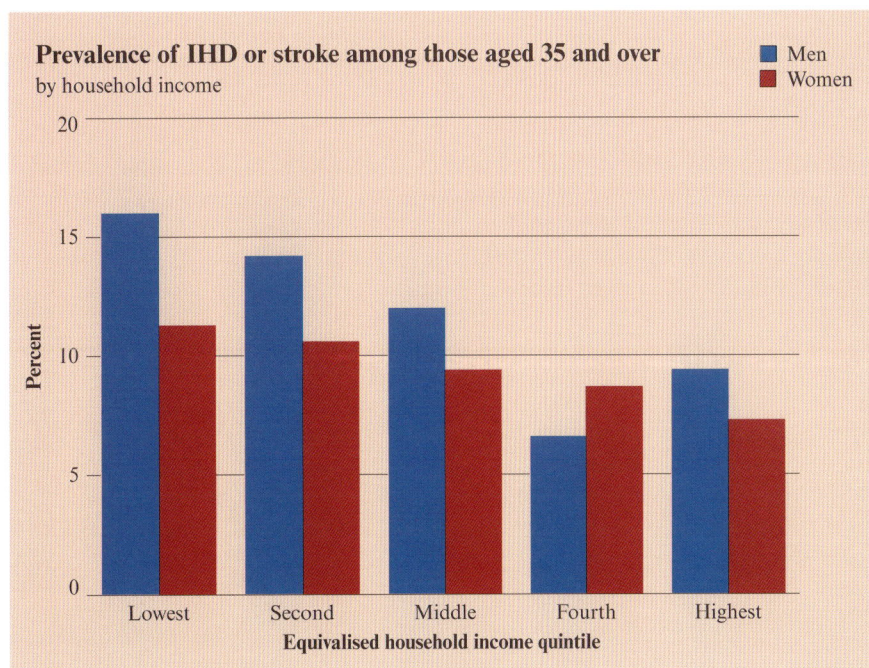

Prevalence of IHD or stroke among those aged 35 and over
by household income

Percent

■ Men
■ Women

Equivalised household income quintile

Age standardised

Alcohol consumption and cigarette smoking

Alcohol consumption did not show any significant change among men from 1994 to 1998, but rose among women. But in 1998, on average men were still drinking well over twice as much as women.

The proportion of women usually drinking more than 14 units of alcohol a week increased from Social Classes IV and V to Social Classes I and II. For men, variation by social class did not follow a clear pattern.

Of men who had an alcoholic drink in the past week, the proportion who had drunk at least 8 units of alcohol on at least one day in the past seven increased progressively from Social Class I to Social Class V. The proportion of women drinkers who had drunk at least 6 units followed a closely similar pattern.

In spite of the higher criterion chosen for men (8 units instead of 6 units), the proportion of 'past week drinkers' drinking more than the stated amount was much higher for men than women.

28% of men and 27% of women reported smoking cigarettes. Previous Health Surveys have shown that cigarette smoking prevalence in both sexes increases markedly from Social Class I to Social Class V. The chart shows that prevalence also varies greatly by equivalised household income, being lowest where income is highest and vice versa.

Weekly alcohol units consumed by men and women, and highest daily amount consumed by those who drank in the past week
by social class

- Men: usual consumption over 21 units/week
- Women: usual consumption over 14 units/week
- Men drinkers: over 8 units on at least one day in past week
- Women drinkers: over 6 units on at least one day in past week

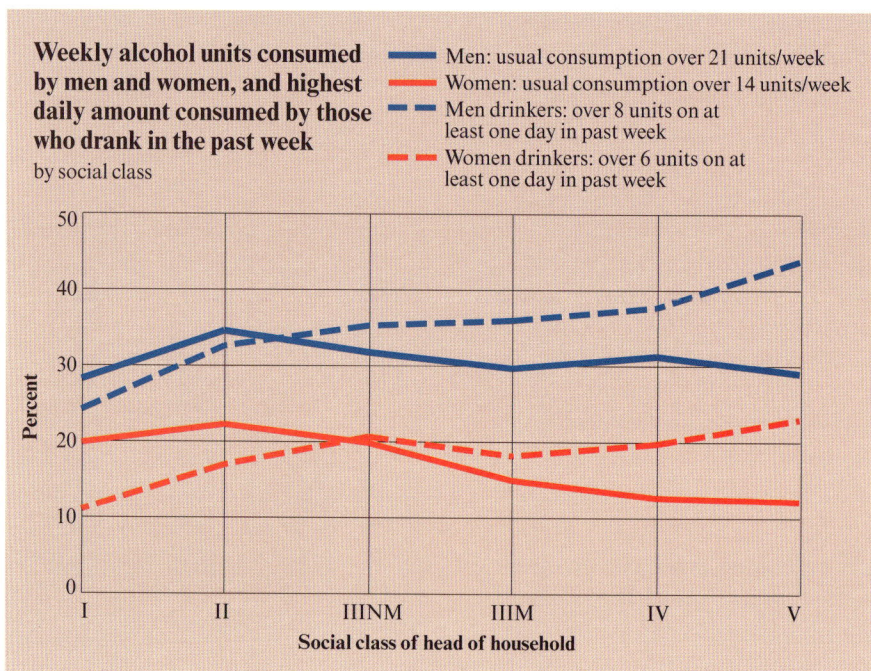

Social class of head of household

Age standardised

Cigarette smoking prevalence
by household income

- Men
- Women

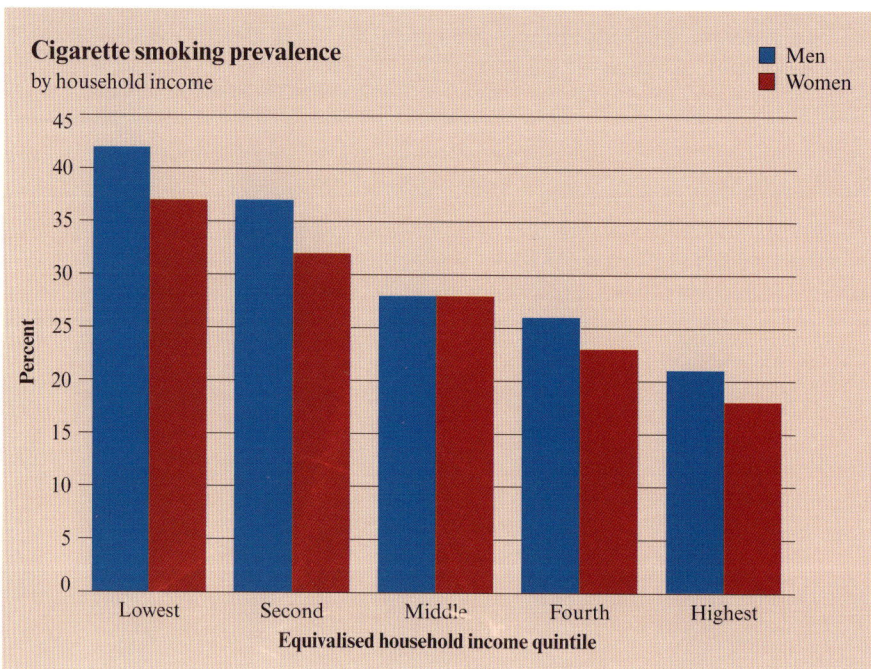

Equivalised household income quintile

Age standardised

Eating habits

Information was collected on the frequency of consumption of various types of food, and scores for fat and fibre consumption were derived using a modified version of the Dietary Instrument for Nutrition Education (DINE).

Low fibre consumption was more prevalent among women than men, while men had a higher prevalence of high fat consumption than women. There was a clear socio-economic gradient in age-standardised high fat and low fibre intakes: in both sexes, the prevalence of high fat and low fibre intake was higher in manual social classes and in lower income households.

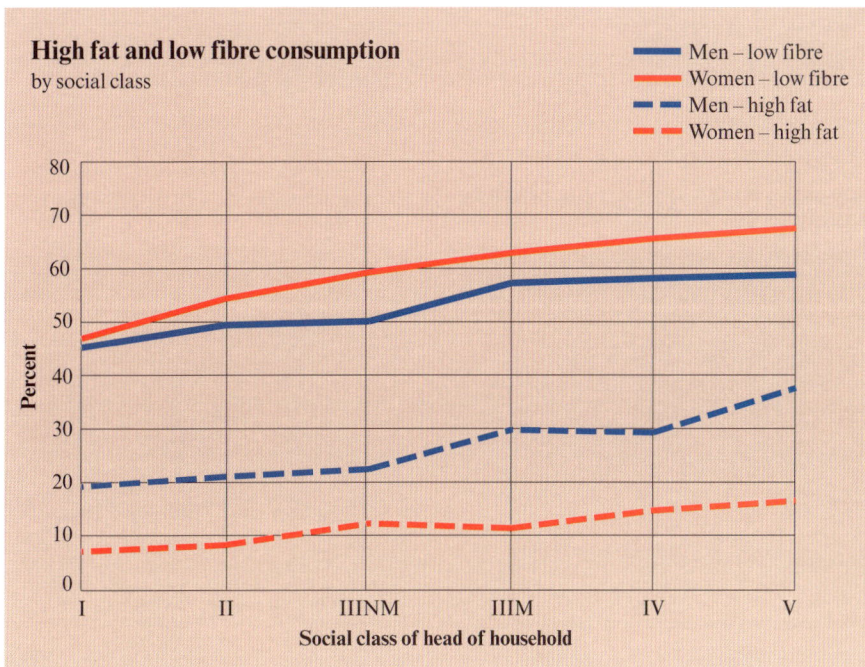

High fat and low fibre consumption
by social class

Men – low fibre
Women – low fibre
Men – high fat
Women – high fat

Age standardised

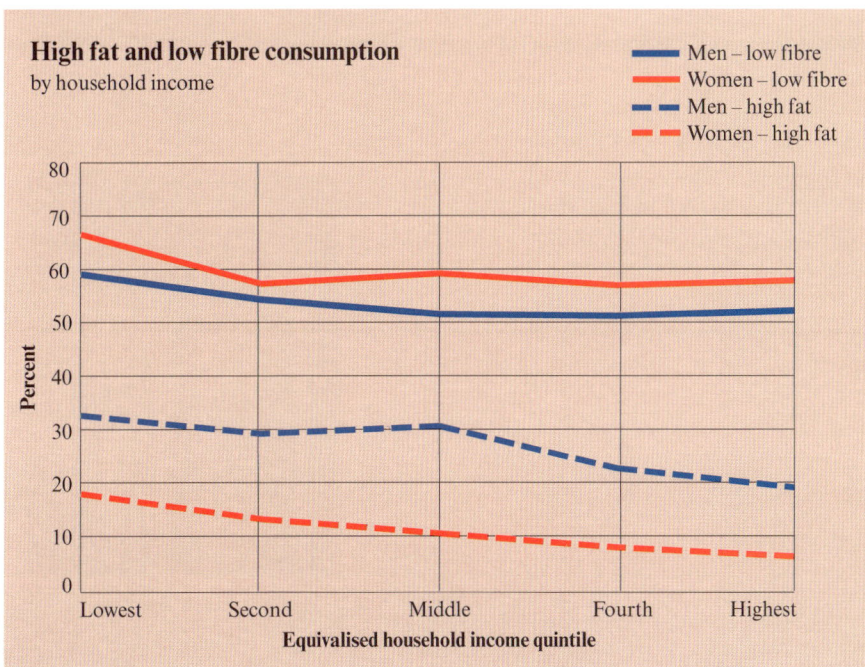

High fat and low fibre consumption
by household income

Men – low fibre
Women – low fibre
Men – high fat
Women – high fat

Age standardised

Physical activity

The chart shows the proportion of men and women participating in three major physical activities, sport/exercise, heavy housework and walking. Levels of participation in sport/exercise were much higher among young men than young women, and decreased more rapidly with age.

Levels of participation in heavy housework, in contrast, were much higher among women than men until converging among those of pensionable age. Relatively low in the youngest age group, women's participation in heavy housework increased to a peak at age 25-34 and declined slowly thereafter.

The other chart classifies informants into one of three activity groups, of which Group 3 is the level that fulfils the current activity guidelines, which are that adults should take part in physical activities of at least moderate intensity and of at least 30 minutes' duration, on most days (at least five days a week). The chart plots the marked decline of men's physical activity with increasing age. Women's activity levels were much lower than men's in the younger age groups, and did not decline much until after about age 55.

Mean days' participation in selected activities in past four weeks
by age

Sports and exercise
Heavy housework
Walking

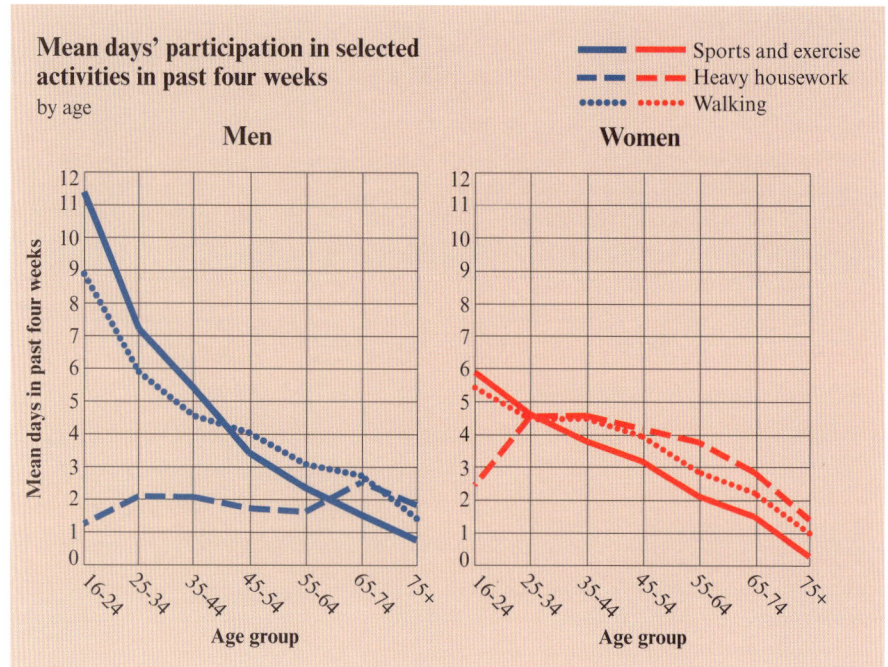

Men

Women

Activity levels
by age

Group 1 – low
Group 2 – medium
Group 3 – high

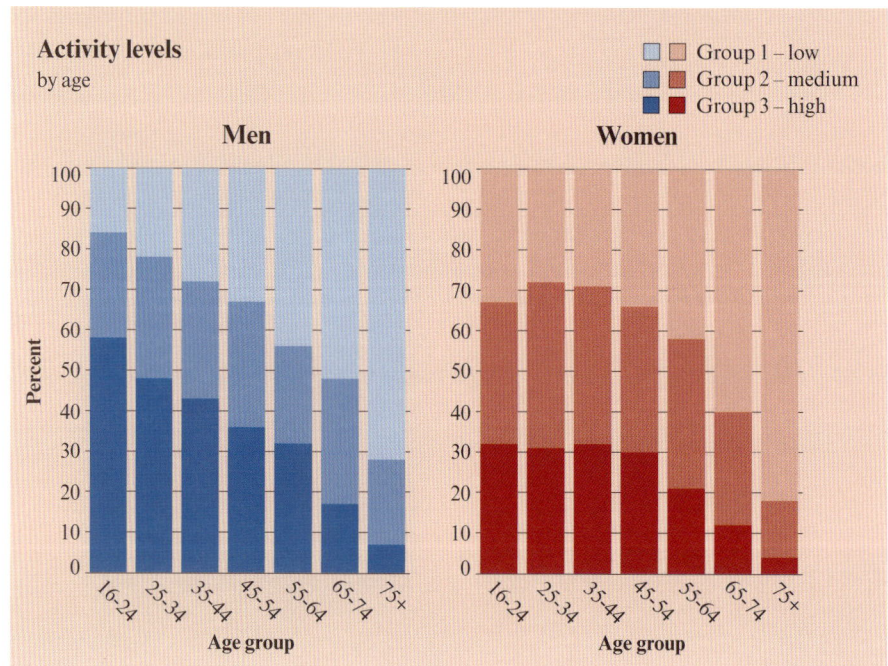

Men

Women

These two charts show only the proportion in activity Group 3. The first chart shows the proportion in Group 3 by age, bringing out clearly the different pattern of men's and women's activity levels.

The second shows that the (age-adjusted) proportion of men in activity Group 3 was considerably higher in manual than non-manual social classes. In contrast, the corresponding proportion of women did not vary much by social class.

Proportion reaching 5x30 minutes guideline (Group 3)
by age

■ Men
■ Women

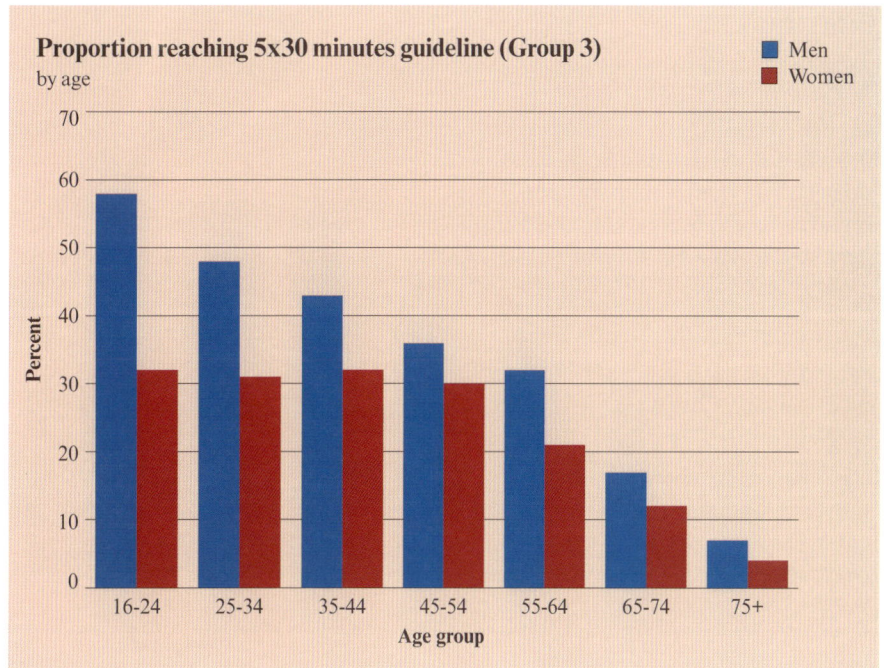

Proportion reaching 5x30 minutes guideline (Group 3)
by social class

■ Men
■ Women

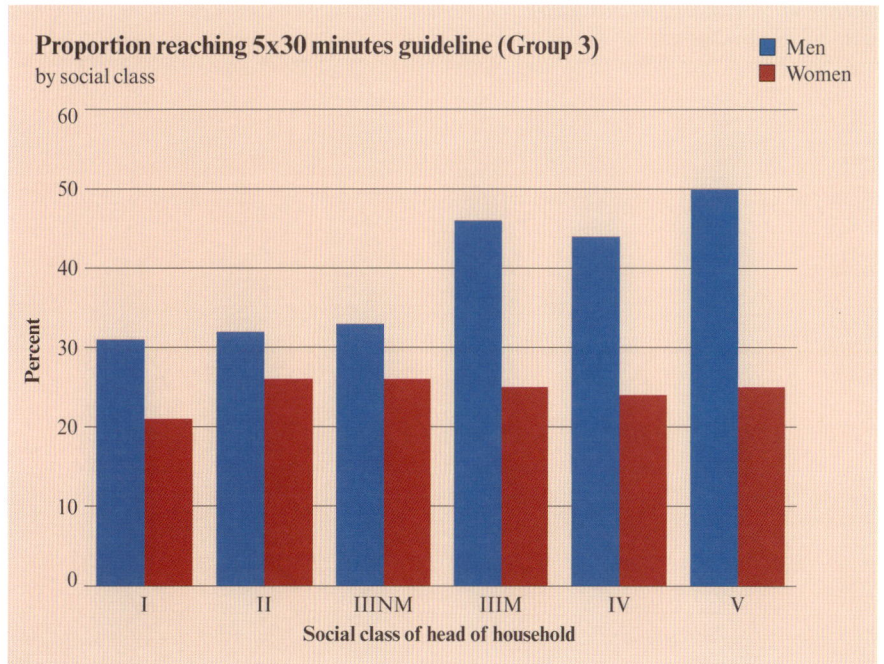

Age standardised

Body mass

Obesity was defined as a body mass index (BMI) greater than 30 kg/m², and overweight as greater than 25 kg/m² but not above 30 kg/m².

Combining the two categories (overweight and obese), prevalence was higher in men than in women. But the prevalence of obesity was higher in women than in men.

The proportion who were either obese or overweight increased between 1994 and 1998 – in the case of men from 58.1% to 62.8%, and for women from 48.7% to 53.3%.

The proportion who were obese increased more rapidly over the same period: men from 13.8% to 17.3%, women from 17.3% to 21.2%.

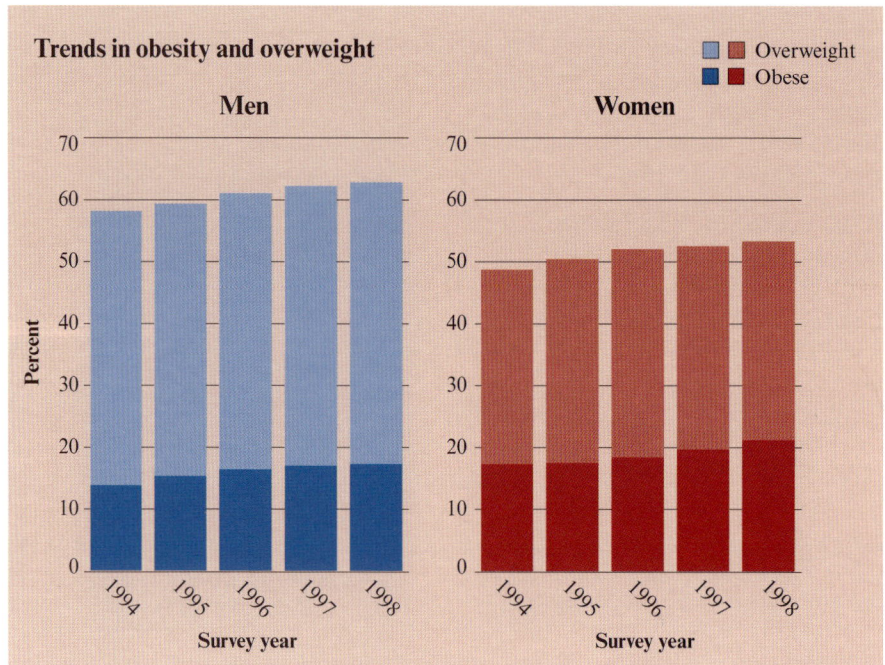

Trends in obesity and overweight

Overweight
Obese

Men

Women

Percent

Survey year

Survey year

The prevalence of overweight and obesity showed socio-economic differences, more marked in women than in men. The age-standardised proportion of women who were obese increased from Social Class I to Social Class V, as did the proportion who were either overweight or obese. There was a similar increase from the highest household income quintile to the lowest. For men the patterns of difference were not so clear-cut.

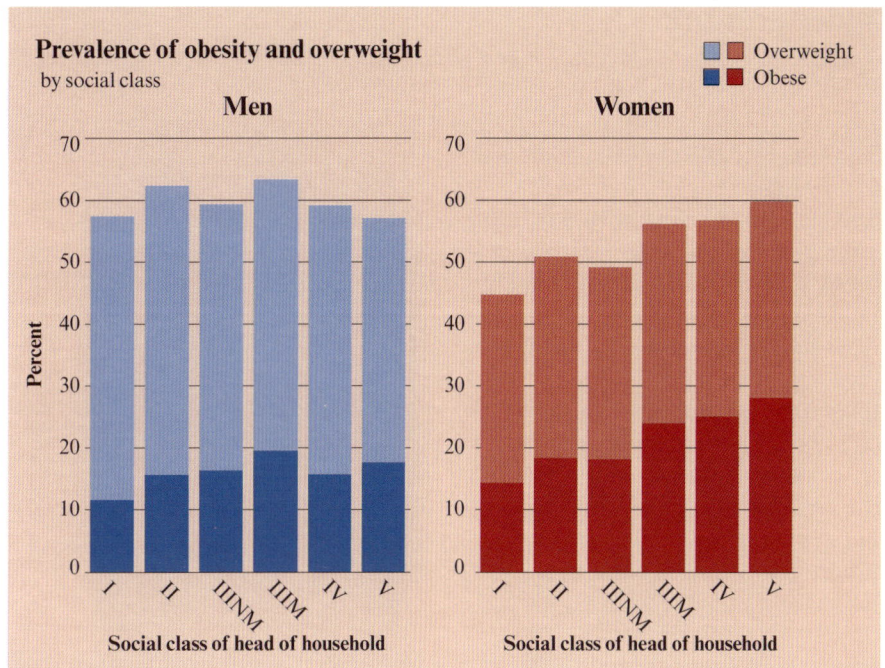

Prevalence of obesity and overweight
by social class

Overweight / Obese

Men — **Women**

Social class of head of household

Age standardised

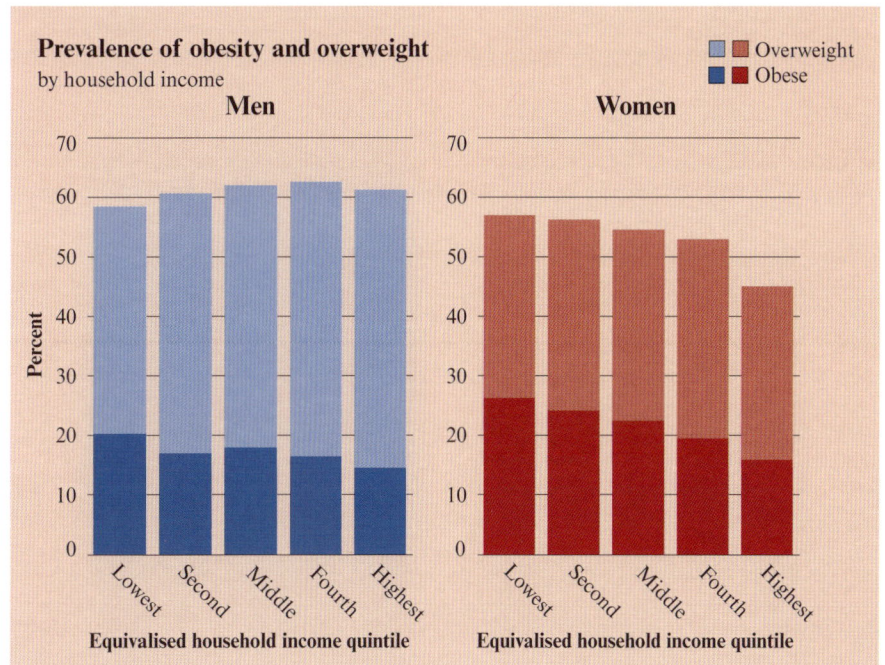

Prevalence of obesity and overweight
by household income

Overweight / Obese

Men — **Women**

Equivalised household income quintile

Age standardised

Blood pressure

The term high blood pressure referred in previous surveys to those with a systolic blood pressure (SBP) of 160 mmHg or more, or a diastolic blood pressure (DBP) of 95 mmHg or more, or taking antihypertensive drugs, regardless of the reason for which they were prescribed. The chart uses this definition to permit comparison of 1998 data with earlier years. There is no evidence of a trend over time in the prevalence of high blood pressure, but it is worth noting that the proportion with high blood pressure not taking antihypertensive medication (ie hypertensive untreated) decreased in both sexes between 1994 and 1998.

Hypertensive categories 1994-98

Legend:
- Hypertensive untreated
- Hypertensive treated
- Normotensive treated

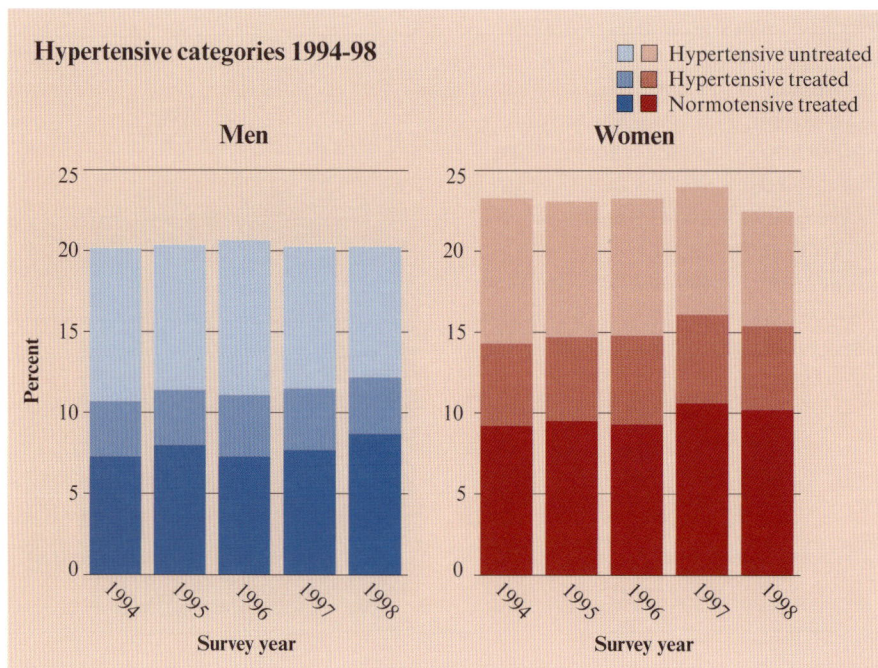

Men

Women

Percent

Survey year

Except for the purpose of making the above comparison, the definition of high blood pressure was changed in 1998, in accordance with the latest guidelines on hypertension management, to refer to those with a SBP of 140 mmHg or more, or a DBP of 90 mmHg or more, or taking drugs prescribed for high blood pressure. The prevalence of high blood pressure using the old definition was 18.4% in both men and in women. Using the new definition, prevalence more than doubled among men, at 40.8%, and almost doubled among women (32.9%). The change in definition has thus resulted in considerably more men than women overall being classified as having high blood pressure, whereas on the previous definition there was no difference between the sexes.

Under the new definition, as under the old, the prevalence of high blood pressure was higher in men than in women up to age 55-64, while in the older age groups the opposite was true.

The prevalence of high blood pressure (new definition) was examined by quintiles of equivalised household income. Among women, the prevalence of high blood pressure decreased as income increased. Among men there was no consistent pattern of variation by income in the prevalence of high blood pressure.

Prevalence of high blood preassure
by age

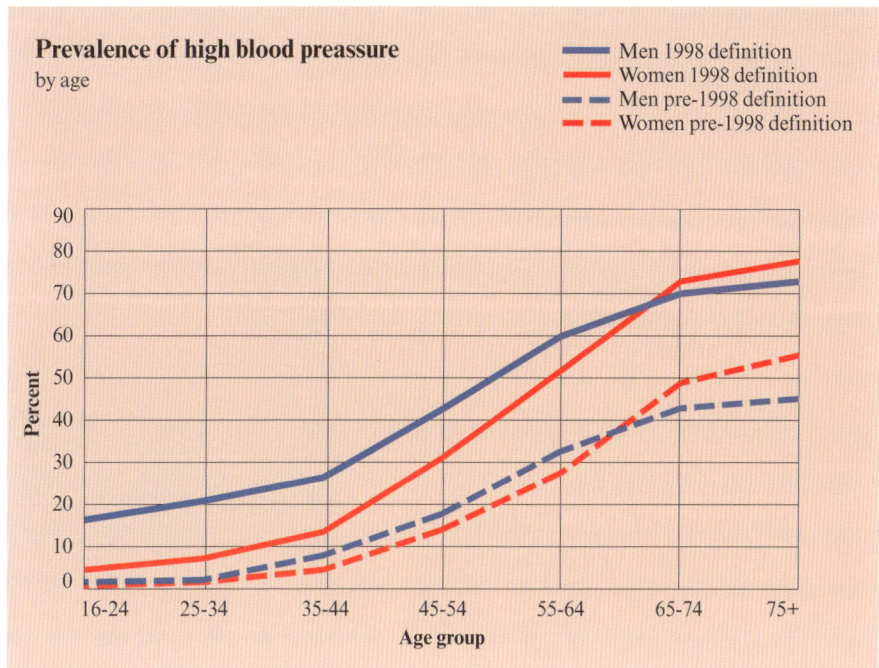

Legend:
— Men 1998 definition
— Women 1998 definition
-- Men pre-1998 definition
-- Women pre-1998 definition

Prevalence of high blood preassure
by household income

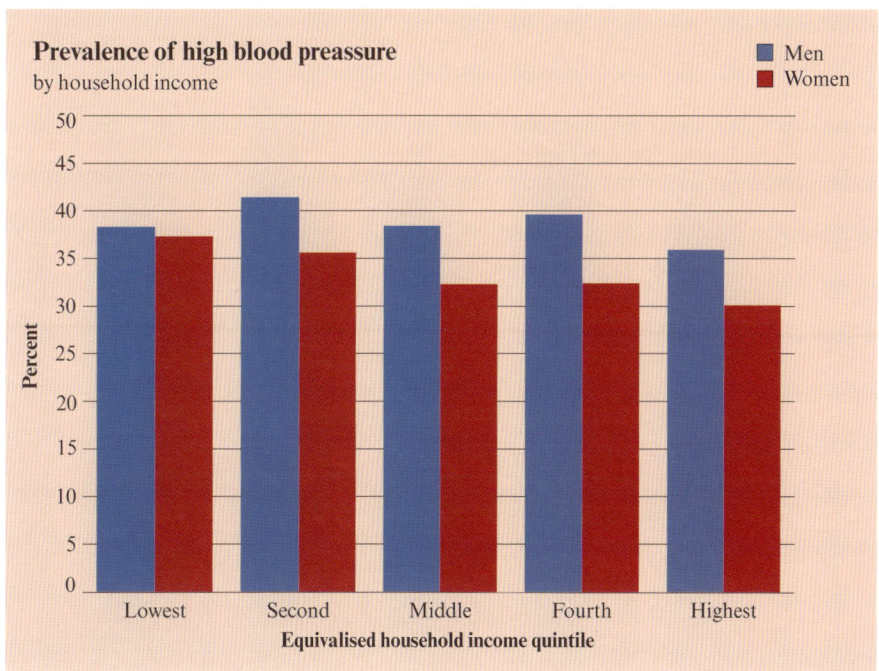

Legend:
■ Men
■ Women

Age standardised

Blood analytes

The blood analytes included in the survey were: total cholesterol, high-density lipoprotein cholesterol (HDL-cholesterol), C-reactive protein and fibrinogen, which are all recognised to be independently associated with cardiovascular disease and are therefore important in the determination of cardiovascular risk profile.

It has been demonstrated that a reduction in total cholesterol, whether by diet or drugs, decreases the risk for coronary artery disease. For the purpose of this survey cholesterol was considered to be raised at a level of 6.5 mmol/l or over. Total cholesterol showed little variation by socio-economic status. Among men the age-standardised prevalence of raised cholesterol was higher in the two lowest income quintiles than in the others, while among women there was no clear pattern.

HDL-cholesterol is a component of total plasma cholesterol, accounting on average for approximately 20% of it. Several studies have shown that reduced plasma levels of HDL-cholesterol are associated with increased risk of coronary heart disease. For the purpose of this survey a level of 0.9 mmol/l or less was considered low, and therefore an indicator of risk.

Prevalence of total cholesterol 6.5 mmol/l or more
by household income

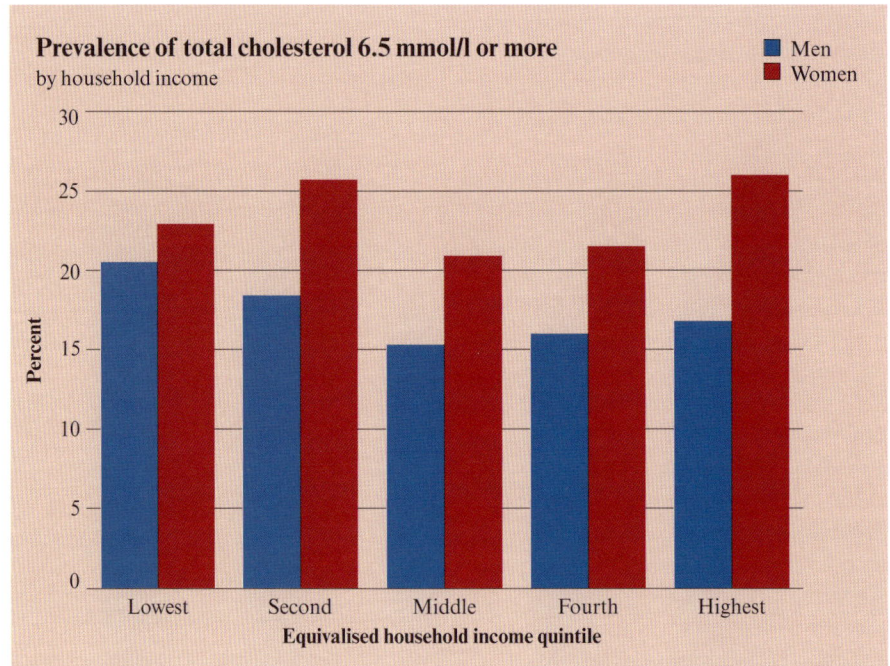

Age standardised

Prevalence of HDL-cholesterol 0.9 mmol/l or less
by household income

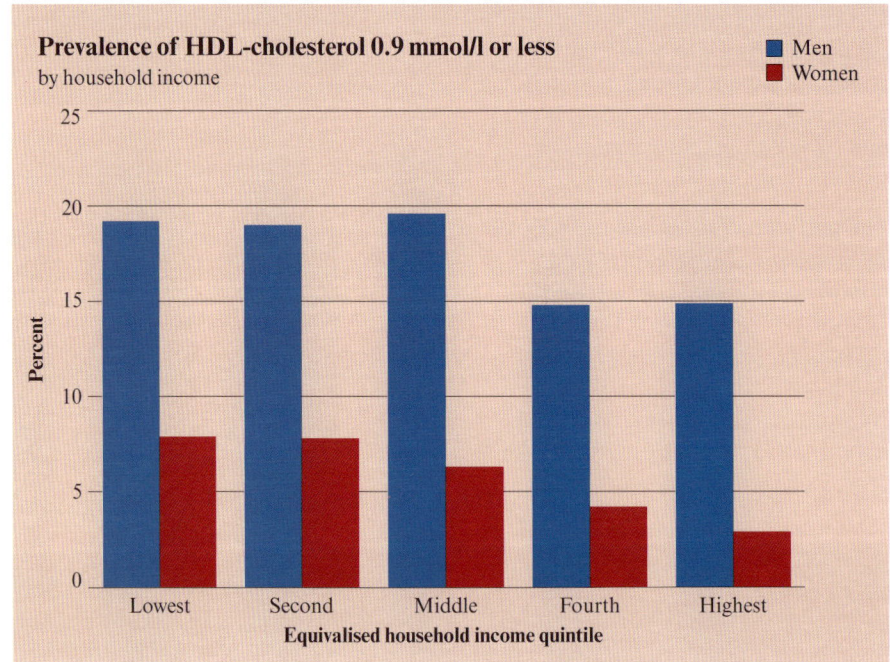

Age standardised

The prevalence of low HDL-cholesterol among women decreased from 7.9% in the lowest income quintile to 2.9% in the highest income quintile. Among men prevalence was lower in the two highest income quintiles than among lower income households.

Raised C-reactive protein is associated with subsequent risk of CVD. In the literature there is no recommendation for a C-reactive protein threshold, and the chart defines having 'high' C-reactive protein as being in the top quintile, that is, having a level of C-reactive protein among the overall top 20% (calculated separately for men and women). It shows that the proportion in the top C-reactive protein quintile increased as income decreased, being highest in the two lowest income groups.

Prospective population studies have demonstrated that fibrinogen is an important predictor for ischaemic heart disease and stroke. Mean fibrinogen increased steadily with age in both men and women. In all age groups, levels were higher for women than men. The difference however was more marked among younger groups, the increase with age thus being more marked with men than with women. The mean among men increased from 2.2 g/l at age 16-24 to 3.1 g/l at age 75 and over. For women the corresponding increase was from 2.5 g/l to 3.2 g/l.

Proportion in top quintile of C-reactive protein
by household income

Legend:
- Men over 3.7 mg/l
- Women over 4.9 mg/l

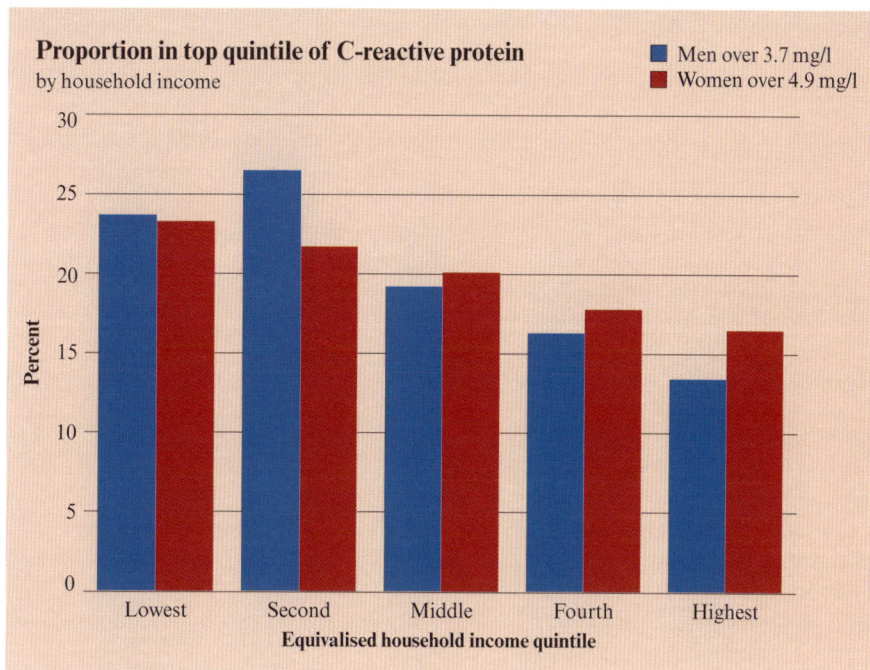

Age standardised

Mean fibrinogen
by age

Legend:
- Men
- Women

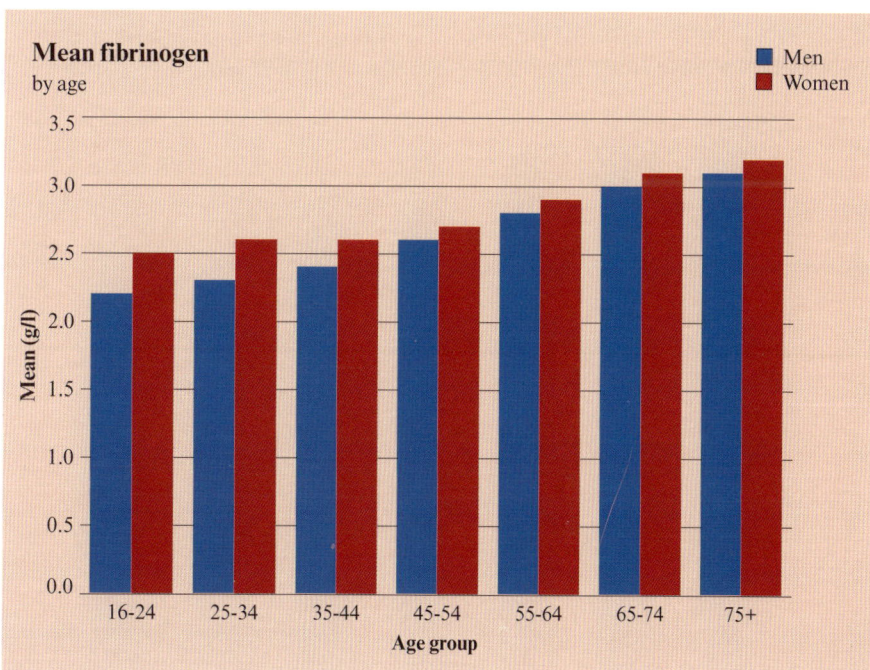

Self-assessed health

The chart shows an increase from 1994 to 1998 in all three measures shown – having a longstanding illness, having been sick in the past two weeks, and assessing one's own health as bad or very bad. For self-assessed health and longstanding illness most of the increase appears to have been in the earlier years of these five.

The left-hand section of the second chart shows, for men, a negative relationship between these health measures and income. For all three, the proportion increased steeply as equivalised household income decreased. In the right hand section, women are seen to follow a similar, but less marked, pattern for longstanding illness and self-reported bad or very bad health.

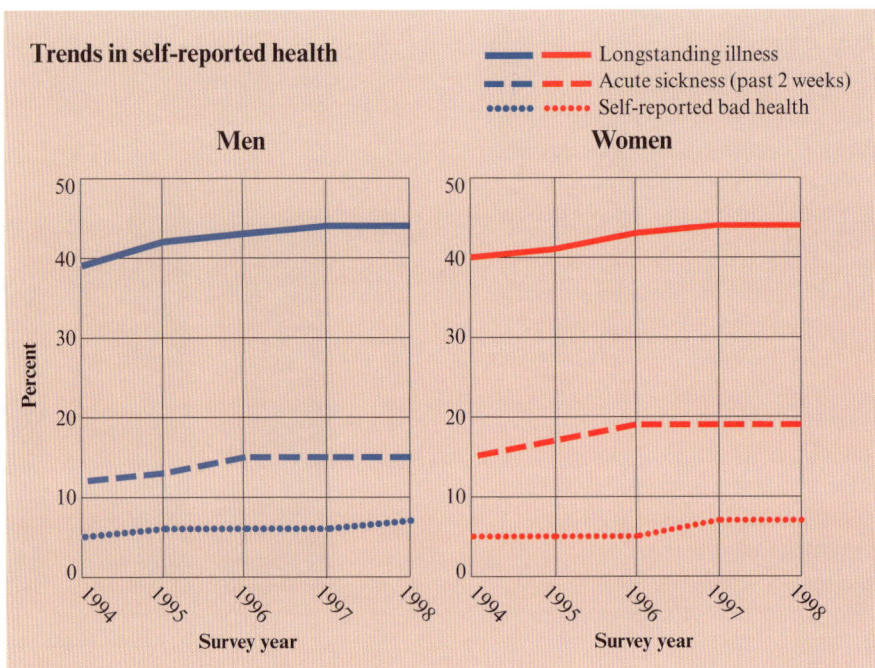

Trends in self-reported health

Longstanding illness — Acute sickness (past 2 weeks) ---- Self-reported bad health ·····

Men / Women

Percent / Survey year

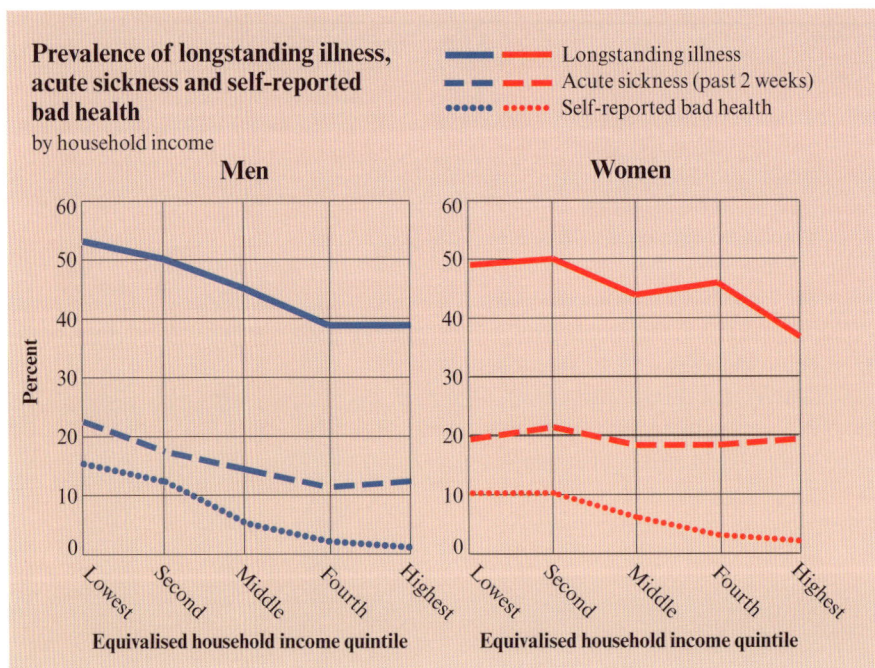

Prevalence of longstanding illness, acute sickness and self-reported bad health

by household income

Longstanding illness — Acute sickness (past 2 weeks) ---- Self-reported bad health ·····

Men / Women

Percent / Equivalised household income quintile

Lowest, Second, Middle, Fourth, Highest

Age standardised

These two charts present results for two psychosocial indicators, a high score (4 or more) on the General Health Questionnaire (GHQ12), which is an indicator of possible psychiatric morbidity, and a perceived 'severe lack of social support', using a scale measuring the level of support that the person concerned feels they have from family and friends.

A higher proportion of women than of men had a high GHQ12 score. Some tendency is seen, in both men and women, for the proportion with a high GHQ12 score to increase from Social Classes I and II to Social Class V, but the pattern is not very marked or consistent. The proportion with a high GHQ12 score decreased with increasing income, particularly among men.

In contrast to high GHQ12, the proportion with a severe lack of social support was higher among men than women. It also exhibited a closer relationship with social class and equivalised household income, increasing from Social Class I to Social Class V and from high incomes to low incomes.

Proportion with high GHQ12/severe lack of social support
by social class

Men – high GHQ12
Women – high GHQ12
Men – severe lack of social support
Women – severe lack of social support

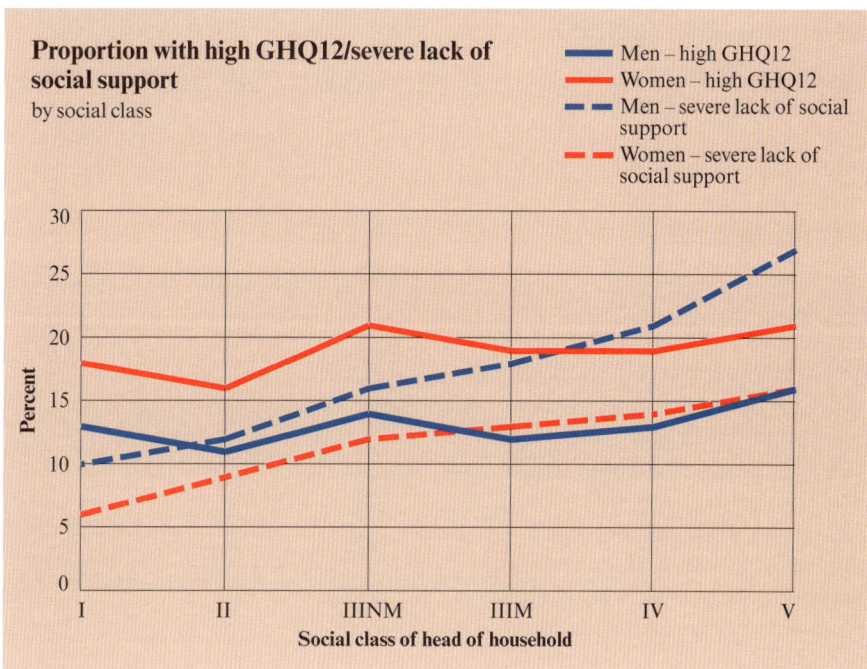

Social class of head of household

Age standardised

Proportion with high GHQ12/severe lack of social support
by household income

Men – high GHQ12
Women – high GHQ12
Men – severe lack of social support
Women – severe lack of social support

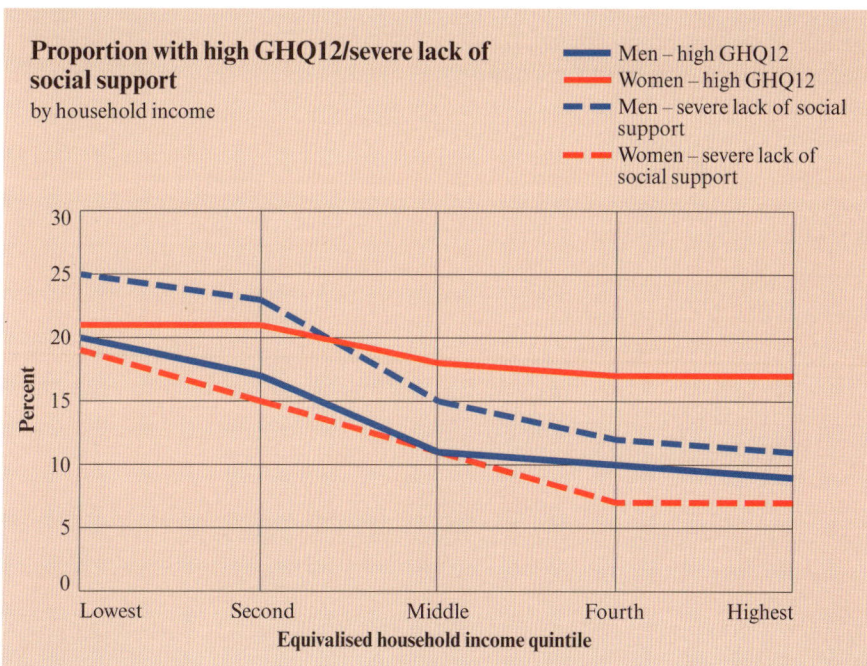

Equivalised household income quintile

Age standardised

Hormone Replacement Therapy (HRT)

Women aged 16 and over were asked whether they were currently on hormone replacement therapy (HRT) or had used it in the past.

Overall, 9% of women aged 16 and over were on HRT when interviewed and 6% had been users in the past. As the chart shows, these proportions varied greatly with age, rising steeply from age 40 onwards. About half of all women between the ages of 50 and 55 had used HRT, two in three of these being current users. Thereafter, the proportion currently using HRT decreased with increasing age, but the proportion who had ever used HRT, either currently or in the past, remained high into the early sixties, though decreasing rapidly thereafter. The fact that the proportion who have ever used HRT does not increase cumulatively with age indicates the presence of a cohort effect , with progressively higher rates of HRT uptake in younger cohorts.

Of those who were current or past users of HRT, 36% had had a hysterectomy, 39% were post-menopausal, and the remainder (25%) reported that they were still menstruating.

Present and past HRT use
by single year of age

Legend:
- Used HRT in past
- Currently on HRT

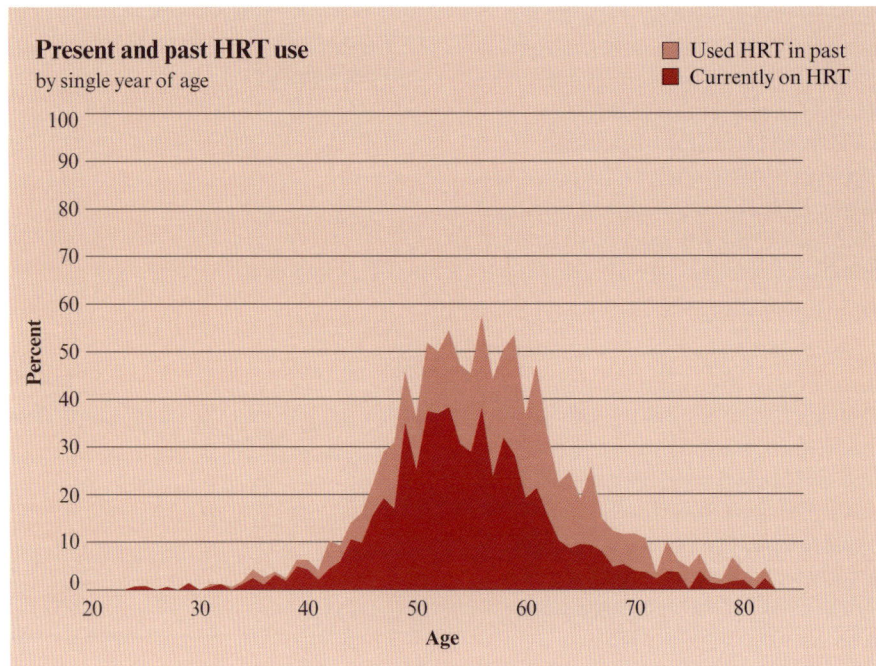

62% of users in the sample started on HRT between the age of 45 to 54 years, although a quarter (26%) started at a younger age. The median age at which women started was 48 years. On average women spent five years on the therapy, with women who started younger spending more years on HRT.

HRT use varied by the social class of the head of the household. On an age-standardised basis, HRT use (past or present) was reported by a higher proportion of women living in households in Social Class I (31%) than of women in households in Social Class V (20%).

HRT use was inversely related to equivalised household income. Again on an age-standardised basis, one in three women living in households in the highest income quintile had used HRT, compared with only one in five in households in the lowest income quintile.

Percentage of women aged 35-74 who had ever used HRT
by social class

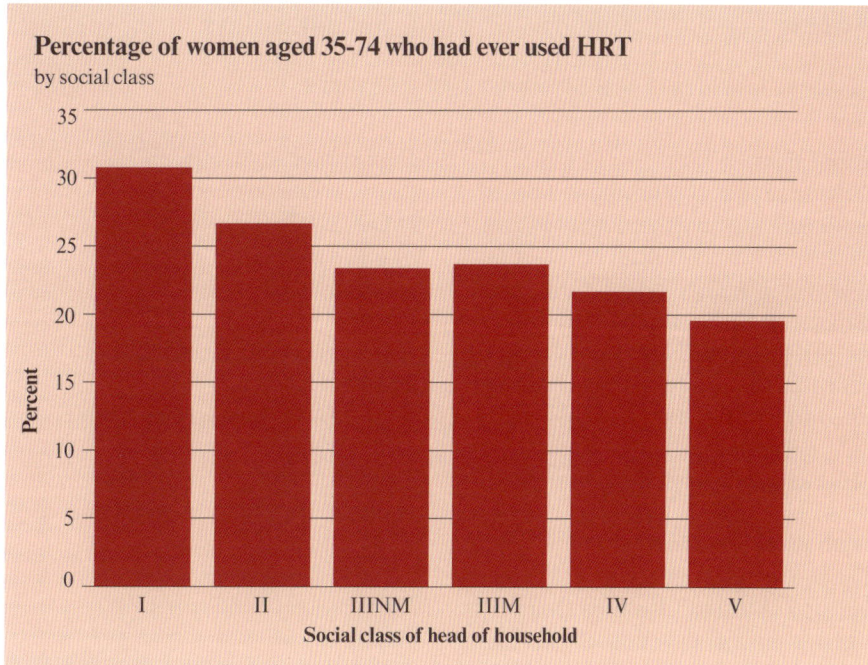

Age standardised

Percentage of women aged 35-74 who had ever used HRT
by household income

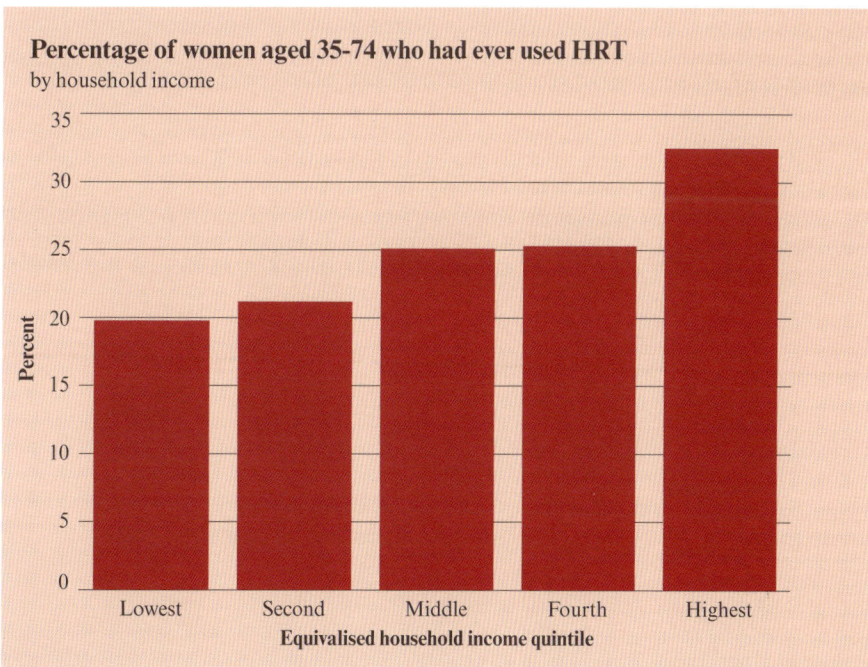

Age standardised

Notes

Contact points

Social class
The social class classification is based on the occupation of the head of the informant's household. The abbreviations IIINM and IIIM refer respectively to Social Class III Non-manual and Social Class III Manual. Analyses by social class have been age standardised to remove the effect of differences in age distributions between social classes.

Equivalised household income
The income classification is based on the total income of the household which is adjusted for household size and composition using the McClements equivalence scale. For analysis purposes households were ranked by equivalised income and grouped into quintiles. All individuals in each household were allocated to the equivalised income quintile to which their household had been allocated. Analyses by household income have been age standardised.

Additional table output
Tables containing additional data, including tables presenting 1998 survey results for children, together with selected trends for both children and adults, will be found on the Department of Health website (address below).

Department of Health
(Survey Section)
Room 451C
Skipton House
London Road
London SE1 6LW
Telephone 0171 972 5675
Fax 0171 972 5662
Website www.doh.gov.uk/public/
summary/htm

National Centre for Social Research
35 Northampton Square
London EC1V 0AX
Telephone 0171 250 1866
Fax 0171 250 1524
Website www.natcen.ac.uk

Department of Epidemiology and Public Health at the Royal Free and University College Medical School
1-19 Torrington Place
London WC1E 6BT
Telephone 0171 391 1733
Website www.ucl.ac.uk/epidemiology/
jhsu/jhsu.html

ESRC Data Archive
University of Essex
Wivenhoe Park
Colchester
Essex CO4 3SQ
Telephone 01206 872001
Fax 01206 872003
Website dawww.essex.ac.uk

Findings in this booklet are taken from:

Health Survey for England : Cardiovascular Disease '98

A survey carried out on behalf of the Department of Health

Edited by Bob Erens and Paola Primatesta

Principal authors: Madhavi Bajekal, Richard Boreham, Bob Erens, Emanuela Falaschetti, Vasant Hirani, Paola Primatesta, Gillian Prior, Clare Tait

The National Centre for Social Research (formerly SCPR)
The National Centre for Social Research is an independent institute specialising in social survey and qualitative research for the development and evaluation of public policy. Research is in areas such as health, housing, employment, crime, education and political and social attitudes. Projects include ad hoc and continuous surveys, using face-to-face, telephone and postal methods; many use advanced applications of computer assisted interviewing. The Centre has over 180 staff, a national panel of over 1,100 interviewers, and 300 nurses who work on health-related surveys.

| National Centre *for* Social Research

Department of Epidemiology and Public Health at the Royal Free and University College Medical School
Including the International Centre for Health and Society, the Department houses around 55 scientists in medicine, dentistry, statistics, economics, sociology and psychology, plus post-graduate students, research assistants and support staff. Its research programme is concerned particularly with social factors in health and illness. The research includes longitudinal studies of cardiovascular disease (Whitehall studies); international studies of cardiovascular disease and diabetes; the socio-dental indicators of need; nicotine dependence; dietary practices; and the socio-economic and policy implications of an ageing population.

UCL

ISBN 1 84182 138 1

Futher copies of this Summary are available from:

Department of Health, PO Box 777, London SE1 6XH
Fax: 01623 724 524. Email: doh@prologistics.co.uk

Full reports of the Health Survey for England are available from:

The Stationery Office Publications Centre
(Mail, fax and telephone orders only)
PO Box 276, London, SW8 5DT
Telephone orders 0171 873 9090, Fax orders 0171 873 8200
The Stationery Office bookshops and agents (see Yellow Pages)
and through good booksellers

10383 1p 5.3k (SWI)

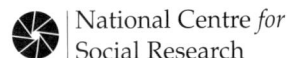